Research and Biostatistics for Nurses

Research and Biostatistics for Nurses

(As per INC Syllabus)

R Sudha MSc (N) PhD
Professor-cum-Principal
MA Chidambaram College of Nursing Voluntary Health Services Campus
(Affiliated to the Tamil Nadu Dr. M.G.R. Medical University)
Taramani, Chennai, Tamil Nadu, India

Foreword
S Ani Grace Kalaimathi

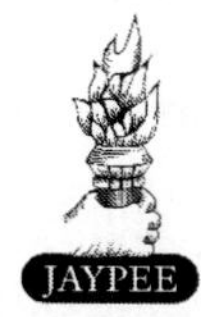

JAYPEE BROTHERS MEDICAL PUBLISHERS
The Health Sciences Publisher
New Delhi | London

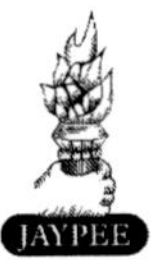

Jaypee Brothers Medical Publishers (P) Ltd

Headquarters
EMCA House
23/23-B, Ansari Road, Daryaganj
New Delhi 110 002, India
Landline: +91-11-23272143, +91-11-23272703
+91-11-23282021, +91-11-23245672
E-mail: jaypee@jaypeebrothers.com

Corporate Office
4838/24, Ansari Road, Daryaganj
New Delhi 110 002, India
Phone: +91-11-43574357
Fax: +91-11-43574314
E-mail: jaypee@jaypeebrothers.com

Overseas Office
J.P. Medical Ltd
83 Victoria Street, London
SW1H 0HW (UK)
Phone: +44 20 3170 8910
E-mail: info@jpmedpub.com

EU GPSR Authorised Representative
Logos Europe, 9 rue Nicolas Poussin
17000, La Rochelle, France
Phone: +33 (0) 6 67 93 73 78
E-mail: contact@logoseurope.eu

Website: www.jaypeebrothers.com
Website: www.jaypeedigital.com

Inquiries for bulk sales may be solicited at: jaypee@jaypeebrothers.com

Research and Biostatistics for Nurses

First Edition: 2017

Reprint: **2026**

ISBN 978-93-86150-97-4

Printed in India

Dedicated to

My students who inspired me, my teachers who provided me wisdom, my friends and colleagues who motivated me and my parents and family members who encouraged and supported me.

Foreword

Most people are unaware that nurses conduct research, but now I am sure people are aware about it.

Nurses and midwives have always had a passion for delivering better care in an ever-changing world. Research-based practice is now the new reality, with nursing knowledge at the core of professionalization. Delivering modern, high-quality care to patients now relies increasingly on routine reference to scientific papers and journals, rather than traditional textbook learning. Acquiring the skills to appraise nursing and medical research papers is a daunting task.

This book is short, readable and useful, without becoming overly bogged down in the mathematical detail that frankly puts so many of us off the subject. I commend this book to all health care professionals. It covers all the ground necessary to critically evaluate the statistical elements of research papers in a friendly and approachable way.

I congratulate the author for her wonderful effort.

Prof Dr S Ani Grace Kalaimathi
RN RM MSc (N) PhD
Registrar (FAC)
Tamil Nadu Nurses and Midwives Council
Chennai, Tamil Nadu, India

Preface

In my experience, I have seen students fearing about the course in research and statistics. Many undergraduate and postgraduate students have their concerns and doubts as to whether they could easily do away with the research projects assigned to them or not. This confusion results in a nightmare for most of them. Also the students correlate statistics with mathematics and have a preconception about the subject as to whether they would be able to get through the final exam. Learning materializes only when the mind is fearless, open and relaxed. A receptive mind receives the concepts well and facilitates faster learning.

This book has been written specifically to meet the needs of the nursing students and to draw their interest towards nursing research. It has been organized into two sections—***Section 1: Research*** and ***Section 2: Biostatistics***. In Research section, the chapters are arranged according to the steps of research process and each chapter explains every step in a simple way to help the students learn the concepts easily. In Biostatistics section, the chapters are sequenced from simple to complex concepts, i.e. descriptive to inferential statistics, each with adequate exercises and lot of examples. This book would get the learners involved, keep them on track and help them reach the final destination with great confidence.

One of the learning outcomes of the students learning the subject on research and biostatistics is to undertake a research project and to write the research report. The task of the selection of the right problem for investigation to the completion of report-writing in the form of final project or dissertation is cumbersome for the students and they need proper guidance from their supervisors. This book would help the students in all stages of their research work.

Writing this book was completely a challenging task which required commitment, time and dedication. Utmost care has been taken to avoid errors and the readers are requested to point out the errors, if any, in the text matter and offer suggestions for improvement.

R Sudha

Acknowledgments

I wish to remember and thank all my postgraduate students who have showed keen interest to learn the concepts of Research and Biostatistics and the endless queries and discussions with them motivated me to write this book.

My heartfelt thanks to Prof Dr S Ani Grace Kalaimathi, Registrar, Tamil Nadu Nurses and Midwives Council, my teacher, guide and well-wisher for writing a foreword for this book.

I would like to express my gratitude to all my teachers in the field of nursing, who provided me the due knowledge and guidance. My special thanks to Dr Beulah Shekhar, my PhD guide, for her guidance and support in my growth.

I would like to express my gratitude to all my friends and colleagues, who had helped me by having read-through, offered comments and talked things over to groom this book.

Special thanks to Shri Jitendar P Vij (Group Chairman), Mr Ankit Vij (Group President), Ms Chetna Malhotra Vohra (Associate Director–Content Strategy) and Mr Tarun Duneja (Director–Publishing). I would also like to thank for the wonderful work done by Ms Samina Khan (Executive Assistant to Director–Publishing), Ms Payal Bharti (Project Manager), Ms Ruby Sharma (Project Manager) and the team of Jaypee Brothers Medical Publishers, New Delhi, India. The team is very prompt in its work, untiring in its following up and reverting back, which served as a driving force towards the completion of this task.

My sincere thanks to all my family members, especially my parents Mr P Radhakrishnan and Mrs R Rajalakshmi; my husband Mr C Arumugam; my daughters AS Neya and AS Dhaya, who have supported me, spared me for my long work and patiently accepted me for my commitment to complete this book.

INC Syllabus

NURSING RESEARCH AND STATISTICS

Placement: 4th Year
Internship

Hours of Instruction
Theory: 45 Hours
Practical: 45 Hours
Total: 90 Hours

Course Description: The Course is designed to enable students to develop an understanding of basic concepts of research, research process and statistics. It is further, structured to conduct/participate in need-based research studies in various settings and utilize the research findings to provide quality nursing care. The hours for practical will be utilized for conducting individual/group research project.

Unit	Time (Hrs)	Learning Objectives	Content	Training Learning Activities	Assessment Methods	Chap
I	4	• Describe the concept of research, terms, need and areas of research in nursing. • Explain the steps of research process.	**Research and Research Process** • Introduction and need for nursing research • Definition of research and nursing research • Steps of scientific method • Characteristics of good research • Steps of research process—overview	• Lecture Discussion • Narrate steps of research process followed from examples of published studies	• Short answer • Objective type	Sec 1: Ch 1
II	3	• Identify and state the research problem and objectives	**Research Problem/ Question** • Identification of problem area • Problem statement • Criteria of a good research problem • Writing objectives	• Lecture discussion • Exercise on writing statement of problem and objectives	• Short answer • Objective type	Sec 1: Ch 2
III	3	• Review the related literature	**Review of Literature** • Location • Sources	• Lecture discussion • Exercise on reviewing	• Short answer • Objective type	Sec 1: Ch 3

Unit	Time (Hrs)	Learning Objectives	Content	Training Learning Activities	Assessment Methods	Chap
			• Online search; CINAHL, COCHRANE, etc. • Purposes • Method of review	one research report/article for a selected research problem • Prepare annotated bibliography		
IV	4	• Describe the research approaches and designs	**Research Approaches and Designs** • Historical, survey and experimental • Qualitative and quantitative designs	• Lecture Discussion • Explain types of research approaches used from examples of published and unpublished research studies with rationale	• Short answer • Objective type	Sec 1: Ch 5
V	8	• Explain the process • Describe the methods of data collection	**Sampling and Data Collection** • Definition of population, sample, sampling criteria, factors influencing sampling process, types of sampling techniques • Data—why, what, from whom, when and where to collect • Data collection methods and instruments: – Methods of data collection – Questioning, interviewing – Observations, record analysis and measurement	• Lecture Discussion • Reading assignment on examples of data collection tools • Preparation of sample data collection tool • Conduct group research project	• Short answer • Objective type	Sec 1: Ch 6, 7 and 8

Unit	Time (Hrs)	Learning Objectives	Content	Training Learning Activities	Assessment Methods	Chap
			– Types of instruments – Validity and reliability of the instrument – Pilot study – Data collection procedure			
VI	4	• Analyze, interpret and summarize the research data	**Analysis of Data** • Compilation, tabulation, classification, summarization, presentation, interpretation of data	• Lecture Discussion • Preparation of sample tables	• Short answer • Objective type	Sec 1: Ch 10, Sec 2: Ch 11 and 12
VII	15	• Explain the use of statistics, scales of measurement and graphical presentation of data • Describe the measures of central tendency and variability and methods of correlation	**Introduction to Statistics** • Definition, use of statistics, scales of measurement • Frequency distribution and graphical presentation of data • Mean, median, mode, standard deviation • Normal probability and tests of significance • Coefficient of correlation • Statistical packages and its application	• Lecture Discussion • Practice on graphical presentations • Practice on computation of measures of central tendency, variability and correlation	• Short answer • Objective type	Sec 2: Ch 11 and 13 to 26
VIII	4	• Communicate and utilize the research findings	**Communication and Utilization of Research** • Communication of research findings – Verbal report – Writing research report	• Lecture Discussion • Read/ presentations of a sample published/ unpublished research report	• Short answer • Objective type • Oral presentation	Sec 1: Ch 10

Unit	Time (Hrs)	Learning Objectives	Content	Training Learning Activities	Assessment Methods	Chap
			– Writing scientific article/paper - Critical review of published research - Utilization of research findings	• Writing group research project	• Assessment of group research project	

Contents

Section 1: Research

Section 2: Biostatistics

Section 1

Research

1. Introduction to Nursing Research
2. Problem Statement
3. Review of Literature
4. Conceptual Framework
5. Research Approaches and Designs
6. Population and Sample
7. Data Collection
8. Pilot Study
9. Research Ethics
10. Interpretation, Communication and Utilization of Research Findings

1 Introduction to Nursing Research

OBJECTIVES

After reading this chapter, you will be able to:

- Explain the sources of knowledge
- Explain scientific method and problem-solving
- State the meanings and definition of research and nursing research
- List the characteristics of good research
- Enlist the principles of research
- Explain the purposes of research and nursing research
- Explain the scope of nursing research
- Describe the types of research
- Explain the steps of research process
- Explain the role of a nurse in the promotion of nursing research.

INTRODUCTION

Research is undertaken within all professions and in all discipline. More than a set of skills, it is a way of thinking—examining critically the various aspects of one's professional work. It is a habit of questioning what we do, and a systematic examination of the observed information to find answers with a view to instituting appropriate changes for a more effective professional service. Research is a process of collecting, analyzing and interpreting information to answer questions. The foundation for effective research is the strong desire and motivation to do research.

Nursing research involves a systematic process which aims to inquire about issues related to nursing. The aim of research in any discipline is to gain new knowledge, verify and clarify the concepts and existing facts. Nursing is a discipline with its own body of knowledge that focuses on promotive, preventive, curative and rehabilitative care of the individual and the group. According to the Flexner's criteria of a profession, and discipline in order to be a profession, it should have its own body of knowledge. Research is one such important aspect which helps to create and develop own body of knowledge for any discipline.

Research is a systematic inquiry into a specific subject or problem that uses various methods, approaches or techniques. Research involves finding out the solutions for problems, discover new knowledge, verify or clarify the existing facts. Research follows specific principles and steps of procedure.

Research is search for knowledge, it is rediscovering existing knowledge and it adds to the existing knowledge or theory. The art of scientific investigation could be termed as research. It is a careful investigation or inquiry specially through search for new facts in any branch of knowledge or discipline. As human beings are endowed with thinking, questioning and various other brain activities, he uses this capacity for the welfare of self and others. He gains knowledge through various mental functions. At the same time, men are never satisfied with whatever knowledge they possess. They are interested and curious to know more and more. Further vistas of knowledge are mastered by them as a result of this urge to know, to explain, control and predict. This means the human mind will always search for facts and knowledge. Men acquire knowledge through various methods/sources ranging from totally unreliable to reliable sources.

METHODS/SOURCES OF ACQUIRING KNOWLEDGE

The methods adopted by men for acquiring knowledge can be categorized under the following heads:

Authority

Appeal to authority and seeking authority's advice was a well-established method of solving problem, even in the earliest civilizations. Even now we seek advice from authorities for the solution of the problem faced by us. The authorities may be the persons who have had long experience related to the problem. When factual evidence cannot be obtained to solve a problem, one may have to rely upon authoritative opinion temporarily as the only possible method for solution. In such cases, care must be employed in choosing authorities. In nursing, we seek senior nurses in the hospital for overcoming problem related to clinical issues and we seek the help of principal in an educational institution to solve problems related to academic issues.

Tradition

Closely related to authority is tradition, upon which man depends for solutions to many of his problems. Man unquestioningly accepts many traditions of his forefathers or culture, such as the way of dressing, food, speech, etc. In clinical setting, nurses follow many techniques and procedures which are being practiced years together. Although automatic acceptance of tradition and custom is often necessary, one should not always assume that everything that has customarily been done is right and valid. If we look into the past, we could find that many theories and concepts based upon tradition, which prevailed for years, were later found to be erroneous and had to be rejected. One should, therefore, evaluate custom and tradition carefully before it is accepted as a truth.

Experience

Our own personal experience or that of others is the most primitive and yet most familiar and fundamental source of knowledge. When confronted with a problem, man often tries to seek its answers from his own personal experience or from others with which he is familiar. A junior nurse consults with the senior nurse for solving problems or to gain new knowledge believing that the senior nurse is more experienced and can contribute toward problem-solving or learning.

Trial and Error

Learning by trial and error is another way of gaining knowledge. This method of learning is practical, but it is unsystematic and may or may not result in desirable outcome. Making mistakes or repeatedly trying various ways of accomplishing something will eventually result in problem-solving. Nursing is a science which deals with patient care where trial and error is not an appropriate way of acquiring new knowledge.

Intuition: It is power of knowing without recourse to inference or reasoning. It is a frequently used method of problem-solving. Intuition is a leap of understanding, grasping of a larger concept unreachable by other intellectual means, yet still it is fundamentally an intellectual process. Intuition and practical reasoning form the base of all reasoning including the scientific reasoning and creation of scientific knowledge.

Deductive Reasoning

A significant contribution towards the development of a systematic method for obtaining reliable knowledge was made by the ancient Greek philosophers like Aristotle and his followers. Aristotle developed the syllogism which can be described as a thinking process in which one proceeds from general to specific statements by deductive reasoning. It provides a means of testing the validity of any given conclusion or idea by proceeding from the known to unknown.

The syllogistic reasoning consists of:

- A major premise based on a self-evident truth or previously established fact or relationship.
- A minor premise concerning a particular case to which the truth, fact or relationship invariably applies.
- A conclusion. If the major and minor premises can be shown to be true, the conclusion arrived at is necessarily true. This can be understood with the following example:
    - All living things are mortal
    - Lion is a living thing
    - Therefore, lion is mortal, i.e. lion will die.

The conclusion of a syllogism is always derived from the content of the premises. So, if one of the premises is erroneous, the conclusions arrived at will not be valid. The limitation of the deductive reasoning is its dependence upon verbal symbolism. Though it proceeds from known to unknown, but it cannot be relied upon as a self-sufficient method for securing reliable knowledge.

Inductive Reasoning

The conclusions derived from generalities and from statements of presumed authorities by deductive reasoning are true only if they are based upon true premises. To determine whether the premises are true, Francis Bacon stressed the need for formulating premises based upon direct observations. This is known as inductive reasoning that is moving from the particular to general. Rather than accepting premises laid down by authorities as absolute truths, Bacon advised man to observe nature closely to experiment to understand all the facts, to study these facts in order to reach minor generalizations and then to proceed from minor generalizations to greater ones.

In deductive reasoning, the premises or generalizations must be known before a conclusion can be reached. On the other hand, in inductive reasoning, a conclusion is reached by observing instance and generalizing from instances to the whole phenomenon. In order to be absolutely certain of an inductive conclusion, all instances must be observed. But practically, it is not possible to observe all instances. One may arrive at a generalization by observing only some instances that make up the phenomenon. This is the limitation of inductive reasoning.

SCIENTIFIC METHOD

The exclusive use of Bacon's inductive method resulted in the accumulation of isolated bits of information which made little contribution to the advancement of human knowledge. Moreover, inductive reasoning alone could not solve many problems. So, the scientific method emerged which generally attributed to Charles Darwin. According to this method, man first operates inductively from known or observed information towards a meaningful whole or hypotheses and then deductively from suggested whole or hypothesis to the particular parts in order to find valid relationships. Scientific method involves working inductively from observations to hypotheses and then deductively from the hypotheses to the logical implications of the hypotheses in relation to what is already known.

Good and Hatt defined ***science*** as a method of approach to the entire empirical world. It is said to be more an approach, which does not aim at persuasion, at knowing the ultimate truth. It refers to the body of systematic and organized knowledge which makes use of the scientific method to advance knowledge in a particular field of enquiry. It refers to clear concepts, theory and other accumulated knowledge developed by scientific method and the best of hypothesis. It may be treated as a 'method of approach to the entire empirical world.' The scientific method is a method of systematic analysis leading to observations, propositions and testing of hypotheses and contributes to the organized body of knowledge. Facts and theories are the two sides of the same coin, which is the scientific method. A consistent interaction between these two elements results in scientific knowledge. The collection of facts and their theoretical treatment are the tools of the scientific method. Theory provides the basis for the scientific method. Theory-based studies are strong in conceptual framework and classification of facts, enabling the research to crystallize the problem and choose the data relevant to it. The possibility for extrapolation from the known to the unknown is the result of a strong theoretical base.

George A Lundberg defined scientific method which consists of systematic observation, classification and interpretation of data.

L L Bernard defined science as six major processes that take place within it. These are testing, verification, definition, classification, organization and orientation which includes prediction and application. The scientific method is systematic method of investigation, evaluation, experimentation, interpretation and theorizing.

Bases of scientific methods are as follows:

Scientific method is a set of rules consisting of certain assumptions, attitudes, goals and procedures for creating and answering questions about nature.

- ***Reliance on empirical evidence:*** Scientific method relies upon the observable evidence, the real facts or truth. The conclusion is drawn only based on the evidence obtained from the use of appropriate methods, such as observation and experimentation. Evidence must be empirical, meaning learned by observation.
- ***Problem to solve:*** Every inquiry must have a definite problem and enquiry without problem is of no use. The problem should be verifiable, observable, replicable and be useful to humanity.
- ***Verifiability:*** The results drawn out of scientific methods should be verifiable at any point of time. This indicates that phenomenon is capable of being observable and measurable. Verification can be done by replication under similar conditions to check its accuracy, to modify or to invalidate them.
- ***Generality:*** The scientific method tries to achieve a rational interconnection of facts. It attempts to establish general propositions. Science seeks to ascertain the common characteristic of types of objects and general laws or conditions of events.
- ***Predictability:*** Scientific results can be predicted with sufficient accuracy. Scientific method assures the predictability of the phenomenon, events or incidents.
- ***Objectivity:*** Objectivity is the willingness and ability to examine evidence dispassionately. Objectivity is that everyone should arrive at the same conclusion about the phenomenon. Science requires objectivity. This means that ideally a researcher's personal biases, attitudes or subjective impressions do not influence the observations or conclusions. Any measurement should be as empirical, objective and precise as possible.
- ***Systematic nature:*** Systematic means that observations are obtained in a methodical step-by-step fashion. The results out of scientific method are arrived out of systematic method. It is only under these conditions that the results can be verified. Scientific method involves accepted method of investigation and the results are accurate.
- ***Control:*** Evidence must be obtained under controlled conditions.

The scientific approach has two components, namely the procedural and the personal. The procedural component involves the major steps as given below:

The personal component involves the abilities and skills of the scientist, such as scientific imagination, resourcefulness, manipulative skill and pursuance to carry through the experiment, knowing what is essential and nonessential and scientific reasoning. The scientist must have sincerity, honesty, integrity and perseverance. He must possess the spirit of independence and the spirit of originality.

The procedural component consists of following five definite steps:

1. ***Identification and definition of the problem:*** A scientific inquiry starts with the identification of a problem that is in need of solution. The problem identified must be defined in such a manner that observation or experimentation in the natural world can provide a solution.
2. ***Formulation of a hypothesis:*** Once the problem is defined, the next step is to formulate the hypothesis, which provides an intelligent guess for the solution of the problem. It requires a critical review of the knowledge or information related to the problem.
3. ***Implications of hypothesis through deductive reasoning:*** The next step after the formulation of a hypothesis is to deduce the implications of the suggested hypothesis that is what would be observed if the hypothesis is true.
4. ***Collection and analysis of evidence:*** Collecting relevant evidence related to them through observation, testing and experimentation tests the deduced implications of the hypothesis.
5. ***Verification, rejection or modification of hypothesis:*** Once the evidence has been collected and analyzed, the result is also analyzed in order to verify whether the evidences support the hypothesis. It may be noted that the characteristics of scientific method are not to prove the hypothesis in terms of absolute truth but to conclude that the evidence does or does not support the hypothesis.

Research and Problem-solving

Research is the scientific investigation of the problem whereas problem-solving involves informal application of methods to solve a problem. Problem-solving may not follow scientific techniques. Problem-solving is a systematic approach to the solution or alleviation of problem by undertaking following activities:

- Identification of the problem
- Defining the problem and its elements
- Gathering relevant information regarding the problem
- Analysis, synthesis and interpretation of the collected facts
- Deciding on the various possible solutions to the problem
- Selecting specific course of action to solve the problem
- Implementation of the course of action
- Observation and evaluation of the course of action.

MEANING AND DEFINITION OF RESEARCH

Research is the scientific investigation of phenomena which includes collection, presentation, analysis and interpretation of facts that lines an individual's speculation with reality. The word ***research*** is used to describe a number of similar and often overlapping activities involving a search for information. Research involves scholarly or scientific investigation or inquiry.

The word 'research' is composed of two syllables, 're' and 'search'. 'Re' is a prefix meaning 'again', 'anew' or 'over again' and 'search' is a verb meaning 'to examine closely and carefully', 'to test and try', or 'to probe'. Together they form a noun describing a careful, systematic, patient study and investigation in some field of knowledge, undertaken to establish facts or principles. It is a systematic investigation to establish facts or principles or to collect information on a subject. It is the systematic investigation into and study of materials and sources in order to establish facts and reach new conclusions

The word 'research' is derived from the Middle French 'recherche', which means 'to go about seeking', the term itself being derived from the Old French term 'recerchier', a compound word from 're-' + 'cerchier', or 'sercher', meaning 'search'. The earliest recorded use of the term was in 1577.

A broad definition of research is given by Martin Shuttleworth. In the broadest sense of the word, the definition of research includes any gathering of data, information and facts for the advancement of knowledge.

Another definition of research is given by Creswell which states that 'Research is a process of steps used to collect and analyze information to increase our understanding of a topic or issue'. It consists of three steps: Pose a question, collect data to answer the question and present an answer to the question.

The Merriam Webster Online Dictionary defines research in more detail as 'a studious inquiry or examination' especially, investigation or experimentation aimed at the discovery and interpretation of facts, revision of accepted theories or laws in the light of new facts, or practical application of such new or revised theories or laws.

According to Cambridge Dictionaries Online, 2003, 'Research is a detailed study of a subject, especially in order to discover (new) information or reach a (new) understanding'.

According to John Best, 'Research is the systematic and objective analysis and recording of controlled observations that may lead to the development of generalizations, principles, or theories, resulting in prediction and possibly ultimate control of events'.

Research is an abstraction and selection from an infinite variety of possible things that one might study (Godwin and Milman).

Research is a careful enquiry or examination in seeking facts or principles, a deligent investigation to ascertain something (Clifford Woody).

Research is a process which systematically searches for new facts and relationships (Notter).

Research is a systematic, formal, rigorous and precise process used to gain solutions to problems or discover and interpret new facts and relationships (Waltz and Bausell, 1981).

Research is a process in which observable, verifiable data are collected from the empirical world to describe, explain, predict or control events (Seaman, 1987).

Research is systematic enquiry that uses disciplined methods to answer or solve problems. The ultimate goal of research is to develop, refine, and expand a body of knowledge.

Nursing research is a systematic inquiry designed to develop knowledge about issues of importance to the nursing profession, including nursing practice, education, administration and informatics.

Characteristics of Research

- ***Need-based:*** A research should be need-based. There should be a strong need supporting the study.
- ***Usability:*** Any research should benefit the humanity. The ultimate aim of any research should be for the welfare of human beings.
- ***Empirical:*** Research is based on the direct experience or observation by the researcher.
- ***Logical:*** Research is based on valid procedures and principles.
- ***Objectivity:*** It refers to scientific nature of the inquiry process which is free from personal bias of the researcher.
- ***Scientific:*** Any research is scientific when it follows scientific methods, principles and procedures.
- ***Cyclical:*** Research is a cyclical process because it starts with a problem and ends with a problem.
- ***Ethical:*** The methods and steps of research should be ethically sound, and follows the principles of research ethics. It should not be harmful in any way to the research participants.
- ***Rigorous:*** Researcher must be scrupulous in ensuring that the procedures followed to find answers to questions are relevant, appropriate and justified. Again, the degree of rigor varies markedly between the physical and social sciences and within the social sciences.
- ***Critical:*** Critical scrutiny of the procedures used and the methods employed is crucial to a research enquiry. The process of investigation must be foolproof and free from drawbacks. The process adopted and the procedures used must be able to withstand critical scrutiny.
- ***Controlled:*** In real-life experience, there are many factors that affect an outcome. In research, there are variables or factors that influence our study variables. The controlled factors or variables should have to be controlled rigorously so as to get accurate results. In pure sciences, it is very easy to control such elements because experiments are conducted in laboratory but in social sciences, it becomes difficult to control these factors because of the nature of research.
- ***Analytical:*** Research utilizes statistical methods such as descriptive and inferential statistics in order to analyze and interpret the data gathered. Research needs careful and precise judgement to find the solution to the problem.

- ***Methodical:*** Research should be conducted in a methodical manner without bias.
- ***Systematic:*** Research is an organized activity which involves using systematic methods and procedures.
- ***Feasibility:*** Research should be practical in nature and it should use possible methods and procedures.
- ***Economic:*** It should be cost-effective in terms of men, money and material used in conducting research.
- ***Problem-solving:*** Research is directed towards solution of a problem.
- ***Replicability:*** It refers to the ability of a research being repeated by other researchers. The research design and procedures are replicated or repeated to enable the researcher to arrive at valid and conclusive results.
- ***Reliability:*** A research is reliable when it yields similar results each time it is undertaken with similar population and with similar procedures. The more the results are similar, the more the reliability is present in the research. It shows the consistency of the methods and procedures used.
- ***Validity:*** Validity determines the applicability of research. A research which is valid will be applicable and generalizable to the population.
- ***Verifiability:*** It is another nature of research. Most of the researches carried on human behavior are of verification type only. The principles, generalizations, theories arrived at based on research under natural and controlled conditions are tested and found to be true and workable in empirical conditions.
- ***Credibility:*** Credibility is obtained with the use of best source of information and best procedures in research.
- ***Accuracy:*** Any research should be accurate in order to obtain the best possible results.
- ***Generalizability:*** It is the extent to which research findings can be applied to larger population. Only when there is wider application, research has social and economic values.

Characteristics of Research according to John Best

- Directed towards solution of a problem
- Emphasizes the development of generalizations, principles or theories
- Based upon observable experiences
- Demands accurate observations and descriptions
- Involves gathering of new data
- Requires carefully designed procedures applying vigorous analysis
- Strives to be objective and logical
- Involves quest for answers to the unsolved problems.

Principles of Good Research

- A research should be need-based. There should be a strong need supporting the study.
- There should be a clear, definite objectives and aims for the study which should be derived from the research problem.

- Research problem should be based on the sound literature review.
- A good research should be ethically sound. A researcher should follow ethical principles, maintain confidentiality and have appropriate documentation, etc.
- Research questions, hypothesis and assumptions formulated should be based on the literature review and existing knowledge.
- Research questions and hypotheses should be testable.
- It follows appropriate methodology, which includes selection of research design, population, sample, sample size, sampling techniques, methods and tools of data collection, etc.
- It uses appropriate statistical methods for analysis.
- From the beginning, the research should have appropriate and sufficient resources in terms of people, time, transport, money, etc. allocated to it.
- The people conducting the research should have adequate knowledge in research. In general, research is carried out personally by the researcher or anybody recruited for this purpose. In any case, they should have knowledge in relation to research problem, research issues, setting, data collection methods and research methodology.
- A good research is utilizable, applicable and transferable.
- Research should be beneficial to the humanity.

Purposes of Research

- ***Description:*** Research is conducted to describe situations and events. Descriptive work aims to gather information that illuminates relationships, patterns and links between variables. The researcher observes and then describes what he or she observed. One example of descriptive social research is the census. The goal of the census is to describe accurately and precisely several characteristics of the population, including race/ethnicity, age, sex, household size, income, etc.
- ***Speculation:*** Research is conducted to speculate the future problems and identify the possible solutions for it. Sometimes research is implemented strategically, where researchers take account of current situations and speculate as to their future implications.
- ***Explanation:*** A third major purpose of research is to explain things. While descriptive studies attempt to answer the *what, when, where,* and *how,* explanatory studies attempt to answer the *why.* For example, reporting the maternal mortality rates of different states is descriptive. Identifying the variables that explain why some states have higher maternal mortality rates than others involves explanation. Likewise, reporting the frequency of patient attendance to various outpatient departments is descriptive, but reporting why some people attend some OPDs of the Government Hospitals while others do not is explanatory. Explanatory research aims to show why relationships, patterns and links occur.
- ***Exploration:*** A great deal of social research is conducted to explore a topic or familiarize oneself with a topic. This typically occurs when a researcher becomes interested in a new topic or when the subject of study itself is

relatively new. This type of research investigates an area or issue on which little previous work has been carried out. In an organizational setting, it may be used to discover whether or not a problem exists. Exploratory studies are typically done for three purposes:
- To satisfy the researcher's curiosity and desire for better understanding
- To test the feasibility of undertaking a more extensive study
- To develop the methods to be employed in any subsequent studies.

- ***Prediction and control:*** Research is also conducted to forecast things. The purpose of this type of research is to predict the likely course of events that can occur in particular circumstances or with given intervening variables. Control is an important facet of research in which a deductive approach is used, such as experimental studies. The researcher uses control in order to prove the outcome of the study.
- ***Evaluation:*** Research is done to evaluate the impact of something; for example, a new policy, event, law, treatment regime, teaching program or the introduction of a new system. It also helps us to analyze the effectiveness of some intervention or protocol used in the research.

Why Nurses Should Read and Conduct Research?

The need to conduct a research can be discussed under two headings. One is the purpose for which any researcher or investigator undertakes a research.

The reasons for the student or beginner researcher may be to fulfill a requirement for getting a degree, or one of the requirements in the course itself. For anybody who had already undertaken the course on research, the reasons may be many. These are:

- To further learn and strengthen the research knowledge by conducting various researches
- To fulfill the requirement in postgraduate or doctoral programs
- To study the issues of importance to nursing by conducting research and also publish many empirical studies so as to make oneself visible in the profession
- To advance oneself in career ladder, research is conducted
- To undertake research project by obtaining research grants/fellowship from University Grants Commission and various other funding agencies. This is mainly to develop new knowledge for the profession
- To promote evidence-based nursing practice by studying the various problems related to nursing.

Importance of Research in Nursing

- For evidence-based practice
- To make clinical decisions
- For cost containment
- To improve health care outcomes
- To understand varied dimensions of profession

- To control the occurrence of undesired outcomes
- To promote desired client behavior
- To provide a scientific basis for the nursing profession
- To develop and evaluate new techniques for delivering patient care
- To provide solutions to problems concerning health care
- To prepare students to be a diligent practitioner of research
- To generate knowledge for nursing
- To fill the gaps in the knowledge and practice
- Providing/identifying new measures in nursing practice
- Helps to improve the standards of nursing education
- Discover and evaluate nursing theories.

Significance of Research

- For students of any discipline who are to write Masters or PhD thesis research meaning fulfilling a requirement which helps them to complete course and earn degree. Thus, it helps them to choose their career.
- For professionals in research, research is a source of livelihood.
- For philosophers and thinkers, research may mean the outlet for new ideas and insights.
- For educated men and women, research may mean the development of new styles and creative work.
- For analysts and intellectuals, research may mean the generalizations of new theories.

Scope of Nursing Research

The scope of nursing research is as wide and as deep as the humanity is concerned. The research in nursing can be conducted on the following areas.

Based on major areas of nursing

- Nursing education
- Nursing administration
- Nursing practice
- Nursing informatics
- Nursing research.

Based on specialty in nursing

- Medical surgical nursing
- Community health nursing
- Child health nursing
- Mental health nursing
- Maternity nursing.

Based on the developmental stages of human beings

Nursing research can be conducted in:

- Infants including newborn
- Children of various age groups
- Adolescents
- Adults
- Old age.

Based on the areas of health

- Nursing research in preventive areas
- Nursing research in promotive areas
- Nursing research in curative areas
- Nursing research in rehabilitative areas.

Based on the settings

Nursing research can be conducted among human beings in various settings, such as:

- Hospital
  Outpatient departments
  Inpatient departments
  General wards
  Palliative care areas
  Intensive care units
- Community areas
  - Urban
  - Rural
- Schools and colleges
- Industry of various types
- Natural and artificial or laboratory settings.

Types of Research

Research can be classified from three perspectives:

1. Application of research study
2. Objectives in undertaking the research
3. Inquiry mode employed.

Application

From the point of view of application, there are two broad categories of research:

- Pure or basic research
- Applied research.

Pure, fundamental or theoretical research is basic or original in nature. It is said that it is undertaken for the sake of knowledge without formal intention of applying it in practice. Pure research involves developing and testing theories and hypotheses that are intellectually challenging to the researcher but may or may not have practical application at the present time or in the future. The knowledge produced through pure research is sought in order to add to the existing body of research methods. Gathering knowledge for knowledge's sake is termed 'pure' or 'basic' research. Research concerning some natural phenomenon or concerning human behavior carried on with a view to make generalizations about human behavior are also examples of fundamental or pure research.

Applied research is done to solve specific, practical questions, and for policy formulation, administration and understanding of a phenomenon. It aims at finding a solution for an immediate problem facing a society or an organization. It can be exploratory, but is usually descriptive. It is almost always done on the basis of basic research.

Objectives

From the viewpoint of objectives, a research can be classified as:

- ***Descriptive research:*** It attempts to describe systematically a situation, problem, phenomenon, service or program, or provides information about any variables under study, e.g. living condition of a community, or describes attitudes toward an issue.
- ***Correlational research:*** It attempts to discover or establish the existence of a relationship/interdependence between two or more aspects of a situation or variables of a research.
- ***Explanatory research:*** It attempts to clarify why and how there is a relationship between two or more aspects of a situation or phenomenon.
- ***Exploratory research:*** It is undertaken to explore an area where little is known or to investigate the possibilities of undertaking a particular research study (feasibility study/pilot study). The objective of the exploratory research is the development of hypotheses rather than their testing. In practice, most studies are a combination of the first three categories.

Inquiry Mode

From the process adopted to find answers to the research questions – the two approaches are:

- Structured approach
- Unstructured approach.
- ***Structured approach:*** The structured approach to inquiry is usually classified as quantitative research. Quantitative research is based on the measurement of quantity or amount. It is applicable to phenomena that can be expressed in terms of quantity. In quantitative research, objectives, design, sample, and the tool to collect data from respondents are predetermined. It is more appropriate to determine the extent of a problem, issue or phenomenon by quantifying the variation, e.g. how many people have a particular problem? How many people hold a particular attitude?
- ***Unstructured approach:*** The unstructured approach to inquiry is usually classified as qualitative research. This is especially important in behavioral sciences where the aim is to discover the underlying motives of human behavior. This approach allows flexibility in all aspects of the research process. It is more appropriate to explore the nature of a problem, issue or phenomenon without quantifying it. The main objective is to describe the variation in a phenomenon, situation or attitude, e.g. description of an observed situation, the historical enumeration of events, an account of different opinions different people have about an issue, description of working conditions in a particular industry.

STEPS OF RESEARCH PROCESS

The entire research process can be discussed under five major headings or components. There are many substeps or activities under each component. These are:

- Problem statement
- Review of literature
- Planning research design and methods
- Data collection
- Data analysis, interpretation and utilization.
- ***Problem statement***
  - Determining the research need
  - Identifying and formulating the research problem/questions
  - Review of literature
  - Gathering background information
  - Refining research problem and statement of hypothesis and objectives.
- ***Review of literature***
  - Reviewing the literature
  - Preparing conceptual framework.
- ***Planning research design and methods***
  - Selecting a research design
  - Deciding on population and samples
  - Selecting sampling techniques and methods
  - Deciding on setting for the study
  - Deciding on methods and preparation of tool for data collection
  - Deciding on the methods of analysis
  - Verifying on research ethics
  - Conducting pilot study.
- ***Data collection***
  - Collecting data
  - Preparing data for analysis.
- ***Data analysis, interpretation and utilization***
  - Analyzing and interpreting findings
  - Utilizing research findings
  - Communicating and disseminating research findings.

Problem Statement

- ***Determining the research need:*** In general, to undertake any activity, there must be a reason behind it. We do not do things simply. As professionals, nurses must have a strong need to perform any professional activity. All nursing interventions are based on a patient's need and there is a rationale behind it. The same way, a nurse should identify the need to undertake any research activity. The need arises from the problem experienced by the researcher. A research problem, in general, refers to some felt difficulty which the investigator experiences in the context of the theoretical or practical situation and for which he feels the urge to solve. A research problem is a situation or circumstance that requires a solution to be described, explained or predicted. The research problem identifies the knowledge gap that needs to be filled. The felt difficulty or the problem to solve is the need to conduct the study.

- ***Identifying and formulating the research problem/questions:*** A research study begins as a question that a researcher would like to answer or as a problem that a researcher would like to solve. A research problem is the first step and the most important requirement in the research process. It serves as the foundation of a research study. According to Kerlinger, in order for one to solve a problem, one must know what the problem is. The large part of the problem is knowing what one is trying to do. A well-formulated problem is already a half-solved problem. A proper definition of research problem will enable the researcher to be on the track whereas an ill defined problem may create hurdle. Thus, proper definition of a research problem is a prerequisite for any study and is a step of the highest importance. The research problem can be written as a statement or as a research question.
- ***Review of literature:*** Research studies are undertaken within the context of an existing knowledge base. A careful review of existing resources, such as journals, books, thesis and other related literature is one of the major steps in any research study. It allows the researcher to acquaint and familiarize himself with current knowledge in the area where he proposed to conduct research. A literature review surveys scholarly articles, books and other sources (e.g. dissertations, conference proceedings) relevant to a particular issue, area of research, or theory, providing a description, summary, and critical evaluation of each work. The literature review is done in the initial process for identification and selection of research problem as well as to gather relevant information on the selected problem.
- ***Gathering background information:*** By careful reviewing of the literature, one could get adequate information regarding existing work on a particular problem and the gaps in previous research. In this step, the researcher can broaden his knowledge on the selected problem, bring clarity and focus to the research problem and delimit the problem. He can search for information from primary and secondary sources.
- ***Refining research problem and statement of hypothesis and objectives:*** The background information about a research problem helps in refining the research problem and objectives. The research problem should be stated in such a way that it would lead to analytical thinking on the part of the researcher with the aim of possible concluding solutions to the stated problem. Research problems can be stated in the form of either questions or statements. The research problem should always be formulated grammatically correct and as completely as possible. Meaningless words should be avoided. It is important to keep in mind that the clearer the research objectives, the more actionable the research findings will be. Aims are broad statements of desired outcomes, or the general intentions of the research. Aims and objectives should be presented concisely and briefly

and be interrelated. The aim is what the investigator wants to achieve, and the objectives describe how the investigator is going to achieve that aim. The objectives of a research are derived from the problem statement which simplifies the step to be followed in a research. It communicates to the readers what the researcher intends to achieve by the study. These objectives should be closely related to the research problem.

The general objective of a study states what researchers expect to achieve by the study in general terms. The specific objectives are the logical steps formulated from the general objectives which explain what the researcher will do in her study.

The next step after defining the problem is to formulate a tentative explanation or solution of that problem in the form of a proposition. The tentative explanation or solution, the validity of which is still to be tested, is called the hypothesis. It is an informed/educated guess. It explains the researcher's expectation of a relationship existing between the variables. It indicates the expectations of the researcher regarding certain variables. While selecting a research problem, the topic or subject which is overdone should not be chosen in general. It will be difficult to throw any new light related to the problem. Also, controversial topics should preferably be avoided. It is not too late for one to decide any changes or modification of the selected problem.

Review of Literature

- ***Reviewing the literature:*** It can be understood in two different meanings. One is the process of searching for specific content in available literature and the second one is the written summary of the searched content.
  - In the first context, 'review of literature' refers to the process of extensive, exhaustive and systemic examination of publications relevant to a specific topic. It is a broad, comprehensive, in-depth, systematic and critical review of scholarly publications, unpublished scholarly print materials, etc.
  - In the second context, 'review of literature' refers to a written report of information gathered from various sources/literature related to a selected topic. This report should be of an evaluative and critical nature and not simply copying from the sources. Such a well-written analytical report forms the theoretical base for any research. The primary purpose of writing the report is to personally understand as well as to convey to the reader what is already established on a topic and what are its strengths and weaknesses. It gives an overview of the key findings and key authors, the prevailing theories and hypotheses and methods and methodologies used. In order to write a relevant literature review, the person who writes should remember the research objectives, the problems or issues to be researched. Rather it should not be a descriptive summary of the available information. The researcher searches for information from the primary and secondary sources and finally makes a complete report of the review.

- ***Preparing conceptual framework:*** A framework is a structure composed of many concepts proposed to serve as a support or guide for the building of something that expands the structure into something useful and meaningful. It is a broad overview, outline, or skeleton of interlinked concepts or items which support a major theme or overall concept. In nursing research, the conceptual/theoretical framework forms an important element. Conceptual framework is used in research to outline possible courses of action or to present a preferred approach to an idea or thought. Conceptual frameworks (theoretical frameworks) are a type of intermediate theory that attempt to connect to all aspects of inquiry (e.g. problem definition, purpose, literature review, methodology, data collection and analysis). Conceptual frameworks can act like a map that explains the logic to empirical inquiry. It clarifies the concepts on which the study is built. It specifies the relationship among the concepts. It identifies and states the assumptions and hypotheses underlying the study. It explains why a research is conducted in a particular way. It guides the researcher in the further course of action.

Planning Research Design and Methods

- ***Selecting a research design:*** Research design is the researcher's overall plan to obtain answer to the problem. In order to obtain solution to the problem, the researcher follows the best possible technique among the alternatives available. Research approach is a broad term which explains how a problem can be approached. 'Research design' is a more specific term which explains how a problem is solved using a specific approach. The selection of research design is influenced by the research approach. The research design is a plan of action indicating the specific steps that are necessary to provide answers to those questions, test the hypotheses, and thereby achieve the research objective that is the outcome of the study. Research design is a conceptual structure or plan of how a research is conducted. The research design is the plan, structure and strategy of investigation conceived so as to obtain answers to research questions and to control variance. The research design constitutes the blueprint for the collection, measurement and analysis of data. In general. research approaches are either quantitative or qualitative. Quantitative approach to research uses experimental, quasiexperimental and nonexperimental designs, whereas qualitative approach to research uses case study, phenomenology, ethnography and grounded theory.
- ***Deciding on population and samples:*** Population is generally a large collection of individuals or objects that is the main focus of a scientific query. It is for the benefit of the population that researches are done. Collection of data is an essential part of the research process. In order to collect data for any research problem, the researcher has to select a representative sample from the population so as to enable him to draw conclusions from the sample, which will hold good for the population. A sample is selected since it is neither possible nor feasible to gather data

for the whole population. By correctly drawing a sample from a specific population, a researcher can analyze the sample and make inferences about population characteristics. However, due to the large sizes of populations, researchers often cannot test every individual in the population because it is too expensive and time-consuming. If the sample is representative of the population from which it is drawn, the researcher can have confidence in concluding that the results are generalizable to the entire population and setting studies. Sampling is done to save time and money. The target population refers to the entire group of individuals or objects to which researchers are interested in generalizing the conclusions. The accessible population is the population in research to which the researchers can apply their conclusions. This population is a subset of the target population and is also known as the study population. It is from the accessible population that researchers draw their samples. Accessible population is feasible for the researcher to access. The researcher can finalize the population and sample.

- ***Selecting sampling techniques and methods:*** The sample refers to those individuals or units or elements who are selected for a study. A sample is simply a subset of the population. The concept of sample arises from the inability of the researchers to test all the individuals in a given population. The sample must be representative of the population from which it was drawn and it must have good size to warrant statistical analysis. Sampling is the process of selection of samples from a population. A sample design is a definite plan for obtaining a sample from the sampling frame. It refers to the technique or the procedure the researcher would adopt in selecting some sampling units from which inferences about the population are drawn. Sampling design is determined before any data are collected. There are two major types of sampling techniques. They are probability and nonprobability sampling techniques. The researcher selects an appropriate method of sampling technique based on his research problem.
- ***Deciding on setting for the study:*** A setting is a place where a researcher can have access to the population. Setting may be a hospital, community, school or college, etc. A researcher has to get prior permission to select samples from the setting. A study can be conducted in a natural setting or in an artificial setting. Many laboratory experiments are conducted in other disciplines too. Setting can be selected based on the feasibility of conducting research and he should check whether he could select adequate samples for the study.
- ***Deciding on methods and preparation of tool for data collection:*** Data collection is an important aspect of any type of research study. Inaccurate data collection can impact the results of a study and ultimately lead to invalid results. Collection of data is the first step in the statistical treatment of a problem. Data may be primary and secondary data. Primary data are original in character and it is collected for the first time. Secondary data refer to those which have been collected already by previous researchers and have gone through the process of standardization. The researcher has

to decide about the data that should be collected during his investigation. A researcher may have to collect primary data or secondary data or both based on the requirement of his research. Data can be collected using three major data collection methods, such as self-report, observation and biophysiological measurements. A researcher can use variety of tools, such as interview schedule, questionnaire, rating scale, checklist, video camera, etc. to collect data. The method and tool selected should be an appropriate one, which would help the researcher to elicit the information for his study.

- ***Deciding on the methods of analysis:*** A researcher has to have a plan of analysis. The analysis is based on the research problem, objectives and hypothesis. He should have a clear idea about what descriptive methods and inferential statistical method he is planning to use to analyze data.
- ***Verifying on research ethics:*** The word 'ethics' means 'moral principles'. 'Ethical' means 'morally correct'. Ethics in nursing research can be defined as 'the set of moral principles which the researcher has to follow while conducting nursing research to ensure the rights and welfare of persons and communities which are the subjects of his/her study'. Research ethics involve the application of fundamental ethical principles to a variety of topics involving scientific research. These include the design and implementation of research involving human experimentation and animal experimentation. Nursing research relies on the collaborations and partnerships based on mutual trust. When that trust is breached, the damage is irreversible. Honesty, openness, respect and sensitivity to others provide the cornerstones for ethical research. It is important that all nursing research is undertaken from a clear ethical stance, with ethical concerns.
- ***Conduct pilot study:*** Pilot study is the study carried out at the end of the planning phase of research, in order to explore and test the research elements. It is a small-scale study that precedes as if it were the actual study, except for the fact that subjects who will participate in the actual study are not used. However, they may be selected at this point. The primary objective of the pilot study is to test as many elements of the research proposal as possible, in order to correct any part that does not work well. For example, the pilot study tests whether the variables defined by operational definition are actually observable and measurable. Pretesting of instrument is also carried in the pilot study. A pilot experiment, also called a pilot study, is a small-scale preliminary study conducted in order to evaluate feasibility, time, cost, adverse events, and effect size (statistical variability) in an attempt to predict an appropriate sample size and improve upon the study design prior to performance of a full-scale research project. It is smaller version of a larger study that is conducted to prepare for that study. A pilot study is an initial investigation to give information that will be necessary when designing a future trial or study. A pilot or feasibility study is a small experiment designed to test logistics and gather information prior to a larger study, in order to improve the latter's

quality and efficiency. A pilot study can reveal deficiencies in the design of a proposed experiment or procedure and these can then be addressed before time and resources are expanded on large scale studies. There should be an outline of the future study for which the pilot is being used to gather information. As the sample size of a pilot study is seldom sufficient to draw reliable conclusions, the pilot should not be an end in itself.

Data Collection

- ***Collecting data:*** In this step, the researcher collects information using predetermined methods and tools. He identifies the population, selects samples and collects data as tested in pilot study. It is an implementation process of the research.
- ***Preparing data for analysis:*** Once data is collected, he has to prepare the data for analysis. This step involves editing, cleaning of the data, classification, coding, and transformation of data. Editing of data is a process of examining the collected raw data (specially in surveys) to detect errors and omissions and to correct these when possible. Editing involves a careful scrutiny of the completed questionnaires and/or schedules. Coding refers to the process of assigning numerals or other symbols to answers so that responses can be put into a limited number of categories or classes. Such classes should be appropriate to the research problem under consideration. A transformation is a mathematical procedure for systematically converting a set of scores into a different set of scores. One reason to transform data is to make different kinds of scores comparable. However, by transforming each score to a percent of total, we are no longer comparing apples to oranges. Second, we transform data because it makes scores easier to work with. Classification is the process of arranging the available data into various homogenous classes and subclasses according to some common characteristic or attribute or objective of an investigation. Tabulation or classification is the process by which data of long series of observation are systematically organized and recorded so as to enable analysis and interpretation.

Data Analysis, Interpretation and Utilization

- ***Analyzing and interpreting findings:*** After collecting and analyzing the data, the researcher has to accomplish the task of drawing inferences. Interpretation refers to the task of drawing inferences from the collected facts after analysis. In fact, it is a search for broader meaning of research findings. Interpretation helps in establishment of some explanatory concepts. After analysis of data, we want to draw conclusions for the population. Drawing conclusion involves generalization of the findings for the population. Interpretation is essential for the simple reason that the usefulness and utility of research findings lie in proper interpretation. Through interpretation, the researcher can link his findings with that of others. The interpretation of the findings of exploratory research study often results into hypotheses for experimental research and, as such, interpretation is involved in the transition from exploratory to experimental research. Since an exploratory study does not have a hypothesis to start with, the findings of such study have to be interpreted on a post factum basis in which case the interpretation is technically described as 'post factum' interpretation. In case of studies aimed at hypothesis testing, the researcher either rejects or accepts the hypothesis.

- ***Utilizing research findings:*** It refers to the use of some aspect of a scientific investigation in an application unrelated to the original research. The research findings are utilized by the investigator herself or any other who is interested in utilizing the findings. The dissemination (knowledge transfer) is the step prior to the utilization, which also varies from person to person. The nurse researcher's duty not only rests with conducting research, it also includes promotion for effective utilization, otherwise her research work is meaningless. By recognizing the difference between the dissemination and utilization, she can prepare model for utilization by which one can encourage effective utilization. Evidence-based practice (EBP) involves making clinical decisions on the basis of the best possible evidence. Usually, the best evidence comes from rigorous research, but EBP also uses other sources of credible information.

A nurse who wants to utilize or shows interest in research utilization undergoes the continuum ranging from receiving information without internalization to application of received information.

Stage 1: A nurse receives information but no internalization occurs.

Stage 2: A nurse receives information and internalization occurs but rejects or ignores to apply.

Stage 3: A nurse receives information, internalizes and partially applies or rejects.

Stage 4: A nurse receives information, internalizes and fully replicates.

Stage 5: A nurse receives information, internalizes, and fully adapts for application.

- ***Communicating and disseminating research findings:*** Research study is complete only when the findings have been shared with others. It is of no value unless the research finding is disseminated to the people. It is the researcher's responsibility to ensure that the research study, and its findings/recommendations are disseminated to as wide an audience as possible. Scientific communication takes place in many ways, including archival publication in scholarly journals and informal communication among groups of scientists, known as invisible colleges. For this, a report of entire study should be written by the researcher. The writing of research report necessitates specific methods depending on the purpose for which it is to be written and skill on the part of the researcher to write a report on one's own work. The purpose of writing a research report is to document the research findings, to share the results with other interested groups, and to apply the results in practice. It is a challenging job and requires imagination, creativity and resourcefulness. The research report aims at telling the readers the problems identified, investigated and methods adopted, the results found and the conclusion reached. Research outcome needs to be shared with other professionals, regardless of the study's outcome.

There are many ways of communicating one's research findings. These are:

- Writing dissertation
- Writing for publication in scholarly journals/books/newspapers
- Writing and presenting at conferences
- Writing for funding agencies
- Preparing and doing poster presentation
- Verbal report/presentation at meetings
- Presentation at journal clubs
- Presentation at continuing nursing education programs.

ROLES OF A NURSE RESEARCHER

A nurse researcher plays various roles and performs many functions in research-related activities. The roles and functions of a nurse researcher are as follows:

- ***Critical thinker:*** Critical thinking is the rational examination of ideas, inferences assumptions, principles, arguments, conclusions, issues, statements, beliefs and actions (Bandman and Bandman, 1998). She should possess critical thinking ability which will help her to do a better job in all works of research. Research requires thinking more than doing.
- ***Disseminator/Communicator:*** To fulfill this role, a nurse researcher has to:
    - Communicate the problem faced in the work area
    - Communicate the need for undertaking any research
    - Communicate the progress of research to the concerned people, such as the research committee, or the management, etc.
    - Communicate the limitations, recommendations and findings
    - Communicate to peers in the journal club and also write for publication in journal
    - Present the findings in the conferences and seminars
    - Write to a professional organization for change of practice or implementation of newer skills.
- ***Educator:*** The nurse researcher has to educate the research methodologies, preparation of measurement tools, importance of evidence-based practice, process of research utilization, etc. to other nurses. She can educate and offer consultation services to novice nurse researchers. She has to involve herself in educating the participants or subjects involved regarding the changed practice as well as nurses for evidence-based practice.
- ***Motivator:*** She has to motivate the peers, novice researchers and others to undertake research. She can motivate them to select an appropriate researchable problem which will be of clinical significance. She has the responsibility of motivating them to communicate and disseminate findings.

- ***Advocate:*** As an advocate, she gets approval from the research committee. She checks for the feasibility to conduct the research study. She gets permission from the appropriate agency/person to conduct the study in the selected setting. She acts as a liaison between the subjects and the approval agency. She voices out for the rights of the subjects if, in case, violated.
- ***Strong believer of ethics:*** A nurse researcher, as a strong believer of ethics, has to perform certain functions:
  - She understands and analyzes the ethical issues pertaining to the research problem
  - She prepares and gets informed consent from the participants
  - She maintains confidentiality of the subjects
  - She sets the rules and regulations in conducting the specific study
  - She maintains morale in data collection and analysis
  - She avoids plagiarism during the whole process of research
  - She ensures benefits for the participants and community.
- ***Problem-solver:*** She avoids unnecessary confusions in the research process. She is clear and precise in conducting the study. She follows research principles and methods. She is acquainted with the ethical concerns to avoid obstacles in the process of research.
- ***Research problem creator:*** She is well-versed in finding out the research topic. She thinks about the pros and cons of each action-oriented research. She expects the possibilities of moving with the difficult situations (inadequacy of samples, miscommunication between the participants, delays in the process). She identifies the potential areas of research and the gap in the theory practice areas. She has ability in selecting appropriate research problems.
- ***Evaluator:*** She analyzes the research findings. She evaluates the extent of involvement of each participant in the research process. She analyzes the work of the entire team (group project). She assesses the need for further research, awareness programs and communication of research findings and also evaluates the need for research utilization.
- ***Critique:*** A nurse researcher should develop the ability to evaluate research critically for which one must have critical reading skills. As a critique, the nurse researcher:
  - Performs the research critique
  - Understands that critiquing is not finding fault and being objective in critiquing
  - Identifies appropriate evidence after critiquing for utilization
  - Critiques a research study for evidence-based practice
  - Identifies the major drawbacks in her study as well as in others.
- ***Change agent:*** The nurse researcher, as a change agent:
  - Identifies the areas which need change
  - Introduces appropriate strategies for change
  - Selects the strategies based on scientific principles
  - Supports people during the change process
  - Motivates people to accept the changes.

- ***Evidence-seeker:*** The nurse researcher:
  - Seeks actively evidence for practice
  - Participates in the research process
  - Reviews literature constantly
  - Updates herself with current information
  - Updates herself technically.
- ***Other roles a nurse researcher plays are as follows:***
  - As a trendsetter
  - As a role model
  - As a leader
  - Uses newer scientific methods
  - As a futuristic nurse.

SUMMARY

- Research is a process of collecting, analyzing and interpreting information to answer questions. The foundation for effective research is the strong desire and motivation to do research. Nursing research involves a systematic process aimed to inquire about the issues related to nursing.
- Nursing research is systematic inquiry designed to develop knowledge about issues of importance to the nursing profession, including nursing practice, education, administration and informatics.
- The methods adopted by man for acquiring knowledge are authority, tradition, experience, inductive and deductive reasoning and scientific methods.
- The purpose of conducting research is to describe, speculate, explain, explore, evaluate and do prediction and control.
- The scope of nursing research is as wide and deep as far as the humanity is concerned. The research in nursing can be conducted in the following areas such as based on the major areas of nursing, specialty areas, various developmental age groups of human beings, preventive, promotive, curative and rehabilitative areas. Research can also be conducted in various settings.
- Research can be categorized into pure or basic research and applied research based on its application.
- Pure research involves developing and testing theories and hypotheses that are intellectually challenging to the researcher but may or may not have practical application at the present time or in the future.
- Applied research is done to solve specific, practical questions for policy formulation, administration and understanding of a phenomenon.
- Research can be classified from the viewpoint of objectives, as descriptive, correlational, explanatory and exploratory research. From the process adopted to find answers to research questions—the two approaches are structured approach and unstructured approach. The structured approach to inquiry is usually classified as the quantitative research whereas the unstructured approach is classified as the qualitative research.
- The major steps in research process are problem statement, reviewing of literature, planning research design and methods, data collection and data analysis, interpretation and utilization.

2 Problem Statement

OBJECTIVES

After reading this chapter, you will be able to:

- State the meaning of research problem
- State the importance of formulating the research problem
- List the sources of research problem
- Explain the steps involved in formulating research problem
- Explain the writing of problem statement
- List the essential elements of research problem
- Describe the critiquing of research problem
- Explain the method of stating research objectives, hypothesis and assumptions.

INTRODUCTION

In the process of research, the first most important step is the selection and statement of the research problem. The research problem is often argued as the heart of the research process, without which no research process can take place. The researcher should formulate it in such a way that it becomes workable or lends itself for investigation. Research is a cycle, it starts with a problem and ends with a solution to the problem. The problem statement is therefore the axis on which the whole research revolves around because it explains in short the aim of the research. A research study begins as a question that a researcher would like to answer or as a problem that a researcher would like to solve.

RESEARCH PROBLEM

A research problem is a question or an issue or a doubt or a situation which makes the person to think deeply, concentrate and focus on and which demands an answer, or solution or clarification etc. A research problem causes the researcher to feel uneasy, confused and he is disturbed till he finds an answer. A research problem in general refers to some felt difficulty which the investigator experiences in the context of the theoretical or practical situation and for which he feels the urge to solve. A research problem is a situation or circumstance that requires a solution to be described, explained or predicted. The research problem identifies the knowledge gap that needs to be filled. It involves the demarcation of a problem with reference to WHO or WHAT, the WHERE, the WHEN and the WHY of the problem in a specific context. The apprehension or the felt difficulty gives rise to the problem to be researched which has to be expressed or stated in a proper way. The problem which is stated as a declarative form is the problem statement or which is asked as a question is known as ***research question***.

Importance of Formulating the Research Problem

According to Kumar (2005) research problem statement is like the identification of a destination before undertaking a journey. As in the absence of a destination, it is impossible to identify the shortest or indeed any route in the absence of a clear research problem, a clear economical plan is impossible. A research problem is the first step and the most important requirement in the research process. It serves as the foundation of a research study. According the Kerlinger, in order for one to solve a problem, one must know what the problem is. The large part of the problem is knowing what one is trying to do. A well formulated problem is already a half-solved problem. A research problem is also expressed as a general question about the relationship between two or more variables. The formulation of a problem introduces the necessity of defining clearly all concepts used and of determining the variables and their relationships. A research problem is like the foundation of a building. The type and design of a building is dependent upon the foundation of a building. A proper definition of research problem will enable the researcher to be on the track whereas an ill defined problem may create hurdle. Thus, proper definition of a research problem is a pre-requisite for any study and is a step of the highest importance.

Sources of Research Problem

Kumar (2005) writes that most research in the humanities revolves around 'four Ps' thus People, Problems, Programs and Phenomena. There are many problem situations that may give rise to research. The sources usually contribute to problem identification are as follows:

Experience

Own experience or the experience of others may be a source of problem supply. The nurses everyday experience provides a rich supply of problems for investigation. Nurses working in various settings such as educational institution, hospitals, community, etc. might experience issues and problems and their experience serves as a source of research problem. For example, the Nursing Superintendent may come across the problem of staff turnover in spite of good remuneration and perks. She must be worried about this problem and may try to analyze the situation and find a solution for this problem. This can be done by undertaking a research. The increased incidence of nosocomial infection in the hospital might serve as problem for a nurse to research on.

Literature

A second source could be scientific literature. We may read about certain findings and notice that a certain field was not covered. This could lead to a research problem. Ideas for research projects often come from reading the nursing literature. Published research reports may suggest problem areas indirectly by stimulating the reader's imagination and directly by explicitly stating the types of additional research that are needed. For example, we knew that over the past half-century, the mass media, including video games, have become important socializers of children. Playing video games is now a major leisurely pursuit among children in many parts of the world. Over the past three decades, a number of studies have looked at the effects of video games on children and adolescents. These studies were conducted mostly in developed high income countries. Several of these studies have shown that violent video game exposure increases aggressive thoughts, angry feelings, physiological arousal, aggressive behaviors and physiological desensitization to violence in the real world. Research evidence has accumulated over the past half-century stating that exposure to violence on television, movies and most recently in video games increased the risk of violent behavior on the viewer's part just as growing up in an environment filled with real violence.

We could find and read many studies on the impact of playing violent video games among children in the developed countries. Developed countries have regulatory mechanisms such as rating of violent video games and specific rules and regulations for selling video games to children. These games are introduced in India and we are not aware of the information regarding the rating. Videogame playing is equated to computer learning. Studies on playing violent video games are very less in India and the short-term and long-term effects of playing violent video games is an unexplored area. The problem for a research emerges from this and one can decide to assess the knowledge/awareness or its long-term and short-term effects on children or the kind of regulatory mechanism we have in controlling and monitoring.

Newspapers, Government reports give lot of information related to health and diseases. Abuse of children and women, report of communicable diseases and non communicable diseases, any specific problems in a particular area were reported often. This could also serve as a source for a research problem.

Theories

Theories could be a third source. Theoretical schemes and conceptual framework that have been developed in nursing and other related disciplines give many ideas through a process of deduction that can be tested. Shortcomings in theories could be researched. Research can thus be aimed at clarifying or substantiating an existing theory, at clarifying contradictory findings, at correcting a faulty methodology, at correcting the inadequate or unsuitable use of statistical techniques, at reconciling conflicting opinions, or at solving existing practical problems.

For example, in the social learning theory, proposed by Albert Bandura explained that human aggression is largely learned by watching other people behave aggressively, either in person or in television/films. It is also learned when we are rewarded for aggression. There are two important principles underlying this theory. In this hypothesis, aggression is initially learnt from social behavior and it is maintained by other conditions. There are a variety of proposed methods through which aggression is learnt and maintained. One method of learning aggressive behavior is through simple operant conditioning. If after performing an aggressive act an animal or human receives a positive reinforcement (such as food or a toy), they are likely to repeat the behavior in order to gain more rewards. From this concept, one can pick up a problem for a research. We can formulate few questions that what is the impact of watching aggression/violence in visual media? Are we rewarding aggressive acts in children in real life situations? What are the factors contributing in the development of aggression in children?.

Ideas from External Sources

External sources can sometimes provide the impetus for research ideas. In some cases, a research topic may be given to students as a direct suggestion. In other cases, ideas for studies may emerge as a result of a brainstorming session or from discussion with other nurses, researchers or nursing faculty.

Research in Social Sciences Revolves Around four Ps

People include a group of individuals with or without problems. Any research is conducted ultimately for the benefit of humanity. Many times, the researcher is interested to study the problems of the people, by the people and for the people. There is no individual without problems. Even if there are no problems or issues, studies are conducted to observe their healthy practices, behaviors, culture, etc. to understand, analyze and modify.

Problems denote the existence of certain issues. Many inventions are evolved out of the problem faced by the humanity. Problems pose threat to the individual/organization/Nation according to its severity. Problems help us to develop new strategies, equip us with new knowledge and facilitate us to face challenges. People and problem are inseparable. Research can be undertaken to ascertain attitude of a group of people towards an issue or how a societal problem is perceived by the people or what impact it may create on the people.

Programs are specific intervention carried out for a specific purpose. There are many programs planned, implemented, revised and modified by the Government and private sector. Programs are devised with specific objectives and lot of input in the form of men, money and material is involved in order to achieve specific objectives. For example, Pulse Polio Programs, Universal Child Immunization and various other welfare programs were formulated for the welfare of the people. We can analyze whether are these programs effective or successful? How effectively can it be carried out? Whether does any program need revision or modification? We can analyze the input vs output, evaluate structure, process and outcome, conduct customer satisfaction surveys, etc.

Phenomena are the appearance, manifestation or experience of something. Sometimes we may observe that certain phenomena may manifest itself regularly or something might be a rare occurrence. Study of phenomena of interest is important particularly to understand the phenomena itself, its nature and its impact. Research can be conducted to establish certain phenomena, evaluate its impact on health and well-being.

In practice, most research studies are based upon at least a combination of two Ps.

Every research study has two aspects:

1. Study population
   - ***People:*** Individuals, organizations, groups, communities (Either they provide us with the information or we collect information about them)
2. Subject area
   - ***Problems:*** Issues, situations, associations, needs, profiles
   - ***Program:*** Content, structure, outcomes, attributes, satisfactions, consumers, service providers, etc.
   - ***Phenomenon:*** Cause-and-effect relationships, the study of a phenomenon itself.

Steps Involved in Formulating a Research Problem

The major steps involved in formulation of a research problem are as follows:

- Identification of a broad area of interest
- Dissection of the broad area into sub-areas
- Selection of the sub-area for the research through the process of elimination
- Writing a problem statement or research questions
- Reviewing and finalizing the problem statement.

Identification of a Broad Area of Interest

In general when we want to do a research we should select a broad area of our own interest. Suppose an investigator wants to undertake research on some specific issues related to child health then this becomes the broad area of interest. Though we study many subjects, we have some preference towards a particular area than other. It is always good to limit ourselves to the area of interest.

Dissection of the Broad Area into Sub-areas

If child health is selected as a broad area which can be dissected into many sub-areas by asking oneself. In child health, one can study on the health of children of various developmental age groups such as newborn, infants, toddler, preschooler, school ager and adolescents. We can study children based on gender difference, health status, i.e. sick or normal children, health dimensions such as physical health, mental health, social health, etc. and also can undertake research on preventive promotive, curative and rehabilitative aspects of children.

Selection of the Sub-area for the Research Through the Process of Elimination

From among the many sub-areas, one can select one particular sub-area through the process of elimination for various reasons. The reasons may be familiarity, interest, feasibility in terms of accessibility to samples, tools/equipments or measuring instruments, finance, time and duration of data collection, permission from the setting, etc. For example, by thinking and analyzing all those factors, an investigator can limit herself to the research on mental health of the adolescents.

Writing a Problem Statement or Research Questions

After selecting the sub-area, one should identify exactly what she wants to study. The major variables of interest should be identified. In the sub theme of mental health of the adolescents, there are many variables which can be studied. For example, knowledge on mental health, assessment of mental health, factors promoting/hindering mental health in adolescents, influence of media on mental health, etc. The researcher should select one or two major variables of interest and should write the proper problem statement or research questions.

Reviewing and Finalizing the Problem Statement

Once the problem statement is formulated, the investigator has to review and check for all the elements of a research problem.

One need not to follow the steps mentioned above in order to write the problem statement. It may be of more use for the novice researcher. An experienced researcher would be able to formulate problem statement based on the need for research. The investigator would be able to identify the need for the research which usually arises from their day to day experience, critical observations made, critical thinking done on issues concerning nursing, etc. It is a known fact that any research should evolve from the specific need. The writing of need for a study needs critical thinking and analytical writing.

1. Example of a need stated in a research on 'A study to assess the psycho-physiological effect of playing violent video games among children in Chennai.'

   Videogames were introduced in India in late1990s. Children were highly fascinated towards playing video games. In the United States, many researchers and psychologists had conducted many researches on the effect of playing violent video games among children. In US, there is a nongovernmental organization called ***ESRB***, the Entertainment Software Rating Board which rates all video games and prescribes regulation to monitor and sale of video games to children. Many studies in this regard, proved that playing violent video games cause the children to exhibit aggression and hostile behavior and also they resort to physical violence against others. Violent video game playing by children result in poor school performance and the reason was explained by the displacement theory. This 'displacement hypothesis' suggests that electronic media can influence learning and social behavior by taking the place of activities such as reading, family interaction, and social play with peers.

The studies related to the effect of playing violent video games in Indian context are very scarce. Little is known about the preference towards games, playing habits, hours of playing, duration of playing, amount spent in playing, the content or theme of the game and the perception by the children and the parents. The need was felt to assess the prevalence and the effect of playing violent video games among children in Chennai.

2. Example of a need stated in a research on 'A study to assess the food practice as expressed by the adolescent boys in Chennai.'

   The eating habits of the adolescent children are changing. The introduction of fast food/ready to eat food/easy to cook food has influenced the eating habits of the adolescent children. The boys especially during adolescence are under peer influence and they prefer to eat outside and their food choices are not the traditional one. They pose lot of demands on the parents and even the parents may not be able to insist on good eating habits. Adolescents need adequate calorie, protein, fat, mineral and vitamins for their growth and a balanced diet could give all these nutrients adequately. Adolescents have the habit of skipping breakfast and they restrict the intake of fruits and vegetables. If they skip breakfast, they tend to buy it outside. When they select food from outside, they do not choose to eat meals instead they choose a junk food and a bottled drink. The fast food may be tasty but they contain more of calorie, fat and salt. This may lead to under nutrition and obesity in many children. The adolescents study about the importance of nutrition in their school subjects. Also their parents and teacher insist on good eating habits. With all that they end up with unhealthy eating habits. With this background information, this study was conducted to assess the food practice of the adolescent boys in Perungudi, Chennai.

3. Gormely, DK & Kennerly, S (2011) on their study on 'Predictors of Turnover Intention in Nurse Faculty,' the need for the study was stated as follows:

   Turnover of nurse faculty is receiving increasing attention in schools and college of nursing as the available number of qualified faculty declines. Understanding factors that contribute to turnover and designing interventions to retain nurse faculty in existing positions is specially important, given that the nursing profession is facing a critical shortage of qualified faculty. The shortage of doctorally prepared nurse faculty has major consequences for the nursing profession. The insufficient number of qualified nurse faculty has already begun to limit the number of students who can be educated. Doctorally prepared faculties are required in academia to conduct nursing research and disseminate knowledge. Because of the inadequate numbers of doctorally prepared nurses in academia, the ability to advance the scientific knowledge base of the profession will be compromised.

Precautions to be Taken while Selecting a Research Problem

- The topic or subject which is overdone should not be chosen in general. It will be difficult to throw any new light related to the problem.
- Controversial topic should preferably be avoided.
- The topic selected should be familiar and feasible.

Writing Problem Statement

Writing problem statement involves questioning skills and critical thinking skills.

1. In general a research problem is stated by starting 'A Study to'.
2. Then the investigator has to decide what she wants to do in her research. She has to ask herself whether she wants to assess, compare, evaluate, identify, etc. It is good to have an outcome based verb at or near the beginning of the problem statement. Some good outcome based verbs are:
   - identify
   - relate
   - describe
   - formulate
   - compare
   - analyze
   - assess
   - categorize
   - evaluate.

   Verbs such as 'understand', 'explore', 'investigate', 'examine' and 'discuss' are poor verbs as they describe processes, not outcomes.
3. After deciding the outcome verb, the researcher can question herself to know what outcome she wants. For example, 'A study to assess ......' In this, one can question herself to know what she wants to assess that is knowledge or practice or impact or effectiveness, etc.
4. The next question is what knowledge/practice/impact or effectiveness she wants to assess. One can answer by the following ways:
   - A study to assess the knowledge on prevention of accidents in children
   - A study to assess the impact of poor eating on growth
   - A study to assess the hand washing practices followed
   - A study to assess the effectiveness of Structured Teaching Program on knowledge.
5. The next step is to decide among whom the investigator wants to assess. It is the samples of the study from whom the data will be collected.
6. The final step is to decide the setting from where the investigator can have access to those samples.

For example:

- A study to + assess + the knowledge on prevention of accidents in children + mothers of under five children + Adayar, Chennai
- A study to assess the knowledge on prevention of accidents in children among mothers of under five children at Adayar, Chennai

- A study to + assess + the impact of eating habits on growth + adolescent girls + selected community setting, Chennai
- A study to assess the impact of eating habits on growth among adolescent girls in selected community setting, Chennai
- A study to + assess + the hand washing practices + nurses + selected hospitals, Chennai
- A study to assess the hand washing practices of nurses working in selected hospitals, Chennai.

Research Question

The research question can also be formulated as follows:

- What is the level of knowledge on prevention of accidents in children among mothers of under five children?
- What is the impact of poor eating on growth among adolescent girls?
- Is there any relationship between the television watching and school performance?

Examples of research questions formulated in research studies

McNiesh, SG (2011) conducted a study on 'The lived experience of students in an accelerated nursing program: Intersecting factors that influence experiential learning.'

The research questions formulated by the researcher were as follows:

- How did previous life experiences, education, and career choices influence the experience of second-degree students?
- What were the potential effects on learning of condensing and accelerating the curriculum as is requisite in second degree programs?

Metz, AM, Cech EA Babcock, T and Smith, JL (2011) on their study on 'Effects of Formal and Informal support structures on the motivation of native American students in nursing' stated research questions as follows:

- What social support factors are most important in predicting Native American student success?
- Does perceived unfairness measurably impact Native American nursing students' success?

Problem statements may be worded in a number of ways. Many research textbooks recommend that research problems be stated in the interrogative form. It has advantage of simplicity and directness. Questions invite an answer and help to focus the researcher's and the readers' attention on the kind of data that would have to be collected to provide that answer. Frequently, researchers state their research problem in the declarative form. Research originates from a need that arises. A clear distinction between the problem and the purpose should be made. The problem is the aspect the researcher worries about, thinks about, and wants to find a solution for. The purpose is to solve the problem, i.e. find answers to the question(s). If there is no clear problem formulation, the purpose and methods are meaningless.

The research problem should be stated in such a way that it would lead to analytical thinking on the part of the researcher with the aim of possible concluding solutions to the stated problem. Research problems can be stated in the form of either questions or statements. The research problem should always be formulated grammatically correct and as completely as possible. Meaningless words should be avoided. There should be no doubt in the mind of the reader what the investigator's intentions are.

Essential Characteristics of a Problem Statement

- The key variables
- The population
- The setting.

Variables and Constants

Characteristics of persons or objects that vary from person to person or object to object are called ***variables*** whereas characteristics that remain constant from person to person or object to object are called ***constants***. Whether a characteristic is designated as a variable or a constant depends on the course of the study in question.

Example 1:

Identify the variable and constant in a study of Hemoglobin level of adolescent girls in a selected community area.
Variable: Hemoglobin level
Constant: Gender and community
Identify the variable and constant in a study of assessment of knowledge on menstrual hygiene among adolescent girls studying in school X.
Variable: Knowledge on menstrual hygiene
Constant: Gender and School.

Population

Population in a research problem means to whom the findings are to be generalized. Without population, a problem statement is incomplete.

Setting

Setting is the place or area where the population is available. From the population, samples are taken for a research.

Example 2:

Identify the variables, population and setting in the problem statement.

1. A study to assess the handwashing practice of nurses working in selected hospitals in Chennai.
   Variable: Handwashing practices
   Population: Nurses
   Setting: Selected hospitals in Chennai.
2. A study to assess the impact of eating habits on growth among adolescent girls in selected community setting, Chennai.
   Variable: Eating habits (Independent variable) and Growth (Dependent variable)
   Population: Adolescent girls

contd...

contd...

Setting: Selected community area, Chennai.

3. A study to assess the knowledge on prevention of accidents in children among mothers of under five children at Adayar, Chennai.
   Variable: Knowledge on prevention of accidents in children
   Population: Mothers of under five children
   Setting: Adayar, Chennai.
4. A study to assess the effectiveness of Structured Teaching Program on knowledge regarding balanced diet among mothers of under five children residing at Porur, Chennai.
   Variable: Structured Teaching Program (Independent variable) and Knowledge (Dependent variable)
   Population: Mothers of under five children
   Setting: Porur, Chennai.

Factors to be Considered while Choosing the Problem for the Research

A researcher needs to consider various factors before finalizing a problem for the research. They are as follows:

1. ***Significance to nursing:*** An investigator has to first satisfy herself that the problem chosen for the research is significant to nursing. The following question can help her in deciding a problem based on its contribution to nursing:
   - Does the problem contribute to nursing education, practice, administration and research?
   - Does this help to add to the body of knowledge for nursing?
   - Does this problem has any practical relevance?
   - Does it have any specific implications to nursing practice?
   - Is the problem an important one?
2. ***Strength of the Researcher:*** The researcher must have insight about his own strength and weaknesses. He must be familiar with the research methodology and the problem chosen should be of his own interest. He must ensure that he had the necessary training and knowledge before proceeding into any research.
3. ***Researchability:*** A problem should be amenable for investigation. There are certain areas which are not amenable for testing. The selection of a problem must be preceded by a preliminary study in case it is less done or no such existing study. But when the field of enquiry is similar to one that already been done, the preliminary study may not be necessary. Too narrow and too vague problems should be avoided.
4. ***Feasibility:*** Feasibility of a study can be assessed by checking the following:
   - ***Time:*** The problem selected must be one which can be studied within the time period available.
   - ***Availability of samples:*** Samples for a specific study must fulfill some criteria. The researcher must ensure whether the adequate number of samples would be available with some specific characteristics within the time frame allocated for the study.

- ***Budget:*** The conduction of research involves money. Money is needed for the purchase of equipments, printing, transportation, etc. Sometimes a research may be funded or the cost may be borne by the researcher herself. One should ensure whether adequate budget is available to complete a study.
- ***Availability of tool for data collection:*** The researcher must ensure that she has the necessary equipments or tool to collect the data. She must be familiar with the tool or equipment and know how to operate it or use it. Tool can be prepared by the researcher herself or standardized tool can be used with necessary permission from the author. In case of mechanical instruments, the researcher must purchase or has to hire for rent. While purchasing, care must be taken to identify a standardized tool which should be valid as well as reliable.
- ***Permission from the setting:*** A study can be conducted in various settings such as hospitals, community areas, schools, etc. The researcher has to check whether the head of the organization would allow or grant permission to conduct study, is it feasible to collect the data in that setting and collecting data would not affect the routine functioning.
- ***Cooperation from all concerned:*** It is not easy to complete a study without the cooperation from the subjects and their relatives, people in the settings and all those either directly or indirectly related to research.
- ***Ethical considerations:*** A research problem may not be feasible if a study addressing the problem would pose unfair or unethical demands on the participants.

Critiquing of a Research Problem

The below written questions will help the researcher to think, analyze and critique the research problem. This aids in reviewing and finalizing problem statement.

- Does the problem contribute to nursing education, practice, administration and research?
- Does this help to add to the body of knowledge for nursing?
- Does this problem have any theoretical or practical value or relevance?
- Does it have any specific implications to nursing practice?
- Is the problem an important one?
- Is the problem statement clearly and concisely articulated?
- Is the problem statement objective and feasible to study?
- Is the problem logical?
- Is the problem too narrow or vague?
- Is the problem complex to study?
- Is the scope of the problem delimited?
- Does the problem statement consist of all elements such as key variables, population and setting?
- Does the problem statement sensible and justifiable?

- Does the problem feasible in terms of time, availability of samples and permission from the setting and budget?
- Is the research free of any ethical problems and limitations?

Difference between the Problem Statement and Title of a Research

The problem statement and title of a research is different. The title is a brief heading of the research whereas the problem statement explains the problem completely with all its elements. The title unlike a problem statement needs not to have all the elements and it is like a title of a book. It should attract the reader, quickly convey the major subject/area of research and it should make the reader to read what is inside. A title should be catchy, neither too lengthy nor too short, simple, related to the research conveying the major area of research. The table 2.1 gives the difference between the problem statement and title of a research.

Table 2.1: Difference between problem statement and title of a research

S. No.	Problem statement	Title of a research
1.	It is one of the components of the research	Title is a brief heading of the research
2.	It consists of some important elements such as the problem, population and place	A title need not to have all the elements
3.	It should be complete otherwise it is meaningless	It conveys meaning even if it is incomplete
4.	Problem statement is the axis with which the whole research revolves around	The title is a mere heading and of no use to build further research
5.	It conveys the reader about the exact problem, among whom it is conducted and the place where the samples are to be selected	Title conveys the major area of research. It may not give information on the population and the setting
6.	It is comparatively lengthy. It is ideal to limit the problem statement within 18–20 words	It is comparatively shorter in length. It may be 10–12 words
7.	**Example:** • A study to assess the psychophysiological effect of playing violent video games among adolescents in Chennai	**Example:** • Adolescents and violent video game playing • Violent video game playing—a study among adolescents in Chennai

RESEARCH AIMS AND OBJECTIVES

It is important to keep in mind that the clearer the research objectives, the more actionable the research findings will be. Aims are broad statements of desired outcomes, or the general intentions of the research. Aims and Objectives should be presented concisely and briefly and be interrelated. The aim is what the investigator wants to achieve and the objectives describe how the investigator is going to achieve that aim.

The objectives of a research are derived from the problem statement which simplifies the step to be followed in a research. It communicates to the readers what the researcher intends to achieve by the study. These objectives should be closely related to the research problem.

The general objective of a study states what researchers expect to achieve by the study in general terms. The specific objectives are the logical steps formulated from the general objectives which explain what the researcher will do in her study.

Purpose of Writing Research Objectives

- It directs the researcher to focus on his study
- It communicates the major activities to be done in the research
- It helps to develop the methodology of research
- It will help to decide on the method of data collection, analysis and interpretation of data
- It enables the researcher to report his findings in a systematic way

Statement of Objectives

- Objectives are stated in achievable, outcome-based terms
- It should be presented as concise statements that describe what the researcher plans to accomplish by research activities
- Objectives should be specific and realistic
- Appropriate action verbs should be used. The examples of action verbs are to assess, to compare, to correlate, to associate, etc.
- Vague and nonaction verbs such as to appreciate, to understand, etc. should be avoided
- Writing too many objectives and too less objectives should be avoided. Too many objectives will lead to overlapping of the content and too less objectives lead to omission of certain areas of study
- It should be written logically and in an orderly way.

Example of Problem of Statement, Aims and Objectives of the Study

1. ***Problem statement:*** A study to assess the psychophysiological effect of playing violent video games among children in Chennai.

   Aim of the study: The major aim of the study was to assess the prevalence and the psychophysiological effect of playing violent video games among children in Chennai.

   Objectives of the study:

   - To assess the prevalence of violent video game playing among children
   - To assess the psychological effect of playing violent video games among children
   - To associate the psychological effect of playing violent video games with the selected demographic variables.
2. ***Problem statement:*** A study to assess the awareness and attitude towards anti-ragging among students studying in selected arts and science college in Chennai.

Aim of the study: The aim of the study was to assess the level of awareness regarding anti-ragging measures among college students and their attitude towards anti-ragging and also to correlate the knowledge and attitude towards anti ragging.

Objectives of the study:

- To assess the level of awareness regarding anti-ragging measures among students studying in selected colleges in Chennai
- To assess the level of attitude regarding anti-ragging measures among students studying in selected colleges in Chennai
- To correlate the awareness and attitude regarding anti-ragging.
- To associate the level of awareness regarding anti-ragging measures with the demographic variables of the students
- To associate the level of attitude regarding anti-ragging with the demographic variables of the students.

3. McNiesh, SG (2011) conducted a study on 'The lived experience of students in an accelerated nursing program: Intersecting factors that influence Experiential learning'.
   The aim of the study as written by the researcher was as follows:
   The overall goal of this interpretive phenomenological study was to articulate the lived experience of students in an accelerated MSN entry program learning the practice of nursing within a clinical setting.
4. Gormely, DK & Kennerly, S (2011) on their study on 'Predictors of Turnover Intention in Nurse Faculty' the purpose was stated as follows:
   The purpose of the study was a secondary analysis of data examining the predictors of turnover intention in nurse faculty working in departments and college of nursing in Carnegie Doctoral/Research Universities—Extensive, public and private, not-for-profit institutions. The original study examined the relationships between organizational climate, role conflict, role ambiguity, faculty work roles, organizational commitment and turnover intention.
5. Nguyen, DN, Zierer, B & Nguyen, HQ (2011) in their study on 'A survey of nursing faculty needs for training in use of new technologies for education and practice' stated the purpose as follows:
   The purpose of this study was to conduct a needs assessment for faculty training in integrating new technologies into nursing education to inform the development of faculty training programs. The primary aim of the study was to describe nursing faculty's use, knowledge and training needs associated with distance learning, simulation, telehealth, and informatics tools. A secondary aim was to examine both individual and institutional factors associated with use and knowledge of distance learning and simulation tolls in nursing education.
6. Metz, AM, Cech, EA, Babcock, T & Smith JL (2011) on their study on 'Effects of formal and informal support structures on the motivation of native American students in nursing' stated the purpose as follows:
   The purpose of this study was to identify which social support factors influence the success of Native American students in an undergraduate nursing curriculum.

HYPOTHESIS

The next step after defining the problem is to formulate a tentative explanation or solution of that problem in the form of a proposition. The tentative explanation or solution, the validity of which is still to be tested is called the ***hypothesis***. It is an informed/educated guess. It explains the researcher's expectation of a relationship existing between the variables. It indicates the expectations of the researcher regarding certain variables.

'Hypo' means less than and 'thesis' means a 'generally held view'. Hypothesis is a less than generally held view. It is an assumption or proposition whose tenability is to be tested. The other explanation given was less than or less certain than a thesis.

A hypothesis is the formal statement of the expected relationship(s) between two or more variables (Burns and Groove).

According to Polit 'A hypothesis is a tentative prediction or explanation of the relationship between two or more variables'.

A hypothesis is a conjectural statement of the relationship between two or more variables (Kerlin, 1986).

It is a tentative assumption or preliminary statement about the relationship between two or more things that needs to be examined (Welman et al, 2005).

Hypothesis is a statement capable of being tested and thereby verified or rejected (Rummel and Balline).

It is a proposition that is stated in a testable form and that predicts a particular relationship between two (or more) variables.

The Difference Between a Hypothesis and a Problem

Both a hypothesis and a problem contribute to the body of knowledge which supports or refutes an existing theory. A hypothesis differs from a problem in the following ways (Refer table 2.2).

Table 2.2: Difference between the research problem and hypothesis

S. No.	Research problem	Hypothesis
1.	It conveys what the researcher wants to study	It conveys what the researcher wants to prove or disprove
2.	It originates from the need	It is derived from the research problem
3.	A problem cannot be directly tested	Hypothesis can be directly tested and verified
4.	It is a problem to be researched	It is a suggested solution to a problem
5.	The scope of a research problem is wide.	It is more specific and suggests the relationship between the variables

When Hypothesis is Formulated?

A hypothesis is an expected answer to a research question, it provides direction to the research study. A hypothesis in reality determines the focal point of the study, in the absence of a valid and testable hypothesis the researcher cannot concentrate on one direction. Many new researchers face the problem of summing up their research question in a precise and concise manner. The reason behind this problem is mainly lack of hypothesis or presence of irrelevant hypothesis.

A hypothesis is formulated after the problem has been stated and the literature review has been done. It is formulated when the researcher is totally aware of the theoretical and empirical background of the problem.

It should however be remembered that the formulation of a hypothesis though advisable is not absolutely necessary in all types of studies. Exploratory and preliminary studies often do not use hypothesis. A researcher may be interested in learning more about some phenomenon and thus may engage in a fact-finding investigation. It is least crucial where the study is exploratory in nature. But it is must where the study is experimental in nature. In experimental studies, formulation of hypotheses is mandatory since hypotheses are the predictions about the outcome of an experiment. In case of historical, descriptive and other fact finding study, hypotheses need not be formulated. Also when there is no prediction possible, a hypothesis need not be formulated.

Advantages of Hypothesis

Hypotheses are important for bringing clarity, specificity and focus to a research study:

- It gives direction to an investigation
- It helps the researcher to focus on the variables to be studied
- It enables the researcher to decide on the data to be collected, method of research including research design and population to be studied
- It directs the measurement of variables and statistical analysis
- It states the relationships between the variables that can be empirically tested
- It furnishes proof that the researcher has sufficient background knowledge
- A good hypothesis enriches the theory
- Hypotheses may only add to the formulation of theory after they have been proven to be true
- Testing hypothesis is a means of generating knowledge through testing of theoretical propositions.

Characteristics of a Good Hypothesis

- It should have elucidating power
- It should strive to furnish an acceptable explanation of the phenomenon
- It should be as simple as possible
- It should be specific but not trivial
- It must be conceptually clear
- It must be verifiable or testable
- It must be formulated in simple, understandable terms
- It should correspond with existing knowledge
- It should be consistent with known facts
- Lastly it should be operationalizable thus expressible in terms that can be measured.

Sources of Hypotheses

- May be based on a hunch that the researcher is interested in studying
- Researcher's own beliefs and insights about the problem
- It can be based on smart observation of some phenomenon
- It can be a restatement of a hypothesis that has been tested previously
- Existing theory related to the problem
- It may be the beliefs of others who have knowledge about the problem.

Elements of Hypotheses

The elements of a hypothesis are:
- The variable(s)
- Relationship and direction
- Population
- Level of significance.

Variables

Variables are anything which varies from person to person. Any hypothesis consists of minimum of two variables. Variables are major focus of the study in a research.

For example, the variables in the hypothesis 'Children with increased frequency of playing violent video game show a significant increase in the level of aggression' are frequency of playing violent video game and the aggression.

Relationship and Direction

Hypothesis is a tentative statement which shows the relationship between two or more variables. It is good if the researcher states the direction of relationship between the variables.

Types of Relationship

- ***Associative relationship:*** It includes research variables and states the covariation of these variables in the real world.
  Example for associative relationship. There is an association between violent video game playing and aggression in children.
- ***Causal relationship:*** It includes independent variable and dependent variable. The independent variable is manipulated by the researcher in order to examine the effects on the dependent variable.

The knowledge score on balanced diet is high in mothers of experimental group receiving Structured Teaching Program than the mothers of control group who do not receive.

In this, knowledge is the dependent variable and the Structured Teaching Program is the independent variable.

Population

Hypothesis is a statement about the relationship between the variables which will be measured in the samples. The samples are selected from the population.

Children are the population in the hypothesis, 'There is an association between violent video game playing and aggression in children.'

Mothers are the population in the hypothesis, 'The knowledge score on balanced diet is high in mothers of experimental group receiving Structured Teaching Program than the mothers of control group who do not receive.'

Adolescent girls are the population in the hypothesis, 'the level of hemoglobin is more in adolescent girls who are non-vegetarian than the vegetarian.'

Level of Significance

It is always good to mention the confidence level with which a researcher would like to test the hypothesis. The level of significance usually set is P = 0.05, 0.01, 0.001 level. It is implied that a hypothesis is to be tested at 0.05 level of significance even if it is not expressed in the hypothesis.

Types of Hypotheses

Hypotheses can be classified as follows:

Based on the Number of Variables

Simple Vs. complex hypotheses: A simple hypothesis states the relationship between two variables. A complex hypothesis predicts the relationship between more than two variables.

Example of simple hypothesis: Children playing violent video game score more on aggression inventory than who play non-violent video game. Boys spend more hours of playing violent video games than girls.

Example of complex hypothesis: As age of the children advances, the frequency, duration, total hours of playing violent video game increases. There is no difference between the male and female children's exposure to violent video game and level of aggression and stress. The violent video game playing is influenced by the age, gender, economic status and the peer influence of the children.

Based on the Direction

Non-directional vs directional hypotheses: A non-directional hypothesis states that a relationship exists but does not predict the exact nature of the relationship. A directional hypothesis states the specific nature of the relationship between two or more variables. The use of such terms as less, more, increase, decrease, greater and smaller indicates the direction of relationship in hypotheses.

Example of directional hypothesis: Children with increased frequency of playing violent video game show a significant increase in the aggression.

As the frequency of playing violent video game increases the level of aggression increases in children. As the duration of playing violent video game decreases the level of aggression decreases. Children attending special coaching score greater than those who do not attend the special coaching.

Example of non-directional hypothesis: There is a relation between the level of knowledge and attitude of children regarding personal hygiene.

There is a difference in the income generated by the transgenders living in urban and rural area.

Based on the Concept of Acceptance or Rejection

Research Hypotheses

Research hypotheses otherwise known as ***scientific hypotheses***. It indicates what the outcome of the study is expected to be. It is also either directional or non-directional. Research hypotheses may be of two types: descriptive and relational. Descriptive hypotheses are those propositions which tentatively state the existence, size, form or distribution of some variable, subject to verification by research. Relational hypotheses are those propositions which state the relationship between two variables. In relational hypotheses there always exist two variables, the independent variable and the dependent variable. Phrases such as 'greater than', 'less than', 'positively or negatively' and 'difference in' states the direction in the hypotheses. The nature of the relationship either causal or associative is also implied by the hypothesis. A causal relationship is one where the researcher is able to predict that the independent variable causes a change in the dependent variable.

Example of research hypothesis

- There is an association between the dietary intake and weight of the children
- There is an association between the intelligence and scholastic performance of the children
- There is a difference in the self-esteem in children from violent and non-violent family
- There is a correlation between the height and weight of the adolescent children
- Structured Teaching Program is effective in increasing the knowledge of mother of under five children on balanced diet
- Relaxation therapy is effective in reducing the stress of patients admitted in acute care ward.

Metz, AM, Cech, EA, Babcock, T & Smith JL (2011) on their study on 'Effects of formal and informal support structures on the motivation of native American students in nursing' stated hypothesis as follows:

Greater amounts of social support would positively predict success.

(Success was defined as identification with, interest in, valuation of, and motivation to pursue nursing as a career).

Negative experiences that undermine support, such as perceptions of institutional unfairness and racism, would adversely affect Native American Nursing students' success.

Null Hypothesis (Ho)

It is referred to as a statistical hypothesis. A null hypothesis is used for the purpose of statistical testing and interpreting statistical outcomes. It is usually formulated for the purpose of being rejected. The null hypothesis states that there is no difference between two variables. The level of significance for rejection or acceptance of the null hypothesis is arbitrarily determined before head by the researcher. Even if the null hypothesis is not stated, it is implied, because it is the converse of the research hypothesis.

Null hypothesis is akin to the legal principle that a man is innocent until he is proved guilty. It constitutes a challenge and the function of research is to give the fact a chance to refute (or fail to refute) this challenge. This type of hypothesis is especially useful in tests of statistical significance. It is also formulated in situations where there is inadequate theoretical or empirical information to state a research hypothesis.

A null hypothesis can be simple or complex, associative or causal. An associative null hypothesis states: There is no relationship between the variables. A causal null hypothesis states that: There is no effect of one variable on another.

Example of null hypothesis

- There is no association between the dietary intake and weight of the children
- There is no association between the intelligence and scholastic performance of children
- There is no correlation between the height and weight of adolescent children
- There is no significant difference in the self-esteem in children from non-violent family and violent family
- Structured Teaching Program is not effective in increasing the knowledge on balanced diet among mothers of under five children
- Relaxation therapy is not effective in reducing the stress of patients admitted in acute care ward.

Hypotheses Formulation for Different Types of Research

The purpose of hypothesis formulation and the method by which it has to be formulated is different for different research studies. Basically there are four types of research studies; purpose of hypothesis testing in each type varies. In general, writing hypothesis requires inductive and deductive thinking. The researcher has to decide the number of variables to be studied which ultimately tells whether a simple or complex hypothesis needs to be formulated. The research problem and purpose guides the researcher to write either an associative or causal relationship is to be studied. The number of hypothesis to be formulated for a research depends on the complex nature of the problem and the expertise of the researcher. There is no set guidelines as how many hypotheses to be formulated for a research. In some studies, though, hypothesis is not required and a valid as well as reliable study can be conducted in the absence of hypothesis. These studies do not require testing of interaction between variables. In most of the other studies this is not so. In addition, a single hypothesis can be enough for many studies but some may require formulation of more than one hypothesis. Such studies are as much valid, reliable and generalizable as studies that have single hypothesis but it takes more time to test more than one hypothesis.

Experimental Studies

The purpose of hypothesis formulation in experimental studies is to build a proposition or to give possible reason for any phenomena that occurs. On the basis of this proposition hypothesis is tested to find out whether a particular phenomena occurs due to this reason or not. In the absence of any suitable hypothesis the experimenter has to test various possible reasons for the phenomena to be interpreted. It should be noted that possible rejection or acceptance of the hypothesis does not influence the credibility of hypothesis. It rather concludes that the reason to be tested was true or false. In case the hypothesis does not proved to be true the researcher gets new ideas or new directions for further research.

Descriptive Research Studies

These studies often do not have any hypothesis because the purpose of the study is to describe a fact, figure, phenomena, situation or a person.

Exploratory Research Studies

Exploratory and preliminary studies often do not use a hypothesis. The purpose of exploratory research is to develop better understanding of phenomena to be tested in future. Exploratory research studies are pure research rather than applied research which can be applied to the population at the current time. Actually these research studies help researcher in formulating hypothesis in future research.

Explanatory Research Studies

The explanatory studies use hypotheses since it determine cause and effect relationship. They explain why there is a correlation between two or more than two phenomena. While experimental studies explain what is the relationship or which two phenomena are related, explanatory studies determine why there is a relationship and test these kind of hypothesis.

Testing of Hypothesis

The steps involved in testing of hypothesis are given in the Fig. 2.1. To test a hypothesis, a study is designed and conducted. Data is collected and subjected to statistical analysis. A hypothesis is evaluated with statistical analysis. The hypothesis that states a causal relationship is analyzed using inferential statistics; it is the null hypothesis that is tested. The level of significance ($P = 0.05, 0.01, 0.001$) is set following the generation of the causal hypothesis.

If the hypothesis states the associative relationship, then correlational analysis are done to determine the existence, type and degree of the relationship between the variables studies.

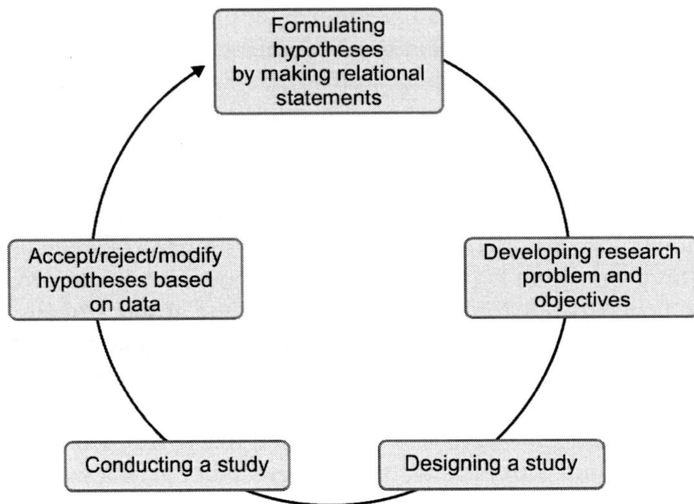

Fig. 2.1: Steps in testing of hypotheses

Hypotheses with causal relationship is analyzed through the use of statistics that examine differences such as 't' test, ANOVA, etc. are used.

For association, chi-square is used and for relationship correlation analysis is used. Hypotheses are not proved 'true' or 'false' by the findings from the study. If the researcher is testing a null hypothesis, the hypothesis is either rejected or accepted. Research hypotheses are described as being supported or not supported in a study.

ASSUMPTIONS

The word assumption means something taken for granted; a supposition: a correct assumption. The synonyms for the word assumption are presupposition; hypothesis, conjecture, guess, postulate, theory.

Assumptions are those things we take it granted in the study. Assumptions are considered as facts or truth though they are not tested scientifically. These are statements by the researcher that certain elements of the research are understood to be true. While assumed, they should still be explicitly stated in the research.

Assumptions are made about (a) the theory under investigation, (b) the phenomenon under investigation, (c) the instrument, (d) the methodology, (e) the analysis, (f) the power to find significance, (g) the participants in the study and (h) the results.

One cannot assume anything as she likes. They are made based on accepted facts/truths, theories, previous research findings and nursing practice.

DELIMITATIONS

Delimitation is a process by which the researcher tries to narrow down his problem. On the other hand, limitation refers to factors which the experimenter cannot control. These are restrictions/bounds that researchers impose prior to the inception of the study to narrow the scope of the study. For example, a study might be delimited to schools located in South Chennai. The delimitations are determined by the conscious exclusionary and inclusionary decisions that were made throughout the development of the proposal. Among these are the choice of objectives and questions, variables of interest, etc.

LIMITATIONS

Limitations are conditions that restrict the scope of the study or may affect the outcome and cannot be controlled by the researcher. Limitations are matters and occurrences that arise in an experiment that are totally out of the researcher's control. It may decrease the generalizability of the findings. They limit the extensity that a study can go to, sometimes affecting the end result of the investigation. An example of a limitation is that a school district might only allow the researcher to collect data during a certain time of the school year, or that selected participants might not answer truthfully or at all.

SUMMARY

- A research problem in general refers to some felt difficulty which the investigator experiences in the context of the theoretical or practical situation and for which he feels the urge to solve.
- A research problem is like the foundation of a building. The type and design of a building is dependent upon the foundation of a building. A proper definition of research problem will enable the researcher to be on the tract whereas an ill defined problem may create hurdle. Thus, defining research problems properly is a prerequisite for any study and is a step of the highest importance.
- Research is a cycle. It starts with a problem and ends with a solution to the problem. The problem statement is therefore the axis which the whole research revolves around, because it explains in short the aim of the research.
- The most research in the humanities revolves around four Ps thus People, Problems, Programs and Phenomena. The major sources of the research problem are experience, theories, literature and ideas from the external sources.
- The major steps involved in formulation of a research problem are identification of a broad area of interest, dissection of the broad area into sub-areas, selection of the sub-area for the research through the process of elimination, writing a problem statement or research questions and reviewing and finalizing the problem statement.
- Essential characteristics of a problem statement are the key variables, the population, the setting and the empirical evidence. Factors to be considered while choosing the problem for the research are significance to nursing, strength of the researcher, researchability and feasibility in terms of time, money, materials, samples, tool and setting.
- The problem statement and title of a research is different. The title is a brief heading of the research whereas the problem statement explains the problem completely with all its elements.

- The objectives of a research are derived from the problem statement which simplifies the step to be followed in a research. It communicates to the readers what is to be achieved by the study. These objectives should be closely related to the research problem.
- The general objective of a study states what researchers expect to achieve by the study in general terms. The specific objectives are the logical steps formulated from the general objectives which explain what the researcher will do in her study.
- A hypothesis is the formal statement of the expected relationship(s) between two or more variables. A hypothesis is formulated after the problem has been stated and the literature review has been done. It is formulated when the researcher is totally aware of the theoretical and empirical background of the problem.
- Hypotheses can be classified based on the number of variables as Simple vs Complex hypotheses; based on the direction as Non-directional vs directional hypotheses and based on the concept of acceptance or rejection as Research vs Null hypothesis.
- Assumptions are those things we take for granted in the study. These are statements by the researcher that certain elements of the research are understood to be true.
- Delimitation is a process by which the researcher tries to narrow down his problem. These are restrictions/bounds that researchers impose prior to the inception of the study to narrow the scope of the study.
- Limitations are conditions that restrict the scope of the study or may affect the outcome and cannot be controlled by the researcher. Limitations are matters and occurrences that arise in an experiment that are totally out of the researcher's control. It may decrease the generalizability of the findings.

EXERCISE

- The problem statements are mentioned below. Identify the elements of a research problem:
  - A study to assess the knowledge on child abuse among mothers residing at Perungudi, Chennai
  - A study to identify the factors influencing academic achievement among students studying in selected nursing colleges, Chennai
  - A study to compare the effectiveness of hot vs cold application in reducing pain among patients diagnosed with Arthritis attending selected hospitals, Chennai.
  - A study to evaluate the effectiveness of refresher program on job satisfaction among staffs working in selected hospitals, Chennai
  - A study to assess the quality of life of mothers of children with autism attending selected special schools, Madurai
  - A study to compare the quality of life of father and mother of children with mental retardation attending selected special schools, Chennai
  - A study to assess the problems perceived by the teachers in handling students with Attention Deficit Hyperactive Disorder working at selected schools, Chennai.
  - A study to assess the knowledge and attitude on healthy behavior among adolescents studying in selected schools, Chennai.
- Identify which element of the research problem is missing:
  - A study to assess the knowledge on prevention of accidents in children in selected community areas in Chennai
  - A study to explore the problems of the mothers of diabetic children in selected hospitals in Chennai

- A study to evaluate the Effectiveness of Structured Teaching Program among mothers of adolescent girls residing at Perungudi, Chennai
- A study to evaluate the Video Assisted Teaching Programme on personal hygiene in selected schools in Chennai
- A study to identify the risk factors among old age people residing at selected community area in Chennai.

- The hypotheses are given below. Identify the type, and its elements:
  - There is an association between the selfesteem and family income of the adolescents
  - The adolescent boys with fewer problems have high selfesteem than the boys with more problems
  - The self-concept of the adolescents decreases as their peer acceptance decreases
  - There is no association between the physical appearance and the self-concept of the adolescents
  - The mothers of children with autism would experience more psychological distress than the mothers of children with mental retardation
  - The parents with more stress experience less marital satisfaction
  - The parents with high annual income experience less stress than those with low annual income
  - The adolescents in the experimental group show high emotional stability than those in the control group.
- From the below mentioned statements, identify the limitation and delimitation:
  - The period of study is 6 weeks
  - The sample size is restricted to 50 samples
  - The hospital authority did not permit for second meeting of the sample to collect data
  - The samples are restricted to teachers working in school X
  - While the samples were taking the nutrition supplementation (intervention), the local government has introduced a new scheme of nutrition supplementation
  - The results of the study is generalizable to teachers working in school X
  - In the study of selfesteem among adolescents, the samples before post test attended an session on values for life conducted by the church authorities
  - The study is restricted to assessment of nursing skills in students in acute care ward.
- Identify which of the following statements are assumptions or hypothesis:
  - Mothers may have adequate knowledge on child abuse
  - The knowledge on child abuse will be influenced by the educational status of the mother
  - The knowledge on child abuse is high among educated mothers than uneducated mothers
  - The teachers may perceive problems while handling children with attention deficit hyperactive disorder
  - The quality of life of fathers is greater than the mothers of children with mental retardation
  - Both father and mother may have poor quality of life
  - There is an association between the job satisfaction and performance outcome of the employees working at selected hospitals, Chennai

- The perceived problems of teachers handling children with attention deficit hyperactive disorder is more than the teachers handling children with mental retardation.

- Identify which statistical analysis can be used to test the following null hypothesis:
  - There is no association between the job satisfaction and staff retention
  - There is no association between the job satisfaction and performance outcome of the employees working at selected hospitals, Chennai
  - There is no difference in the problems perceived by the father and mother of children with mental retardation
  - There is no difference in the scholastic performance of the children studying School X and School Y
  - There is no correlation between the height and weight of the adults residing at selected community area.

3 Review of Literature

OBJECTIVES

After reading this chapter, you will be able to:

- State the meaning of literature review
- List the purposes of literature review
- Explain the levels of evidence in research
- List the sources of literature review
- Explain the search of literature on the internet
- Explain the practical steps in reviewing the literature
- Enlist the factors to be remembered in doing literature review.

INTRODUCTION

Research can never be done in isolation. Any research is either directly or indirectly related to the existing concepts or work done earlier. A fresh research is theoretically not possible since any research problem is somehow related to the existing concepts. Research studies are undertaken within the context of an existing knowledge base. A careful review of existing resources, such as journals, books, thesis and other related literature is one of the major steps in any research study. It allows the researcher to acquaint and familiarize himself with current knowledge in the area where he proposed to conduct research. A literature review surveys scholarly articles, books and other sources (e.g. dissertations, conference proceedings) relevant to a particular issue, area of research, or theory, providing a description, summary and critical evaluation of each work. The purpose is to offer an overview of significant literature published on a topic.

Meaning of Literature Review

Review of literature can be understood in two different meanings. One is the process of searching for specific content in available literature and the second one is the written summary of the searched content.

In the first context, 'Review of literature' refers to the process of extensive, exhaustive and systemic examination of publications relevant to a specific topic. It is a broad, comprehensive, in-depth, systematic and critical review of scholarly publications, unpublished scholarly print materials, etc.

In the second context, 'Review of Literature' refers to a written report of information gathered from various sources/literature related to a selected topic. This report should be of an evaluative and critical nature and not simply copying from the sources. Such a well-written analytical report forms the theoretical base for any research. The primary purpose of writing the report is to personally understand as well as to convey to the reader what is already established on a topic and what are its strengths and weaknesses. It gives an overview of the key findings and key authors, the prevailing theories and hypotheses and methods and methodologies used. In order to write a relevant literature review, the person who writes should remember the research objective, the problems or issues to be researched. Rather, it should not be a descriptive summary of the available information.

Purposes of Literature Review

A literature review may constitute an essential chapter of a thesis or dissertation, or may be a self-contained review of writings on a subject. Reviewing literature can be time-consuming, daunting and frustrating, but is also rewarding. In either case, its purpose is to

- delimit and define the problem
- bring clarity and focus to the research problem
- broaden the knowledge
- know and explain what is already done
- identify any gaps in the previous research
- formulate hypotheses and assumptions
- develop a theoretical and conceptual framework
- decide on research methodology
- develop tool for data collection
- describe the relationship of each work to others under consideration
- identify areas of prior scholarship to prevent duplication of effort
- contextualize the study findings
- identify of experts in the field who could be used as consultants
- to plan intervention or protocol
- to understand and reveal aspects which have and have not been researched
- to understand and overcome problems faced by other workers
- to calculate sample size from previously published data
- to plan for data analysis and statistical methods to be used.

Levels of Evidence

In the process of literature search, we search for the existing evidences or research findings related to the problem of interest. The evidences can range from lowest level to the highest level. It is the researcher who has to decide based on his research problem what level of evidence he has to seek for his problem.

Levels of Evidence in Medical Research

In general, much of the medical research focuses on techniques, drugs and vaccines. It is usually tried on animals and later the efficacy of new drug or vaccine is checked by undertaking randomized controlled trial by comparing with placebo or else with the standard one. Any newer technique or intervention is tried on individual basis and later into a large samples. In nursing, we do not engage in drug trial or test any invasive procedures (Fig. 3.1). The evidence for nursing research can range from case series to meta-analysis (Fig. 3.2).

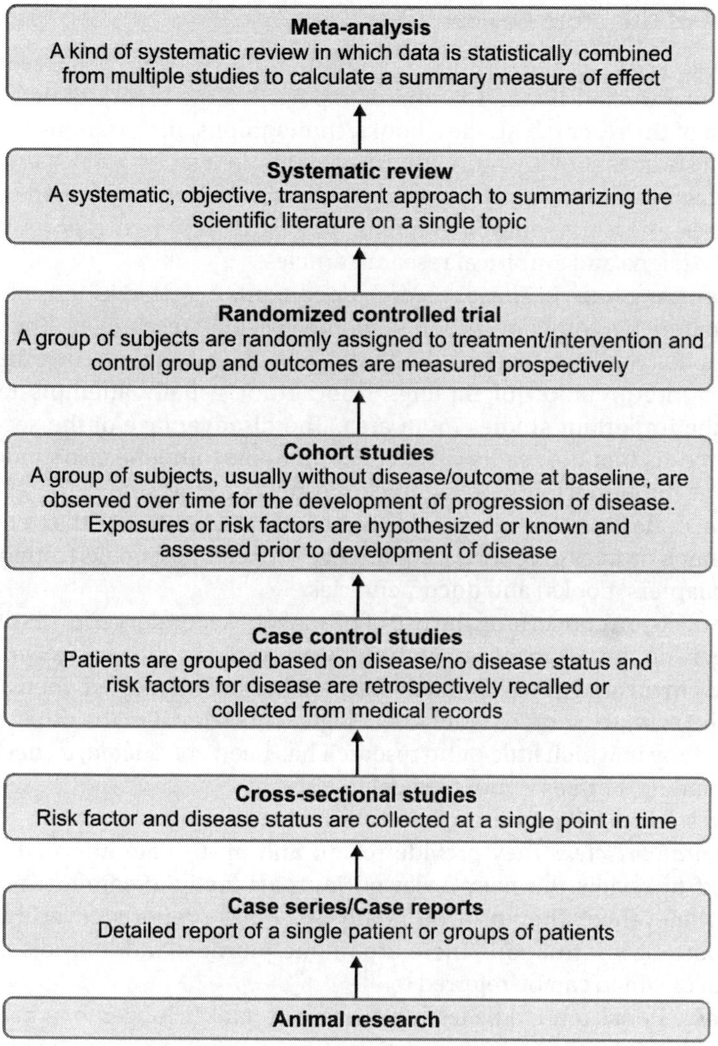

Meta-analysis
A kind of systematic review in which data is statistically combined from multiple studies to calculate a summary measure of effect
Systematic review
A systematic, objective, transparent approach to summarizing the scientific literature on a single topic
Randomized controlled trial
A group of subjects are randomly assigned to treatment/intervention and control group and outcomes are measured prospectively
Cohort studies
A group of subjects, usually without disease/outcome at baseline, are observed over time for the development of progression of disease. Exposures or risk factors are hypothesized or known and assessed prior to development of disease
Case control studies
Patients are grouped based on disease/no disease status and risk factors for disease are retrospectively recalled or collected from medical records
Cross-sectional studies
Risk factor and disease status are collected at a single point in time
Case series/Case reports
Detailed report of a single patient or groups of patients
Animal research

Fig. 3.1: Level of evidence in medical research

Meta-analysis
Systematic review
Experimental studies
Descriptive/correlational studies

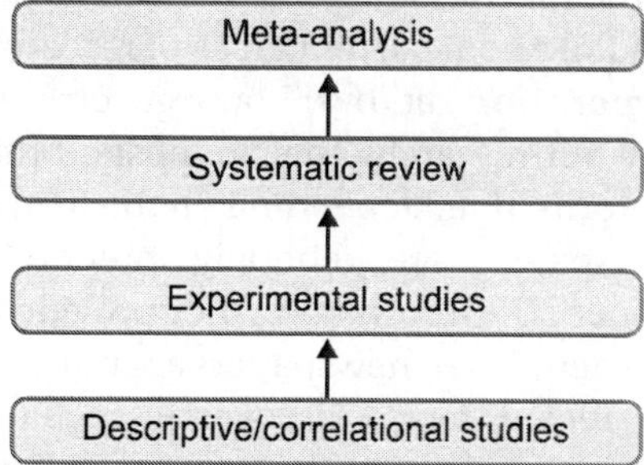

Fig. 3.2: Level of evidence in nursing research

Sources of Literature Review

- ***Primary source:*** They are descriptions of studies written by the researchers who conducted them. The author reports his own work directly in the form of the research articles, books, monographs, dissertations or theses. Such sources provide more information about a study since it is author's own work. The examples of primary sources are letters/correspondence, diaries, memoirs, autobiographies, official or research reports, patents and designs and empirical research articles.
- ***Secondary source:*** These research documents are descriptions of studies prepared by someone other than the original researcher. The author compiles and summarizes the findings of the work done by others and gives interpretation of findings. The author usually attempts to cover all the important studies in an area. The disadvantage of the secondary sources is that the reader has to depend upon someone else's judgments about the important and significant aspects of the study. The examples of secondary sources are academic journal articles (other than empirical research articles or reports), conference proceedings, books (monographs or chapters' books) and documentaries.

  The decision concerning the use of primary or secondary sources depends largely on the nature of research study proposed by the researcher. If it is a study in an area in which much research has been reported, then a review of the primary sources would be a logical first step. On the other hand, if the study in which little or no research has been conducted, a check of the secondary sources is more logical.

Various sources of literature are as follows:

- ***Journal articles:*** They provide recent and up-to-date information. It is good to review the peer-reviewed journals for its credibility, reliability and relevance. They provide relatively concise reports covering all the important information. There are online journals and journals in print, both of which can be referred to.
- ***Books:*** Books tend to be less up-to-date as it takes longer for a book to be published than for a journal article. Books which are recently published with latest edition are reviewed. E-books are also available on the internet.
- ***Conference proceedings:*** These can be useful in providing the latest research, or research that has not been published. They are also helpful in providing information about current areas of research.
- ***Government/Corporation reports:*** Many government departments and corporations carry out research. Their published findings can provide a useful source of information, depending on the field of study.
- ***Newspapers:*** Newspapers are generally intended for a general (not specialized) audience. The information they provide will be of very limited use for literature review. Often newspapers are more helpful as providers of information about recent trends, discoveries or changes, e.g. announcing changes in government policy, epidemics of any diseases, but one should then search for more detailed information in other sources.

- ***Theses and dissertations:*** These can be useful sources of information. However, it has its disadvantages. It is not a published work and is available only in the libraries. It is written by students who may not be experienced researchers and, therefore, the findings have to be treated with more caution than published research.
- ***Internet:*** It is the fastest-growing source of information. Anyone can post information on the internet so the quality may not be reliable and the information found may be intended for a general audience. It may be less detailed and not be suitable for inclusion in literature review. At the same time, more and more refereed electronic journals (e-journals) are appearing on the Internet, if they are refereed, it means that there is an editorial board that evaluates the work before publishing it in their e-journal. So, the quality is more reliable.
- ***CD-ROMs:*** These provide kind of specialized, detailed information about academic research and are mostly available for use in academic libraries. So, they can be a very valuable tool in searching for the information we need.
- ***Magazines:*** They provide news or general information about new discoveries, policies, problems, etc. which are intended for a general audience. As newspapers, they can be referred to but detailed information to be collected from various sources. Some specialized magazines may be more useful.

Searching for the Review on the Internet

A researcher can search information using search engines in the internet. A search engine is an information retrieval system designed to help find information stored on a computer system. The search results are usually presented in a list and are commonly called ***hits***. Search engines are programs that search documents for specified keywords and returns a list of documents where the keywords were found. These search engines enable users to search for documents on the World Wide Web. Web search engines work by sending out a spider to fetch as many documents as possible. Another program, called an ***indexer*** then reads these documents and creates an index based on the words contained in each document. The examples of search engines are as follows:

- Google
- Yahoo
- Bing
- Altavista
- Go
- Ask
- Aol
- mywebsearch
- info
- Webopedia

A database is an organized collection of data. A structured set of data held in a computer, specially one that is accessible in various ways. Examples of databases:

PubMed

MEDLINE (Medical Literature Analysis and Retrieval System Online, or MEDLARS Online) is a bibliographic database of life sciences and biomedical information. It includes bibliographic information for articles from academic journals covering medicine, nursing, pharmacy, dentistry, veterinary medicine and health care. It is compiled by the United States National Library of Medicine (NLM) at the National Institutes of Health (NIH). MEDLINE is freely available on the Internet and searchable via PubMed and NLM's National Center for Biotechnology Information's Entrez system. PubMed is a free search engine accessing primarily the MEDLINE database of references and abstracts on life sciences and biomedical topics.

MeSH is the acronym for 'Medical Subject Headings.' It is a list of vocabulary terms used for analysis of biomedical literature by the NLM. MeSH vocabulary is used for indexing journal articles for Index Medicus® and MEDLINE and is also used for cataloging books and audio-visuals. One must know about the Boolean logic. Boolean logic symbolically represents relationships between entities. There are three Boolean operators:

1. And
2. Or
3. Not

It can be used in the following ways in advanced search at PubMed. Suppose we enter 'diarrhea and dehydration' in the search column in the PubMed, the search details appear as follows:

(diarrhea [All Fields] OR diarrhea [MeSH Terms] OR diarrhea [All Fields]) and (dehydration [MeSH Terms] OR dehydration [All Fields]) and (Clinical Trial[ptyp] and 2004/01/01 [PDat]: 2013/12/28 [PDat])

Suppose if we enter 'diarrhea or dehydration' in the search column, the search details appear as follows:

(diarrhea [All Fields] OR diarrhea [MeSH Terms] OR diarrhea [All Fields]) OR (dehydration [MeSH Terms] OR dehydration [All Fields]) and (Clinical Trial[ptyp] and 2008/12/30 [PDat]: 2013/12/28 [PDat])

Suppose if we enter 'diarrhoea' and not 'adults,' the search details appear as follows:

(diarrhea [All Fields] OR diarrhea [MeSH Terms] OR diarrhea[All Fields]) NOT (adult [MeSH Terms] OR adult [All Fields] OR adults [All Fields]) and (Clinical Trial [ptyp] and 2008/12/30 [PDat]: 2013/12/28 [PDat])

We can use filters in advanced search. The articles can be filtered based on:

Article Type

- Clinical trial
- Review

- Systematic reviews
- Bibliography
- Journal articles, etc.

Text Availability

- Abstract available
- Full text available
- Free full text available.

Publication Dates

- 5 years
- 10 years
- Custom range (One can select the period during which all the articles indexed can be accessed).

Species

- Human
- Animal.

Language

- English
- Other languages.

Sex

- Male
- Female.

Ages

- Child
- Infant
- Adult
- Aged.

There are a few other additional filters one can use in the PubMed advanced search.

Cochrane Library

The ***cochrane library*** is a collection of six databases that contain different types of high-quality, independent evidence to inform healthcare decision-making, and a seventh database that provides information about groups in the Cochrane Collaboration. The Cochrane Database of Systematic Reviews (CDSR) is the leading resource for systematic reviews in health care. The ***CDSR*** includes all Cochrane Reviews (and protocols) prepared by Cochrane Review Groups in the Cochrane Collaboration. Each Cochrane Review is a peer-reviewed systematic review that has been prepared and supervised by a Cochrane Review Group (editorial team) in the Cochrane Collaboration according to the ***cochrane handbook for systematic reviews of interventions or cochrane handbook for diagnostic test accuracy reviews***. The topic can be browsed by topics or other browse options.

MedIND

MedIND has been produced under an ICMR-funded project—'National Databases of Indian Medical Journals.' Its purpose is to provide free access to full text of articles published in selected Indian Biomedical Journals indexed in IndMED or PubMed.

Apart from these databases, there are paid/free online journals which can be accessed freely without any subscription. The ***BMJ*** (formerly the British Medical Journal) is an international peer-reviewed medical journal and a fully 'online first' publication. All articles will appear on bmj.com before being included in an issue of the print journal. The website is updated daily with the ***BMJ***'s latest original research, education, news, and comment articles, as well as podcasts, videos, and blogs.

Steps in Searching Literature on Internet

Develop a Search Strategy

The researcher has to develop a search strategy before beginning the search. A search strategy is a plan that helps us to look for the information we need. Start with a focused, answerable question. We can use PICO format.

P Patient or Problem
I Intervention
C Comparison and
O Outcome

Select a High-yield Database

The researcher can choose PubMed, cochrane library, MedIND, etc.

Identify the Key Concepts or Key Words

Determine the alternative terms for these concepts, if needed. Terms like MeSH can be used to search for the sources.

Use Filters

Refine search to dates, study groups, etc. as appropriate. Filters in advanced search can be used to narrow down the search which will be more focused.

Practice Helps

Strategies and styles will differ according to personal choice and professional discipline. Practice facilitates faster search. One must be familiar with the techniques and facilities available in each search engine and databases.

Steps in Reviewing Literature

The major steps involved in reviewing the literature are as follows:

1. ***Identification of the topic or concepts to be reviewed:*** This requires the researcher to decide on the topic(s)/concept(s) or the content to be reviewed, which is usually related to the research problem. Literature review on the broader area of interest helps the investigator in selection and refining the problem and once the problem is stated, it helps in the review of specific concepts related to the problem being studied.
2. ***Search for the literature:*** This step involves in finding the sources/materials relevant to the subject being explored. The investigator can search from various sources both primary and secondary from journals, books, newspapers, magazines, dissertations, thesis, internet, etc. In doing so, one must:
   - Prepare a list of journals and books to be reviewed
   - Locate the books and journals
   - Select the latest issue, examine its contents page to find the articles relevant to the study
   - Look at the index of research abstracts in the relevant field to identify and read the articles.
   - Take photocopies wherever necessary.
   - Writing annotated bibliography helps the researcher in identifying the content in the books and journals.
3. ***Data evaluation:*** As the investigator goes through the data from various sources, she has to analyze the credibility of the data, its geniuneness, reliability and accuracy. The investigator can check for the following:
   - ***Authority:*** Who is the author? What are his/her credentials? What is his/her area of expertize?
   - ***Provenance:*** What are the author's credentials? Are the author's arguments supported by evidence?
   - ***Objectivity:*** Is the author's view objective or prejudiced? Is contrary data considered or is certain pertinent information ignored to prove the author's point?
   - ***Persuasiveness:*** Which of the author's information are most/least convincing?
   - ***Significance:*** Are the author's arguments and conclusions convincing? Does the work ultimately contribute to an understanding of the subject?
   - ***Accuracy:*** Whether the information seems to be accurate and consistent with the other reports?
   - ***Usefulness:*** How is this source related to the topic? How current or relevant it is to the topic?
   - ***Reliability:*** Does the information come from a reliable, trusted source, such as an academic journal?
4. ***Analysis and reporting of the data:*** There are many information available in relation to a particular concept. The information may be in support of or in opposition of or may offer alternative ideas. All the available information related to a concept(s) are analyzed and interpreted for the purpose of understanding and communication. This is written as a report

which includes how each work is similar to and how it varies from the others.

In a nutshell, the researcher must:

- Write a summary and record it for reference for later use
- Record the main findings with respect to the theme in question
- List the main themes that have emerged while reading literature
- Convert them into subheadings. These subheadings should be precise, descriptive of the theme in question and follow a logical progression
- Pay attention to methodology, its soundness, the testing procedures, subjects and materials used in the study
- Note conflicting theories, methodologies and results. Check for any assumptions being made by most/some researchers
- Evaluate and synthesize the findings and conclusions.

Points to be remembered in reviewing literature: When reviewing the literature:

- Remember the purpose
- Read with a purpose
- Write with a purpose.

Some traps to avoid:

- Trying to read everything
- Reading but not writing
- Not keeping bibliographic information.

Sample Review of Literature

De, De Bruijn, De Weert-van Oene and Strivers (2010) conducted a prospective study to analyze the internet and game behavior of secondary school children. This study investigated the internet and game use of secondary school children, the compulsiveness of their use and the relationship with other health behaviors. It also evaluated the preliminary results of a recently developed school health promotion program, implemented at a secondary school in the Netherlands in January 2008. This program was one of the first to combine seven health behaviors in one educational program and was a pilot project for a case-control study. A total of 475 secondary school children completed an extensive questionnaire before and a year after starting the program. Of these children, 367 were in first, second and third grades; the grades in which the lessons about internet and game behavior were implemented. Questionnaires contained questions about personal information, internet and game use (Compulsive Internet Use Scale), and other health behaviors (alcohol use, physical activity, psychosocial well-being and body mass index, BMI).

The study findings revealed that heavy internet use was significantly associated with psychosocial problems and heavy game use was significantly associated with psychosocial problem and less physical activity. No relationship was found with alcohol use or body mass index. The time spent on internet (hours/day) and the number of pathological internet users increased during the study. The number of game users decreased but heavy game use increased. The study concluded that there was an association between heavy internet use and psychosocial problems and between game use and psychosocial problems and less physical activity. They further suggested that a case-control study is needed to further assess the program-induced changes in internet and game behavior of school children.

Devis-Devis, Peiro-Velert, Beltran-Carrillo and Tomas (2009) examined the Screen Media Time Usage (SMTU) of 12–16-year-old Spanish school adolescents (N = 323) and the effects of personal and socioeconomic factors, season and type of day. The research design adopted was a cross-sectional survey, in which an interviewer-administered recall questionnaire was used. Statistical analyses included repeated measures analysis of variance, analysis of covariance and structural equation models. Results showed an average of 2.52 hours per day of total SMTU and partial times of 1.73 hours per day in TV viewing, 0.27 hours per day in computer/video games, and 0.52 hours per day in mobile use.

Four significant predictors of SMTU emerged in this study. Firstly, the type of school was associated with the three media of the study, particularly students from state/public school spent more time on them than their private-schools' counterparts. Secondly, older adolescents (14–16-years-old) were more likely to use computers/video games and mobile phones than younger adolescents. Thirdly, the more accessibility to household technology, the more probably computers/video games and mobile phones were used. Additionally, results revealed that adolescents seemed to be using TVs and computers/video games in autumn than in winter, and more TVs and mobile phones on weekends than on weekdays, specially among state school students.

SUMMARY

- Review of literature refers to an extensive, exhaustive and systemic examination of publications relevant to the research project. It is a broad, comprehensive, in-depth, systematic and critical review of scholarly publications, unpublished scholarly print materials, etc.
- In the process of literature search, we search for the existing evidences or research findings related to the problem of interest. The evidences can range from the lowest level to the highest level.
- There are primary and secondary sources for reviewing the literature. The primary sources are descriptions of studies written by the researchers who conducted them. The author reports his own work directly in the form of the research articles, books, monographs, dissertations or theses. Such sources provide more information about a study since it is author's own work.
- The secondary source documents are descriptions of studies prepared by someone other than the original researcher. The author compiles and summarizes the findings of the work done by others and gives interpretation of findings.
- The various sources are journal articles, books, conference proceedings, Government/ Corporation reports, newspapers, theses and dissertations, internet, CD-ROMs and magazines.

- A researcher can search information using search engines in the internet. A search engine is an information retrieval system designed to help find information stored on a computer system. The search results are usually presented in a list and are commonly called hits.
- A database is an organized collection of data. Pubmed and Cochrane Library are the examples of databases.
- The major steps involved in reviewing the literature are identification of the topic or concepts to be reviewed, search for the literature, data evaluation, analysis and reporting of the data.

EXERCISE

- Select a topic of interest and review the literature. Write a report of the review.
- Identify various online databases and review the literature on a selected topic of interest.

4 Conceptual Framework

OBJECTIVES

After reading this chapter, you will be able to:

- State the meaning and definition of conceptual framework
- Explain the purposes of writing conceptual framework
- Explain the method of writing conceptual framework for a research.

INTRODUCTION

We all know that the framework of a human body is our skeletal system which gives shape and structure. The pillars and columns gives the shape and structure for the building without which the building cannot exist. A framework is a structure composed of many concepts proposed to serve as a support or guide for the building of something that expands the structure into something useful and meaningful. It is a broad overview, outline, or skeleton of interlinked concepts or items which supports a major theme or overall concept. It explains the approach to a specific objective and serves as a guide that can be modified as required by adding or deleting items or concepts. In nursing research, the conceptual/theoretical framework forms an important element. Conceptual framework is used in research to outline the possible courses of action or to present a preferred approach to an idea or thought. Conceptual frameworks (theoretical frameworks) are a type of intermediate theory that attempt to connect to all aspects of inquiry (e.g. problem definition, purpose, literature review, methodology, data collection and analysis). It can act like a map that explains the logic to empirical inquiry.

THEORY

Theory is a statement that accounts for or characterizes some phenomena (Stevens, 1984). Theory is a general statement that explains the interrelationships among observed facts and propositions (Seaman, 1987).

It is a set of interrelated constructs (concepts) definitions and propositions that present a systematic view of phenomena by specifying relations among variables with the purpose of explaining and predicting the phenomena (Kerlinger, 1986).

Chinn and Kramer (2004) defined theory as 'a creative and rigorous structuring of ideas that projects a tentative, purposeful and systematic view of phenomena.' The word creative means imaginative and innovative and these concepts try to explain the phenomena. In their views, theories are tentative and as such are open to revision as new evidence emerges. Concepts are building blocks of theories. Concepts must be defined precisely and explicitly. The concepts are defined constitutively and operationally. Concepts are connected by statements called ***propositions***. The hypothesis is a postulate containing operationally defined terms. Hypotheses are not a part of theory but are derived from it. The theory is the explanation of relations between concepts; this explanation is tested through the test of hypotheses. The components of theories are as under:

- Concepts
- Assumptions
- Contexts within which the theory is placed
- Identified relationships between and among the concepts.

Theory provides a structure for the interpretation of individuals' behavior and of events. Many theories are required to account for the multitude of experiences encountered by human beings. They state what something is, how something happens or why it happens. Their function therefore, is to describe, explain, or predict specific aspects of reality. The primary goal of theory is to provide a framework that links research and practice and contributes on making scientific findings meaningful and generalizable.

Functions of Theory

- It provides structure for interpreting observed behavior, situations and events. For example, theory of psychosexual and psychosocial development provides explanations about the childrens' behavior. Maslow's hierarchy of needs explains what and why of human priority of needs.
- It serves as a source to generate the hypotheses that predict what will be found when data are collected and analyzed. Theory explains, why and what will occur in a specific context. For example, theory of cognitive development explains what is expected to certain age groups. We can test in real situation whether something said in the theory is observable in human being.
- It serves as a framework for guiding research. Theory forms the base for a research which helps us to understand the concepts and predict something.
- It also serves as a guide in selecting the appropriate method to answer the research question and in interpreting the results.
- It is a source of professional autonomy. Theory guides the nurses' thinking and provides a basis to describe, explain or predict factors that influence nursing care. It enables nurses' to explain nursing actions and their outcomes.

When we link or connect our research with the theories, the power of the study increases. Because a research guided by a theory has a strong foundation. Theory, research and practice were strongly related. As stated, the function of theory is to explain, predict and describe the nursing phenomenon. The function of research is to generate and test theory that will influence the nursing practice either directly or indirectly. Theory is tested on human being by conducting research in nursing practice. The three are strongly interrelated and one cannot isolate them.

Types of Theories

Grand theories are the most abstract type of theories. They embody the beliefs, traditions, goals and values of the discipline. It mainly deals with the phenomenon central to nursing such as person, health, environment and nursing. They broadly define these four concepts and link them through relationship statements reflective of the theorist's view of the discipline.

Middle range theories are in between the most abstract concepts and the concrete concepts. They are less abstract than grand theories and more broader than the practice theories. They deal with the limited aspects of nursing phenomenon. They contain well-defined concepts and propositions.

Practice theories are narrower in scope and more specific than middle range theories. Concepts are specifically and narrowly defined and its utility in practice is more when compared to grand and middle range theories. They provide clear directions for practice.

Building Blocks of Theories

- ***Concepts:*** It is a mental image of a phenomenon, an idea or a construct in the mind about a thing or an action. They are abstract entities that represent broad general ideas that are not directly observable in the real world. However, they are formed from the real world observations of objects or things. For example, beauty is a concept and everyone has some idea or construct about beauty in their mind. The concept of beauty varies from individual to individual and hence, it should be defined accordingly so that one can observe in the research.
- ***Constructs:*** They are concepts specified in such a way that they are observable in the real world. Making a concept potentially observable facilitates testing of the idea. For example, knowledge is a concept, which is specified in a research, so that one can assess or measure the knowledge.
- ***Variables:*** Anything which varies from person to person is a variable. Variables are concepts that are observable, measurable and have a dimension that can vary. Knowledge is a variable which may be high or low in a person. Pulse is a variable which may be normal in rate or either increased or decreased. There are different types of variables one may come across in a study (Table 4.1).

Table 4.1: Types of variables

S. No.	Variables	Explanations and examples
1.	Binary/Discrete variable, Dichotomous variable	Observations that occur in one or two possible states, often labeled zero and one. e.g. 'improved/not improved' variable having only integer values
2.	Categorical/ Nominal Variable	Observation based on some classification such as gender (male or female), marital status (married, single, divorced, widowed). The categories are often assigned numerical values used as labels, e.g., 0 = male; 1 = female
3.	Confounding variable	A variable that obscure the effects of another variable, for example, intelligence obscures the school performance. Educational status obscures the knowledge and attitude
4.	Continuous variable	A variable that is not restricted to particular values. For example, weight and height are continuous variable
5.	Control variable	An extraneous variable that an investigator does not wish to examine in a study. Thus, the investigator controls this variable and also called a covariate
6.	Criterion variable	The presumed effect in a non-experimental study is known as criterion variable
7.	Dependent variable	The presumed effect in an experimental study. The values of the dependent-variable depend upon another variable, the independent-variable. Hemoglobin(dependent-variable) depend upon the dietary intake(independent-variable)
8.	Independent / Manipulated variable	The presumed cause in an experimental study. Structured teaching program is an independent-variable
9.	Intervening variable	A variable that explains a relation or provides a causal link between other variables. Physical activity or sports activity is an intervening variable between physical growth and dietary intake
10.	Latent variable	An underlying variable that cannot be observed. Growth Potential or heredity is a latent variable of height
11.	Manifest variable	An observed variable assumed to indicate the presence of a latent variable, also known as an indicator variable. We cannot observe intelligence directly, for it is a latent variable. We can look at indicators such as vocabulary size, success in one's occupation, IQ test score, ability to play complicated games well, writing ability and so on
12.	Moderating variable	A variable that influences, or moderates, the relation between two other variables and thus, produces an interaction effect
13.	Ordinal variable	A variable used to rank a sample of individuals with respect to some characteristics, but differences (i.e., intervals) and different points of the scale are not necessarily equivalent. For examples, anxiety might be rated on a scale 'none', 'mild', 'moderate,' and 'severe', with numerical values of 0, 1, 2, 3.

contd...

contd...

S. No.	Variables	Explanations and examples
		A patient with an anxiety score of 1 is ranked as less anxious than a patient with a score of 3, but patients with scores 0 and 2 do not necessarily have the same differences in anxiety as patients with scores of 1 and 3
14.	Outcome variable	The presumed effect in a non-experimental study. Synonym for criterion variable
15.	Polychotomous variables	Variables that can have more than two possible values. Strictly speaking, this includes all except binary variables. The usual reference is categorical variables with more than two categories. Example, marital status (married, single, divorced, widowed)
16.	Predictor variable	The presumed 'cause' on a non-experimental study. Often used in correlational studies. Smoking is a presumed cause of lung cancer. Violent video game playing is a presumed cause of aggressiveness.

- ***Relational statement:*** It is a proposition describing a specific relationship between two or more concepts. Propositions are statements of proposed relationships between two or more concepts in a theory. Propositions link concepts by relational statements so that a theory explains, predicts or describes something. Hypothesis is a form of relational statement which explains the relationship between two or more concepts. A hypothesis may be directional or nondirectional. It may be simple or complex. Hypotheses advance nursing knowledge by confirming or refuting the theoretical propositions from which they are derived. Developing and testing theory requires conceptualization.
- ***Conceptualization:*** It refers to the process of developing and refining abstract ideas. It is a process of thinking and organizing ideas that grows from the learning of facts and events to concepts to theory development.

CONCEPTUAL MODEL/THEORETICAL FRAMEWORK

A model is a simplified representation of a theory or of certain complex events, structures or systems. The example for a model of structure is model of kidney or heart. A model is a hypothetical representation of something that exists in reality. The purpose of a model is to attempt to explain a complex reality in a systematic and organized manner. An institution's organization chart is a model that attempts to demonstrate the interrelationships of the various levels of the organization's administration.

Conceptual Model

It is a group of concepts or ideas that are related but the relationship is not explicit. Conceptual models have a 'set of concepts' however, the relational statement explaining the connections between the concepts are obscure.

Framework

It is a structure that serves to hold parts together, e.g. skeleton forms the framework of our body.

Conceptual Framework

A written or visual presentation that explains either graphically, or in narrative form, the main things to be studied—the key factors, concepts or variables and the presumed relationship among them. (Miles and Huberman, 1994).

Theoretical Framework

A structure composed of concepts related to form a whole (Chinn and Kramer). It consists of a set of defined concepts and relational statements linking them. In general, nursing theories are developed based on the following methods:
- Inductive process
- Deductive process
- Borrowing from other disciplines.

Theoretical frameworks are brief descriptions of a theory, or portions of a theory, to be tested in a research. It describes a basic structure of ideas, essentially the concepts within which the study is conducted and the results are interpreted.

Purposes of a Conceptual Framework

- It clarifies the concepts on which the study is built
- It specifies the relationship among the concepts
- It identifies and states the assumptions and hypothesis underlying the study
- It explains why a research is conducted in a particular way
- It acts as a filtering tool for selecting appropriate research questions and related data collection methods
- It can also help us to understand and use the ideas of others who have done similar things
- It is a set of coherent ideas or concepts organized in a manner that helps in communication to others
- It directs the thinking process about how and why an empirical research and how we understand its activities
- It forms the basis for thinking about what we do and what it means, influenced by the ideas and research of others
- It also acts as a reference point/structure for the discussion of the literature, methodology and results
- The conceptual framework is like a travel map. The investigator prepares and uses to reach a destination which also understood by others.

Relationship between conceptual model and theoretical framework

- Conceptual model is not a theory
- Conceptual model is highly abstract
- Theory contains more concrete concepts
- A conceptual model embodies the world view, the paradigm of a discipline or a school of thought
- Each theory derived from a model explains some or all of the paradigm's phenomena but only within a limited range
- A theory is more precise and limited in scope than its parent conceptual scheme
- The conceptual framework serves as a stepping stone for the formulation of the 'theoretical framework' which comprises established explanations, theoretical principles and suggested theoretical relations in preparation of a more specific inquiry.
- The conceptual framework in quantitative and qualitative study is unique (Refer table 4.2).

Table 4.2: The relationship between the conceptual framework and other components in quantitative and qualitative study

Elements/components	Quantitative study	Qualitative study
Research problem	The issue of theoretical or practical interest	
Paradigm	The philosophical assumptions about the nature of the world and how we understand it	
	Positivism	Interpretivism
Aims and objectives	What we want to know or find out?	
Research questions	Specific questions related to the issue of theoretical or practical interest that requires answers	
Literature review	A critical and evaluative review of the work done by others	
Conceptual framework	Formulated based on literature and personal experience before the study. Provides the structure/content for the whole study	Not formed before the study
Data collection and analysis	Methodology, methods and analysis	
Interpretation of the results	Making sense of the results and the questions are answered	Conceptual framework develops as participants' views and issues are gathered and analyzed
Evaluation of the research	Revisiting of the conceptual framework	

Steps in Developing a Conceptual Framework

- State the problem as clearly as possible
- Identify the keywords or concepts or variables of the study

- Review the literature for theories, theoretical generalizations, empirical generalizations, and systematized facts related to the phenomenon of interest (problem)
- Review the existing conceptual or theoretical framework already used to guide professional activities
- Write the relational statements, and organize these into a study framework
- Draw a visual model of concepts and known or proposed relationships.

To develop a conceptual framework one must clearly state the problem to be investigated. Once the problem is clearly defined, the major concepts or variables must be identified and defined. Concepts, no matter what their level of abstraction, must be defined unambiguously as possible, so that they can be easily communicated to others. A conceptual definition conveys the general meaning of the concept, as does a dictionary definition. Operational definition is written by adding operationalization to the conceptual definition by delineating the procedures or operations required to measure the concept. An operational definition provides specificity and direction for constructs to guide the development of the research study. Once the construct or concept is operationalized (made measurable), it is termed as ***variable***.

After identification and definition of the variable, a possible relationship between these variables must be explored. Writing relational statement is an extremely important ingredient in any attempt to build a scientific body of knowledge. It must be formulated before explanation or predictions can be made. The statement can be relational or nonrelational. The relational statement declares relationship of some kind between two or more concepts whereas nonrelational statement asserts the existence of the concept or it may be a definition. Relational statement either asserts association or causality. The association may be positive, negative or no association. The causality declares the cause and effect relationship. Nonrelational statement serves as adjuncts to relational statements. The assertion 'there is a phenomenon known as maternal attachment is an existence statement.

The way in which the concepts are linked is limited only by the investigator's imagination. One way of making the connections between concepts is to draw a picture of how the concepts are believed to fit together. The connections made between the concepts should make sense. The investigator can make these connections based on the existing knowledge and she should know to what extent these relations are explored already (Fig. 4.1).

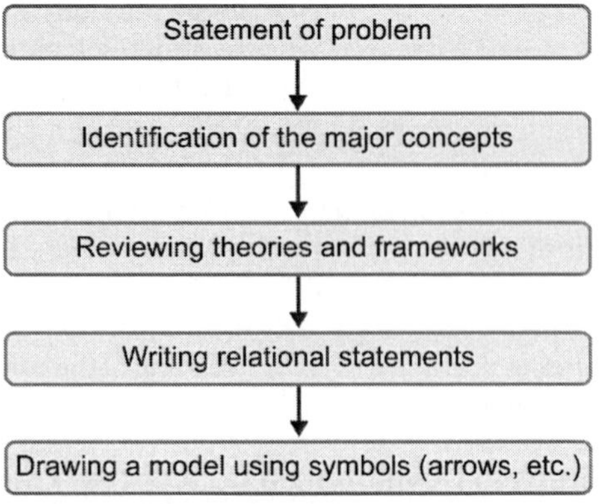

Fig. 4.1: Steps in developing a conceptual framework

Writing a framework requires that the investigator exercises creativity in all the steps and she should explain the basis on which it is developed, so that others will be able to understand. She can use flowcharts, triangles, circles and mind maps to explain. The purpose of the study is dictated by the framework which has indicated the current level of knowledge about the phenomenon of interest.

When developing a conceptual framework for nursing research studies, knowledge is acquired through two approaches. Either it is developed primarily in disciplines other than nursing and borrowed for the purpose of answering questions or it is derived by asking questions about phenomenon that are unique to nursing.

The framework formulated may be a process framework or content framework. Process framework explains the process of research and sets out the stages through which an action moves from initiation to the end. For example, research studies using the Von Bertalanffy's General System Theory explains the process of the research. The theory's major concepts are the input, throughput and output. The content framework explains the variables and the relationships between the variables. The process framework answers how each action works and what are its effects whereas the content framework answers why there is a relationship between the variables, its nature and strength.

Whether it is a process framework or content framework, it can be formulated as follows:

- Flowcharts (Fig. 4.2)
- Tree diagrams (Fig. 4.3)
- Mind maps (Fig. 4.4)
- Shape based diagrams—triangles, concentric circles, overlapping circles (Fig. 4.5)
- Soft systems.

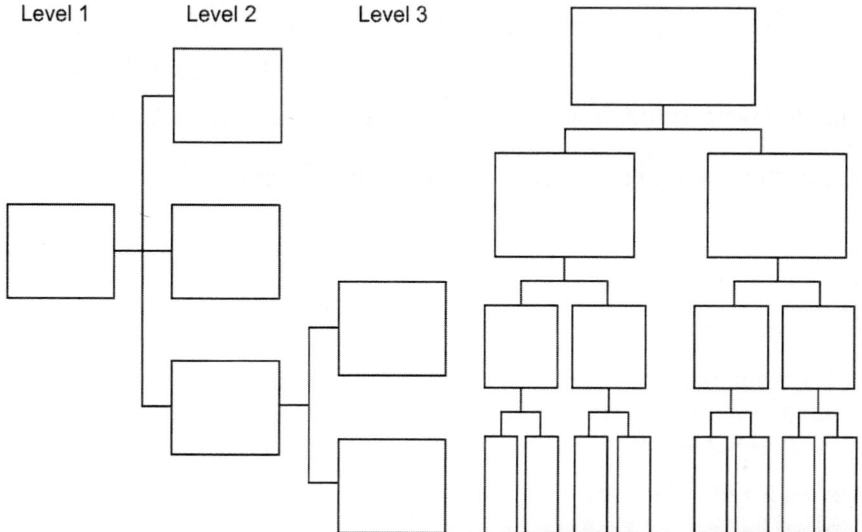

Fig. 4.2: Example of flow diagram

Fig. 4.3: Example of tree diagram

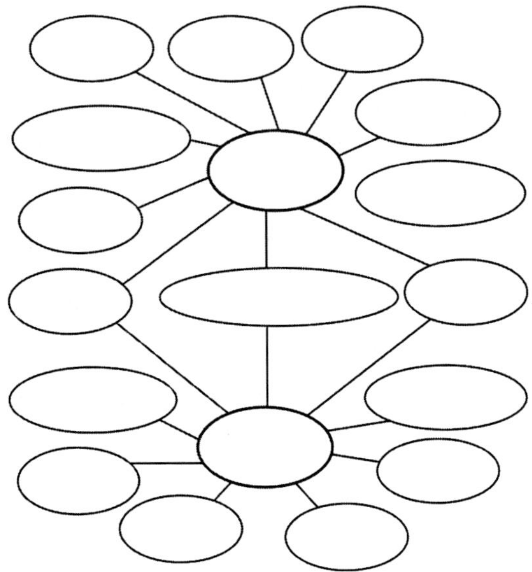

Fig. 4.4: Example of mind map

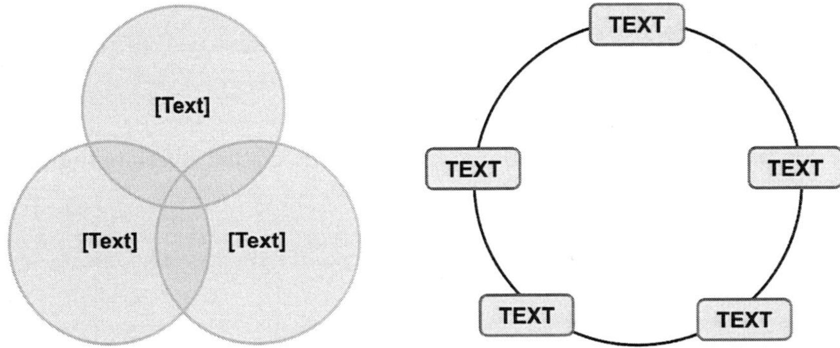

Fig. 4.5: Example of overlapping circles

Fig. 4.6: Example of cycle diagram

Use of Nursing and Non-nursing Frameworks/Theories

A researcher can use nursing theories as well as non-nursing theories to form a base of his research. There are many nursing theories developed by nurse theorists. Examples of nursing theories are as follows:

Grand Theories

- Roy's adaptation model
- Roger's model: Science of unitary human being
- Betty Neuman's systems model.

Middle Range Theories

- Pender's theory of health promotion
- Jessor's problem behavior theory.

Practice Theories

- Theory of interpersonal relationship
- Theory of non-nutritional infant sucking.

There are lot of non-nursing theories as theories in psychology such as theories of personality, intelligence, etc. such as theories of leadership, theories of management, theories of growth and development, genetic theories, social theories, etc. A research should decide which theory is best suits his research problem and it can be adopted for his study. For example, if a researcher wants to study the coping of hospitalized children, he can base his problem on theories of growth and development, cognitive theories, theories of pain, etc. and which theory to be selected is purely a researcher's choice. It is not selecting a correct or incorrect theory for investigation. Rather, it is the ability of the researcher to see the logical links and relational statements explained in a theory and utilize these concepts and test it in his study. In case of burrowed theories, such as theories not related to nursing and originally from other discipline, its utilization is acceptable until it is able to explain the concepts and phenomena related to nursing.

Conceptual Framework in a Quantitative Research

Conceptual framework is formulated in a quantitative research in the beginning of the study. Formulation of conceptual framework requires the researcher to review literature and his experience on the issue(s) of interest facilitate the development of the framework. One can adopt the existing theories or model and the concepts can be fit into the model. The researcher must have the knowledge of nursing theories and the major components of those theories. By adopting existing models or theories, one can test the theories (Refer table 4.2).

Conceptual Framework in a Qualitative Research

Normally, qualitative work is described as starting from an inductive position, seeking to build up theory, with the conceptual framework being 'emergent', because existing literature/theories might mislead. However, Miles and Huberman (1994) note that researchers generally have some idea of what will feature in the study, a tentative rudimentary conceptual framework and it is better to have some idea of what we are looking for/at even if that idea changes over time. This is particularly true for inexperienced and/or time constrained researchers. Yin (1994) explained about pattern matching and explanation building. Pattern matching starts with existing theory and tests its adequacy in terms of explaining the findings. Explanation building starts with theory and then builds an explanation while collecting and analyzing the data.

Inputs Required for the Development of a Conceptual Framework

The following inputs are required for the novice and experienced researchers and their supervisors:

- The knowledge of existing theories, models and concepts
- Technical knowledge of how a conceptual model is formulated

- Research experience
- Critical thinking and reasoning skills
- Data from the literature review-related studies can be reviewed to understand the concepts and relationships between the concepts
- Data from the research study in case of qualitative study.

Limitations of Conceptual Framework

- It is influenced by the experience and knowledge of the investigator. There is a chance for the subjective bias (initial bias)
- Once developed will influence the researcher's thinking and may result in some things being given prominence and others being ignored (ongoing bias)
- The solution is to revisit the conceptual framework, particularly at the end when evaluating one's work.

MODEL OF PROCESS FRAMEWORK

Example 1:

Satish L (2012) has developed a conceptual framework based on General systems theory proposed by Ludwig Von Bertalanffy (1968) in his study on assessment of effectiveness of Video Assisted Teaching Program (VATP) on knowledge on basic life support among students studying in polytechnic colleges in Chennai.

General system theory is a holistic theory that describes a complex system by examining the interactions between its components, rather than by analyzing the detailed structure of each components. General system theory serves as a model for viewing people as interacting with environment. All living systems are open in which there is a continuous exchange of energy, matter and information with the environment from which the system receives input and gives back output in the same form of energy, matter and information. Ludwig Von Bertalanffy described living organisms as 'open systems' that interacts comprehensively with their environment. Next, he recognized that complex systems have emergent properties that cannot be predicted by knowing the properties of its components. In addition, he observed that such a system can also exert control over its components, such as in homeostasis, by using feedback loops (Fig. 4.7).

A system is a complex of interacting elements. It can be open or closed. ***Open system*** are open for the exchange of matter, energy and information with their environment from which the system receives input and gives back output. Open system theory mainly consists of three elements such as:

1. Input
2. Throughput
3. Output

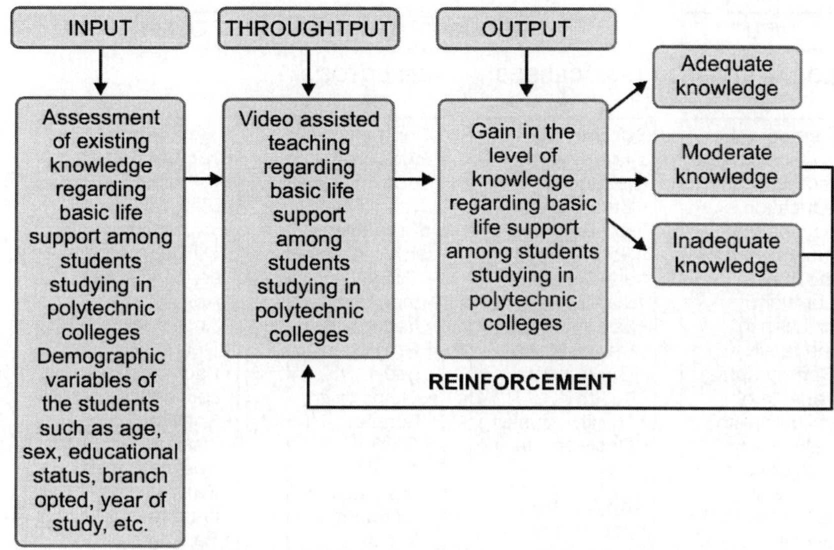

Fig. 4.7: Conceptual framework based on general system theory (Ludwig Von Bertalanffy), 1968

Input refers to the stimuli and imported materials from the external environment. The system uses input through self-regulation to maintain the equilibrium or homeostasis. Inputs are used always in their original state whereas other process requires complex transformation. In this study, the input is assessment of existing knowledge using structured questionnaire regarding basic life support among students studying in polytechnic colleges.

Throughput refers to the use of different operational procedures implemented within the process of system. In this study, it refers to the video assisted teaching that is planned for a duration of 30 minutes which includes introduction, incidence, indications and the technique of performing basic life support among students studying in polytechnic colleges.

Output refers to the resulting response to the ultimate outcome of the study. In this study, the output is gain in the level of knowledge regarding basic life support, which will be assessed by the same structured questionnaire. If the output is moderate or inadequate, it would suggest that the students studying in polytechnic colleges are in need of strengthening their throughput hence reinforcement is given through the video assisted teaching once again.

Example 2:

Divya T (2013) has developed a conceptual framework based on modified sister Callista Roy's adaptation model for her study on assessment of the psychosocial problems and coping measures adopted by the mothers of children with autism in selected special schools in Chennai. This theory views mothers as an adaptive system and need for the adaptation is triggered by the various stimuli.

The Roy's adaptation model consist of 3 aspects, such as input, throughput and output (Fig. 4.8).

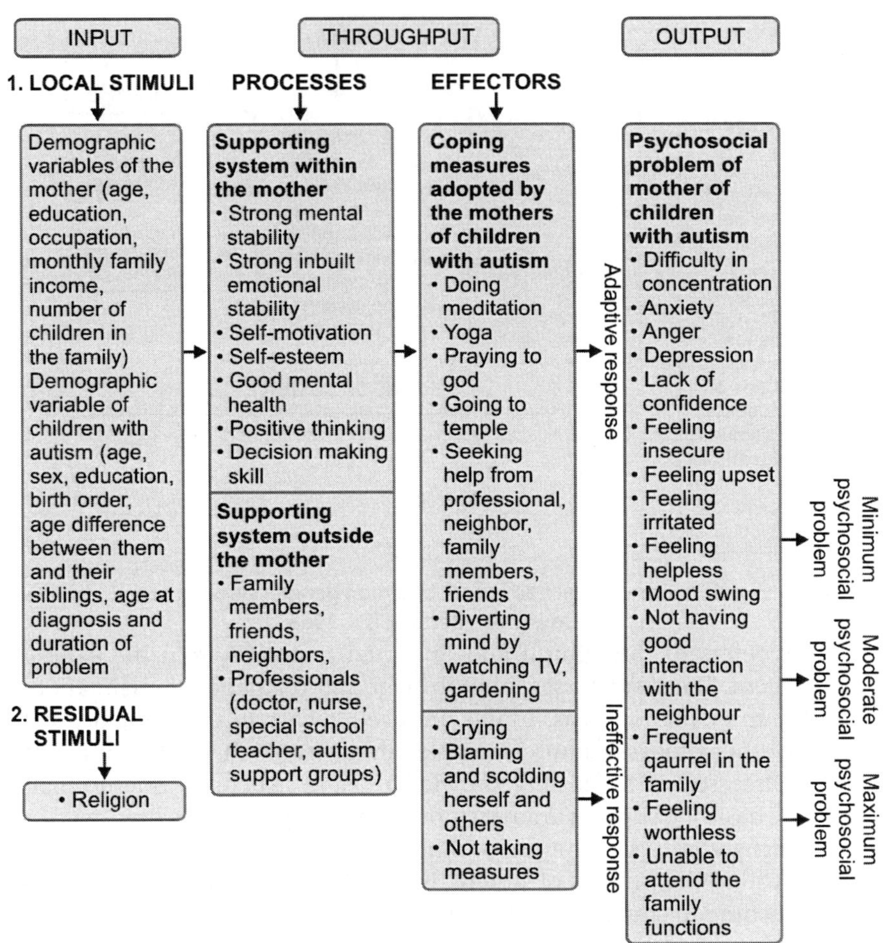

Fig. 4.8: Conceptual framework based on sister Callista Roy's adaptation

Input: In her study, the local stimuli were the demographic variables of mothers of children with autism like age, education, occupation, monthly family income, type of family, number of children in the family and demographic variables of child with autism like age, sex, education, birth order, age difference between child with autism and its siblings, age at diagnosis and duration of problem. Residual stimuli is religion.

Throughput: Throughput makes use of person's process and effectors. Processes refer to the defense mechanism and effectors refer to the process involved in adaptation. Here, person's processes are defense mechanism within the mother like strong mental stability, strong emotional inbuilt stability, self- esteem, self-motivation, good mental health, positive thinking, decision making skills and defense mechanism outside the mother like family members, friends, neighbors and professionals. Here, effectors refers to the measures adopted by the mothers of children with autism like doing meditation, yoga, crying, praying to god, going to temple, keeping silent, blaming themselves, blaming and scolding others, seeking help from friends, family members, neighbours and professionals, diverting mind by watching television and gardening.

Output: It is the outcome of the system when the system is a person, output refers to person's behaviors. Output is categorized as adaptive responses (those that promote a person's integrity) and ineffective responses (those that do not promote goal achievement). Here, the adaptive responses results from doing meditation, yoga, praying to god, going to temple, gardening, seeking help from family members, friends and professionals, etc. The ineffective responses such as not taking measures, crying, blaming themselves and scolding others lead to psychosocial problems like difficulty in concentrating, anxiety, anger, depression, lack of confidence, feeling of insecurity, upset, feeling of helplessness, feeling of worthless, irritation, mood swing, not having good interaction with the neighbors, frequent quarrels in the family and not able to attend family function, etc. It is graded as maximum, moderate and minimum psychosocial problems. Output provides feedback for the system. Here, strengthening and reinforcement of the supporting system present within the mother and outside the mother.

MODEL OF CONTENT FRAMEWORK

Example 3:

Sneha Mercy R (2013) in her study on assessment of knowledge on early identification and prevention of behavioral problems in children among teachers in selected schools in Chennai, developed a conceptual framework, based on Rosenstock's Health Belief Model. The model consists of three major factors:

(i) ***Individual perceptions:*** The teachers might have perception on the susceptibility of behavioral problems in children with their existing knowledge. The knowledge can differ from individual to individual and it may depend on the demographic variables.

(ii) ***Modifying factors:*** It refers to the demographic variables like age, sex, educational status, income, religion, type of school, years of experience, age group of students and subjects taught are presumed to influence the behavior and knowledge on early identification and prevention of behavioral problems in children.

(iii) ***Likelihood of action:*** The likelihood of a sample following the process of early identification and prevention for behavioral problems in children depends on perceived benefits and barriers to action (Fig. 4.9).

Example 4:

Oli Pushpha OS (2013) has developed a conceptual framework in her study on assessment of the effectiveness of specified oral hygiene routine on oral health of patients undergoing chemotherapy in selected hospital settings. A modified and adopted prescriptive theory 'Helping Art of Clinical Nursing' proposed by Ernestine

contd...

contd...

Wiedenbach was used. This study is based on the concept that specified oral hygiene routine will improve the oral health of the patients undergoing chemotherapy and enhances their well-being. The prescriptive theory directs action towards an explicit goal. The factors involved in prescriptive theory are central purpose, prescription and realities:

- Central purpose is the overall goal towards what a nurse strives or what the nurse wants to accomplish. In this study, the central purpose is to improve the oral health of the patients undergoing chemotherapy.
- Prescription refers to the plan of care for a patient. It is based on central purpose; the nurse can implement it through the nursing care plan. Here, the prescription is the instructions given regarding specified oral hygiene routine to patients undergoing chemotherapy.
- Realities refer to the physical, psychological, emotional and spiritual factors that come into play in a situation involving nursing actions. The five realities identified by Wiedenbach are agent, recipient, goal, means and framework. Agent is the practicing nurse, recipient is the patient, goal is the nurse's desired outcome, means are the activities and devices used by the nurse to achieve goal and framework is the facilities where the nursing interventions are put into practice.

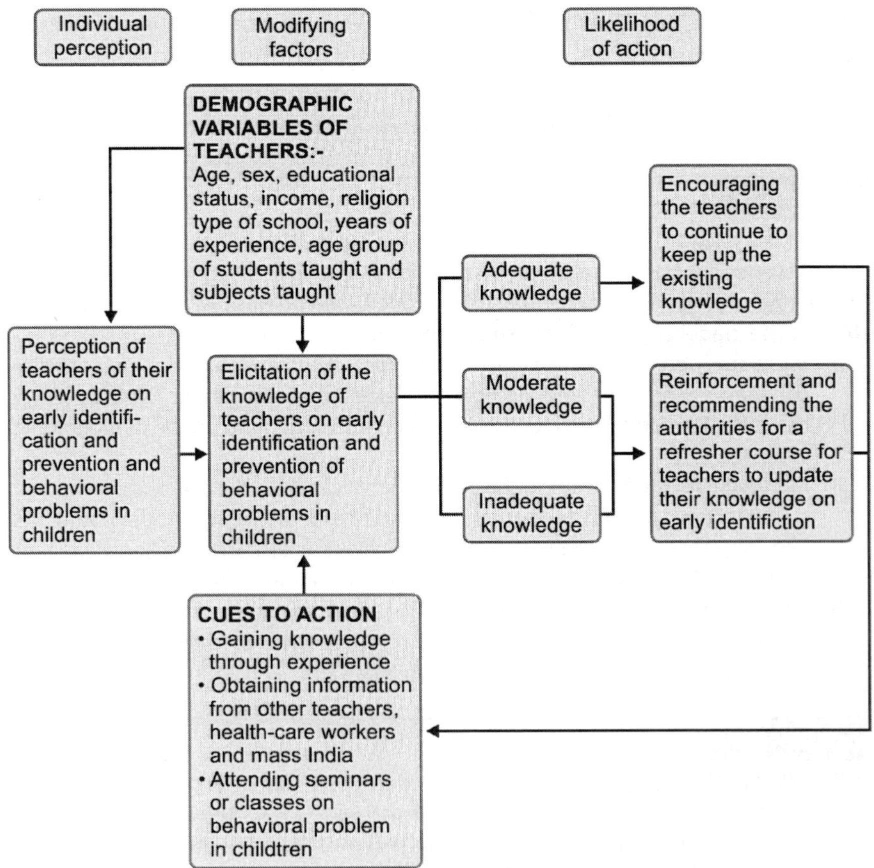

Fig. 4.9: Conceptual framework based on the Rosenstock's health belief model (1974)

Agent is the investigator who collects the data from the samples and teaches the specified oral hygiene routine to the patients undergoing chemotherapy. Recipients are the patients undergoing chemotherapy in selected hospital settings. Goal is to promote the level of oral health among the patients undergoing chemotherapy. Means is the teaching given on specified oral hygiene routine among the patients undergoing chemotherapy. Framework is the selected hospitals in Chennai where patients were taking treatment.

Central purpose, prescription, realities components of prescriptive theory is interdependent on one another as depicted. The prescription was derived by the investigator for her central purpose and is affected by the realities of the situation. The investigator develops prescription based on her central purpose, which is implemented in the realities of the situation. Together these components constitute the substance of Ernestine Wiedenbach's prescriptive theory (Fig. 4.10).

Wiedenbach's vision of nursing practice closely parallels the assessment, implementation and evaluation steps of the nursing process. Factual and speculative knowledge, judgment and skills are necessary for effective nursing practice. According to Wiedenbach, nursing practice consists of:

- Identifying a patient's need for help
- Ministering the needed help
- Validating that the need for help was met.

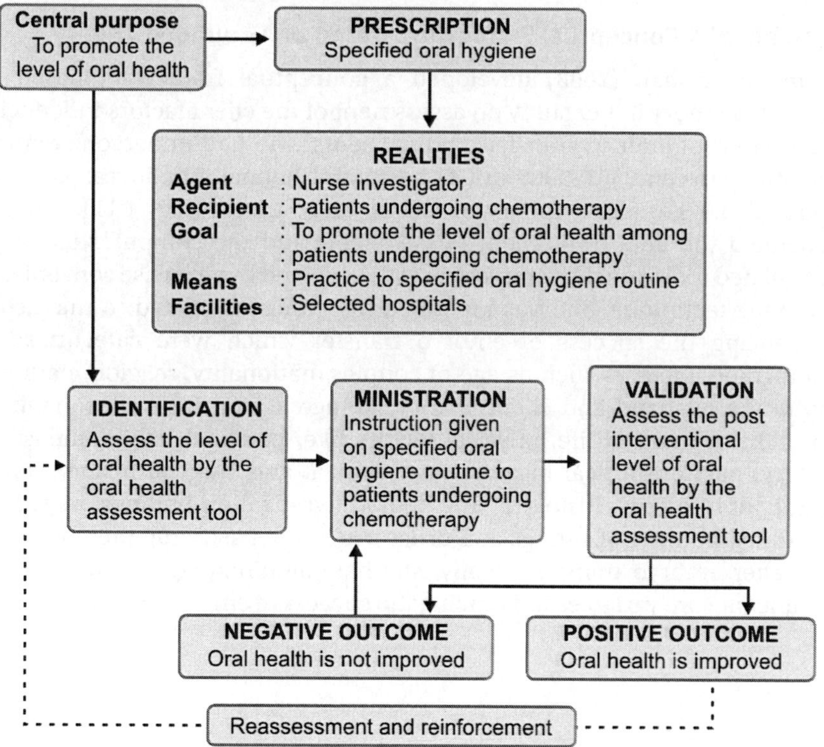

Fig. 4.10: Conceptual framework based on Wiedenbach's helping art of clinical nursing theory (1964)

1. ***Identification:*** It determines a patient's need for help based on the existence of a need, whether the patient realizes the need, what prevents the patient from meeting the need and whether the patient cannot meet the need alone. In this study, the need was identified by assessing the existing level of oral health among the patients undergoing chemotherapy by using the oral health assessment tool.
2. ***Ministration:*** It refers to provision of needed help. In this study, the investigator taught about the practice of specified oral hygiene routine and advised the patients to practice regularly.
3. ***Validation:*** It refers to the collection of evidence that shows one's need to be met and functional ability to be restored as a result of the nurse's actions. In this study, the validation was met by assessing the post interventional level of oral health of patients undergoing chemotherapy using oral health assessment tool.

The outcome could be either positive or negative. A positive outcome represents that the oral health is improved for the patients who practiced specified oral hygiene routine regularly and the negative outcome represents that the patient's oral health is not improved even after practicing specified oral hygiene routine regularly and thus the intervention has to be repeated or reassessed for its success.

Example of a Conceptual Framework Based on Grounded Theory

Prema Janardhan (2008) developed a conceptual framework based on grounded theory in her study on assessment of the client factors influencing the success of embryo transfer among clients who had undergone embryo transfer between 2003–2005 in GG hospital, Chennai. The investigator has adopted the grounded theory of Glaser and Strauss (Fig. 4.11). She has generated the data from client's case sheets and the computer using the formulated tool from the samples(records) selected by year wise convenience sampling technique. She has identified the concepts related to the factors influencing the success of embryo transfer which were categorized as demographic factors such as age of couples, nationality, religion, nature of job of the husband and client factors like age at marriage, consanguinity, duration of married life, physical factors like, personal habits, menstrual history, past obstetrical history, past medical and surgical history, family history of infertility, history of any injury, investigation findings, reason for infertility, number of sittings and drugs use in the past, drug therapy before and after embryo transfer. Finally, she has identified significant and non significant core variables influencing the success of embryo transfer.

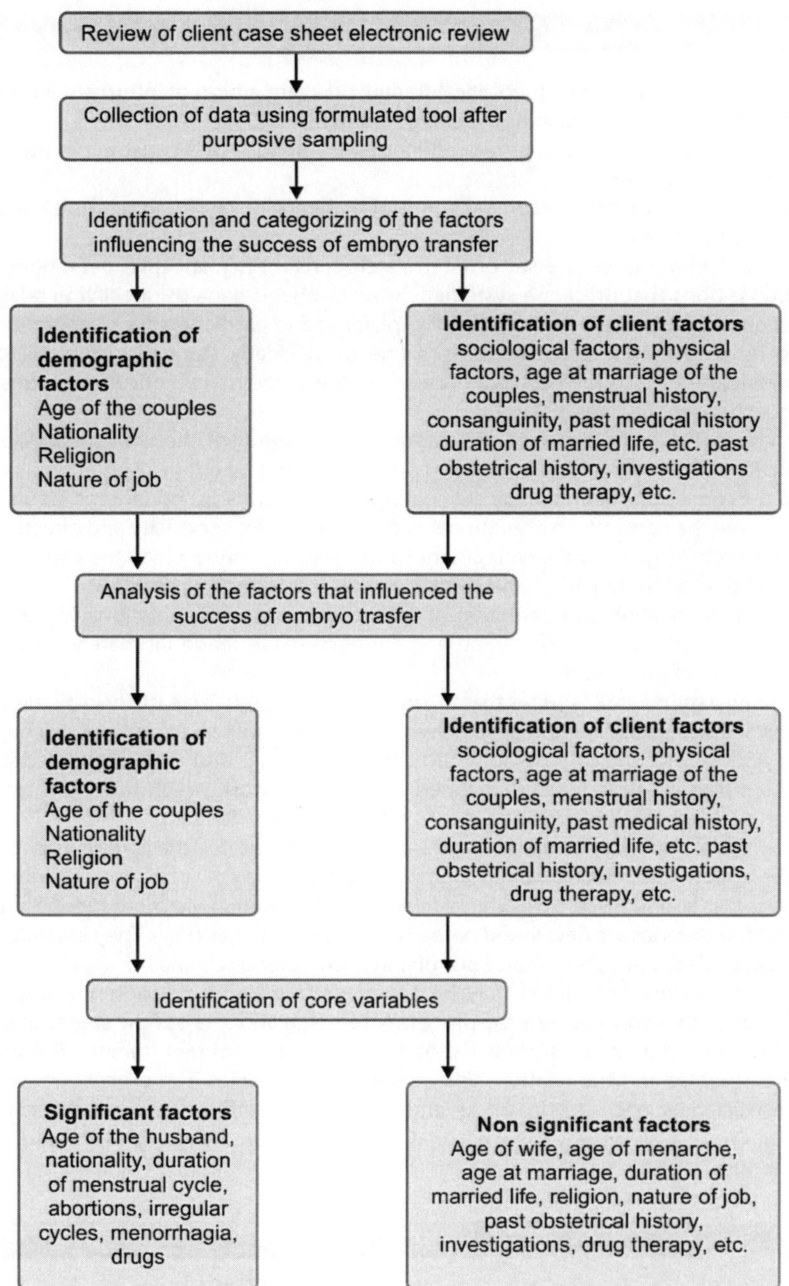

Fig. 4.11: Modified grounded theory of Glaser and Strauss

SUMMARY

- Conceptual frameworks (theoretical frameworks) are a type of intermediate theory that attempt to connect to all aspects of inquiry.
- A concept is a mental image of a phenomenon, an idea or a construct in the mind about a thing or action.
- A model is a simplified representation of a theory or of certain complex events, structures or systems.
- A conceptual model is a set of interrelated constructs (concepts) definitions and propositions that present a systematic view of phenomena by specifying relations among variables with the purpose of explaining and predicting the phenomena.
- To develop a conceptual framework one must clearly state the problem to be investigated. Once the problem is clearly defined, the major concepts or variables must be identified and defined.
- A conceptual definition conveys the general meaning of the concept, as does a dictionary definition. Operational definition is written by adding operationalization to the conceptual definition by delineating the procedures or operations required to measure the concept. An operational definition provides specificity and direction for constructs to guide the development of the research study. Once the construct or concept is operationalized (made measurable), it is termed as ***variable***.
- After identification and definition of the variable, a possible relationship between these variables must be explored and connection are made ultimately leading to formation of framework.
- Writing a framework requires that the investigator exercises creativity in all the steps and she should explain the basis on which it is developed so that others will be able to understand. She can use flowcharts, triangles, circles and mind maps to explain. The purpose of the study is dictated by the framework which has indicated the current level of knowledge about the phenomenon of interest.
- The conceptual framework serves as a stepping stone for the formulation of the 'theoretical framework' which comprises established explanations, theoretical principles and suggested theoretical relations in preparation of a more specific inquiry.
- Nursing theories are developed based on the following methods. They are inductive process, deductive process and burrowing from other disciplines.
- The framework formulated may be a process framework or content framework. Process framework explains the process of research and sets out the stages through which an action moves from initiation to the end. The content framework explains the variables and the relationships between the variables. The process framework answers how each action works and what are its effects whereas the content framework answers why there is a relationship between the variables, its nature and strength.

EXERCISE

- Identify the major concepts in the conceptual framework. Derive the research problem and objectives. Think of fitting the same concepts in other theories (Figs 4.12 and 4.13).
- For the given research problem (problem statement) or questions, what existing theory/model do you think will fit into?
  - A study to assess the psychophysiological effect of playing violent video games among children in Chennai.

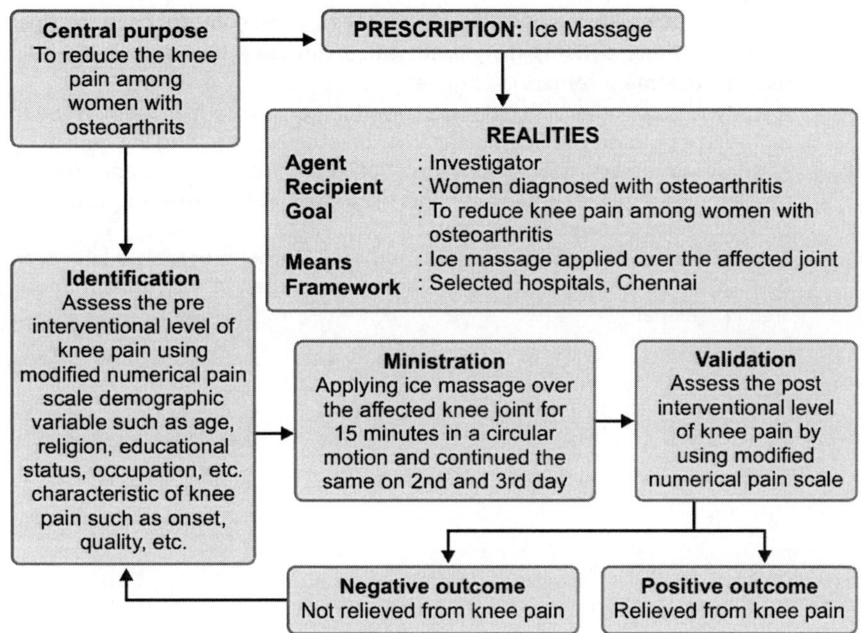

Fig. 4.12: Conceptual framework based on Wiedenbach's helping art of clinical nursing theory (1964)

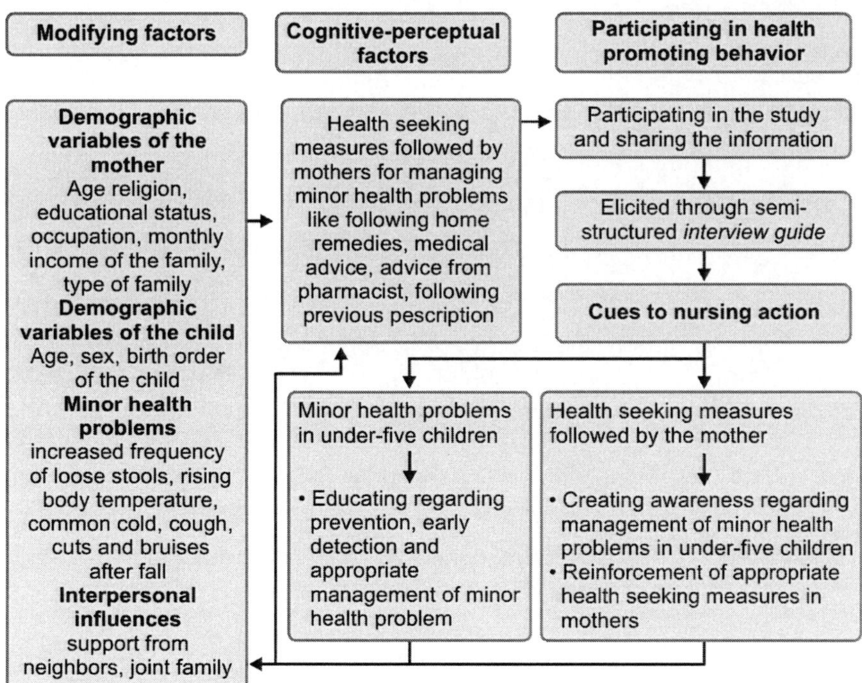

Fig. 4.13: Conceptual framework based on Pender's health promotion model

- A study to assess the compliance and reasons for non compliance to treatment regimen among patients diagnosed with pulmonary tuberculosis attending selected treatment centers in Chennai.
- A study to assess the difficulties perceived in home care management by the mothers of children with Mental Retardation at selected setting in Chennai.
- A study to assess the effectiveness of Breathing exercises on selected physiological variables among patients diagnosed with hypertension attending OPD, at selected hospitals, Chennai.
- A study to assess the effectiveness of Mother to Mother program on knowledge on child abuse among mothers of under-five children at selected community area in Chennai.

5 Research Approaches and Designs

OBJECTIVES

After reading this chapter, you will be able to:

- State the meaning of research approaches and designs
- Differentiate the research approach and design
- Explain various research approaches used in nursing research
- Explain various research designs used in nursing research
- Describe the selection of research approaches and designs for a research study.

INTRODUCTION

Research design is the researcher's overall plan to obtain answer to the problem. In order to obtain solution to the problem, the researcher follows the best possible technique among the alternatives available. 'Research approach' is a broad term which explains how a problem can be approached. 'Research design' is a more specific term which explains how a problem is solved using a specific approach. The selection of research design is influenced by the research approach. The research design is a plan of action indicating the specific steps that are necessary to provide answers to those questions, test the hypotheses and, thereby, achieve the research objectives that is the outcome of the study.

Meaning and Definition

We travel to many places. Suppose, if we want to go to a city, we think of what are the possible ways to reach the city. It may be by road, air, water or by train. The selection of the mode of transport depends upon the purpose of reaching a city, that is, the time availability, cost involved and many other factors. After selecting a mode, we may further decide about our travel to reach the destination. Same way, a researcher has to select a particular approach and design, which will best suit his research problem (Table 5.1).

Research design is a conceptual structure or plan of how a research is conducted. The research design constitutes the blueprint for the collection, measurement and analysis of data.

- According to David J Luck and Ronald S Rubin, 'A research design is the determination and statement of the general research approach or strategy adopted for the particular project. It is the heart of planning. If the design adheres to the research objective, it will ensure that the client's needs will be served.'

- According to Kerlinger, 'Research design is the plan, structure and strategy of investigation conceived so as to obtain answers to research questions and to control variance.'
- According to Green and Tull, 'A research design is the specification of methods and procedures for acquiring the information needed. It is the overall operational pattern or framework of the project that stipulates what information is to be collected, from which source and by what procedures.'
- A research design is the arrangement of conditions for collection and analysis of data in a manner that aims to combine relevance to the research purpose with economy in procedure (Claire Selltiz and others).

Table 5.1: Difference between research approach and research design

S. No.	Research approach	Research design
1.	Explains how a problem is solved or destination is reached	Explains how a problem is solved or destination is reached using a particular approach
2.	Broad in scope	Narrow in scope
3.	Selected based on the objective or purpose of the research.	Selected based on the approach to solve a problem.

Advantages of Selecting a Research Design

- It saves a lot of researcher's time, energy and effort
- It provides direction as how to proceed
- It ensures time schedule
- It enables resource planning and forecasting
- It helps to predict the future activities
- It helps to check the progress
- It reduces error
- It provides a sense of fulfillment and satisfaction.

Research Approaches (Fig. 5.1)

The three main approaches to research are:

1. Quantitative approach
2. Qualitative approach
3. Pragmatic approach

Quantitative approach to research aims at quantifying the variables of a study. It includes the collection of data pertaining to research variables and converting it into numerical form in order to subject them to statistical analysis. It involves the generation of data in quantitative form, which can be subjected to rigorous quantitative analysis in a formal and rigid fashion. The

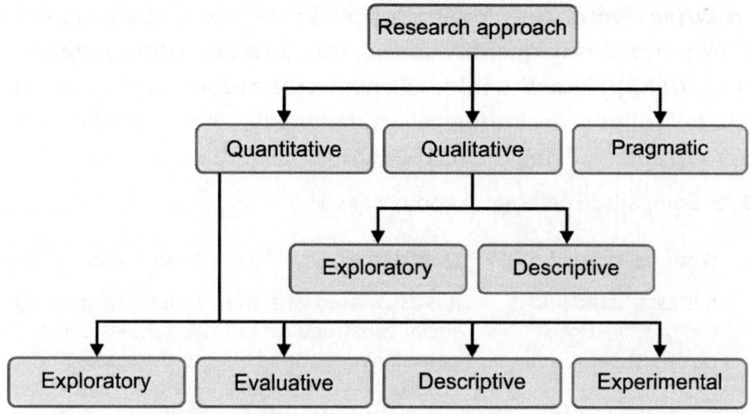

Fig. 5.1: Classification of research approaches

conclusions are drawn from the statistical analysis. Information is obtained to generalize the findings to the population (Table 5.2).

Qualitative approach to research is associated with the understanding of the human behavior and experience. It is concerned with subjective assessment of attitudes, opinions and behavior. Research in such a situation is a function of researcher's insights and impressions. The aim is not to quantify, instead to explore the deeper meaning of various behaviors and human experiences. It involves recording, analyzing and attempting to uncover the meaning and significance of experience and behavior, including contradictory beliefs and emotions (Table 5.2).

Pragmatic approach to research ***(mixed methods):*** The pragmatic approach to science involves using the method which appears best suited to the research problem and not getting caught up in philosophical debates about which is the best approach. Pragmatic researchers, therefore, grant themselves the freedom to use any of the methods, techniques and procedures typically associated with quantitative or qualitative research. They recognize that every method has its limitations and that the different approaches can be complementary (Table 5.2).

Experimental approach is characterized by much greater control over the research environment and, in this case, some variables are manipulated to observe their effect on other variables.

Exploratory approach to research is used when the researcher wants to know how and why certain phenomenon occurs. The purpose of exploratory research is to know the unknown. The objective of exploratory research is to generate/discover new ideas. The secondary/published data can be used for exploratory research as such data are easily available. It is primarily done for the purpose of finding anything new in any subject arena and always tries to shed some light in the unknown domain of knowledge.

Evaluative approach to research aims at evaluating the variables of the study. The purpose is to quantify, assess, categorize and draw inference.

Descriptive approach to research involves the description of the variables of the study. It aims at describing the characteristics of a particular individual, or of a group and studying the relationship among the variables.

Table 5.2: Comparison of research approaches

S. No.	Quantitative	Qualitative	Pragmatic
1.	It is associated with the positivist/post positivist paradigm	It is associated with the social constructivist paradigm which emphasizes the socially constructed nature of reality	It uses the method which best suits to the research problem associated with quantitative or qualitative research
2.	It will have one or more hypotheses	Qualitative researchers do not base their research on pre-determined hypotheses	It may or may not have hypotheses
3.	It requires clearly defined plan of action	It allows for greater flexibility than in quantitative research	It is both flexible and rigid wherever necessary
4.	Data is collected using self-report, questionnaire, etc. and is quantified.	Data is collected in textual form on the basis of observation and interaction, focused and in-depth interviews	It uses both quantitative and qualitative data. So, it uses various techniques and tools
5.	Involves larger number of samples	Often involves a smaller number of participants	The number of samples depends upon the problem
6.	Limits freedom and participants are forced to select from the responses most of the time	Give participants a certain degree of freedom and permit spontaneity rather than forcing them to select from a set of pre-determined responses	It gives freedom to participants when required and the same time it limits the freedom to the participants when required
7.	Statistical analyses are carried out	It is not converted into numerical form and is not statistically analyzed	Statistical analyses are carried out
8.	More objective. Less bias	More subjective	It is both subjective as well as objective

contd...

contd...

S. No.	Quantitative	Qualitative	Pragmatic
9.	The main emphasis of quantitative research is on deductive reasoning which tends to move from the general to the specific	The approach adopted by qualitative researchers tends to be inductive, which means that they develop a theory or look for a pattern of meaning on the basis of the data that they have collected. This involves a move from the specific to the general	Triangulation is a common feature of mixed method studies. It involves, data triangulation, investigator triangulation, theory triangulation and methodological triangulation
10.	Attempts to generalize	Does not attempt to generalize	It attempts to generalize wherever necessary
11.	This is sometimes referred to as a top down approach.	It is sometimes called a bottoms-up approach.	It uses both the approaches.

Need for Research Design

- It facilitates the researcher to function smoothly
- It maximizes the input and minimizes the time, money and effort
- It demands good planning, thereby promoting a better output
- It helps the researcher organize his ideas and proceed further.

Features of Good Design

- Flexible
- Appropriate
- Efficient
- Economical.

EXPERIMENTAL RESEARCH DESIGNS

Experimental designs are either true experimental or quasiexperimental studies (Fig. 5.2). In order to be a true experiment, a research has to fulfill certain principles. The principles of experimental designs are as follows:

- ***Principle of Control:*** Control refers to the extent to which different factors or variables in an experiment are accounted for. Researcher uses control to show the outcome with confidence. Control is achieved in an experimental study by manipulating and randomizing, by carefully preparing the experimental protocols, and by using a control group. Researcher uses control in order to prevent that any factor or variable other than the independent variable influencing the dependent variable, so that the effect of independent variable on the dependent variable can be measured. High degree of control is achieved in the laboratory settings, whereas it is not possible in social setting and other natural settings.

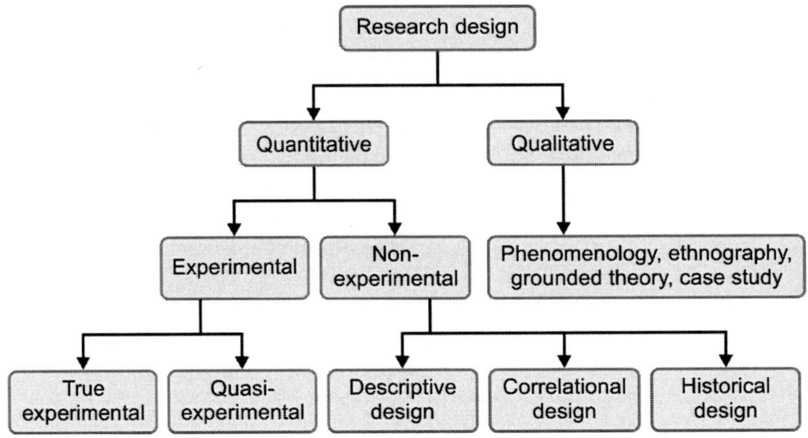

Fig. 5.2: Classification of research design

The term 'control group' refers to a group of subjects whose performance on a dependent variable is used to evaluate the performance of the experimental group or treatment group (the group that receives the intervention) on the same dependent variable. There are methods of controlling inter-subject differences. They are random assignment of subjects to groups, subject-to-subject matching, matching for mean and standard deviation (in case of groups), ranking of subjects on the matching variable and using subjects as their own controls.

- ***Principle of Manipulation:*** Manipulation refers to a deliberate operation of the conditions by the researcher. In the process of manipulation, a predetermined set of varied conditions are imposed on the subjects selected for the experimental group. It involves doing something to study participants. The introduction of that something (i.e. the experimental treatment or intervention) constitutes the independent variables. The experimenter manipulates the independent variable by administering a treatment to some subjects and withholding it from others (or by administering some other treatment). The experimenter, thus, consciously varies the independent variable and observes the effect on the dependent variable.
- ***Principle of Randomization:*** Randomization (also called 'random assignment') involves placing subjects in groups at random. Random essentially means that every subject has an equal chance of being assigned to any group. If subjects are placed in groups randomly, there is no systematic bias in the groups with respect to attributes that could affect the dependent variable.

Experimental designs enable the researcher to test hypothesis. Besides fulfilling the principles of experimental designs, the researcher must ensure three important criteria before proceeding into the experimental research. These are as follows:

Appropriateness

The design selected should be appropriate for testing of hypothesis. There are various true and quasiexperimental research designs and the investigator should select the appropriate design for his experiment.

Control

The design must provide adequate control so that the effect of independent variable on the dependent variable can be measured. The adequate control of the extraneous variable helps to isolate and measure the impact of independent variable on the dependent variable.

Controlling Extraneous Variables

Instructions to participants help in controlling extraneous variables. Automation, that is using electronic or mechanical devices to present stimuli and to measure and record responses helps to control extraneous variable. The demand characteristics should be controlled in a study. Demand characteristics is an extraneous cue that guides or biases a participants behavior. Demand characteristics are cues that bias subjects, resulting in responses that are not valid, reliable reactions to our variables.

Types of Demand Characteristics

- Reactivity is the bias in responses that occurs because participants are aware that they are being observed
- Hawthorne effect refers to the influence on participants' performance—usually an improvement that occurs due to the novelty of being in a study
- Social desirability occurs when people provide what they consider to be the socially acceptable response
- ***Experimenter expectation:*** Participants are very sensitive to the expectation of the experimenter.

Controls for Demand Characteristics

- ***Single- and double-blind procedure:*** In single-blinding, participants may not be aware of the manipulation. Whereas in double-blinding both the participant and the researcher may not be aware. The principal investigator must train others to collect data. A double-blind procedure keeps both the researcher and the participant blind to the conditions so that their expectations do not influence the results
- ***Habituation:*** By habituation, we familiarize participants with a procedure before beginning actual data collection
- ***Unobtrusive measure:*** It means we measure participants' behavior without making them aware the measurement is being made. To keep demand characteristics constant, control groups are given placebo. A placebo is given to control groups so that they experience the same demand characteristics as experimental groups.

Validity

Validity refers to worth. Here the validity refers to validity of the research design in conducting an experiment. In general, validity is of two types. These are internal and external validity.

Internal Validity

It refers to ensuring that only the independent variable has influenced the dependent variable and no other extraneous variables contributed to the effect on the dependent variable. There are certain factors contributing to the threat to internal validity. They are as follows:

- ***History:*** Apart from experimental treatment, the researcher should control any specific events related to experiment that could influence the dependent variable.
- ***Maturation:*** It is possible that the subjects in the experiment undergo changes over a period of time during experimentation. These changes might affect the dependent variable.
- ***Pretesting:*** The exposure of the subjects to the pretest may serve as the learning experience and, therefore, it may affect their post-test performance.
- ***Measuring instruments:*** Different measuring instruments, scorers, raters, interviewers or the observers used at the pre and post testing may account for differences in the scores or measures of the dependent variable.
- ***Statistical regression:*** The individuals or groups chosen based on the extreme scores may move or regress towards the common mean on subsequent measures. This may operate to produce an effect that could be interpreted as an effect due to experimental treatment.
- ***Differential selection of subjects:*** If subjects of both groups are not homogenous and significantly differ on variable related to the dependent variable even before the application of the experimental treatment, the results are influenced.
- ***Experimental mortality:*** The loss of subjects from the comparison groups may affect the findings of the study.
- ***Interaction of selection and maturation and selection and history:*** When two comparison groups have the same scores in pretest but due to interaction, one group may score higher than the other not because of experimental variable but due to the interaction of other variables.

External Validity

It refers to determining the extent to which the study findings are generalizable. There are two types of external validity. They are ***population validity*** and ***ecological validity***. ***Population validity*** refers to the extent to which the findings based on the samples are generalizable to the population. ***Ecological***

validity refers to the extent to which the findings can be generalizable to the other environmental conditions.

Types of Experimental Designs

There are various experimental designs. They vary in complexity and adequacy. Based on the objectives, nature and purpose of the experiment, a particular design is selected.

Pre-experimental Designs

Pre-experimental designs provide little or no control of extraneous or situation variables. There are two types of pre-experimental designs. These are:

1. ***One Group Pre-test/Post-test design***

   Pre-test *Intervention* *Post-test*

   In this design, a researcher measures the dependent variable before and after the independent variable is applied. The difference is measured and this is taken as the amount of change as a result of the application of the independent variable or treatment.

Limitations

- There is no control group. So, the investigator cannot assume that difference is only due to the experimental treatment
- History and maturation are two major extraneous variables that are controlled in this design
- Since post-test is a repeated test, a sample's performance in post-test is influenced by the exposure to the pre-test
- Once pre-test is administered, there may be reactivity among samples (i.e. the sample might refer or clarify some themes in the pre-test with others) which will bring the change in the post-test apart from the treatment.

Example 1:

Sowndaram (2013) has conducted a research to test the effectiveness of psycho-social intervention on mental health of the 30 adolescent school children from a selected school in Mysore. The adolescents were selected using purposive sampling method and their mental health was assessed by using Mental Health Scale initially. Then the intervention package was given for a period of one month with the help of the teachers. The intervention package consisted of selected physical tasks, like walking, jogging, yoga, etc. and cognitive behavior therapy, talk therapy, creative expressions, establishing positive relationships, with the family members and with the peer groups. Bhagavad Gita recitation, dance and music therapy also given. Again the mental health was assessed by using the same scale. The results revealed that there was a statistically significant difference in mental health status seen before and after intervention and they concluded that the intervention helped in promoting the mental health of the group.

Sample	Pre-test	Intervention	Post-test
30 adolescents school children selected using purposive sampling technique	Assessment of mental health using mental health status scale by Sharma (1996)	Intervention package given for one month. First week, as a group intervention, it was given by the researcher and then followed by the class coordinator and the parents	Assessment of mental health using mental health status scale by Sharma (1996)

Example 2:

Bharathi (2012) conducted a study to assess the use of positive therapy to enhance the general well-being among prisoners. A group of prisoners was collected and administered a pretest to assess the level of anxiety, stress and general well-being. Positive therapy was given to prisoners. It consisted of relaxation therapy, counseling, exercise and behavioural assignments. It was given as 1-hour session on alternate days for 6 sessions spread over 2 weeks. Post-test was conducted using the same pre-test quesionnaire.

Sample	Pre-test	Intervention	Post-test
Group of prisoners	Assessment on level of anxiety, stress and general well-being	Positive therapy was given to prisoners. It consisted of relaxation therapy, counseling, exercise and behavioral assignments. It was given as 1-hour session on alternate days for 6 sessions spread over 2 weeks	Assessment of level of anxiety, stress and general well-being

Example 3:

Dal and Sarpakaya (2013) did a study to determine the cardiopulmonary resuscitation (CPR) knowledge and skill levels of nursing students in North Cyprus. Eighty-three third-year students of nursing participated in the study. A questionnaire was applied to the students before the CPR lecture. Then the students were informed about adult CPR by the researchers and all the students practiced CPR on a Resusci-Anne manikin. One and six months after this training, the same questionnaire and skills checklist of CPR were applied.

2. ***Two Groups Static Design:*** To overcome the limitations of the one group pre-test and post-test design, two groups are used and only one group is exposed to the experimental treatment and the other group is not given any experimental treatment. The other group is used as a control group for comparison. Post-test is conducted for both the groups after the experimental treatment for the experimental group alone. The basic assumption is that both the groups are equivalent and the experimental group performs better than the control group in post-test. Then the

researcher can confidently say that the independent variable (experiment/treatment) is responsible for the change in the dependent variable.

Experimental group	Intervention	Post-test
Control group	No intervention	Post-test

Limitations

Two equal group (experimental and control) formations are difficult. The researcher has to use either randomization or matching.

True Experimental Designs

1. ***Two groups, Randomized subjects, Post-test only design:*** This design helps to overcome the limitation of the previous two groups' static design. The samples are randomized and assigned to experimental and control groups. After the application of experimental treatment to the experimental group, post-test is conducted for both the groups.

Experimental group	Treatment/Intervention	Post-test
Control group	No treatment	Post-test

A study that tested the effect of gentle massage on the pain levels of elderly nursing home residents. This example illustrates a simple design that is sometime referred to as an after-only design because data on the dependent variable are collected only once–after random assignment is completed and the experimental treatment has been introduced.

Advantages

- Randomization is used
- No pre test is conducted. So there is no effect of history, maturation, pre testing and reaction effect
- This design is useful where pretest is unnecessary.

Limitations

- The use of this design seriously restricts the external validity (population and ecological validity)
- Randomization may be difficult in some situations.

2. ***Two groups, Randomized matched subjects, Post-test only design:*** The investigator, in addition to randomization, should use the technique of matching the subjects for experimental and control groups.

Advantages

- It is useful where the previous design is not applicable
- Matching adds strength to the design
- It controls or reduces inter-subject differences.

Limitation

- Not possible to locate the appropriate match.

3. ***Randomized Groups, Pre-test-post-test design:*** This design, because of its two measurement points, is referred to as a before-after design or

a pre-test/post-test design. In such designs, the initial measure of the dependent variable is often referred to as the baseline measure and the post-test measure of the dependent variable may be referred to as the outcome measure, i.e. the measure that captures the outcome of the experimental interventions.

Experimental group	Pre-test	Intervention	Post-test
Control group	Pre-test	No intervention	Post-test

The subjects are assigned to two groups, i.e. experimental and control group after randomization. Both the groups are administered pre-test and treatment or experimental intervention is given only to the experimental group. Then post-test is conducted for both the groups.

The difference in the test measures helps the investigator to conclude whether the treatment brought the changes in the post-test and having the control group to compare, the researcher can confidently say that the changes brought are due to the experimental treatment alone.

Advantages

- Random assignment
- Reaction effect and pre-testing effect are checked
- It controls history and maturation too.

Limitation

- There is an interaction between the pre-test and the experimental treatment. The interaction may change or sensitize the subjects.

Example 4:

Narayanan (2013) conducted an experimental study to assess the impact of group counselling intervention on knowledge on reproductive health among adolescent girls studying in a selected school in Chennai. In this study, 100 adolescent girls were randomly assigned to experimental and control groups. Pre-test was conducted on assessment of knowledge on reproductive health using structured questionnaire consisting of 25 items related to menstruation, female reproductive system, pregnancy, conception, causes and prevention of HIV/STD to both the groups. The group counseling was given by a gynecologist and a social worker to the experimental group. After a week, post-test was conducted using the same questionnaire for both the groups.

Sample	Pre-test	Intervention	Post-test
Experimental group—50 adolescent girls assigned using random technique	Structured questionnaire consisting of 25 items related to menstruation, female reproductive system, pregnancy, conception, causes and prevention of HIV/STD	Group counseling was given by a gynecologist and a social worker on reproductive health	Structured questionnaire consisting of 25 items related to menstruation, female reproductive system, pregnancy, conception, causes and prevention of HIV/STD

contd...

contd...

Sample	Pre-test	Intervention	Post-test
Control group—50 adolescent girls assigned using random technique	Structured questionnaire consisting of 25 items related to menstruation, female reproductive system, pregnancy, conception, causes and prevention of HIV/STD	No intervention given	Structured questionnaire consisting of 25 items related to menstruation, female reproductive system, pregnancy, conception, causes and prevention of HIV/STD.

Example 5:

Sudha (2002) conducted a study to evaluate the effectiveness of structured teaching program on knowledge on management of malnutrition in children among mothers of malnourished underfive children in two selected villages at Porur, Chennai.

Sample	Pre-test	Intervention	Post-test
Experimental group—30 mothers of malnourished under-five children using simple random sampling technique	Structured questionnaire on prevention and management of malnutrition in under-five children	Structured teaching and demonstration was given to the mothers of malnourished under-five children	Structured questionnaire on prevention and management of malnutrition in under-five children
Control group—30 mothers of malnourished under-five children using simple random sampling technique	Structured questionnaire on prevention and management of malnutrition in under-five children	No intervention given	Structured questionnaire on prevention and management of malnutrition in under-five children.

Example 6:

Wu, HU, McCoy and Effrd (2014) conducted a study to evaluate the effects of a breastfeeding self-efficacy intervention on short-term breastfeeding outcomes among primiparous mothers in Wuhan, China. An experimental pre-test and post-test, two-group design was used in the study. A total of 74 participants were recruited to the study from a tertiary hospital in Central China. Participants were randomly assigned to an intervention or reference group. An individualized, standardized nursing intervention was delivered to enhance mothers' breastfeeding self-efficacy, breastfeeding duration and exclusivity at 4–8 weeks postpartum. Participants in the intervention group received three individualized, self-efficacy-enhancing sessions. Participants in the reference group received standard care.

4. ***The randomized solomon three-groups design:*** It uses three groups with random assignment of subjects to groups. There are two control groups, one group receives treatment, whereas the other group does not receive any treatment. Among these two control groups, pre-test is administered to one group and the other group does not receive any pre-test. This design checks the effect of pretesting and the interactive effect of pre-testing and experimental manipulation.

Experimental Group	Pre-test	Treatment	Post-test
Control Group	Pre-test	No intervention	Post-test
Control Group	No pre-test	Treatment	Post-test

Advantages

- Randomization is done
- It controls the extraneous variable
- The second control group provides control over the interactive effect of pre-testing and experimental treatment.

5. ***The randomized solomon four-group design:*** The samples are assigned to four groups by random assignment. The experimental group and one of the control groups are administered pre-test. The other two control groups are not pre-tested. This design enables the experimenter to control and measure both the main and interaction effects of testing.

Experimental group	Pre-test	Treatment	Post-test
Control group	Pre-test	No treatment	Post-test
Control group	No Pretest	Treatment	Post-test
Control group	No pretest	No treatment	Post-test

Advantages

- Randomization is done
- It controls the extraneous variable
- The control group provides control over the interactive effect of pre-testing and experimental treatment
- It gives the researcher greater confidence in his findings.

Limitations

- It is difficult to carry out in a practical situation
- It involves more time and effort.

6. ***Factorial design:*** This factorial design permits the testing of multiple hypotheses in a single experiment. It enables the researcher to evaluate or manipulate two or more variables simultaneously in order to study the effects of number of independent factors singly as well as the effects due to interactions with one another. Factorial designs vary according to the degree of complexity depending upon the nature and purpose of the experiment. They include two or more independent variables and each one is manipulated into two or more ways to assess both their separate and their combined effects. A cross-cover design (also known as a repeated measures design) involves the exposure of the same subjects to more than one experimental treatment.

Example 7:

Retal (2013) conducted feasibility study of an optimized person-centered intervention to improve mental health and reduce antipsychotics amongst people with dementia in care homes. The study design is a cluster-randomized 2 × 2 × 2 factorial design with two replications in 16 care homes. Each cluster includes a minimum of 12 participants (depending upon the size of the care home, the number of people with dementia and the number consenting). Each cluster receives a randomly allocated intervention for a minimum of nine months. Each care home is randomized to receive one of the eight possible permutations of the four key interventions, with each possible combination delivered in two of the 16 homes.

Example 8:

Ketal (2009) conducted a factorial randomized trial to ascertain the feasibility of a full trial of a nurse-led weight-management program in general practice in UK. A total of 123 adults with body mass index (BMI) > or = 27 kg/m recruited from eight practices were randomized to receive structured lifestyle support (n = 30), structured lifestyle support plus pedometer (n = 31), usual care (n = 31), or usual care plus pedometer (n = 31) for a 12-week period. A total of 103 participants were successfully followed-up. The adjusted mean difference in weight in structured support compared to usual care groups was –2.63 kg (95% confidence interval [CI] = – 4.06 to –1.20 kg), and for pedometer compared to no pedometer groups, it was –0.11 kg (95% CI = –1.52 to 1.30 kg).

Example 9:

Defeyter and Russo (2013) conducted a study to evaluate the effectiveness of breakfast cereal consumption on adolescents' cognitive performance and mood. The short-term effects of cereal consumption on cognition were investigated using a cross-over design in which 40 adolescents were given a ready-to-eat breakfast cereal or no breakfast cereal. According to treatment, all participants were provided with 35 g low-GI breakfast cereal or no breakfast. Adolescents were tested prior to consumption of breakfast (baseline) and then 120 min post start of breakfast consumption. The order of breakfast consumption and breakfast omission was fully counterbalanced, so that half of the children consumed breakfast on the first test day and omitted breakfast on the second test day while the remaining children were presented with the same conditions but in the reverse order. Half of the participants completed the low cognitive load tests followed by the high cognitive load tests, and the remaining participants completed the high cognitive load tests followed by the low cognitive load tests. Thus, participants acted as their own controls.

Quasiexperimental Research Design

There are many experimental situations in which it is not possible for the experimenter to assign subjects randomly to two groups. In such situations, he uses quasiexperimental designs. Quasiexperiments, like true experiments, involve the manipulation of an independent variable, that is, an intervention. However, quasiexperimental designs lack randomization to treatment groups, which characterizes true experiments.

1. ***Non-randomized control group pre-test/post-test design:*** The most frequently used quasiexperimental design is the nonequivalent control

group pre-test/post-test design, which involves an experimental treatment and two groups of subjects observed before and after its implementation.

Experimental group	Pre-test	Intervention	Post-test
Control group	Pre-test	No intervention	Post-test

(Two groups are not randomized)

Advantages

- The reactive effects of experimentation are more easily controlled
- It is easily conducted in many settings.

Limitation

- This design poses major threat to internal validity.

Example 10:

Yoo, Jeon and Kim (2013) conducted a study to determine the effects of a fall prevention program on falls, physical function, psychological function, and home environmental safety in frail elders living at home in rural communities. The design of this study was a nonequivalent control group pre posttest design. The study was conducted with 30 participants in the experimental group and 30 in the control group. The prevention program on falls consisted of laughter therapy, exercise, foot care and education. The program was provided once a week for 8 weeks and each session lasted 80 minutes. Results show that the risk score for falls and depression in the experimental group decreased significantly compared with scores for the control group. Compliance with prevention behavior related to falls, knowledge score on falls, safety scores of home environment, physical balance, muscle strength of lower extremities and self-efficacy for fall prevention significantly increased in the experimental group compared with the control group.

Example 11:

Lin (2013) conducted a study to explore the effectiveness of an anti-smoking program on urban aboriginals in Taiwan. A quasi-experimental study design with purposeful sampling was employed. A total of 125 aboriginal subjects were recruited from two local churches and they were divided into an experimental group (n = 64) and a control group (n = 61). Both took pre-tests in order to set baseline values, and only the experimental group participated for 3-weeks in the anti-smoking program classes. Both groups took post-tests immediately after the intervention in order to evaluate the immediate effects of the teaching program and a follow-up test was conducted four weeks after the intervention.

2. ***One group time series design:*** In this design, information is collected over an extended period and an intervention is introduced during that period. The researcher takes a number of measurements and exposes the group to the treatment and then again takes the post-interventional measurements.

   T1 T2 T3 T4 Treatment T5 T6 T7 T8

Advantage

- Multi-testing provides some checks on internal validity.

Limitations

- It fails to control the effects due to history
- Repeated testing may lead to some interaction effect.

Example 12:

Waller (2010) conducted a study using time series design to evaluate the effectiveness of an intervention program. People with advanced cancer and their caregivers completed bimonthly telephone interviews over a period of up to 18 months to assess unmet needs, anxiety and depression, quality of life, satisfaction with care and service utilization. The intervention, introduced after at least two baseline phone interviews, involved training medical, nursing and allied health professionals at each recruitment site on the use of the Palliative Care Needs Assessment Guidelines and the Needs Assessment Tool. Changes in outcomes were compared pre- and post-intervention.

3. ***Control group time series design:*** A time series nonequivalent control group design would involve collecting data over an extended period.

Experimental group	T1	T2	T3	T4	Treatment	T5	T6	T7	T8
Control group	T1	T2	T3	T4	No treatment	T5	T6	T7	T8

Advantage

- Control group enables comparison.

Limitations

- It fails to control the effects due to history
- Repeated testing may lead to some interaction effect.

Example 13:

Jang and Kim (2010) investigated the effects of breastfeeding education and support services on rate of breastfeeding three and six months after birth, and the effect on infant's growth (weight, height, BMI). The experimental group which had both education and support services was compared with the control group which had only breastfeeding education. This study was a quasiexperimental study with a time-series design. The participants were 39 mothers who were hospitalized for childbirth. Twenty mothers were assigned to the experimental group and 19 mothers, to the control group. The breastfeeding education was done during hospitalization, and support services were provided once a week after discharge for a month (a total 4 times) by a maternity ward nurse. Data regarding breastfeeding rate at one month after childbirth was collected by phone calls; the breastfeeding rates at three and six months after childbirth were collected in a visit to the families. The child's weight and height were also measured during the visit.

HISTORICAL DESIGN

The word 'History' is derived from the Greek word 'historia' meaning 'inquiry', knowledge acquired by investigation. History includes discovery, collection, organization and presentation of information about the past events. Scholars who write about history are called ***historians***. History is a meaningful and an organized record of the past events.

The historical method of investigations may be used to ascertain the meaning and reliability of past facts encountered in everyday life and in all disciplines. The main purpose of historical research is to arrive at an account of the past so as to gain a clearer perspective of the present.

The historical method is employed by researchers who are interested in reporting events and/or conditions that occurred in the past. It is the procedure supplementary to observation in which the researcher seeks to test the authenticity of the reports or observations made by others.

Importance of Historical Research in Nursing

- It helps us to understand how nursing has evolved
- It gives opportunity to look at events in the past
- It helps us to understand and interpret events happened in the past and appreciate it
- It gives meaning and texture to the care provided by the nurses
- It suggests the ways and recommends modification in the educational preparation of nurses
- It aids in comparison of the past, present and the future
- It helps in the development of nursing as a profession.

Traditions of Historical Research Method

The positivistic or neopositivistic historians take a more quantitative posture and their main focus is on reducing history to universal laws. They use data to verify information and they strongly exhibit cause-effect relationships.

The idealist historians are most concerned with getting inside an event while considering the time, place and situations and they are more closely aligned with the values of qualitative research.

Historical Research Methods

- ***Biographical history:*** It is the study of an individual and it uses the story of a person's life to understand the values, expectations, tensions and the conflicts of the time and culture within which he or she lived. A biographical history of Mahatma Gandhi is one such example.
- ***A social history:*** It explores a particular period and attempts to understand the prevailing values and beliefs by examining the everyday events of that period. It explores into the lives of people and provides a richer understanding of events.
- ***An intellectual history:*** It is the method of exploring the ideas of an individual considered to be an intellectual thinker of a period. For example, Florence Nightingale's thoughts and concepts on nursing have influenced the development of nursing education and practice.

Sources of Information for Historical Research

- Original documents
- Relics
- Remains
- Artifacts

- Textbooks
- Encyclopedias
- Newspapers and periodicals
- Review of research and other references.

Steps in Historical Research

- Formulating the problem.
- Collecting the source materials.
- Formulating hypotheses to explain events or conditions.
- Interpreting and reporting findings.

Formulating the Problem

Historical research begins when the past is questioned. When we review the material or record which explains something that happened in the past, that becomes the source for the research problem for the historical design. The historical design investigates the individuals, institutions, organizations, structures and processes.

Collecting the Source Materials

In order to collect data, the investigator goes deep into the relevant sources of the past. There are primary and secondary sources of data that the investigator reviews in order to collect information about the past. The researcher tries to obtain the best evidence from primary sources. This includes the witness to past events and the actual objects used in the past that could be directly examined. The primary sources form very vital evidence in historical studies. Though primary sources are important, secondary sources also provide information. Secondary sources are information given by a person other than the original witness. The secondary sources should be handled with care and bias. Some of the sources are:

- ***Official records:*** Administrative, legislative, policy and judicial documents prepared by the central, state and local governments, organizations, laws, charters and court proceedings and decisions, vital statistics, all provide information. Minutes of meetings, various committee reports, special directives, surveys, various records maintained by all organizations including hospitals provide information about the past.
  The information from the following sources are useful for the historian since it explains the culture, way of living and community life, civilization, language, hobbies, food habits, rituals, festivals, their faith, religious activity, etc.
- ***Personal records:*** Diaries, autobiographies, letters, wills, deeds, contracts, original drafts of speeches, etc. provide information about a person and organization.
- ***Oral traditions:*** Myths, folk tales, family stories, dances, games, ceremonies, reminiscences by eyewitnesses to events and recordings provide information about the culture, way of living and the community life.

- ***Pictorial records:*** Photographs, movies, microfilms, drawings, paintings, coins and sculpture.
- ***Published materials:*** Newspaper, pamphlet and periodicals, literary and philosophical works.
- ***Mechanical records:*** The recordings of interview and meetings, phonograph records of pupil's speech or reading efforts.

  Apart from the records, reports and words of others, the historian can actually view or handle objects of the past that have been preserved. These remains or relics which are handed down from the past without the specific intent of imparting facts or information constitute an unconscious testimony of incidents in the lives of the people.
- ***Physical remains:*** Buildings, facilities, furniture, equipment, awards and skeletal remains.
- ***Printed materials:*** Policy documents, newsletters, circulars, intimation letters, textbooks, contracts, attendance forms, report cards and newspaper advertisements.
- ***Handwritten materials:*** Manuscripts of the nurse leaders, nurses, heads of the institutions, local communications, pupil manuscripts, drawings and exercises.

Criticizing Source Materials

An investigator can subject the source materials to internal and external criticism in order to avoid bias.

- ***External criticism:*** It involves checking for the genuineness and integrity of the source material, such as originality, ownership, accuracy, publication details, etc. External criticism is concerned with establishing the time, place, and authorship of the document and restoring the original form and language employed by the author.
- ***Internal criticism:*** It is concerned with ascertaining the meaning and trustworthiness of the data within the document. It involves checking for the meaning, credibility of the content and to determine the intention of producing such document, the validity of the intellectual premises upon which the writer proceeded and the correct interpretation of the data.

  Researchers make many judgments while evaluating records and other sources. The principles of criticism according to Woody are worth studying.
- Do not judge the author ignorant of certain events because he failed to mention them in his records.
- Do not underestimate or overestimate a record.
- Read the documents of the same period for the information regarding an event, etc. Neither reading earlier document nor the later document is useful.
- Establish objectivity and confirm the accuracy by checking the various sources, such as witnesses documents, records, etc.

- Identical errors prove the dependence of sources on each other or a common source.
- If witnesses contradict each other on a certain point, one or the other may be true, but may be in error.
- Direct, competent, independent witnesses, who report the same central fact and also any peripheral matters in a casual way, may be accepted for the points of their agreement.
- Official testimony, oral or written, must be compared with unofficial testimony whenever possible, for neither one nor the other is alone sufficient.

Formulation of Hypotheses in Historical Study

Hypotheses in historical study provide the direction for the procedure of the study. Different types of hypotheses are used for a variety of purposes:

- Casual hypotheses provide a framework for the entire research.
- The hypotheses must be formulated based on the past events and are investigated that could be accepted or defended.
- The hypotheses can help to formulate conceptual and factual elements and relationships. The assumption made in relation to the study might influence the data collection which must be made visible to the readers.
- Quantitative methods could be used to make the vague qualitative findings clearer and more precise. Hence, probability statistics and other quantitative methods could be used in hypotheses testing in historical research.
- The hypotheses are tested based on the information pooled out of the sources and generalization and predictions are made. Historical methods are very useful in investigating the past. There are several impediments in data gathering and interpretation in historical studies when compared to other studies. A historian should bear this in mind when he conducts a historical research.

Interpreting and Reporting Findings

Once the data have been collected, the researcher interprets and reports the findings in the light of his problem. He should understand the events and establish the relationship with the facts collected. The report can be presented in the logical and chronological order. The facts should be written and organized by giving headings and side-headings. It should be clear, concise and should have clarity.

Advantages

- The research is not physically involved in the situation under study
- No danger of experimenter-subject interaction
- Documents are located by the researcher, data is gathered and conclusions are drawn out of sight

Example 14:

Immonen (2013) did a historical study using narratives, government documents and literature. The study focuses on challenges in nursing care that arose during the war because of war. Interviews with nurses and persons active in health care during World War II constitute the main data of the research. Thematic issues that arise from interviews are analyzed. Primary and secondary written sources are used in analyzing the topics. Because of war activities, deportation and burning of the county, archives were partly destroyed. Central archives can contribute with annual reports, whereas local archives are fragmentary. There are a number of reports written soon after the war, as well as a number of biographical books of newer date.

DESCRIPTIVE DESIGN

Descriptive research is also termed as 'normative research.' The aim of descriptive research is to design in such a way that it obtains precise information about a phenomena and also enables the researcher to draw general conclusion from the facts discovered.

They are conducted not only to fact-finding but may often result in the finding of the solution of significant problems concerning local, state, national and international issues. Descriptive studies are more than just a collection of data; they involve measurement, classification, analysis, comparison and interpretations. They collect and provide three types of information: (1) of what exists with respect to variables or conditions in a situation; (2) of what we want by identifying standards or norms with which to compare the present conditions or what experts consider to be desirable; and (3) of how to achieve goals by exploring possible ways and means on the basis of the experience of others or the opinion of experts.

Major Steps in Descriptive Studies

- Identifying and defining the problem
- Stating the objectives, hypotheses and assumptions
- Selection of subjects and source materials
- Selection or construction of tools for data collection
- Collection of data
- Describing, analyzing and interpreting the data in clear and precise terms
- Drawing significant and meaningful conclusions.

At times, descriptive researcher is not directed towards hypothesis testing. The researcher is merely interested in studying the situation that prevails and attempts no explanation of underlying reasons responsible for such events. It is conducted merely to provide information to assist in decision-making.

Nature of Descriptive Research

- This investigates the phenomena in their natural setting
- They constitute a primitive type of research and do not aspire to develop an organized body of scientific laws
- They provide information useful to the solution of the local problems

- Descriptive research differs from other types of research in purpose and scope
- The historical research deals with the past, whereas the descriptive research deals with the present
- The cause-effect relationships are difficult to establish in descriptive research
- It is less scientifically sophisticated when compared to the experimental research
- No variables are manipulated
- Descriptive studies involve events that have already taken place and are related to a present condition.

Types of Descriptive Studies

There are three types of descriptive studies. They are:

1. Survey studies
2. Interrelationship studies
3. Developmental studies

Survey

Survey is the technique of investigation through direct observation of a phenomena or systematic gathering of data from population. The survey is an important tool to gather evidence regarding certain social problems. Survey research is an organized attempt to analyze, interpret and report the present status of a social institution, group or area. The survey can be conducted by telephone, by mail and personal interview.

The survey method primarily focuses on the present. It is a non-experimental method where the investigator studies a community or a group of people for the purpose of examining the characteristics, opinion, and orientations of the population. Data may be gathered by asking questions, by interview, by observing as to what people are doing, thinking or feeling. Survey is the most appropriate method of gathering information from a large sample. Surveys may be descriptive and specify the properties of phenomena or they may be explanatory and specify interrelationships among variables.

Characteristics of Social Survey

- Surveys are concerned with widely dispersed group of people as against laboratory experiments.
- It is a form of planned collection of data for the purpose of description or prediction or for the purpose of analyzing relationships between certain variables.
- The facts collected in a social survey may form the basis of future social research. It may also form the basis of some hypothesis.
- Sample surveys are carried out to make assertion about the distribution of characteristics in a population.
- A social survey is confined to the study of specific current problems of society, e.g. poverty, unemployment and the purpose of the survey is to remove the social evils.

There are three main types of surveys. They are by telephone, by mail and by personal interview.

The varieties of survey research are as follows:

1. ***Considering surveys by purpose:***
   - ***Descriptive survey:*** The objective of the descriptive survey is description only. This does not mean that they cannot be the basis of extensive implications and actions.
   - ***Evaluative survey:*** It is descriptive but has the additional dimension of one or more criteria by which some evaluative judgement will be made about the respondents, either individually or as group.
   - ***Comparative survey:*** In this, the researcher wishes to obtain data to enable her to decide whether two or more entities are similar or different, again in terms of specific criteria.
   - ***Correlational survey:*** This survey collects data on more than one variable from the group of respondents with the intent of estimating the magnitude of the relationship between the variables.
   - ***General survey:*** The survey conducted for collecting general information about any desired population, institution or phenomena without any particular object or hypothesis is called a general survey. Surveys such as the census of the population are examples of general survey.
   - ***Specific survey:*** This survey is conducted to study specific problems for testing a certain theory or hypothesis.
2. ***Considering surveys by sample base:***
   - ***A.Mass survey:*** A survey which is intended to provide insight into a large population or universe, and which accomplishes this by obtaining data from the entire population or from a sample, carefully selected to represent that population.
   - ***B.Case study:*** A survey based on a sample of one or a few. Given the small sample base, the case study substitutes depth for broad coverage.
3. ***Considering surveys by orientation in time:***
   - ***A.Cross-sectional survey:*** In this, the elements of the survey currently at different points of progress are surveyed at the same point in time and assumed to represent the different points in time or may be employed to study associations between different diseases, but they cannot often determine which disease might have occured first.
   - ***B.Longitudinal surveys:*** These collects data from the same people at different points in time. The major strength of the longitudinal design is that it avoids the assumption of comparability of different groups by using the same respondents at every data collection interval.

Steps in Survey Research

- Planning a survey
  - Identification of the problem
  - Statement of objectives
  - Reviewing of literature

- ❐ Preparation of work schedule and budget
- ❐ Identifying the population, methods and materials
- ❐ Selection, training and supervision of field investigators
- Piloting the research
- Data collection
- Analysis and reporting.

Advantages

- The greater strength of survey research is its flexibility and capacity to meet broad ranges of research needs.
- The amount of information obtained in surveys is quite large.
- It brings the researcher to come face-to-face with the realities of life and see things personally.
- The researcher can observe the activities of the group under study.
- Surveys facilitate the formulation of policy.
- It is useful in testing the validity of many theories.
- It permits greater objectivity, since the data are not influenced by any one man's view or beliefs. The use of large number of field workers removes the possibilities of personal bias.
- It aids in fomulation of hypotheses. It helps in generation of new hypothesis that may be completely outside the scope of the existing theory and may also lead to the new theory.

Disadvantages

- It is expensive, time-consuming and wasteful
- Information obtained in surveys tends to be superficial
- Offers little evidence to support cause-effect relationship
- The survey method lacks flexibility. Any change in research design may mean conducting the fresh survey
- ***Bias:*** The prejudices and the desire of the investigators become unconsciously woven into the fabric of conclusions
- Under survey method, it is very difficult to verify the accuracy of the data collected because it is dependent on honesty, sincerity, personal qualities and unbiased attitude of the numerators and cooperation of the respondents
- If sample surveys are not conducted properly, the results may not be applicable
- There is nonresponse error which occurs when the samples fail to respond.

Interrelationship Studies

Research studies that help to establish relationships between facts that will provide a deeper insight into the phenomena are termed as ***interrelationship studies***. Casual comparative studies, correlation, prediction studies and cross-cultural and comparative studies are examples of interrelationship studies.

Casual Comparative Studies

Sometimes, research studies are conducted to discover not only what a phenomena is like, but, if possible, how and why it occurs. In these studies, the likenesses and differences are compared among phenomena to identify and explore what factors or circumstances contribute to the occurrence of certain events, conditions or practices. Casual comparative studies are employed when a researcher cannot manipulate the independent variable and establish the controls that are required in experiments. In experimental studies, especially in laboratory settings, an investigator controls all variables except the independent variable or the variable which he wants to manipulate and see the outcome. But in social context, one cannot control all the variables which can affect the independent variable and also it may not be possible to manipulate the independent variable. In such cases, casual comparative studies are conducted. The investigator selects the samples according to the criterion, that is, samples with some specific phenomena or characteristics and compares with that of samples who do not possess the same characteristics or phenomena. By doing this, the researcher concludes the likeness and the differences between these groups and can identify what lead them to possess or what factors contributed to develop certain characteristics or experience the phenomena. In these conditions, the researcher need not to manipulate anything in order to identify the factors. These methods are useful when experimental method is impractical or costly in time, money and effort. The limitations of these studies are: (1) lack of control; (2) difficulty in identifying the relevant factors causing a particular condition or phenomenon; (3) difficulty in identifying which is the cause and which is the effect; and (4) problems in selection of samples and dividing them into two groups.

Correlation Studies

Correlation studies are conducted to find out the nature and degree of relationship between the phenomena. Correlation refers to any kind of relationship between variables or phenomena; but in statistical analysis, it refers exclusively to quantifying the magnitude of the relationship between variables. Correlation techniques enable the investigator to ascertain the degree and the direction of the relationship between variables. The direction of the relationship may be negative or positive; the degree of the relationship varies from –1 to +1 and the relationship may be linear or nonlinear. In general, the magnitude of the correlation depends on the extent to which an increase or decrease in one variable is accompanied by an increase or decrease in the other. It is relatively easy to design and conduct. It involves the measurement of two variables and computing the correlation coefficient between these two. The computation states the nature and degree of relationship. Multiple correlation is used when the researcher is interested in determining the relationship between one independent variable and two or more dependent variables. The findings are interpreted based on the correlation coefficient values. Any value nearer +1 indicates positive strong correlation; –1 indicates negative but strong correlation and any value near 0 indicates weak correlation. Besides this, one must see the statistical significance of the magnitude of the relationship in order to draw inference about the population from which the samples are selected. The statistical significance conveys that the relationship does not occur by chance. Sometimes, the coefficient of correlation may be low in magnitude and yet statistically significant.

Prediction Studies

Correlation studies are particularly useful in making predictions. Researchers may conduct psychological, sociological or economic prediction studies. For example, the scores obtained by the students on certain tests may be used to predict how successful the students will be in particular subjects, curricula or fields of specialization. It is possible to predict one variable from the other if we know that there is substantial correlation between two variables.

Cross-cultural and Comparative Studies

These studies are conducted to compare the number of societies or communities or groups of people in terms of their cultural behaviors, practices, norms, values, traditions and folklores. This is to determine the behaviors whether they are cultural-specific or common behavior.

Developmental Studies

These studies are concerned, besides exploring the existing status and interrelationships of phenomena, with changes that take place as a function of time. These include growth studies and trend studies. Both longitudinal and cross-sectional techniques can be adopted to collect data and analyzed to identify trends and make predictions. Longitudinal studies follow the same subject, a group of subjects or an institution over a long period of time. It is a kind of extended case study which involves multiple data collection.

The limitations of the longitudinal studies are:

- Time-consuming
- Difficult to select the samples representative of the population
- Development of bias due to contact with the sample over a period of time
- Difficulty in collecting data from the mobile groups
- Problems related to drop-out
- Cannot make improvement in the tool after the study has been started
- Requirement of extensive facilities, money, preservation of material and personnel.

Because of these limitations, these studies are not conducted by the individuals and are conducted by the organizations as a project. Many of the limitations can be overcome by conducting the cross-sectional studies. This involves collection of data at one point of time from the samples; the phenomena under study are captured during one period of data collection.

Cross-sectional studies are appropriate for describing the status of phenomena or for describing relationships among phenomena at a fixed point in time.

Cohort studies are a particular kind of trend study in which specific subpopulation are examined over time. The samples are usually drawn from specific age-related subgroups. In panel studies, the same people are used to supply data at two or more points in time. The term 'panel' refers to the sample of subjects providing data. Follow-up studies are similar to panel studies, but are usually undertaken to determine the subsequent development of individuals, who have a specified condition or who have received a specified intervention.

Example 15:

Prathima (2013) conducted a study to assess the caregivers' perception on emotional problems in children living with HIV/AIDS. In this, she has selected caregivers of HIV infected children aged 4-16 years. The strength and difficulties questionnaire elicited information on emotional symptoms.

Example 16:

Sundaram and Siddegowda (2013) conducted a cross sectional survey to assess major correlates of language and cognitive development of toddlers. In this survery, the researcher used multistage cluster random sampling technique. All the taluks of rural and urban districts were included for the study. Three villages were selected randomly from each taluk in Bengluru rural district and then hundred households were randomly selected from each village. Similarly, three urban cities were selected from each urban district and then 100 households were selected from each urban city. From these households, those who met inclusion criteria were selected Atleast one of the parents along with their children aged one to three years were participated in the study. Parenting style questionnaire, the infant/toddler home inventory, were used language and cognitive development of the toddlers were assessed.

Example 17:

Sudha and Shekhar (2013) conducted a study to find the correlation between the duration, frequency and favorite video game with the selected physiological variables, such as pulse, respiration, height and weight. 100 samples who met the inclusion criteria were selected using purposive sampling technique. Data on violent video game playing and their physiological variables were assessed.

QUALITATIVE RESEARCH DESIGNS

Tradition of science is uniquely quantitative. The measurements of speed, velocity, weight, mass, volume, etc. are quantitative in nature. Quantitative approach to research aims at measuring, analyzing, replicating and applying gained knowledge. There are certain phenomena which cannot be quantified. The inability to quantitatively measure some phenomena, like values, culture and relationships has led to an emergence of using qualitative research approaches. The tradition of using qualitative studies has been grounded in social sciences, which arose because certain aspects of human values, culture and relationships were unable to be described fully using quantitative research methods. One can understand that the human phenomena/experience cannot be measured and could be understood. The core of nursing is the patient, the individual human being who has to be understood in order to provide better nursing care. The emergence of holistic care demands the nurses to understand the patient in all his dimensions. The changing concept of care from healing to promotion of health of the individual under care requires the nurse to apply the qualitative concepts and use qualitative research approaches to answer the questions of clinical significance. Health care professionals including nurses want to understand the lived-in experience of their clients, to enter into the world of their clients and to understand the basic social processes that lead to health and illness in a human being. Qualitative research is a field of inquiry that crosscuts disciplines and subject matters. Qualitative researchers aim to gather an in-depth understanding of human behavior and the reasons that govern such behavior and also aims to see the world through the eyes of the subjects. The discipline investigates the 'why and how' of decision-making, not just 'what, where and when'. It is concerned with the generation and not testing of hypothesis.

Meaning and Definition of Qualitative Research

Qualitative research designs are any kind of research that produces findings not arrived at by means of statistical procedures or other means of quantification. (Strauss and Corbin, 1990). Qualitative research seeks to understand research problem from perspectives of the people being studied. It is effective in obtaining culturally specific information about values, opinions, behaviors and social contexts of particular populations. Qualitative researchers do not use controlled experimental designs and are flexible. Exploration unfolds and emerges as the field work progresses. Qualitative research involves in finding out what people think and how they feel. It includes feelings and impressions rather than numbers. This kind of information is subjective.

Characteristics of Qualitative Research

- A belief in multiple realities
- Commitment to understanding the phenomena
- Commitment to understanding the research problem from perspectives of the people being studied.
- Emphasis on providing 'holistic' understanding of phenomena
- Relies on a research strategy which is flexible and interactive
- Research is conducted at the natural setting
- No manipulation of variables
- Participants' viewpoint is the prime factor
- Involves respondents as active participants
- Conduction of inquiry aiming at knowing the natural content of the phenomena
- Participation of the researcher in the research process

- Reporting of data in a rich literary style
- No prior conclusion is formed
- No assumption/hypothesis is formulated
- Researcher is the instrument in the research process.

Research Problem in Qualitative Research

In general, qualitative research is conducted when little is known about an area or existing understanding appears inadequate. The approach is used when we want to construct a theory or theoretical framework. This approach helps in making sense of complex situations. The research problem in qualitative research may be oriented towards describing actual behaviors of the individual or eliciting people's beliefs and attitudes.

Hypotheses in Qualitative Research

Researchers usually refrain from formulating hypothesis in a qualitative research since they use an inductive mode of inquiry. At the beginning of data collection, general research questions are typically asked and as they proceed further, more specific questions usually emerge. In qualitative research, data collection and analysis proceeds simultaneously. Hence, the research questions are reframed or modified or 'at times' deleted. The objective of this process is the emergence of a comprehensive, accurate description of the phenomena being investigated from the perspective of those who experience it.

Selection of Participants

- Samples are termed as participants, not subjects
- Participants have active involvement
- They are selected on the basis of first-hand experience with a culture, social process or phenomena of interest
- Purposeful sampling is only used
- Sample size is based on saturation.

Data Collection

The chief data collection devices are observation, interview, narrative and focused groups, using chat rooms, using participant observations, field visits, artifact (i.e. records, documents, etc.), oral histories and specimen records (behavior recorded through observation). Qualitative research data records are typically quite massive. Also, the qualitative researcher is advised to keep fairly detailed records of his or her thoughts, feelings, and behaviors while the data are collected. It is important to determine whether or not the researcher himself or herself a source of bias. These notes also contain changes in the work design and research questions or hypotheses.

In-depth interview means purposeful fact to face interactions between two people focused on one person trying to get information from the other person. It permits the exploration and probing of participants' thoughts to get more in-depth information. It helps in collecting information on sensitive issues. In-depth interview has its own disadvantages. It is time-consuming and expensive. It relies soley on verbal statements which are subject to distortions. While an interview being in progress, a researcher can take notes which is very cumbersome or else he can write it immediately after the interview, which can lead to loss of information. Audio or video recording can be done, which is the preferred method of data collection. An interview guide facilitates data collection. Construction of probes helps in collection of in-depth information. Probes are devices used to prompt a respondent to speak further when an initial question fails to elicit the information. It helps the participant elaborate the information. Informed consent should be obtained from the participants before beginning data collection.

Focus Group Discussion

Focus group discussion is another method of eliciting information from the participant in qualitative research. It is a carefully planned discussion designed to obtain perceptions on a defined area of interest in a non-threatening environment. It is an interview conducted by a trained moderator in a non-structured and natural manner with a small group of respondents. For this, a group of 6–12 people with similar characteristics are gathered to discuss a focused topic of interest. A moderator guides the discussion. A note-taker records the nonverbal aspects of the group. Tape recorded notes are combined with the nonverbal notes and transcribed for analysis.

It helps in obtaining a range of perceptions, opinions or beliefs about an issue and to explore controversial topics. The data collected from this helps in generating hypotheses for further research. The advantages of focused group discussion are many. It is cost-effective. Quality data can be collected. Focus group tends to be enjoyable to participants.

The disadvantages are—the number of questions are restricted; time-consuming; sensitive and highly personal topics cannot be explored; and confidentiality cannot be assured.

Achieving Saturation

It refers to the repetition of discovered information and confirmation of previously collected data. This means saturation of information and not the participants, e.g. saturation can be achieved at the end of 10 interviews or even 20 interviews.

In a qualitative research, phenomena are viewed in its entirety or holistically. It is not possible to reduce complex phenomena into a few interdependent or independent factors. The researcher's role is to record what he or she observes and/or collects from subjects' in their natural environment. Research is done in natural settings and variables are not manipulated. 'Reality' exists as the subjects see it. The researcher is to record fully, accurately and unbiasedly, that reality as seen through the eyes of the subjects. Any prior conclusions are avoided since conclusions emerge from the data.

Data Analysis and Interpretation

Qualitative analysis transforms data into findings. No formula exists for that transformation. It involves the search for patterns and ideas in data that explain why those patterns are there in the first place. Data analysis and collection are iterative. Data must be organized and reduced (data classification and reduction).

Reading is the first step in the qualitative data analysis. It involves in-depth reading of all notes and transcripts and developing relationship with the data by immersing into it.

The next step is the coding. Data are organized by coding. Descriptions of behavior, statements, feelings, thoughts, etc. are identified and coded. Code is a word or short phrase that symbolically assigns a summative essence for a text of the raw data. Coding is not a precise science. It is an interpretive act. It begins after becoming familiar with the data. Coding helps in identification of key themes and patterns within the data.

A researcher can use a deductive or inductive approach to coding. Deductive approach uses categories constructed from theory in order to develop a coding framework. Inductive approach selects code from the data collected using various methods.

Wiersma (1995) identified three types of codes:

1. ***Setting or context codes:*** These codes describe the setting or context descriptors of the phenomenon under study. Given that copious field notes are taken, codes for specific or regularly occurring characteristics contribute to efficient and effective field note production.
2. ***Perception codes:*** These codes are used to accurately record subjects' reported perception, understanding, etc. about relevant people, circumstances, or things.
3. ***Process codes:*** These codes are used to note event or process evolution and factors which cause or contribute to the said evolution.

The specific coding system employed by a researcher usually emerges as the iterative data analysis and interpretative process unfolds. Coding begins after becoming familiar with the data. The coding system employed by the qualitative researcher should be: (1) comprehensive and tailored to his or her needs; (2) accurate in recording what is being observed or reported; and (3) useful in describing and enabling understanding of the phenomenon under study. The coding process involves the creation of codes and categories and from these themes/concepts and theories.

Trustworthiness of Qualitative Research

- Credibility
- Dependability
- Conformability
- Transferability
- The answers to the below mentioned questions will help us to understand the trustworthiness of qualitative research.
- Was data collection systematic? Adequate?
- Is reference made to accepted procedures for analysis?
- Was a systematic inductive approach used?

- Is there adequate discussion of how the themes, concepts and categories were derived from the data?
- Are the researcher's conceptualisations true to the data?
- Are findings presented within a context?
- Is the reader able to apprehend the essence of the experience from the report of findings?
- Is the credibility of the findings addressed?
- Do the conclusions reflect study findings?

Perspectives for Designing the Qualitative Study

- ***Funnel Approach:*** In the working design phase, the researcher has a very general research question or hypothesis which is used to select the initial research site, subjects, data to be collected, etc. Based on results generated from the earlier initiative, the research question or hypothesis becomes increasingly focused. This process is repeated until data collection, analysis, and interpretation focus exclusively on the phenomena under study and produces 'solid' conclusions.
- ***Modified Analytic Induction Approach:*** According to Wiersma (1995), in this approach, the researcher starts with specific research question(s); identifies virtually all instances (or cases) of the phenomenon under investigation; and investigates each case, employing an iterative process, where the research question or phenomenon explanation is revised until he or she arrives at a suitable comprehensive, descriptively rich narrative.

Establishing a Qualitative Study's Validity

Internal validity (i.e. the design integrity of the study) relies on logical analysis; it is virtually impossible to control variables in 'natural' settings. Thus, it is essential that full descriptions of the research site and subjects, data collection devices and procedures, etc. be presented. Two strategies for arguing for internal validity include interpretive validity and trustworthiness.

- ***Interpretive validity:*** It is the degree to which data interpretation and conclusions are considered accurate so as to be reflective of the subjects' or phenomenon's 'reality'. There are four dimensions to interpretive validity. The greater the degree of acceptance by other researchers, the more valid the original researcher's interpretation is perceived (Altheide and Johnson, 1994).
- ***Usefulness:*** Usefulness is determined by the extent the report informs and stimulates further research.
- ***Contextual completeness:*** This refers to the fullness and richness of the description (usually in narrative form) of the report.
- ***Research positioning:*** Qualitative researchers have been referred to as data collection devices, given the centrality of the researcher in qualitative strategies. Thus, the researcher must document his, her, or their direct and indirect effects on the research site(s), participants, etc.

- ***Reporting style:*** This refers to the extent the research report by authors' description is perceived as authentic.
- ***Trustworthiness:*** A study's 'trustworthiness' is increased when data analysis and conclusions are triangulated; subjects' perceptions are verified in a systematic manner; and the project's data chain of evidence is established (Gall, Borg and Gall, 1996).
- ***Triangulation:*** The use of multiple data collection devices, sources, analysts, etc. to establish the validity of findings. Data, method and theoretical triangulation are used.
- ***Member checking:*** Research participants should review findings for accuracy and representativeness.
- ***Chain of evidence:*** The logical relationship between research questions, research procedures, raw data, and results should be such that a reasonably prudent person would arrive at the same or similar conclusions. Five strategies for establishing the data's chain of evidence are:
    1. ***Outlier analysis:*** Highly dissimilar cases should be examined and differences explained. This will contribute to strengthening the findings' integrity.
    2. ***Pattern matching:*** It is comparing two patterns to determine whether they match or do not match. If such are matched, then the argument for 'trustworthiness' is enhanced.
    3. ***Representativeness check:*** This strategy is akin to monitoring used in survey research. An interview or artifact is reviewed to assess its representativeness as compared to other similar interviews or artifacts.
    4. ***Long-term involvement:*** This is similar to trend analysis. If data are collected over the long-term, then situation-specific influences are 'canceled' out.
    5. ***Coding check:*** Here multiple researchers code the data and check for differences. Those differences are then resolved. A high level of agreement between coders is very desirable.

Qualitative Reliability and Generalizability

Where possible, it is wise to use multiple observers and 'run' inter-rater reliability coefficients, if standard rating forms were used. Establish fully developed procedures for resolving disagreements among raters. Documents that present findings which are consistent with those of other investigators conducting similar research establishes the reliability. Draw on the procedures for establishing a study's trustworthiness.

The qualitative researcher does not share the same level of concern for generalizability as does the quantitative researcher. Qualitative external validity concerns itself with comparability (i.e. the ability of other researchers to extend knowledge based on the 'richness and depth' of the description) and translatability (i.e. the extent to which other researchers understand the results, given the theory and procedures underlying the study.

Characteristics of Qualitative Design

- Asks why, how and under what circumstances things occur.
- Seeks depth of understanding
- Provides insights into meanings of decisions and actions
- Often has triangulation
- Flexible and elastic
- Tends to be holistic
- Intense researcher involvement
- Researcher is the research instrument
- Requires ongoing analysis of the data to formulate subsequent strategies
- Uses interpretive and open-ended methods
- Involves respondents as active participants.

Approaches to Qualitative Research

Table 5.3 explains the difference between the qualitative and quantitative research.

- ***Ethnographic research*** is used for investigating cultures by collecting and describing data that is intended to help in the development of a theory. This method is also called ***ethnomethodology*** or ***methodology of the people***. An example of applied ethnographic research is the study of a particular culture and their understanding of the role of a particular disease in their cultural framework.
- ***Critical social research*** is used by a researcher to understand how people communicate and develop symbolic meanings. Ethical inquiry is an intellectual analysis of ethical problems. It includes the study of ethics as related to obligation, rights, duty, right and wrong, choice, etc.
- ***Foundational research*** examines the foundations for a science, analyzes the beliefs and develops ways to specify how a knowledge base should change in light of new information.
- ***Historical research*** allows one to discuss past and present events in the context of the present condition, and allows one to reflect and provide possible answers to current issues and problems. Historical research helps us in answering questions, such as: Where have we come from, where are we, who are we now, and where are we going?
- ***Grounded theory*** is an inductive type of research, based or 'grounded' in the observations or data from which it was developed. It uses a variety of data sources, including quantitative data, review of records, interviews, observation and surveys.
- ***Phenomenological research*** describes the 'subjective reality' of an event, as perceived by the study population. It is the study of a phenomenon.
- ***Philosophical research*** is conducted by field experts within the boundaries of a specific field of study or profession. The best qualified individual in any field of study to use an intellectual analysis, in order to clarify definitions, identify ethics, or make a value judgment concerning an issue in their field of study.

Table 5.3: Difference between quantitative and qualitative research

S. No.	Quantitative research	Qualitative research
1.	Objective	Subjective
2.	'Hard science'	'Soft science'
3.	One reality	Multiple realities
4.	Mechanistic	Organismic
5.	Literature review must be done early in study	Literature review may be done as study progresses or afterward
6.	Seeks to confirm hypothesis	Seeks to explore phenomena
7.	Hypotheses	Research questions
8.	Focus is concise and narrow	Focus is complex and broad
9.	Parts are equal to whole	Whole is greater than parts
10.	Researcher is separate	Researcher is a part of the process
11.	Subjects	Participant
12.	Context-free	Contextual
13.	Highly structured	Semistructured or unstructured
14.	Study design is fixed	Study design is flexible
15.	Descriptive, correlational and experimental designs	Phenomenological, grounded theory, ethnographic study, philosophical and case study
16.	Measurable	Interpretive
17.	Uses instruments	Uses communication and observation
18.	Reports statistical analysis	Report is narrative
19.	Data is numerical	Data is textual
20.	Basic element of analysis is numbers	Basic element of analysis is words/ideas
21.	Reduction-control-prediction	Discovery-description-understanding
22.	Reports on established and predetermined methods	Reports on literary style
23.	Tries to infer for the population.	Describes individual experiences and group norms.
24.	Strives for generalization	Strives for uniqueness

Steps in Planning Qualitative Design

- Select broad framework or tradition to guide a certain decision
- Identify potential study collaborators

- Develop a broad data collection strategy
- Select a site
- Identify any 'gatekeepers'
- Collect written or photographic information about site
- Determine the maximum amount of time available for study
- Identify the types of equipment needed
- Determine the number and type of research assistants
- Arrange for training the assistants
- Identify appropriate informed consent procedures and other procedures requiring ethical consideration
- Develop plans for assessing the trustworthiness of data.

Grounded Theory

Grounded theory is an inductive process used to generate theory from the individual level, which could then be generalized and applied to nursing practice. Grounded theory method was discovered by two sociologists in 1067, Dr Berney Glaser and Dr Anselm Strauss. Grounded theory method is heavily indebted to the discipline of sociology and draws on the 'field research' approach to the discovery of new knowledge. Field research is conducted in naturalistic settings, such as hospitals, outpatient clinics, and nursing homes. The basic assumption is that theories about people's actions or experience can be discovered by observing and interacting with the social group, rather than theorizing from the outside.

Grounded theory is a qualitative research approach used to explore the social processes that present within human interactions (Speziale and Carpenter, 2007). Grounded theory method is an inductive approach involving a systematic set of procedures to arrive at theory about basic social processes. Grounded theory method is typically used to identify the 'patterns of action and interaction between and among various types of social units'. (Denzin and Lincoln, 1998).

The aim of grounded theory is to discover underlying social forces that shape human behavior. This method is used to construct theory where no theory exists or in situations where existing theory fails to explain a set of circumstances. The main purpose of using grounded theory method is to explore social processes with the goal of developing theory.

Research questions are formulated to address issues of basic social process. Research question should have a scope of obtaining in-depth explanation of the phenomenon leading to theory development. The researcher brings some knowledge of the literature to the study and not an exhaustive review of literature. This allows theory to emerge directly from data. Theory remains connected to or 'grounded in' the data. Sample selection involves choosing participants who are experiencing the circumstance and selecting events and incidents related to the social process under investigation. Data are collected through interviews and through skilled observations of individuals interacting in a social setting. Interviews are audio-taped and then transcribed, and observations are recorded as field notes. Open-ended questions are used initially to identify concepts for further focus.

Data collection and analysis occur simultaneously in the grounded theory. It requires systematic, detailed record-keeping using field notes and transcribed interview tapes. Data is collected using various methods, such as interviews, observations, documents or from a combination of these sources. Daily journals, participant observation, formal or semistructured interviews facilitate data collection. As the researcher collects data through interviews, participant observation, field notes and so forth, coding begins. Coding entails line-by-line examination of the data to identify concepts and conceptualize underlying patterns. This type of close analysis of the data is called open-coding and results in many theoretical codes. The code can be a word or phrase taken directly from the data, which is called an 'in vivo' code. Constant comparison is done. Data that represent the similar facets of the same concept are grouped together. Glaser introduced memos as free-form and hand-written. Memos should contain heading, dates include short quotes and references.

Hunches about emerging patterns in the data are noted in memos, and the researcher directs activities in the field of pursuing these hunches. This technique, called theoretical sampling, is used to select experiences that will help the researcher to test ideas and gather complete information about developing concepts. The initial analytical process is called open coding (Strauss, 1987). Data are examined carefully line by line, broken down into discrete parts, and compared for similarities and differences (strauss and Corbin, 1990). Data are compared with other data continuously as they are acquired during research. This is a process called the constant comparative method. Codes in the data are clustered to form categories, which are then expanded and developed or collapsed into one another. Theory is constructed through this systematic process. As a result, data collection, analysis, and theory generation have a direct reciprocal relationship (Charmaz, 2000; Strauss and Corbin, 1990).

- ***Open coding:*** As the initial coding effort, data are deconstructed into the simplest form possible, examined for commonalities and sorted into categories.
- ***Axial coding:*** As the intermediate step, data are reassembled based on logical connections between categories.
- ***Selective coding:*** At this third stage of coding, the 'core' category is determined and the relationships between it and secondary categories are posited. Core and secondary category relationships are later validated. Categories needing further refinement or development are completed.

Two or more related categories (or concepts) give rise to a theory (McMillan and Schumacher, 1993), which is referred to as a proposition (Strauss and

Corbin, 1990). Since several conceptual relationships (i.e. concepts) are required to define a theory, such theories are said to be conceptually dense.

- ***Communicating findings:*** Strauss and Corbin (1990) write that to achieve 'integration', the core category (or concept) is presented as a story line which becomes the lens through which all other categories are examined. The relationships are compared to the data for validation, refinement, or discard.

  Related literature, both technical and nontechnical, is reviewed continuously through data collection and analysis. All literature is treated as data and is compared with the researcher's developing theory as it progresses.

  Grounded theory studies are reported in sufficient detail to provide the reader with the steps in the process and the logic of the method. Reports use descriptive language and diagrams of the process to ensure that the theory reported in the findings remains connected to the data.

Case Study

Case study is about studying the peculiarities and the commonalities of a specific case. In case study, the researcher explores in-depth a program, an event, an activity, a process, or one or more individuals. The cases are bounded by time and activity, and researchers collect detailed information using a variety of data collection procedure over a sustained period of time (Stake, 2000).

Purpose

- Gaining insight into little known problem
- Providing background data for the planning of broader studies
- Developing explanations of social-psychological and social-structural processes
- Offering rich descriptive anecdotes or examples to illustrate generalized statistical findings.

Identifying the Phenomenon

Case studies are constructed to richly describe, explain, or assess and evaluate a phenomenon, e.g. event, person, program, etc. (Gall, Borg, and Gall, 1996). The 'case' is studied onsite within its natural context. The data-gathering process is often interactive as the researcher or researchers associate with persons involved in the 'case' under study. By a single case, designating a focus on an individual, a family, a community, an organization-some complex phenomenon that demands close scrutiny for understanding.

The research question for case study is one that provokes the curiosity of the researcher. Research questions should be developed around issues that serve as a foundation to uncover complexity and pursue understanding.

The researcher uses an interactive process of 'growing questions' in the field, i.e. as data are collected to address these questions. So, research questions evolve over time and recreate themselves in case study research.

When the researcher begins with questions developed around suspected issues of importance, the perspective of the researcher is reflected in the questions, i.e. an etic perspective. As the researcher begins engaging the phenomenon of interest, the story unfolds and leads the way, shifting from an etic (researcher) to an emic (story) perspective (Stake, 2000).

Sample Selection

This is one of the areas where scholars in the field present different views, ranging from only choosing the most common cases to only choosing the most unusual cases.

Data Collection

Data is collected primarily by fieldwork, but secondary data collection is usually employed as well. It is important that the researcher(s) understand the phenomenon from the perspective of the participants. Data are gathered using interview, observation, document review and other methods that enable understanding of the complexity of the case.

Data analysis/describing findings: Data analysis is closely tied to data gathering and description of findings as the case study story is generated. Gall et al (1996) outlined three approaches to case data analysis:

1. ***Interpretational analysis:*** When employing this strategy, the researcher is looking for patterns (threads, constructs, commonalities, etc.) within the data to explain the phenomenon.
2. ***Structural analysis:*** Investigating patterns which may be found in conversations, text, activities, etc. with little or no explication as to pattern meaning.
3. ***Reflective analysis:*** The description and evaluation of the studied phenomenon based on judgment and intuition by a highly qualified expert.

The case narrative richly and fully reports the subject's perceptions about the phenomenon being investigated (Leedy, 1997).

Advantages of Case Study

- Stimulates insight
- Suggests directions for future research
- Provides information that is rich
- Well-suited for studying a process over time.

Disadvantages of Case Study

- Problems with generalizability
- Investigators have no guidelines to help them decide whether they have collected enough data because case studies are based on interviews and observations
- Researcher's bias
- Not adequate for testing casual hypothesis
- Unsuited for scientific cause and effect.

Example 18:

Gayathri, Kumar and Ramakrishnan (2013) conducted a case study on a nine-year-old girl studying 4th standard. She belonged to upper middle class family and was born after 8 years of marital life of her parents after infertility treatment. Born in full-term normal delivery, she had birth cry and her mother denied any problem in milestone development. The father spent only 3 months with the child after her birth and went to abroad for a job. The mother stayed with the child for one year and 3 months and she joined her husband. The child was left under the care of maternal grandparents. The child received priority and grew with lot of attention. The mother visited the child once in three years. She was average in her studies and had scholastic backwardness. She developed adjustment problems with the peer group since she was not given special recognition in the school. When the mother visited the child, she took the child to the hospital for counseling. She had problems, such as school refusal, crying spells, decreased communication with others, sad mood, irritability, sleep disturbances, feeling of helplessness and hopelessness. In the hospital, she was treated with antidepressants and cognitive behavior therapy session was conducted. At the end of the therapy, the patient was symptom-free, vulnerability factors solved in the child's life. The therapist educated the child and mother regarding relapse prevention at the termination of the therapy.

Ethnography

The word ***ethnography***, is derived from the Greek word 'ethnos' meaning 'folk, people, nation' and 'grapho' means 'I write'. An ethnography means to represent graphically and in writing, the culture of a group. The word 'ethnography' means portrait of people. According to Spradley (1980), 'Ethnography is the work of describing culture'. It is factual description and analysis of aspects of the way of life of a particular culture or subcultural group. The outcome of the ethnographic research/report reflects the knowledge and the system of meanings in the lives of a cultural group. Ethnographic researcher collects empirical data on human societies and cultures.

Ethnography is the study of social interactions, behaviors and perceptions that occur within groups, teams, organizations and communities. Great emphasis is given to the relationship between culture and behavior since it involves the description and interpretation of cultural behavior. Ethnography is the process by which the ethnographer inevitably comes to understand a culture. It is a branch of human inquiry associated with the field of anthropology that focuses on the culture of a group of people with an effort to understand the worldview of those under study.

Aim

The central aim of ethnography is to provide rich, holistic insights into people's views and actions, as well as the nature (that is, sights, sounds) of the location they inhabit, through the collection of detailed observations and interviews. As Hammersley states, 'the task of ethnographers is to document the culture, the perspectives and practices of the people in these settings. The aim is to 'get inside' the way each group of people sees the world.' It aims to get at the implicit as well as explicit aspect of culture. By ethnography, they learn the meaning they attach to activities related to events, behaviors, knowledge, artifacts, rituals, lifestyle, values, belief system, language, norms, economics and patterns of social interactions. It attempts to learn from members of a cultural group to understand their worldview as they perceive and live it. In order to understand, the ethnographers use the emic and etic perspectives. An emic perspective refers to the way the members of the culture envision their world. It is the insiders' view. The emic aspect is the local language, concepts or meanings of the group under study to name and characterize their experiences. An etic perspective refers to the outsiders' interpretation of the experiences of that culture. It is the language used by those doing the research to refer to the same phenomena.

Approaches

There are two ethnographic approaches. They are macroethnography and microethnography. ***Macroethnography*** deals with the broadly defined culture whereas ***microethnography*** deals with the narrowly defined exhaustive, fine-grained studies of either small units in a group or culture (e.g. culture of hostellers).

Classification

- Classical ethnography deals with description and demonstration of behavior, why and under what circumstances the behavior took place
- Systematic ethnography defines the structure of culture
- Interpretive or hermeneutic ethnography discovers the meaning of observed social interactions
- Critical ethnography focuses on issues of injustice and social oppression.

Characteristics

- Ethnography is a holistic approach to the study of cultural systems
- It is the study of the sociocultural contexts, processes and meanings within cultural systems
- It is the study of cultural systems from both emic and etic perspectives and cultural immersion is mandatory
- It is a process of discovery, making inferences, and continuing inquiries in an attempt to achieve emic validity
- It is an interative process of learning episodes
- It is an open-ended emergent learning process and not a rigid investigator-controlled experiment
- It is a highly flexible and creative process
- It is an interpretive, reflexive and constructivist process
- It requires the daily and continuous recording of fieldnotes during the fieldwork
- It presents the world of its host population in human contexts
- It requires the researcher as an instrument
- Cyclic nature of data collection and analysis facilitates collection of rich information
- Reflexivity (tension between as researcher and as cultural member).

Key Features

- A strong emphasis on exploring the nature of a particular social phenomenon
- Necessitates direct engagement and participant observation
- A tendency to work primarily with 'unstructured data'—that is, data that have not been coded at the point of data collection as a closed set of analytical categories
- Investigation of a small number of cases (perhaps even just one case) in detail
- Analysis of data that involves explicit interpretation of the meanings and functions of human actions; the product of this analysis primarily takes the form of verbal descriptions and explanations
- Key issues emerge from the data
- Data analysis is done by inductive process
- Ethnographers immerses themselves in the setting.

Cultural Systems Paradigm (CSP)

- The CSP began to emerge in the early 1980s to respond to two methodological needs.
- The lack of adequate models for interpreting the complex data generated by ethnoraphy
- The frequency with which ethnographic inquiry yielded narrative answers from informants which expressed a range of concerns outside the research questions but which appeared to be of extreme importance to those being studied.

The major categories of CSP are:

- The individual human organism and its biological status, psychological make-up, personality and intelligence and skill levels, etc.
- The social systems or units of social relationship, which individuals interact within, are influenced by and have influence on (residential units, extra-residential networks and dyads, and community or societal organizations and agencies)
- Individual and shared (with others in select social systems) behavioral patterns
- The significant idea systems (knowledge, attitudes, beliefs, values and symbolisms or units of meaning) held by individual and social systems
- Expressive culture as represented in such forms as language, music, art, etc.
- Technologies and man-made material objects or material culture
- The physical environments in which humans interact
- Needs that humans must meet in order to achieve the level of physical functioning necessary to the survival of the individual and group
- The human group's shared history of significant events and processes.

Following are some different settings that have been studied by ethnographers:

- Bars
- Churches
- Playgrounds
- Gymnasiums
- Beauty parlors
- Discos
- Farmers' markets
- Sports events
- Food activities (dinner, feast)
- Festivals
- Shopping malls
- Jails/prisons
- Parks
- Court rooms
- A family's settings
- Industry or work settings
- Slaughter houses
- School rooms
- Cafeterias
- Swimming pools
- Grocery stores
- Hospitals
- City halls
- Agencies
- Main streets
- Busy neighborhoods
- Town meetings
- Office meetings
- Parties
- Airport/bus terminals
- Barber shops
- Mental health institutions.

Steps in Conducting Ethnographic Research

- Do participant observation
- Make ethnographic record
- Make descriptive observations
- Make domain analysis
- Make focused observation
- Make taxonomic analysis
- Make selected observations
- Make componential analysis
- Discover cultural themes

- Take cultural inventory
- Write an ethnography report.

Ethnographers typically bring a strong cultural perspective to their studies and this perspective shapes their initial field work.

Data Collection

Several levels of clearance and consent are essential. Key informant or liaison person is essential as gatekeeper. Ethnographic research is very labor- and time-intensive, involving extensive fieldwork in a natural setting. Usually, a general research question(s) is (are) identified. Once entry is gained and rapport (or trust) is established, the research questions are continually refined, becoming more focused. The researcher uses the below-mentioned techniques to collect data.

- **Participant observation:**
  - Complete observer
  - Observer as participant
  - Participant as observer
  - Complete participant
- Interviewing
- Supplementary data sources

Here, the researcher may participate in the phenomenon under study to varying degrees. Observation runs a continuum from detached observer to complete participant observer. The researcher must take great care to be as objective as possible. He or she is the single greatest source of bias within this strategy. The researcher will usually record his or her thoughts, feelings, etc. when developing field notes so as to guard against bias when interpreting the collected data. Ethnography involves a secondary data collection strategy, which typically includes unofficial documents, official documents, objects, etc. which provide insight into the lives, experiences, and perceptions of subjects.

He uses field notes, writes verbatim, condensed notes and interview notes. He transcribes, writes codes and analyzes the data. After analyzing the data, the researcher categorizes it. While analyzing data, the researcher compares, contrasts, analyzes and synthesizes the data. Research report is written in a narrative, literary style to preserve the flavor of original cultural scene. It includes multiple abstraction, and inclusion of maps, diagrams and labels also can be done. Ethnographic researchers use multiple data collection devices so that interpretations may be grounded and triangulated. Reliability is established by ensuring consistency of both the sources of data, i.e. informants and researchers. Validity is also established by checking for the face validity of informant and content validity through verification as cultural informant.

Data collection methods are meant to capture the 'social meanings and ordinary activities' of people (informants) in 'naturally occurring settings' that are commonly referred to as 'the field.' The goal is to collect data in such a way that the researcher imposes a minimal amount of their own bias on the data. Multiple methods of data collection may be employed to facilitate a relationship that allows for a more personal and in-depth portrait of the informants and their community. These can include participant observation, field notes, interviews, and surveys. Interviews are often taped and later transcribed, allowing the interview to proceed unimpaired of note-taking, but with all information available later for full analysis. Secondary research and document analysis are also employed to provide insight into the research topic.

In order to make the data collection and interpretation transparent, researchers creating ethnographies often attempt to be 'reflexive'. Reflexivity refers to the researcher's aim 'to explore the ways in which (the) researcher's involvement with a particular study influences, acts upon and informs such research'. Despite these attempts of reflexivity, no researcher can be totally unbiased, which has provided a basis to criticize ethnography.

Traditionally, the ethnographer focuses attention on a community, selecting knowledgeable informants who know the activities of the community well. These informants are typically asked to identify other informants who represent the community, often using chain sampling. Ethnography relies greatly on up-close, personal experience. Participation, rather than just observation, is one of the keys to this process.

Observation is made by the ethnographer in relation to:

- People
- Place they live
- Activities performed by the people in the place
- Related activities in the place
- Peoples' felt and expressed emotions
- Things people wanted to achieve
- Objects present in the place
- Time at which the events occur
- Sequencing of the events.

During their observations, ethnographers routinely use informal or conversational interviews, which allow them to discuss, probe emerging issues, or ask questions about unusual events in a naturalistic manner. Because of the 'casual' nature of this type of interview technique, it can be useful in eliciting highly candid accounts from individuals. Ethnographers also gather formal in-depth interviews and documentary data, such as minutes of meetings, diaries, and photographs. Participants or situations are sampled on an opportunistic or purposive basis.

Data Analysis

Data analysis within ethnographic research occurs as data are collected. The researcher codes and classifies data (e.g. events, observations, quotes, etc.) into a meaningful taxonomy. New data are compared and contrasted to old so as to note patterns, etc. This iterative process continues until the researcher is able to make 'assertions' which describe the participants' 'reality' and perspectives.

Analysis of ethnographic data tends to be undertaken in an inductive thematic manner. Data are examined to identify and to categorise themes and key issues that 'emerge' from the data. Through a careful analysis of their data, using this inductive process, ethnographers generate tentative theoretical explanations from their empirical work.

Reflexivity (that is, the relationship a researcher shares with the world he or she is investigating) is a central element of ethnographic work, owing to the relationship the ethnographer shares with participants and the ethical issues that flow from this close relationship. Within research reports, reflexivity is presented in the form of a description of the ethnographer's ideas and experiences, which can be used by readers to judge the possible impact of these influences on a study.

To enhance the quality of their work, ethnographers will often provide a detailed or 'thick description' of the research setting and its participants, which will typically be based on many hours of direct observation and interviews with several key informants.

In addition, ethnographic work commonly uses methodological triangulation—a technique designed to compare and contrast different types of methods to help provide more comprehensive insights into the phenomenon under study. This type of triangulation can be very useful, as sometimes what people say about their actions can contrast with their actual behavior.

'Triangulation' is a term linked to navigation or surveying. People discover their position on a map by taking bearings on landmarks, and where the lines intersect is where they are positioned. Alongwith methodological triangulation, Denzin outlines three other types:

- ***Data triangulation***, which uses different sources of data to examine a phenomenon in several different settings and different points in time or space.
- ***Investigator triangulation***, which uses multiple researchers to generate a complex range of perspectives on the data.
- ***Theory triangulation***, in which researchers approach data with different concepts and theories to see how each helps to understand the data.

Ethnographers often draw upon social sciences theory (for example, interactionism, feminism and postmodernism) to strengthen their research focus and analyzes.

Ethnography and Nursing

- Contributes to describe the theory
- Explains the theory
- Aids in hypotheses development
- Yields insight for examining current nursing practice
- Plan for cultural change to improve nursing practice style
- Presents nursing practice realities
- Addresses the wide range of human problems.

Newer Developments in Ethnographic Inquiry

Auto-ethnography, in which researchers' own thoughts and perspectives from their social interactions form the central element of a study; meta-ethnography, in which qualitative research texts are analyzed and synthesized to empirically create new insights and knowledge; and online (or virtual) ethnography, which extends traditional notions of ethnographic study from situated observation and face-to-face researcher-participant interaction to technologically mediated interactions in online networks and communities.

Advantages

- Ethnography facilitates the ethnographers to gain rich understanding of social action and its subtleties in different contexts.
- Participant observation enables the ethnographers to gather empirical insights into social practices that are normally 'hidden' from the public gaze.
- Generation of holistic social accounts in ethnography leads to identification, exploration, and linking social phenomena which, on the surface, have little connection with each other.

Disadvantages

- Ethnographic research takes a long time for understanding the social process.
- Repeated observations may not be possible or permitted by the participant or an organization.
- Obtaining formal approval from research ethics committees can be complicated.
- The interaction between the ethnographer and the patient may be seen with suspicion since the qualitative studies require more researcher involvement rather detachment.
- It is very difficult to completely capture and record the multifaceted nature of social action and interaction.
- Problem may arise during data collection since the social process may be sometimes unpredictable. It requires the ethnographer to be flexible, patient and persistent.

Evaluation

Richardson (2000) provides five criteria for the evaluation of ethnography:

1. ***Substantive contribution:*** 'Does the piece contribute to our understanding of social life?'
2. ***Aesthetic merit:*** 'Does this piece succeed aesthetically?'
3. ***Reflexivity:*** 'How did the author come to write this text... Is there adequate self-awareness and self-exposure for the reader to make judgments about the point of view?'
4. ***Impact:*** 'Does this affect me? Emotionally? Intellectually? Does it move me?'
5. ***Expresses a reality:*** 'Does it seem true—a credible account of a cultural, social, individual, or communal sense of the real?'

Example 19:

Mull, Agran, Winn and Anderson (1999) conducted a study to explore reasons for high rates of unintentional poisoning among Latino children under 5-years-old. Ethnographic interviews were carried out using a sample of 50 mothers identified via door-to-door canvassing in an area with documented high injury rates among Latino children from low-income neighborhoods of Southern California. Interviews included many open-ended and follow-up questions to elicit a detailed family history and emphasized observation of conditions and behaviors in the homes. Children were exposed to potential poisoning agents in more than 80% of homes. Contributory factors were related to culture-included favorable attitudes toward iron as a healthful substance; extensive use of products that lack child-resistant packaging, such as rubbing alcohol; high prevalence of shared housing; limited familiarity with toxic household chemicals not widely used and inability to read warning labels in English.

Example 20:

Wolf, Ekman and Dellenborg (2012) did a study with the aim to describe the everyday practices of professionals and patients in a coronary care unit, and to analyze how the routines, structures and physical design of the care environment influenced their actions and relationships. Ethnographic fieldwork was conducted over a 16-month period (between 2009 and 2011) by two researchers working in parallel in a Swedish coronary care unit. Observations, informal talks and formal interviews took place with registered nurses, assistant nurses, physicians and patients in the coronary care unit. explored a particular care environment in a coronary care ward. With its architecture and cultural characteristics, the care environment effectively reduced the freedom of both patients and healthcare professionals to work towards achieving their different goals.

Phenomenology

Phenomenology, both as philosophy and research approach, allows nursing to explore and describe phenomenon important to the discipline. Nursing practice depends on the people's experience, it is a well-suited method. Phenomenology is a science whose purpose is to describe particular phenomena, or the appearance of things, as lived experience. Lived experience of the world of everyday life is the central focus of phenomenological inquiry. Phenemenology is as much a way of thinking or perceiving as it is a method. Phenomenology as a research method is a rigorous, critical, systematic investigation of phenomena. The purpose of phenomenological inquiry is to explicate the structure or essence of the lived experience of a phenomenon on the search for the unity of meaning which is the identification of the essence of phenomenon and its accurate description through everyday lived experience (Rose, Beeby and Parker, 1995).

Phenomenology is both a philosophy and a research experience to generate and enhance the understanding of what it means to be human. Phenomenology is a way of viewing ourselves, others and everything else that comes in contact with our lives. In nursing, phenomenology helps to explore and understand the phenomena related to nursing.

Origin

The word 'phenomenology' is derived from the Greek word 'Phainomenon' meaning 'appearance' and Logos meaning 'study'. It refers to 'the study of everyday life as it is actually lived and experienced'. 'What is the meaning of one's lived experience?' The only reliable source of information to answer this question is the person himself. Understanding, human behavior or experience requires that the person interpret the action or experience for the researcher, and then the researcher must interpret the explanation provided by the person.

Steps/Elements

Spigelberg (1965, 1975) identified six core steps or elements central to phenomenological investigations. These are described as follows:

- ***Descriptive phenomenology:*** It involves direct exploration, analysis and description of particular phenomena. The process for descriptive phenomenology includes intuiting, bracketing, analyzing and describing.
    - ***Intuiting:*** It requires the researcher to become totally immersed in the phenomenon under investigation and begin to know about the phenomenon as described by the participants. Intuiting is a process of thinking through the data and in intuiting, researcher becomes absorbed in the phenomenon. 'Researcher as an instrument' in the interview process collects the data and then studies the data as they are transcribed and reviews repeatedly.
    - ***Bracketing:*** Bracketing refers to the process of holding assumptions and presuppositions in suspension to improve the rigour of the research (Holloway, 2005). This means that researchers explore their own assumptions and preconceptions in order to set them aside or keep them in suspension, rather than conceal them, so that they do not interfere with the information given by the participants. The bracketing process is crucial throughout the research process, especially during data analysis. Bracketing requires the researcher to remain neutral with respect to belief or disbelief in the existence of the phenomenon (Streubert, Speziale and Carpenter, 2003).
    - ***Analyzing:*** It involves identifying the essence of the phenomenon under investigation from the data obtained. In the process of analysis, the essence or themes will emerge. It requires the researcher to dwell with the data as long as possible for pure and accurate description.
    - ***Describing:*** It involves communicating, writing and verbal description of the phenomenon. The researcher must avoid premature description of the phenomena.
- ***Phenomenology of essences:*** It involves probing through the data to search for common themes or essences and establishing pattern of relationships shared by particular phenomena.
- ***Phenomenology of appearances:*** It involves giving attention to the ways in which phenomena appear. The researcher pays particular attention to the different ways in which an object presents itself.

- ***Constitutive phenomenology:*** It involves studying the phenomena as they become established or constituted in our consciousness and it means the process in which the phenomena takes shape in our consciousness.
- ***Reductive phenomenology:*** The researcher identifies personal biases, assumptions and presuppositions about the phenomena in order to preserve the objectivity of the phenomenological investigation. This process involves a critical self-examination. It is critical if the researcher wants to achieve pure description. Postponing the review of literature until the analysis is complete facilitates phenomenological reduction.
- ***Hermeneutic phenomenology:*** It is a special kind of phenomenological interpretation, designed to unveil otherwise concealed meanings in the phenomena. There are three main steps in the process of hermeneutic phenomenology:
  - ***First, during the naïve reading:*** The researcher reads the text as a whole to become familiar with the text and begins to formulate thoughts about its meaning for further analysis.
  - ***Second, structural analysis (interpretive reading):*** It involves identifying patterns of meaningful connection.
  - ***Third, interpretation of the whole:*** Ensures a comprehensive understanding of the findings.

Characteristics of Phenomenological Research

It is a rigorous, critical, systematic investigation of a human experience in context. The aim of a phenomenological study is to gain a deep understanding of a nature or meaning of everyday experiences. Phenomenology is always a retrospective reflection on experience.

Indications for the use of Phenomenology

The purpose of phenomenological enquiry is to explicate the structure or essence of the lived experiences. By exploring this, one can identify the meaning they attach with the experience. The meaning which we understand from this methodology help us to identify the essence of phenomena. Qualitative phenomenology is employed for the purpose of:

- Clarifying the nature of being human
- Expanding awareness about a certain phenomenon
- Fostering human responsibility in the construction of realities
- Tightening the bond between experiences and the concepts and theories used to explain those experiences (Streubert, Speziale and Carpenter, 2003).

This is one of the most important research methodologies since nurse researchers have and function on philosophical beliefs about people and profession.

Sample: Purposive sampling is used so that the participants who have lived the experience or phenomena under study can be included and are able and willing to describe it.

Steps in Phenomenology

According to Colaizzi (1978)

- Describe the phenomenon of interest
- Collect participants' descriptions of the phenomenon
- Read all participants' descriptions of the phenomenon
- Return the original transcripts and extract significant statements
- Try to spell out the meaning of each significant statement
- Organize the aggregate formalized meanings into clusters of themes
- Write an exhaustive description
- Return to the participants for validation of the description
- If new data are revealed during the validation, incorporate them into an exhaustive description.

According to Giorgi (1985)

- Read the entire description of the experience to get a sense of the whole
- Reread the description
- Identify the transition units of experience
- Clarify and elaborate the meaning by relating constituents to each other and to the whole
- Reflect on the constituents in the concrete language of the participant
- Transform concrete language into the language of concepts of science
- Integrate and synthesize the insight into a descriptive structure of the meaning of the experience.

According to Streubert (1991)

- Explicate a personal description of the phenomenon of interest
- Bracket the researcher's presuppositions
- Interview participants in unfamiliar settings.
- Carefully read the interview transcripts to obtain a general sense of the experience
- Review the transcripts to uncover the essences
- Apprehend essential relationships
- Develop formalized descriptions of the phenomenon
- Return to participants to validate descriptions
- Review the relevant literature
- Distribute the findings to the nursing community.

Data Collection

- Extracting essences from transcribed descriptions (participant's language). An extracted essence is a complete expression of a core idea described by the participant
- Synthesizing essences (researcher's language)
- Joining the core idea of the synthesized essences from each participant. (preposition)
- An extracted core concept is written in phrase that captures the central meaning of prepositions

- ***Synthesizing a structure:*** It is a statement conceptualized by the researcher joining the core concepts
- Data are collected through a variety of means:
  - Observation
  - Interactive interviews
  - Videotape
  - Written descriptions by subjects.
  - Researcher is an instrument for data collection.

Research Questions

The first step in conducting a phenomenological study is to identify the phenomenon to explore. Next, the researcher will develop research question. Two factors need to be considered in developing the research question:

- What are the necessary constituents of this feeling or experience?
- What does the existence of this feeling or experience indicate concerning the nature of the human being?

Data analysis involves listing each word or phrase (expression) that describes some aspect of the lived experience and grouping similar expressions. Test each expression against two criteria:

A. Does the expression contain an aspect of the experience that may structure the meaning of the experience?

B. If yes, abstract this expression and label it.

- Eliminate any irrelevant expressions.
- Reduce concrete, vague and overlapping expression to more exactly worded descriptive constituents.
- Cluster common descriptive constituents and label the cluster with more abstract expression of the common theme.

Topic Appropriate to Phenomenological Research

- ***Human life experiences:*** For example, happiness, fear, commitment, stress.
- ***Health-related topics:*** For example, meaning of pain, living with chronic illness, end of life issues.

Data Analysis

In phenomenological research, the analysis begins as soon as the first data are collected. The actual data analysis occurs when the researchers read the entire data set. Phenomenology reading is more than casually taking note of the content. The researchers immerse themselves in the data, read and reread, and dwell with the data, in order to achieve closeness to the data and a sense of the whole. The researchers translate and transcribe the tape-recorded interviews, then read and reread the interviews in their entirety, reflecting on the interviews as a whole. Then, the researcher has to summarize the interviews keeping in mind that more than one theme might exist in a set of interviews. Once identified, the themes that appeared to be significant and concepts linking substantial portions of the interviews are written down and entered on computer (Morse and Field, 1996).

Content Analysis

In this analysis, the researcher reads the entire interview, identifying several topics. These topics then become primary categories or category labels. With too many categories, saturation is achieved slowly. Once the categories have ample data, the researcher may select to categorize this data into subcategories of two or more (Morse and Field, 1996). A tree diagram develops with types of the main category. When each category is reasonably full and saturation is reached, the researcher writes descriptive paragraphs about the categories and looks for relationships between categories. These relationships could be concurrence, antecedents or consequences of an initial category (Morse and Field, 1996).

The data analysis process: It is done by following the below-mentioned steps:

- The researcher has to carefully read through all the transcriptions one by one and by making notes of ideas, topics or themes that emerge.
- Then the researcher has to arrange the similar topics or themes in groups. In doing so, one can arrange the transcripts based on the major themes, unique topics and others.
- The collected topics can be given specific codes and also can check if any new codes emerge.
- The topics together can be grouped to form categories based on some relationship between the topics.
- A final decision can be made on each category and the codes can be arranged alphabetically.
- The data material belonging to each category is put together in one place and preliminary analysis performed.
- Recording of the data is done if necessary.

Advantages of Phenomenology

- It is a highly appropriate approach to research human experience.
- As a research method, it is a rigorous, critical, systematic investigation of phenomena (Streubert, Speziale and Carpenter, 2003).

Researcher's Role

Lived experience should be transformed for others to understand. Reinharz (1983) articulated five steps:

1. First, transformation occurs as people's experiences are transformed into language.
2. The researcher transforms what is seen and heard into an understanding of the original experience.

3. He transforms what is understood about the phenomenon under investigation into conceptual categories that are the essences of the original experience.
4. He transforms those essences into a written document that captures what the researcher has thought about the experience and reflects the participants' descriptions or actions.
5. He transforms the written document into understanding that can function to clarify all preceding steps.

Journaling helps in continuing the reductive process. Researchers' use of a journal can facilitate phenomenological reduction.

Example 21:

Hounsgaard, Augustussen, Moller, Bradley and Moller (2013) conducted a study on the topic 'Women's perspectives on illness when being screened for cervical cancer' using phenomenological-hermeneutic approach. They have stated the need for the study based on the information that, in Greenland, the incidence of cervical cancer caused by human papillomavirus (HPV) was 25 per 100,000 women; 2.5 times the Danish rate. In Greenland, the disease was most frequent among women aged 30–40. Systematic screening could identify women with cervical cell changes, which, if untreated, may cause cervical cancer. In 2007, less than 40% of eligible women in Greenland participated in screening.

The objective quoted in the study was to examine Greenlandic women's perception of disease, their understanding of the connection between HPV and cervical cancer, and the knowledge that they deem necessary to decide whether to participate in cervical cancer screening. They conducted 2 focus-group interviews with 5 Danish-speaking women and 2 individual interviews with Greenlandic-speaking women. The analysis involved three levels, such as naive reading, structural analysis and critical interpretation.

Results revealed that women were unprepared for screening results showing cervical cell changes, since they had no symptoms. When diagnosed, participants believed that they had early-stage cancer, leading to feelings of vulnerability and an increased need to care for themselves. Later on, an understanding of HPV as the basis for diagnosis and the realization that disease might not be accompanied by symptoms developed. The outcome for participants was a life experience, which they used to encourage others to participate in screening.

Example 22:

Laavanya (2013) conducted a phenomenological study to assess the adolescents' perception of bodily changes in order to understand how adolescents construct their own meaning of bodily change. The researcher selected five adolescent boys and girls in the age group of 15–17 years, who have experienced bodily changes and who were willing to share their experiences. The study was conducted in Chennai. The major themes emerged from the narrative analysis and discussion were social situation led to the interpretation of bodily change, adolescent girls construct dissatisfied body image and boys construct satisfied body image and adolescent self-regulated behavior as an outcome of their interpretation.

Example 23:

A study was conducted by Hosseini and Abdi (2012) with the aim of describing the experiences of the men who underwent vasectomy. The sample consisted of 14 vasectomized men selected through purposive sampling method. In-depth and open interviews with participants were conducted to collect the data. The results were transcribed and recorded in comprehensive field notes. Colaizzi's method was used to analyze the data. Four themes emerged from the obtained results of the present study, which described the structure of the experiences of men as follows: Opinions about vasectomy, own perceptions about vasectomy, experiences with the procedure and recommendation of vasectomy to others.

Narrative Analysis, Systematic Reviews and Meta-analysis

The health care professionals are moving towards the evidence-based practice. The terms such as Evidence-based Medicine, Evidence-based Nursing and Evidence-based Nursing practice are not new for us. We often rely upon the review articles as a source of summarized evidence on a particular topic. Narrative reviews are the one where experts in a particular field provide what is supposed to be a summary of evidence in that field.

Narrative analysis focuses on story as the object of inquiry to determine how individuals make sense of events in their lives. Narratives are viewed as a type of cultural 'envelope' in which people pour their experiences and relate their importance to others. Narrative analysis focuses on broad conatus of Narrative; stories are not fractured and dissected.

Steps:

- ***Constructing:*** Individuals construct stories when they wish to understand specific events and situations that require linking an inner world of desire and motive to an external world of observable action.
- ***Reconstructing:*** Individuals reconstruct stories by filling the gaps in comprehending the stories.
- ***Narrating:*** Individuals narrate stories to others.
- ***Analyzing:*** Analyzing stories opens up forms of telling about experience and is more than just content. Narrative analysis ask as to why was the story told that ways?

Dimensions of narrative approach:

- People organize significant events in terms of stories and through telling of these stories, they make meaning of their experiences in lives.
- Time and plot are structured properties of Narratives. Events in a story follow a sequence.
- Narratives have a cultural context, they do not occur by themselves.
- Narratives are relational stories told to other people.
- Narratives have power to shape human behavior. Narratives can be used to produce a moral story of how people are supposed to behave.

Narrative reviews are criticized for their risk of bias. Systematic reviews are the preferred methodology rather than the narrative analysis since the use of scientific strategies eliminates the bias.

Narrative analysis	Systematic analysis	Meta-analysis
Narrative analysis focuses on story as the object of inquiry to determine how individuals make sense of events in their lives. Narratives are viewed as a type of cultural 'envelope' in which people pour their experiences and relate their importance to others	A systematic review is a review of a clearly formulated question that uses systematic and explicit methods to identify, select, and critically appraise relevant research, and to collect and analyze data from the studies that are included in the review	Meta-analysis refers to the use of statistical techniques in a systematic review to integrate the results of included studies
There is a high risk of bias	The risk of bias is less	No bias is involved
The recommendations may be inappropriate	The recommendations may be appropriate	The recommendations may be appropriate

A systematic review is a form of research that provides a summary of reports on a specific clinical question. In the process of systematic review, explicit methods are used to search, critically appraise and synthesize the available literature. It is particularly useful in bringing together a number of separately conducted studies, sometimes with conflicting findings, and synthesizing their results (Fig. 5.3).

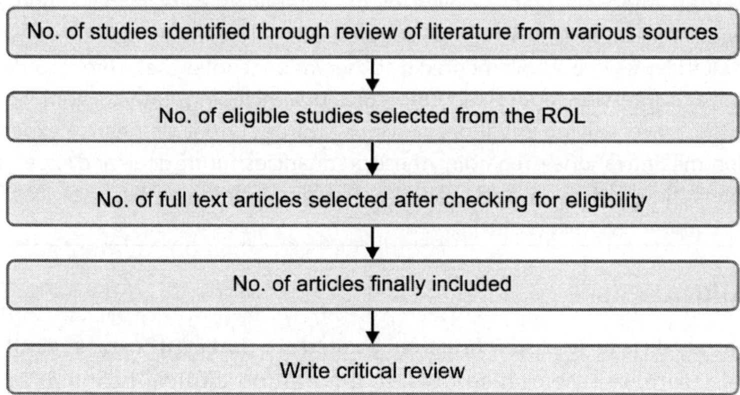

Fig. 5.3: Process of systematic review

Method of doing Systematic Reviews

- Identify and formulate the clinical question which needs to be answered
- State the objective of review
- Formulate eligibility criteria to include the studies for systematic review
- Conduct an exhaustive review of literature to identify the studies, especially primary studies related to the clinical question
- Tabulate characteristics of each study identified and assess its methodological quality

- Appraising critically for its quality, assemble the relevant studies after justifying exclusions
- Prepare a critical summary of the review, stating aims, describing materials and reporting results.

Advantages of Systematic Reviews

- Systematic reviews provide a whole range of relevant findings from research on a particular topic, and not just the results of one or two studies.
- They can be used to establish whether scientific findings are consistent and generalizable across populations, settings, and treatment variations, or whether findings vary significantly by particular subgroups.
- Systematic reviews limit bias and will improve reliability and accuracy of conclusions.

Systematic reviews of randomized controlled trials (RCTs) are considered to be evidence of the highest level in the hierarchy of research designs evaluating effectiveness of interventions in the field of medicine.

Example 24:

The researchers documented 26 pregnancy outcomes among 13 homeless women (aged 18–26) and eight homeless men through interviews and participant-observation. Bulk of the data on the experience of pregnancy came from participant-observation notes and 21 semistructured, transcribed in-depth interviews that followed an interview guide. Eleven of the interviews were with women alone, four with men alone, and five with couples; one interview included two women. These interviews were supplemented by observational notes that were recorded and coded. Each interview addressed core concepts, including path to homelessness, family life, current living situation, previous and/or current pregnancy experience, decision-making rationale regarding these pregnancies, future goals and expectations and interaction with social and health services and opinion of these services [Smid, Bourgois and Auerswald (2011)].

META-ANALYSIS

Meta-analysis is a rigorous statistical procedure that synthesizes results from multiple primary research studies on a common clinical problem or issue. Meta-analysis provides the power to detect differences and effects across studies using similar variables in order to answer questions that a single study could not. Following a systematic review, data from individual studies may be pooled quantitatively and reanalyzed using established statistical methods. This technique is called ***meta-analysis***. The meta-analysis is done with the fact that combining the samples of the individual studies, the overall sample size is increased, thereby improving the statistical power of the analysis as well as the precision of the estimates of treatment effects. It is commonly used in the field of medicine where all randomized controlled trials are pooled together to do meta-analysis.

Method of doing Meta-analysis

Meta-analysis involves a two-stage process:

1. ***Calculation of treatment effect of individual studies:*** In the first stage, treatment effect is calculated with its 95% confidence intervals (CI) for each individual study. In order to calculate the treatment effect, odds ratios (OR), relative risks (RR) and risk differences are used.
2. ***Calculation of overall treatment effect:*** In the second stage of meta-analysis, an overall treatment effect is calculated as a weighted average of the individual study's summary statistics. In the calculation of overall treatment effect, data from the individual studies are not simply combined as if they were from a single study. Greater weights are given to the results from studies that provide more information. The weights are often the inverse of the variance (the square of the standard error) of the treatment effect, which relates closely to sample size. A 'forest plot' is developed from the data on the individual studies.

Forest Plot

It is a visual diagram which shows at a glance the information from the individual studies included into the meta-analysis, and an estimate of the overall results. It also allows a visual assessment of the amount of variation between the results of the studies (heterogeneity). The forest plot helps in deciding whether a particular intervention will produce statistically significant effect on samples.

Advantages of Meta-analysis

- It gives overall treatment effect of many studies conducted on a specific topic
- It combines many studies by which overall sample size is increased; thereby it improves the statistical power of the analysis as well as the precision of the estimates of treatment effects.

Disadvantages of Meta-analysis

- Requires a good deal of time and effort
- Selection bias fosters a continuous threat
- Relies upon the published result of others. If the primary studies were not conducted with scientific rigour, it influences the final outcome.

Example 25:

Wang, Shu, Fetzer and Chang (2014) conducted a meta-analysis to assess the difference in parenting style between women who conceived using *in vitro* fertilization (IVF) and those who conceived naturally. This meta-analysis searched three electronic databases (MEDLINE, PsychInfo, and CINAHL) for relevant articles published between 1978 and 2011. Key words used included parenting, mothering, parent-child relations, child-rearing, infertility, assisted reproductive technique, IVF and intracytoplasmic sperm injection (ICSI). Wang, Shu, Fetzer and Chang (2014) conducted a meta-analysis to

contd...

contd...

assess the difference in parenting style between women who conceived using *in vitro* fertilization (IVF) and those who conceived naturally. This meta-analysis searched three electronic databases (MEDLINE, PsychInfo, and CINAHL) for relevant articles published between 1978 and 2011. Key words used included parenting, mothering, parent-child relations, child-rearing, infertility, assisted reproductive technique, IVF and intracytoplasmic sperm injection (ICSI). Three hundred ninety studies were identified. Fourteen studies met the inclusion criteria. Studies that included women who conceived using a donor egg or sperm for IVF and those that included women who were either surrogates or in homosexual relationships were excluded. The Newcastle-Ottawa Scale was used to appraise the quality of the data. The IVF participants used significantly greater controlling parenting behaviors than their natural conception participant peers ($d = 0.148$, $p < .01$). There was no difference between the two groups in terms of parenting behaviors related to warmth, rejection, or respect for autonomy. The homogeneity test for the effect size of warmth and controlling parenting behavior achieved significance.

Qualitative Outcome Analysis and Secondary Analysis

Outcome analysis is an evaluation of what happens with regard to outcomes of interest after implementing a program or intervention, without using an experimental design to assess net effects.

An evaluation of the effect of a program or intervention on outcomes of interest, net of other factors influencing those outcomes is called the impact analysis. Qualitative research lacks procedural guidelines for moving from theory development to identification and evaluation of specific clinical interventions. The developed procedure is called qualitative outcome analysis. (QOA). It addresses the theory practice gap in qualitative research.

In secondary analysis, the data collected by one researcher are reanalyzed by another investigator to answer new research questions. It focuses on a particular sub-group of the full original sample.

Qualitative researcher collects more data than what is required for analysis. Secondary analysis of qualitative data provides opportunities to exploit rich data sets, although there may be difficulty in identifying a suitable data set. The use of available data from other studies makes it possible to bypass time-consuming and costly steps in the research process. The disadvantage is that the data collected may be deficient in the sample used.

Secondary analysis involves the use of the existing data, in order to pursue a research interest which is distinct from that of the original work; this may be a new research question or an alternative perspective on the original question.

Forms of Secondary Analysis

- ***Additional in-depth analysis:*** A more intensive focus on a particular finding or aspect was undertaken as part of the primary work.

- ***Additional sub-set analysis:*** A selective focus on a sub-set of the sample from the original study (or studies), sharing characteristics which warrant further analysis.
- ***New perspective/conceptual focus:*** The retrospective analysis of the whole or part of a data set from a different perspective, to examine concepts which were not central to the original research.

Advantages of Secondary Analysis

- Limited opportunities for conducting primary research and the costs of qualitative work have prompted researchers to consider maximizing use of the data available to them.
- The advent of software to aid the coding, retrieval and analysis of qualitative data is another development which is likely to facilitate both the archiving and availability of qualitative data for secondary analytic purposes.
- It has been contended that the approach can be used to generate new knowledge, new hypotheses, or support for the existing theories; that it reduces the burden placed on respondents by negating the need to recruit further subjects; and that it allows wider use of data from rare or inaccessible respondents.
- More convenient approach for particular researchers, notably students.

EPIDEMIOLOGICAL STUDIES

Epidemiology is defined as 'the study of the distribution and determinants of health-related states or events in specified populations and the application of this study to the prevention and control of health problems'. The word 'epidemiology' is derived from the Greek words: epi 'upon', demos 'people' and logos 'study'. This broad definition of epidemiology can further be elaborated as follows: Study includes surveillance, observation, hypothesis-testing, analytic research and experiments (Refer Fig. 5.4). Distribution refers to analysis of times, persons, places and classes of people affected. Determinants include factors that influence health, biological, chemical, physical, social, cultural, economic, genetic and behavioral. Health-related states and events refer to diseases, causes of death, behaviors such as use of tobacco, positive health status, reactions to preventive regimes and provision and use of health services. Specified populations include those with identifiable characteristics, such as occupational groups. Application to prevention and control is the aim of public health—to promote, protect and restore health (Last JM, 2001). The studies used in epidemiological investigations are as follows:

Epidemiological studies can be classified as either observational or experimental.

- ***Observational studies:*** Observational studies allow nature to take its course—the investigator measures but does not intervene. They include studies that can be called ***descriptive*** or ***analytical***. A ***descriptive study*** is

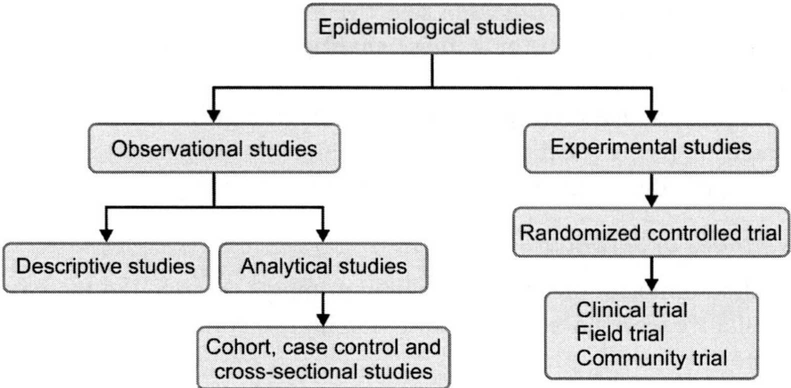

Fig. 5.4: Classification of epidemiological studies

limited to a description of the occurrence of a disease in a population and is often the first step in an epidemiological investigation. An ***analytical study*** goes further by analyzing relationships between health status and other variables. Apart from the simplest descriptive studies, almost all epidemiological studies are analytical in character. Pure descriptive studies are rare, but descriptive data in reports of health statistics are a useful source of ideas for epidemiological studies.

- ***Descriptive studies:*** These are simple description of the health status of a community, based on routinely available data or on data obtained in special surveys. It is often the first step in an epidemiological investigation. In many countries, this type of study is undertaken by National Center for Health Statistics. Pure descriptive studies make no attempt to analyze the links between exposure and effect, they are usually based on mortality statistics and may examine patterns of death by age, sex or ethnicity during specified time periods or in various countries. Ecological (or correlational) studies are useful for generating hypotheses. In an ecological study, the units of analysis are groups of people rather than individuals. Ecological studies can also be done by comparing populations in different places at the same time or, in a time-series, by comparing the same population in one place at different times.
- ***Analytical studies:*** Cohort, cross-sectional, and case-control studies are collectively referred to as observational studies because the investigator simply observes. In observational studies no interventions are carried out by the investigator.
- ***Experimental studies:*** Experimental or intervention studies involve an active attempt to change a disease determinant, such as an exposure or a behavior, or the progress of a disease through treatment and are similar in design to experiments in other sciences. Major experimental study designs include the following:
- randomized controlled trials using patients as subjects (clinical trials)
- field trials in which the participants are healthy people
- community trials in which the participants are the communities themselves.

Observational Studies

Cohort Studies

The term 'cohort' has military roots. A cohort was a 300–600 men unit in the Roman army; ten cohorts formed a legion. The etymology of the term provides a useful mnemonic. A cohort study consists of bands or groups of people marching forward in time from an exposure to one or more outcomes. Cohort studies are used to study incidence, causes, and prognosis. They measure events in chronological order which can be used to distinguish between cause and effect. These are the best methods for determining the incidence and natural history of a condition.

Cohort studies, also called 'follow-up or incidence studies', begin with a group of people who are free of disease, and who are classified into subgroups according to exposure to a potential cause of disease or outcome. Variables of interest are specified and measured and the whole cohort is followed up to see how the subsequent development of new cases of the disease (or other outcome) differs between the groups with and without exposure.

A cohort study follows up two or more groups from exposure to outcome. In its simplest form, a cohort study compares the experience of a group exposed to some factor with another group not exposed to the factor. If the former group has a higher or lower frequency of an outcome than the unexposed, then an association between exposure and outcome is evident. The defining characteristic of all cohort studies is that they track people forward in time from exposure to outcome. Researchers doing this kind of study must, therefore, go forward in time from the present or go back in time to choose their cohorts. Either way, a cohort study moves in the same direction, although gathering data might not.

- ***Prospective cohort studies:*** A group of people is chosen who do not have the outcome of interest (for example, myocardial infarction). The investigator then measures a variety of variables that might be relevant to the development of the condition. Over a period of time, the people in the sample are observed to see whether they develop the outcome of interest (that is, myocardial infarction). In single cohort studies, those people who do not develop the outcome of interest are used as internal controls. Where two cohorts are used, one group has been exposed to or treated with the agent of interest and the other has not, thereby acting as an external control.
- ***Retrospective cohort studies:*** These use data already collected for other purposes. The methodology is the same but the study is performed post hoc. The cohort is 'followed up' retrospectively. The study period may be many years but the time to complete the study is only as long as it takes to collate and analyze the data.

Advantages and Disadvantages

- The use of cohorts is often mandatory as a randomized controlled trial may be unethical; for example, people cannot be deliberately exposed to cigarette smoke or asbestos. Thus, research on risk factors relies heavily on cohort studies.

- As cohort studies measure potential causes before the outcome has occurred, the study can demonstrate that these 'causes' preceded the outcome, thereby avoiding the debate as to which is cause and which is effect.
- A further advantage is that a single study can examine various outcome variables. For example, cohort studies of smokers can simultaneously look at deaths from lung, cardiovascular, and cerebrovascular disease.
- Cohorts permit calculation of the effect of each variable on the probability of developing the outcome of interest (relative risk). However, where a certain outcome is rare, then a prospective cohort study is inefficient.
- Another problem with prospective cohort studies is the loss of some subjects to follow up. This can significantly affect the outcome. Taking incidence analysis as an example (incidence = cases/period of time), it can be seen that the loss of a few cases will seriously affect the numerator and, hence, the calculated incidence. The rarer the condition the more significant is this effect.
- Retrospective studies are much cheaper as the data have already been collected. One advantage of such a study design is the lack of bias because the outcome of current interest was not the original reason for the data to be collected. However, because the cohort was originally constructed for another purpose, it is unlikely that all the relevant information will have been rigorously collected.
- Retrospective cohorts also suffer the disadvantage that people with the outcome of interest are more likely to remember certain antecedents, or exaggerate or minimize what they now consider to be risk factors (recall bias).
- Where two cohorts are compared, one will have been exposed to the agent of interest and one will not. The major disadvantage is the inability to control for all other factors that might differ between the two groups. These factors are known as ***confounding variables***.
- A confounding variable is independently associated with both the variable of interest and the outcome of interest. For example, lung cancer (outcome) is less common in people with asthma (variable). However, it is unlikely that asthma in itself confers any protection against lung cancer. It is more probable that the incidence of lung cancer is lower in people with asthma because fewer asthmatics smoke cigarettes (confounding variable).
- Finally, problems can arise as a result of bias. Bias can occur in any research and reflects the potential that the sample studied is not representative of the population it was drawn from and/or the population at large. A classic example is using employed people, as employment is itself associated with generally better health than unemployed people. Similarly, people who respond to questionnaires tend to be fitter and more motivated than those who do not.

Conducting a Cohort Study

If the data are readily available, then a retrospective design is the quickest method. If high-quality reliable data are not available, a prospective study will be required. The first step is the definition of the sample group. Each subject must have the potential to develop the outcome of interest. Furthermore, the sample population must be representative of the general population if the study is primarily looking at the incidence and natural history of the condition (description). If, however, the aim is to analyze the relation between predictor variables and outcomes (analytical), then the sample should contain as many patients likely to develop the outcome as possible, otherwise much time and expense will be spent collecting information of little value.

Each variable studied must be accurately measured. Variables that are relatively fixed, for example, height in adults, need to be recorded once. Where change is more probable, for example, weight, needs to be repeatedly measured.

All patients entered into the study should also be followed up for the duration of the study. Losses can significantly affect the validity of the results. To minimize this, as much information about the patient (name, address, telephone, etc) needs to be recorded as soon as the patient is entered into the study. Regular contact should be made; it is hardly surprising if the subjects have moved or lost interest and become lost to follow up if they are only contacted at 10-year intervals. Follow-up is usually easier in people who have been exposed to the agent of interest and this may lead to bias.

Example 26:

Jetal (2014) examined the behavioral outcomes of late preterm infants, who were admitted to Neonatal Intensive Care in comparison with late preterm infants, who were not admitted. This cohort study prospectively recruited 225 children born late preterm (34–36+6 weeks gestation) in 2006 in Northern Ireland. Two groups were compared: LPIs who received NIC (study; n = 103) and LPIs who did not receive NIC (control; n = 122). Parents/guardians completed the Child Behavior Checklist. Descriptive maternal and infant data were also collected. LPI children admitted to NIC had higher medical risk than the nonadmitted comparison LPIs admitted to NIC scored higher on the Child Behavior Checklist compared with those who were not admitted indicating more behavioral problems.

Cross-sectional Studies

Cross-sectional studies measure the prevalence of disease and, thus, are often called ***prevalence studies***. Prevalence equals the number of cases in a population at a given point in time. All the measurements on each person are made at one point in time. In a cross-sectional study, the measurements of exposure and effect are made at the same time. It is not easy to assess the reasons for associations shown in cross-sectional studies. The key question to be asked is whether the exposure precedes or follows the effect. If the exposure data are known to represent exposure before any effect occurred, the data from a cross-sectional study can be treated like data generated from a cohort study.

Cross-sectional studies are relatively easy and inexpensive to conduct and are useful for investigating exposures that are fixed characteristics of individuals, such as ethnicity or blood group. In sudden outbreaks of disease, a cross-sectional study to measure several exposures can be the most convenient first step in investigating the cause. Data from cross-sectional studies are helpful in assessing the health care needs of populations. Data from repeated cross-sectional surveys using independent random samples with standardized definitions and survey methods provide useful indications of trends.

Cross-sectional studies are also used to infer causation. At one point in time, the subjects are assessed to determine whether they were exposed to the relevant agent and whether they have the outcome of interest. Some of the subjects will neither have been exposed nor have the outcome of interest. This clearly distinguishes this type of study from the other observational studies (cohort and case controlled) where reference to either exposure and/or outcome is made.

The advantage of such studies is that subjects are neither deliberately exposed, treated, or not treated and, hence, there are seldom ethical difficulties. Only one group is used, data are collected only once and multiple outcomes can be studied; thus, this type of study is relatively cheap. Many cross-sectional studies are done using questionnaires. Alternatively, each of the subjects may be interviewed.

Any study with a low response rate can be criticized because it can miss significant differences in the responders and nonresponders. At its most extreme, all the non-responders could be dead. Strenuous efforts must be made to maximize the numbers who do respond. The use of volunteers is also problematic because they too are unlikely to be representative of the general population. A census is another example of a cross-sectional study.

Conduction of cross-sectional study involves formulating the research question(s) and selecting the sample population. A method for contacting sample subjects must be devised and then implemented. In this way, the data are collected and can then be analyzed.

Advantages and Disadvantages

- The most important advantage of cross-sectional studies is that, in general, they are quick and cheap. As there is no follow-up, less resources are required to run the study.
- Cross-sectional studies are the best way to determine prevalence and are useful at identifying associations that can then be more rigorously studied using a cohort study or randomized controlled study.
- The most important problem with this type of study is differentiating cause and effect from simple association.
- Rare conditions cannot efficiently be studied using cross-sectional studies because even in large samples, there may be no one with the disease. In this situation, it is better to study a cross-sectional sample of patients who already have the disease (a case series).

Example 27:

Goyal Aetal (2014) conducted a cross-sectional study to assess the impact of dental fear on oral health-related quality of life among school-going and non-school-going children in Udaipur city.

The study sample consisted of 279 school children and 257 non-school-going children. The sampling frame comprised of 12–15-year-old children attending two upper primary public schools and non-school-going children working at shops or not working. Information on dental fear and Oral Health Related Quality of Life (OHRQoL) was obtained by personal interviews by a single trained and calibrated examiner through a structured questionnaire. Mean dental fear scores among school-going (35.41 [11.79]) and non-school-going (47.59 [3.80]) children revealed that dental fear was significantly ($P \leq 0.05$) higher among non-school-going children than among school-going children. In school-going children, the likelihood of having poor oral symptoms, functional limitation and poorer social and emotional well-being were significantly ($P \leq 0.05$) lesser as compared with non-school-going children.

Case-control Studies

Case-control studies are very common. They are particularly useful for studying infrequent events. Case-control studies are longitudinal in contrast to cross-sectional studies. Case-control studies have been called ***retrospective studies*** since the investigator is looking backward from the disease to a possible cause. This can be confusing because the terms ***retrospective*** and ***prospective*** are also used to describe the timing of data collection in relation to the current date. In this sense, a case-control study may be either retrospective, when all the data deal with the past, or prospective, in which data collection continues with the passage of time.

Case-control studies provide a relatively simple way to investigate causes of diseases, especially rare diseases. They include people with a disease (or other outcome variable) of interest and a suitable control (comparison or reference) group of people unaffected by the disease or outcome variable. The study compares the occurrence of the possible cause in cases and in controls. The investigators collect data on disease occurrence at one point in time and exposures at a previous point in time.

Case-controlled studies compare groups retrospectively. They seek to identify possible predictors of outcome and are useful for studying rare diseases or outcomes. They are often used to generate hypotheses that can then be studied via prospective cohort or other studies.

In contrast with cohort and cross-sectional studies, case-control studies are usually retrospective. People with the outcome of interest are matched with a control group who do not. Retrospectively, the researcher determines which individuals were exposed to the agent or treatment or the prevalence of a variable in each of the study groups. Where the outcome is rare, case-control studies may be the only feasible approach.

As some of the subjects have been deliberately chosen because they have the disease in question, case-control studies are much more cost-efficient than cohort and cross-sectional studies—that is, a higher percentage of cases per study.

Case-control studies determine the relative importance of a predictor variable in relation to the presence or absence of the disease. Case-control studies are retrospective and cannot, therefore, be used to calculate the relative risk. Case-control studies can, however, be used to calculate odds ratios, which, in turn, usually approximate to the relative risk.

Conduction of case-control study involves deciding the research question to be answered and formulation of hypothesis. Then decision should be made on what will be measured and how. A valid control group is selected. Then both the groups can be compared for the 'exposure' to each variable.

Advantages and Disadvantages

- When conditions are uncommon, case-control studies generate a lot of information from relatively few subjects. When there is a long latent period between an exposure and the disease, case-control studies are the only feasible option.
- In case-control studies, comparatively few subjects are required, so more resources are available for studying each. As a consequence, a huge number of variables can be considered. This type of study is, therefore, useful for generating hypotheses that can then be tested using other types of study.
- This flexibility of the variables studied comes at the expense of the restricted outcomes studied. The only outcome is the presence or absence of the disease or whatever criteria was chosen to select the cases.
- The major problems with case-control studies are the familiar ones of confounding variables and bias.
- ***Bias may take two major forms.***
    - **Sampling bias**. The patients with the disease may be a biased sample or the controls may be biased (for example, volunteers, different ages, sex or socioeconomic group).
    - **Observation and recall bias**, As the study assesses predictor variables retrospectively, there is great potential for a biased assessment of their presence and significance by the patient or the investigator, or both.
- **Overcoming sampling bias**. Ideally, the cases studied should be a random sample of all the patients with the disease. This is not only very difficult but, in many instances, is impossible because many cases may not have been diagnosed or have been misdiagnosed. For example, many cases of non-insulin-dependent diabetes will not have sought medical attention and, therefore, be undiagnosed.
- Selecting the controls is often a more difficult problem. To enable the controls to represent the same population as the cases, one of the four techniques may be used.
    - ***A convenience sample:*** Sampled in the same way as the cases.
    - ***Matching:*** The controls may be a matched or unmatched random sample from the unaffected population. Again the problems of controlling for unknown influences is present but if the controls are too closely matched, they may not be representative of the general

population. 'Overmatching' may cause the true difference to be underestimated. The advantage of matching is that it allows a smaller sample size for any given effect to be statistically significant.

- ***Using two or more control groups:*** If the study demonstrates a significant difference between the patients with the outcome of interest and those without, even when the latter have been sampled in a number of different ways (for example, outpatients, inpatients, GP patients), then the conclusion is more robust.
- ***Using a population-based sample for both cases and controls:*** It is possible to take a random sample of all the patients with a particular disease from specific registers. The control group can then be constructed by selecting age- and sex-matched people randomly selected from the same population as the area covered by the disease register.

Overcoming Observation and Recall Bias

Overcoming retrospective recall bias can be achieved by using data recorded, for other purposes, before the outcome had occurred and, therefore, before the study had started. The success of this strategy is limited by the availability and reliability of the data collected. Another technique is blinding, where neither the subject nor the observer know if they are a case or control subject. Nor are they aware of the study hypothesis. In practice, this is often difficult or impossible and only partial blinding is practicable. It is usually possible to blind the subjects and observers to the study hypothesis by asking spurious questions. Observers can also be easily blinded to the case or control status of the patient where the relevant observation is not of the patients themselves but a laboratory test or radiograph.

Blinding cases to their case or control status is usually impracticable as they already know that they have a disease or illness. Similarly, observers can hardly be blinded to the presence of physical signs, for example, cyanosis or dyspnea. As a result of the problems of matching, bias and confounding, case-control studies, are often flawed. They are, however, useful for generating hypotheses. These hypotheses can then be tested more rigorously by other methods—randomized controlled trials or cohort studies.

The odds ratio is very similar to the risk ratio, particularly if a disease is rare. For the odds ratio to be a good approximation, the cases and controls must be representative of the general population with respect to exposure. However, because the incidence of disease is unknown, the absolute risk cannot be calculated. An odds ratio should be accompanied by the confidence interval observed around the point estimate.

Historical Cohort Studies

Costs can occasionally be reduced by using a historical cohort (identified on the basis of records of previous exposure). This type of investigation is called a historical cohort study, because all the exposure and effect (disease) data have been collected before the actual study begins.

Nested Case-control Studies

The nested case-control design makes cohort studies less expensive. The cases and controls are both chosen from a defined cohort, for which some information on exposures and risk factors is already available. Additional information on new cases and controls, particularly selected for the study, is collected and analyzed. This design is particularly useful when measurement of exposure is expensive.

Selection of Cases and Controls

A case-control study begins with the selection of cases. These cases should represent all the cases in a specified population group. Cases are selected on the basis of disease, not exposure. Controls are people without the disease. A critical and challenging aspect of population-based case-control studies is finding a cost-effective way to identify and enroll control subjects. The most difficult task is to select controls so as to sample the exposure prevalence in the population that generated the cases.

Furthermore, the choice of controls and cases must not be influenced by exposure status, which should be determined in the same manner for both. It is not necessary for cases and controls to be all-inclusive; in fact, they can be restricted to any specified subgroup, such as elderly people, males or females.

The controls should represent people who would have been designated as study cases if they had developed the disease. Ideally, case-control studies use new (incident) cases to avoid the difficulty of separating factors related to causation and survival (or recovery), although studies have often been conducted using prevalence data (for example, case-control studies of congenital malformations). Case-control studies can estimate relative risk of disease, but they cannot determine the absolute incidence of disease. Furthermore, researchers should detail eligibility criteria used for selection, such as age range and location (clinic, hospital, population-based). Finally, they should gather data preferably from incident (new) rather than prevalent (both old and new) cases; since diagnostic patterns change over time, recent diagnoses are likely to be more consistent than those obtained from different periods.

The control group provides the background proportion of exposure expected in the case group. Controls should, therefore, be free of the disease (outcome) being studied, but should be representative of those individuals who would have been selected as cases, if they had developed the disease. In other words, controls should represent the population at risk of becoming cases. Selection of controls must be independent of the exposure being investigated.

Exposure

An important aspect of case-control studies is the determination of the start and duration of exposure for cases and controls. In the case-control design, the exposure status of the cases is usually determined after the development of the disease. The association of an exposure and a disease (relative risk) in a case-control study is measured by calculating the odds ratio (OR), which is the ratio of the odds of exposure among the cases to the odds of exposure among the controls.

Odds Ratio

The odds for a group is defined as the number of patients in the group who achieve the stated end-point divided by the number of patients who do not. For example, the odds of dysmenorrhea reduction during treatment with fish oil capsules in a group of 20 adolescent girls (experimental/treatment group) may be 12–8 (12 with reduction of dysmenorrhea divided by 8 without = 1.5); in a control group the odds may be 6–14 (0.43). The odds ratio, as the name implies, is a ratio of two odds. It is simply defined as the ratio of the odds of the treatment group to the odds of the control group. In our example, the odds ratio of treatment to control group would be 3.5 (1.5 divided by 0.43).

Risk and Relative Risk

Risk, as opposed to odds, is calculated as the number of patients in the group who achieve the stated end-point divided by the total number of patients in the group. Risk ratio or relative risk is a ratio of two 'risks'. In the example above, the risks would be 12 in 20 in the treatment group (12 divided by 20 = 0.6) and 6 in 20 in the control group (0.3), giving a risk ratio, or relative risk of 2 (0.6 divided by 0.3).

Interpretation of odds ratios and relative risk: An odds ratio or relative risk greater than 1 indicates increased likelihood of the stated outcome being achieved in the treatment group. If the odds ratio or relative risk is less than 1, there is a decreased likelihood in the treatment group. A ratio of 1 indicates no difference—i.e. the outcome is just as likely to occur in the treatment group as it is in the control group. As in all estimates of treatment effect, odds ratios or relative risks reported in meta-analysis should be accompanied by confidence intervals.

Using Secondary Data

Pre-existing databases provide an excellent and convenient source of data. There are a host of such databases and the increasing archiving of information on computers means that this is an enlarging area for obtaining data. Such databases enable vast numbers of people to be entered into a study prospectively or retrospectively. They can be used to construct a cohort, to produce a sample for a cross-sectional study, or to identify people with certain conditions or outcomes and produce a sample for a case-controlled study.

Advantages and Disadvantages

These type of data are ordinarily collected by people other than the researcher and independently of any specific hypothesis. The opportunity for observer bias is, thus, diminished. The use of previously collected data is efficient and comparatively inexpensive and moreover the data are collected in a very standardized way, permitting comparisons over time and between different countries. However, because the data are collected for other purposes, it may not be ideally suited to the testing of the current hypothesis. Additionally, it may be incomplete. This may result in sampling bias. Because observational studies are not experiments (as are randomized controlled trials), it is difficult to control many external variables.

Example 28:

Gremigni and Cappelli (2014) did a study with the aim to compare 30 successful (>1 year) kidney transplantation recipients with 30 matched-pair healthy controls on psychosocial well-being. Independent of gender, age and time since transplantation, transplanted patients equalled healthy people in the intrapersonal domains but scored worse in the interpersonal domains of psychosocial well-being.

Example 29:

Shrikshande, Zodpey and Negandhi (2014) conducted a case-control study to examine the association between infectious agents and acute myocardial infarction. The study compared the risk of occurrence of AMI (outcome) if subjects were ever-infected with *Helicobacter pylori* or *Chlamydophila pneumoniae*; and their CRP positivity (exposure). Incident cases of myocardial infarctions in a tertiary care hospital were included as cases. The study recruited 265 cases and 265 controls and detected an odds ratio (OR) of 2.50 (95% confidence interval [CI]: 1.69–3.70) and an OR of 2.50 (95% CI: 1.71–3.65) for *C. pneumoniae* and *H. pylori*, respectively. Raised CRP levels had an OR of 3.85 (95% CI: 2.54–5.87).

Randomized Controlled Trials

A randomized controlled trial is an epidemiological experiment designed to study the effects of a particular intervention, usually a treatment for a specific disease (clinical trial). Subjects in the study population are randomly allocated to intervention and control groups, and the results are assessed by comparing outcomes.

To ensure that the groups being compared are equivalent, patients are allocated to them randomly, i.e. by chance. If the initial selection and randomization are done properly, the control and treatment groups will be comparable at the start of the investigation; any differences between groups are chance occurrences unaffected by the conscious or unconscious biases of the investigators.

Field Trials

Field trials, in contrast to clinical trials, involve people who are healthy but presumed to be at risk; data collection takes place 'in the field', usually among noninstitutionalized people in the general population. Since the subjects are disease-free and the purpose is to prevent diseases that may occur with relatively low frequency, field trials are often logistically complicated and expensive endeavors. Field trials can be used to evaluate interventions aimed at reducing exposure without necessarily measuring the occurrence of health effects.

Community Trials

In this form of experiment, the treatment groups are communities rather than individuals. This is particularly appropriate for diseases that are influenced by social conditions, and for which prevention efforts target group behavior. Cardiovascular disease is a good example of a condition appropriate for community trials, although unanticipated methodological issues can arise in large community intervention trials.

Limitations of Community Trials

A limitation of such studies is that only a small number of communities can be included and random allocation of communities is usually not practicable; other methods are required to ensure that any differences found at the end of the study can be attributed to the intervention rather than to inherent differences between communities. Furthermore, it is difficult to isolate the communities where intervention is taking place from general social changes that may be occurring. Design limitations, especially in the face of unexpectedly large, favorable risk factor changes in control sites, are difficult to overcome. As a result, definitive conclusions about the overall effectiveness of the community-wide efforts are not always possible.

Example 30:

Vermandel, Weyer, De Wachter and Wyndaele (2008) did a randomized controlled trial among healthy young toddlers. They evaluated in a randomized way the comprehensive use of a daytime wetting alarm at home for 5 days in healthy children and compared it with timed potty training. Thirty-nine children, between 20 and 36 months of age, were randomized to wetting alarm diaper training (WAD-T; n=20) or timed potty training (TP-T; n=19). Toilet behavior was observed by parents and independent observers before, at the end, and after 2 weeks of training. Late evaluation at 1 month was done by telephone. The WAD-T group did significantly better than the TP-T group at the end training (p=.041), at 14 days (p=.027), and 1 month after training (p = .027). Independent bladder control was achieved in 88.9% of the WAD-T group.

SUMMARY

- Research design is the researcher's overall plan to obtain answer to the problem. In order to obtain solution to the problem, the researcher follows the best possible technique among the alternatives available.
- Research approach is a broad term which explains how a problem can be approached. Research design is a more specific term which explains how a problem is solved using a specific approach.
- A research design is the specification of methods and procedures for acquiring the information needed. It is the overall operational pattern or framework of the project that stipulates what information is to be collected from which source and by what procedures.
- Research approach may be quantitative, qualitative or pragmatic.
- Quantitative approach to research aims at quantifying the variables of a study. It includes the collection of data pertaining to research variables and converting it into numerical form in order to subject them to statistical analysis.

- Qualitative approach to research is associated with the understanding of the human behavior and experience. It is concerned with subjective assessment of attitudes, opinions and behavior.
- The pragmatic approach to science involves using the method which appears best suited to the research problem and not getting caught up in philosophical debates about which is the best approach.
- The features of good design are flexibility, appropriateness, efficiency and economical.
- The principles of experimental designs are principle of control, principle of manipulation and principle of randomization.
- The experimental designs are classified into pre experimental, true experimental and quasiexperimental designs.
- The historical method of investigations may be used to ascertain the meaning and reliability of past facts encountered in everyday life and in all disciplines. The main purpose of historical research is to arrive at an account of the past so as to gain a clearer perspective of the present.
- Descriptive research is also termed as 'normative research'. The aim of descriptive research is to design in such a way that it obtains precise information about a phenomena and also enables the researcher to draw general conclusion from the facts discovered.
- There are three types of descriptive studies. They are survey studies, interrelationship studies and developmental studies.
- Survey is a nonexperimental method where the investigator studies a community or a group of people for the purpose of examining the characteristics, opinions and orientations of the population.
- Research studies that help to establish relationships between facts that will provide a deeper insight into the phenomena are termed as 'interrelationship studies'. Casual comparative studies, correlation, prediction studies and cross-cultural and comparative studies are examples of interrelationship studies.
- Casual comparative studies are employed when a researcher cannot manipulate the independent variable and establish the controls that are required in experiments.
- Correlation studies are conducted to find out the nature and degree of relationship between the phenomena. Correlation refers to any kind of relationship between variables or phenomena; but in statistical analysis, it refers exclusively to quantifying the magnitude of the relationship between variables.
- Cross-cultural and comparative studies are conducted to compare the number of societies or communities or groups of people in terms of their cultural behaviors, practices, norms, values, traditions and folklores. This is to determine the behaviors whether they are culturally specific or common behavior.
- Developmental studies include growth studies and trend studies. Both longitudinal and cross-sectional techniques can be adopted to collect data and analyzed to identify trends and make predictions.
- Qualitative research designs are any kind of research that produces findings not arrived at by means of statistical procedures or other means of quantification. Qualitative research seeks to understand research problem from perspectives of the people being studied. It is effective in obtaining culturally specific information about values, opinions, behaviors and social contexts of particular populations.
- Grounded theory is a qualitative research approach used to explore the social processes that present within human interactions. The aim of grounded theory is to discover underlying social forces that shape human behavior. This method is used to construct theory where no theory exists or in situations where existing theory fails to explain a set of circumstances.

- Case study is about studying the peculiarities and the commonalities of a specific case. In case study, the researcher explores in depth a program, an event, an activity, a process, or one or more individuals.
- Ethnography is the work of describing culture. It is factual description and analysis of aspects of the way of life of a particular culture or sub-cultural group.
- Phenomenology is both a philosophy and a research experiences to generate and enhance the understanding of what it means to be human. Phenomenology is a way of viewing ourselves, others and everything else that comes in contact with our lives.
- Outcome analysis is an evaluation of what happens with regard to outcomes of interest after implementing a program or intervention, without using an experimental design to assess net effects.
- Epidemiological studies can be classified as either observational or experimental. Observational studies allow nature to take its course, the investigator measures but does not intervene. They include studies that can be called descriptive or analytical.
- A descriptive study is limited to a description of the occurrence of a disease in a population and is often the first step in an epidemiological investigation. An analytical study goes further by analyzing relationships between health status and other variables.
- The term 'cohort' has military roots. A cohort was a 300–600 men unit in the Roman army; ten cohorts formed a legion. The etymology of the term provides a useful mnemonic: a cohort study consists of bands or groups of persons marching forward in time from an exposure to one or more outcomes.
- Cohort studies are used to study incidence, causes, and prognosis. They measure events in chronological order which can be used to distinguish between cause and effect. These are the best methods for determining the incidence and natural history of a condition.
- Prospective cohort studies involve selection of a group of people who do not have the outcome of interest (for example, myocardial infarction). The investigator then measures a variety of variables that might be relevant to the development of the condition. Over a period of time, the people in the sample are observed to see whether they develop the outcome of interest (that is, myocardial infarction).
- Retrospective cohort uses data already collected for other purposes. The methodology is the same but the study is performed post hoc. The cohort is 'followed up' retrospectively.
- Case-control studies provide a relatively simple way to investigate causes of diseases, especially rare diseases. They include people with a disease (or other outcome variable) of interest and a suitable control (comparison or reference) group of people unaffected by the disease or outcome variable.
- Cross-sectional studies measure the prevalence of disease and, thus, are often called 'prevalence studies'. Cross-sectional studies are also used to infer causation.
- A randomized controlled trial is an epidemiological experiment designed to study the effects of a particular intervention, usually a treatment for a specific disease (clinical trial). Subjects in the study population are randomly allocated to intervention and control groups, and the results are assessed by comparing outcomes.

EXERCISE

- Identify the research design used in the below-mentioned context and state the reason.
  - A researcher selected one batch of girls studying in VII standard. A questionnaire on menstrual hygiene was given to them to assess their knowledge. Then self-

instructional module on menstrual hygiene was given to all girls and asked to read them. After 10 days, knowledge was assessed using the same questionnaire.

- In a hospital X, all nurses working in ICU were selected and their knowledge on management of ICU psychosis was assessed. Then structured teaching program was given to them. After 7 days, their knowledge was assessed.
- In a maternity ward of two hospitals, 30 primigravida women who were admitted for labor were selected from each hospital. For women in one hospital, olive oil back massage was given. For both the groups, pain and labor progress was assessed.
- Hospital A was compared with Hospital B for the nurses' job satisfaction. In hospital A, all staff nurses were given additional benefits in addition to their increment. In hospital B, all nurses were given only the increment. The nurse's job satisfaction was assessed twice, that is, after 3 months and after 6 months of increment.
- In a research study, children with cough and cold were selected and were given polyherbal formulation for the management of cough and cold. Their recovery and prognosis were compared with the group of children who received standard care for cough and cold.
- In a dialysis unit in a hospital, 60 samples were selected and assigned to two groups using simple random sampling technique. For one group of patients along with routine care, stretch exercises were prescribed and they were asked to perform during dialysis. For both the groups, information on the development of leg cramps and the pain was assessed.
- In a secondary care stroke unit, 60 samples with the diagnosis of stroke were selected and randomly assigned to two groups. One group was given the standard care by the secondary care unit and the other group was given care based on the stroke specialist's recommendation through telemedicine. Both the groups were followed and assessment was done on their progress at discharge, after one month and 6 months respectively.
- In a postoperative ward, 60 children were selected and they were randomly assigned to two groups and also matched for age and gender. One group of children were given selected nonpharmacologic pain management intervention in addition to standard pain management therapy. The other group was given only the standard pain management therapy. Both the groups were compared for their level of pain, progress, length of hospital stay and any morbidity.
- In an elderly home, 80 elderly women and men were selected and they were randomly assigned to two groups and matched for their age, gender, any physical illness. One group was given selected physical intervention program for one month. At the end of one month, general well-being, flexibility and mobility was assessed for all samples.
- In a research, 100 students studying in polytechnic college were selected and were randomly assigned to two groups. Both the groups were given questionnaire to assess the knowledge on Cardiopulmonary Resuscitation. Then for one group, video-assisted teaching program was given on cardiopulmonary resuscitation. For both the groups, knowledge on cardiopulmonary resuscitation was assessed after 7 days.
- In a village, adolescent girls with mild anemia were selected and were randomly assigned to two groups. For one group, nutritional supplementation in addition to iron and folic acid therapy was given. For the other group, only iron and folic acid therapy was given. After one month, for both the groups, hemoglobin was checked.

- A research selected 90 patients who were diagnosed with asthma and assigned to three groups by simple random sampling technique. For group A, quality of life was assessed and selected interventions along with routine care were given for one month. For group C, intervention was given for one month followed by quality of life assessed. For group B, quality of life was assessed on the same period as that of group A and C.
- In a study, a group of adults with *diabetes mellitus* were selected and were asked to perform moderate physical exercises for 30 minutes once a day for two weeks and twice a day for two weeks. Then they asked to perform selected yoga for 30 minutes once a day for two weeks and twice a day for two weeks. Their blood glucose levels were assessed on alternative days in the morning and evening and the results were compared for four variations.
- In a research, two class students' performance in research and statistics subjects was compared. Individual student's existing cumulative performance in research and statistics subject was calculated. One group/class was given extended coaching on few selected topics under teacher supervision. The other group was given regular coaching on the same selected topics. For both the groups, test was conducted and the results were compared.
- In a research study, patient-centered rehabilitation model was evaluated. 146 patients aged 65 and older with hip fracture participated as patients in the usual care (70) and intervention (patient-centered rehabilitation) group (76). Patient mobility was assessed at admission and discharge.
- In a research study, a group of adolescents who scored high on risk behavior inventory were selected and their baseline risk scores were calculated. They were given group counseling twice with the duration of one month. Their risk behaviors were assessed using the same inventory after 1, 6, 12 and 24 months.
- In a research study, adolescent girls residing at two villages were selected. In both the villages, their dietary intake was assessed. Their height, weight, body mass index (BMI) were also checked for two times with a gap of one month in between. In one village, special nutrition education program was given by the peer educators. For both the groups, dietary intake, height, weight, and BMI were assessed after 3, 6 and 9 months respectively.
- In a study, the researcher assessed the knowledge, attitude and practice of 50 antenatal mothers regarding antenatal exercise in a selected maternity hospital in Chennai.
- In a study, a researcher collected data from adolescents on their violent video game playing habits and level of aggression on aggression inventory with the aim to find correlation between these two. A study was conducted to assess the difficulties in meeting activities of daily living among old-age people residing at the selected old-age home in Chennai.
- The investigator attempted to study the experiential structures of suicidality and of self-determined behavior and tried to describe the possible forms and scopes of lived self-determination in suicidal mental life from the first-person perspective.
- A study was conducted to explore the experiences of the undergraduate students when they come face-to-face with cancer care during their clinical placements. The main objective was to help nursing students understand and interpret their experience. The reflective diaries were used to elicit the research data with a narrative approach (unstructured recordings) that emphasized on the description of the experience through the use of 'texts'.

- The opinions and experiences of directors of nursing in both Ireland and the source countries, as well as the personal experiences and opinions of the overseas nurses themselves, currently working in place X were collected. The aim of this paper is to establish the perceptions and opinions of those involved in the recruitment process on their role and the effects recruitment has on both source and destination countries. Data were collected through in-depth interviews All interviews were audio-taped and transcribed verbatim. A 'bottom up' approach to coding was used. Five main themes were identified: migratory intentions, the effects of recruitment/migration, workforce diversity, alternatives to recruitment, and compensation.
- A study was conducted among health professionals, including nurses, pediatricians and assistant nurses, of their work at a NICU in place X. The aim was to understand how health professionals, who work under stressful conditions in an ethically sensitive ward, can counteract the negative sides of work to such a degree that they experience happiness. The collection of data was based on the fieldwork, and the methods used were participant observation and semi-structured interviews. The professionals evaluated their well-being in line with conventional definitions of happiness.

6 Population and Sample

OBJECTIVES

After reading this chapter, you will be able to:

- State the meaning and definition of population and sample
- List the factors influencing sampling
- List the steps in sampling
- Explain various sampling techniques used in nursing research
- Explain the estimation of sample size for a research study
- List the problems in sampling.
- Explain the probability and sampling error.

INTRODUCTION

Population is generally a large collection of individuals or objects that is the main focus of a scientific query. It is for the benefit of the population that researches are done. Collection of data is an essential part of the research process. In order to collect data for any research problem the researcher has to select a representative sample from the population so as to enable him to draw conclusions from the sample, which will hold good for the population. A sample is selected since it is neither possible nor feasible to gather data for the whole population. By correctly drawing a sample from a specific population, a researcher can analyze the sample and make inferences about population characteristics. However, due to the large sizes of populations, researchers often cannot test every individual in the population because it is too expensive and time-consuming. If the sample is representative of the population from which it is drawn, the researcher can have confidence in concluding that the results are generalizable to the entire population. Sampling is done to save time and money.

Meaning and Definition of Universe, Population and Sample

'Universe' refers to the total of the items or units in any field of inquiry, whereas the term 'population' refers to the total of items about which information is desired. Population is any collection or aggregate of specified group of human beings or non human entities such as objects, time units and others. Thus, all units in any field of inquiry constitute universe and all elementary units (on the basis of one characteristic or more) constitute population. In practice, these two terms such as population and universe, are taken as interchangeable. However, a researcher must necessarily define these terms precisely. Population is the entire group whom you want to generalize the research finding. For example if you want to study the morbidity and mortality pattern of children with Leukemia in Tamil Nadu, the population might be defined as all children with Leukemia in Tamil Nadu. The population may be finite or infinite.

The number of units constituting the population is called the size of population. For example, in the study of socioeconomic conditions of a particular village, all families or houses in the village will be a population. A population comprises all possible cases (persons, objects, events) that constitute a known whole. The population or universe can be finite or infinite. The population is said to be finite if it consists of a fixed number of elements so that it is possible to enumerate it in its totality. For instance, the population of a city, the number of nurses working in Government sectors are examples of finite populations. The symbol 'N' is generally used to indicate how many elements (or items) are there in case of a finite elements.

Types of Population

Finite vs Infinite Population

A population containing a finite number of units, individuals, or member is called a 'finite population' (e.g. the students studying a particular college).

A population containing a infinite number of units, individuals or members is called 'infinite population' (e.g. all stars in the sky). The infinite population cannot be counted.

Real (or) Existent vs Hypothetical Population

Real population: In real population, all potential observations are possible and accessible at the time of sampling. This is otherwise known as existent population which is the population of concrete individuals. Example, Weight of all students in a college.

Conceptual/hypothetical population: It is a population which does not physically exist or potential observations are not accessible at the time of sampling is referred to as the hypothetical population. For example, all possible values of tomorrow's highest temperature or all possible new cases of diabetes mellitus in the next year.

Target Population vs Accessible Population

Target population refers to the entire group of individuals or objects to which researchers are interested in generalizing the conclusions. The target population usually has varying characteristics and it is also known as the 'theoretical population'. For example, we may want to study the problems of adolescents in Chennai. In this case, the target population may be all those adolescents residing at Chennai is our population.

The accessible population is the population in research to which the researchers can apply their conclusions. This population is a subset of the target population and is also known as the 'study population'. It is from the accessible population that researchers draw their samples. For example, in the study of problems of adolescents in Chennai, the researcher may have access to adolescents studying in 8 schools in Chennai. In this case, the adolescents studying in the selected 8 schools in Chennai is the accessible population. Accessible population is feasible for the researcher to access. In a research, the researcher would like to study the children with Leukemia, he cannot have access to all children with Leukemia. He may have access to children who are attending OPD or In patient department of few hospitals. Any of the clients at these few hospitals would constitute the accessible population for the study.

Sample

The sample refers to those individuals or units or elements who are selected for a study. A sample is simply a subset of the population. The concept of sample arises from the inability of the researchers to test all the individuals in a given population. The sample must be representative of the population from which it was drawn and it must have good size to warrant statistical analysis.

According to Goode and Hatt, "A sample as the name applies, is a smaller representative of a large whole". According to Pauline V Young, "A statistical sample is a miniature of cross selection of the entire group or aggregate from which the sample is taken". A sample is a part of the population from which it was drawn.

Sampling

Sampling is the process of selection of samples from a population. According to Bogardus, "Sampling is the selection of certain percentage of a group of items according to a context of funds available for the research study'. It should be such that the results of sample study can be applied, in general, for the universe with a reasonable level of confidence. It should result in small sampling error. Sampling is the process of selecting a group of subjects for a study in such a way that the individuals represent the larger group from which they were selected. This representative portion of a population is called as sample. Sampling may involve the selection of people, events, organizations, periods of time, record and many other phenomena of concern to the field of nursing.

Sampling Frame

Sampling frame is a list of all elements of the population and it is the list from which we draw a sample. Sampling frame can be prepared for the finite population whereas it is impossible in infinite population. The elementary units or the group or cluster of such units may form the basis of sampling process in which case they are called ***sampling*** units is known as ***sampling frame***. Thus sampling frame consists of a list of items from which the sample is to be drawn. If the population is finite and the time frame is in the present or past, then it is possible for the frame to be identical with the population. In most cases they are not identical because it is often impossible to draw a sample directly from population. As such this frame is either constructed by a researcher for the purpose of his study or may consist of some existing list of the population. For instance, one can use telephone directory as a frame for conducting opinion survey in a city. Whatever the frame may be, it should be a good representative of the population.

Ideally, the sampling frame and the population are identical. But practically, it is not possible to include all the units of the population. We may omit few elements or it may be an incomplete list. The goal is to get accurate sampling frame list as much as possible.

Sampling Design or Sampling Technique

A sample design is a definite plan for obtaining a sample from the sampling frame. It refers to the technique or the procedure the researcher would adopt in selecting some sampling units from which inferences about the population is drawn. Sampling design is determined before any data are collected. There are two major types of sampling techniques. They are probability and non probability sampling technique.

Factors to be Considered in Selecting Samples and Sampling

- ***Type of universe:*** A researcher must decide whether the universe is finite or infinite. In case of finite population, preparation of sampling frame is possible. Sampling frame facilitates the job of the researcher in selecting the samples for the study
- ***Sample frame:*** It contains the names or lists of all items of a universe. It should be a representative of the population and should be appropriate, reliable, correct and comprehensive.
- ***Sample unit:*** It is to be decided before selecting the sample. Sampling units may be geographical, constructional, social and individual.
- ***Sample size:*** This refers to the number of items to be selected from a universe to form a sample. Sample size should not be very large or too small. It should fulfill the requirements of reliability, efficiency, flexibility and representativeness. While deciding the size of sample, the researcher must consider the population size, the parameter of interest in research study and the budgetary constraints.
- ***Parameters of interest:*** While determining a sample design, the specific population parameters, which are of interest, must be taken into account by the researcher. For instance, the researcher may be interested in estimating the portion of persons with some characteristic in the population or he may be interested in knowing some average or the other measures concerning the population. A sample design is generally affected by all this. Suppose one may like to study the individuals with rare form of cancers in which case availability of samples itself is very limited.

- ***Budgetary constraints:*** The size as well as the type of sample depends upon the cost consideration.
- ***Sampling procedure:*** Finally the researcher must decide about the techniques to be used in selecting the items for the sample, i.e. he must decide the type of sample. This technique stands for the sample design itself. He should select the sample design in such a way that for a given sample size and for a given cost, the sample design has a smaller sampling error.

Significance (Reason) of Using Sampling

- ***Scientific base:*** It is scientific because the conclusion derived from the study of certain units can be verified from other units. By taking random sample, we can determine the amount of deviation from the norm.
- ***Economy:*** The sampling technique is much less expensive, much less time consuming than the census technique. Sampling can save time and money. A sample study is usually less expensive than a census study and produces results at a relatively faster speed.
- ***Reliability:*** If the choice of sample unit is made with due care and the matter under survey is not heterogeneous, the conclusion of the sample survey can have almost the same reliability as those of census survey.
- ***Detailed study:*** Since the number of sample units is fairly small, these can be studied intensively and elaborately. They can be examined from multiple views.
- ***Greater suitability in most situations:*** Most of the surveys are made by the techniques of sample survey, because whenever the matter is of homogeneous nature, the examination of few units suffices.
- ***Speed:*** The data can be collected and summarized more quickly by studying a sample than by studying the entire universe.
- ***Practicability:*** When the universe is extremely large, sampling is the only practical method for analysis. Sampling remains the only way when population contains infinitely many members. Sampling remains the only choice when a test involves the destruction of the item under study.
- ***Estimation of sampling errors:*** Sampling usually enables to estimate the sampling errors and, thus, assists in obtaining information concerning some characteristic of the population.

Characteristics of Sampling

- Sample design should be such, so that systematic bias can be controlled in a better way
- It should result in a truly representative sample
- It should be viable in the context of funds available for the research study
- It should be such that the results of sample study can be applied, in general, for the universe with a reasonable level of confidence
- It should result in small sampling error.

Steps in Sampling

- Identify the target population
- Identify the accessible population
- Specify sampling frame
- Determine the size of the sample
- Decide sampling plan
- Select the sample.

Sampling Techniques

There are various types of sampling techniques. Basically, they are classified as probability and non probability sampling techniques (Fig. 6.1).

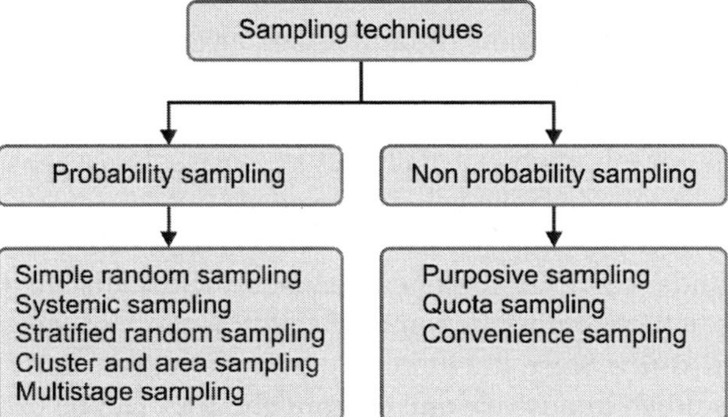

Fig. 6.1: Classification of sampling techniques

Probability Sampling Techniques

In this, every item has equal chance of being included in the sample. It is a lottery method in which individual units are picked up from the whole group by some mechanical process and not deliberately. The results obtained can be assured in terms of probability, i.e. the error of estimation or the significance of results obtained can be measured. Random sampling ensures the law of statistical regulatory which states that if on an average the sample chosen is a random one, the sample will have the same composition and characteristics as the universe. That is why this sampling is considered as the best techniques of selecting a representative sample.

Simple Random Sampling

This type of sampling is also known as chance sampling or probability sampling where each and every item in the population has an equal chance of inclusion in the sample.

Lottery method: In this the number of data are written on sheet of paper and they are thrown into a box. Now a casual observer selects the number of item required in the sample. For this method, it is necessary that sheet of paper should be of equal dimensions. For example, if we have to select a sample of 100 items from a universe of 1,000 items, then we can put the names or numbers of all the 1,000 items on slips of paper and conduct a lottery. Using the random number tables is another method of random sampling. To select the sample, each item is assigned a number from 1–1,000. Then, 100 random numbers are selected from the random table. Since the numbers were placed in the table in a completely random fashion, the resulting sample is random. This procedure gives each item an equal probability of being selected. In case of infinite population, the selection of each item in a random sample is controlled by the same probability and that successive selections are independent of one another.

Advantages

- Due to impartiality, there is possibility of selecting any unit as sample
- Units have the characteristic of universe, hence units are more representative
- Simplicity of method makes no possibility of error
- Error can be known easily
- It saves money, time and labor.

Disadvantages

- The selector has no control over the selection of units. The researcher cannot contact the far situated units
- He cannot prepare the whole field when the universe is vast
- If units have no homogeneity, the method is not appropriate
- There is no question of alternatives. The selected units cannot be replaced or changed.

Systematic Sampling

In some instances the most practical way of sampling is to select every 1st, say example, 10th name on a list, every 10th house on one side of a street and so on. Sampling of this type is known as systematic sampling. An element of randomness is usually introduced into this kind of sampling by using random numbers to pick up the unit with which to start. This procedure is useful when sampling frame is available in the form of a list. In such a design the selection process starts by picking some random point in the list and then every nth element is selected until the desired number is secured.

Advantages

- It can be taken as an improvement over a simple random sampling
- It is an easier and less costlier method of sampling and can be conveniently used even in case of large populations.

Disadvantages

If there is a hidden periodicity in the population, systematic sampling will prove to be an inefficient method. For example, if we take every 4th piece of thermometer in a production unit which is defective, we will get all defective thermometer as our samples.

Stratified Sampling

If the population from which a sample is to be drawn does not constitute a homogeneous group, then stratified sampling technique is applied so as to obtain a representative sample. In this technique, the population is stratified into a number of non overlapping subpopulations or strata and sample items are selected from each stratum. If the items selected from each stratum is based on simple random sampling, the entire procedure, first stratification and then simple random sampling, is known as stratified random sampling.

Process of stratifying: The stratification of domain or data should be with great care, because the success of the technique depends upon successful stratification. Following points should be kept in mind:

- We should process extensive information of all items included in a domain and should know which item make a coherent whole on the basis of similar traits and which others are different from them and why?
- The size of each stratum should be large to enable the use of random sampling technique.
- In stratifying, it must be kept in mind that various strata should have similar relation to the domain and should be themselves homogeneous.
- The various strata which differ from each other should be the same as the proportion of stratum from the domain. Suppose a domain has four strata, accordingly the proportion of each stratum of domain is ¼. Now if the number of total items of the sample is 64, we shall select 16 items from each stratum and thus the proportion of selected items from each stratum will be ¼.

The strata may be formed on the basis of common characteristics of the items to be put in each stratum. This means that various strata be formed in such a way as to ensure elements being most homogeneous within each stratum and most heterogeneous between the different strata. Thus, strata are purposively formed and are usually based on past experience and personal judgment of the researcher. From the strata, samples can be selected using simple random sampling technique or systematic sampling technique. Regarding the number of samples to be selected from each strata, a proportionate sampling can be done, i.e. the samples from different strata are kept proportional to the sizes of the strata.

Example 1:

Suppose, if we want to select 50 samples from 6000 population which is divided into 3 strata of 1000, 2000 and 3000 then the proportionate sample can be selected from each strata as follows:

The number of sample to be selected from the strata one = $\frac{1000}{6000} \times 50 = 8.3 = 8$

The number of sample to be selected from the strata two = $\frac{2000}{6000} \times 50 = 16.66 = 17$

The number of sample to be selected from the strata three = $\frac{3000}{6000} \times 50 = 25$

The total sample size = 8 + 17 + 25 = 50

Proportional allocation is considered most efficient and an optimal design when the cost of selecting an item is equal for each stratum, there is no differences in within stratum variances. But in case if we want to compare the strata, then we have to select equal number of samples from each stratum even if it differs in size.

Advantages

- Neither group nor class of importance is totally neglected as units of each are represented in the sample
- If different classes are divided properly, selection of few units represents the whole group
- On the classification of regional basis, units are not in contact easily. This leads to economy of time and money
- There is a facility in substitution of units. If someone is not contacted easily, the other person of the same class can be substituted for him. Such inclusion will not show any contradicting result.

Disadvantages

- The sample does not become representative if selected sample has more or less units of a class
- If the sizes of different group are different, no equal proportional quality can be viewed
- Non-proportional selection leads to more emphasis in the end. During such time researcher can be biased, hence samples will not be a representative
- If group is not expressed properly, the difficulty is seen about the unit to be kept under which group or class.

Cluster Sampling

Cluster sampling involves grouping the population and then selecting the groups or the clusters rather than individual elements for inclusion in the sample. Suppose a college wishes to sample its alumni members for some purpose and if it has 20,000 alumni members, and the sample size is to be kept say 200. For cluster sampling this list of 20,000 students could be formed into 10 clusters of 100 students each. Two clusters might then be selected for the sample randomly. The clustering approach can, however, make the sampling procedure relatively easier and increase the efficiency of field work, especially in the case of personal interviews.

Advantages

- It is no doubt, reduces cost by concentrating surveys in selected clusters. Cluster sampling is used only because of the economic advantage it possesses; estimates based on cluster samples are usually more reliable per unit cost
- The ***disadvantage*** is that it is less precise than random sampling.

Area Sampling

It is quite close to cluster sampling and is often talked about when the total geographical area of interest happens to be big one. Under area sampling we first divide the total area into a number of smaller non-overlapping areas, generally called 'geographical clusters', then a number of these smaller areas are randomly selected, and all units in these small areas are included in the sample. Area sampling is especially helpful where we do not have the list of the population concerned. It also makes the field interviewing more efficient since interviewer can do many interviews at each location.

Multi-stage Sampling

This is a further development of the idea of cluster sampling. This technique is meant for big inquiries extending to a considerably large geographical area like an entire country. Under multi-stage sampling the first stage may be to select large primary sampling units such as states, then districts, then towns and finally certain families within towns. If the technique of random-sampling is applied at all stages, the sampling procedure is described as multi-stage random sampling.

Non Probability Sampling Techniques

This procedure does not afford any basis for estimating the probability that each item in the population has been included in the sample. Deliberate sampling, purposive sampling and judgment sampling are non probability sampling methods. In this type of sampling, there is always a danger of entering personal element into the selection of the sample. The investigator may select a sample which will yield results favorable to his point of view. If such things happen, then the entire inquiry may get spoiled. If the investigator is impartial, and if work without bias, then the results of selected sample may be tolerably reliable. The sampling error cannot be estimated in this method.

Purposive Sampling

It is otherwise known as deliberate sampling. In this method the investigator has complete freedom to choose his sample according to his wishes and desire. This sampling method involves purposive or deliberate selection of particular units of the universe for constituting a sample which represents the universe. To choose or leave an item for the purpose of study depends entirely upon the wishes of investigator and he will chose items or units which in his judgment are representative of the whole data. This is a very simple technique of choosing the samples and is useful in cases where the whole data is homogeneous and the investigator has full knowledge of the various aspects of the problem.

Judgment Sampling

Purposive sampling is otherwise known as judgmental sampling, uses the researcher's expertise and knowledge of the population to hand pick the cases to be included in the sample. The researcher usually selects participants who are considered to be typical of the population of interest.

In judgment sampling the researcher's judgment is used for selecting items which he considers as representative of the population. For example, a judgment sample of mothers of children with autism might be taken to study their coping strategies. Judgment sampling is used quite frequently in qualitative research where the desire happens to be to develop hypotheses rather than to generalize to larger populations.

Expert Sampling

Expert sampling is a type of purposive sampling used in Delphi technique. Sample of experts on a particular phenomena is selected based on the belief that they are the expertise in those field.

Convenience Sampling

Convenience samples involve selection on the basis of ease or convenience. When population elements are selected for inclusion in the sample based on the ease of access, it can be called 'convenience sampling'. At times such a procedure may give very biased results particularly when the population is not homogeneous.

Advantages

- More representation is possible in this method
- As sample is small in size, the method is less expensive and less time consuming
- The utility of this method increases when few units of universe have special importance
- When units are less in number, sample is profitable.

Disadvantages

- Units are selected by researcher at his will. Hence sample is biased
- The error of the sample cannot be detected
- Researcher is unable to understand the whole group
- Those hypotheses on which inference of error of sample is attributed, are less used.

Quota Sampling

In stratified sampling the cost of taking random samples from individual strata is often so expensive that interviewers are simply given quota to be filled from different strata, the actual selection of items for sample being left to the interviewer's judgment. This is called 'quota sampling'. The size of the quota for each stratum is generally proportionate to the size of that stratum in the population. Quota sampling is thus an important form of non-probability sampling. Quota samples generally happen to be judgment samples rather than random samples.

In practice, several of the methods of sampling described above may well be used in the same study in which case it can be called 'mixed sampling'. It may be pointed out here that normally one should resort to random sampling so that bias can be eliminated and sampling error can be estimated. But purposive sampling is considered desirable when the universe happens to be small and a known characteristic of it is to be studied intensively. Also, there are conditions under which sample designs other than random sampling may be considered better for reasons like convenience and low costs. The sample design to be used must be decided by the researcher taking into consideration the objectives, availability and feasibility, time and the cooperation of the others.

Deciding on the Size of the Sample

The usual question that many researcher asks is 'How big should my sample be?' Using as large a sample as possible is better. The reason is larger the sample, the better it represents the population. But if the sample size is too large, then the value of sampling—reducing time and cost of the study—is negligible. Then what is the minimum number of subjects to study effectively? The size of the samples depends on certain factors. They are:

- Availability of resources
- Cost
- Accuracy
- Nature of research
- Method of sampling
- Homogeneity of the population.

L R Gay suggests 10% of large populations and 20% of small populations as minimums.

Dr John Curry, Professor of Educational Research, North Texas State University (now retired), provided his research students (fall, 1984) with the 'rule of thumb' on sample size.

Size of population	Sampling percent (%)
0–100	100
101–1,000	10
1,001–5,000	5
5,001–10,000	3
10,000+	1

Factors to be Considered in Determining the Sample Size

Size of the sample should be determined by a researcher keeping in view the following points:

- ***Nature of universe:*** Universe may be either homogenous or heterogeneous in nature. If the items of the universe are homogenous, a small sample can serve the purpose. But if the items are heterogeneous, a large sample would be required. Technically, this can be termed as the dispersion factor.

- ***Number of classes proposed:*** If many class-groups (groups and sub-groups) are to be formed, a large sample would be required because a small sample might not be able to give a reasonable number of items in each class-group.
- ***Nature of study:*** If items are to be intensively and continuously studied, the sample should be small. For a general survey, the size of the sample should be large, but a small sample is considered appropriate in technical survey.
- ***Type of sampling:*** Sampling technique plays an important part in determining the size of the sample. A small random sample is apt to be much superior to a larger but badly selected sample.
- ***Probability value or alpha level:*** In general, we keep the alpha value as 0.05. When it is small, we need larger sample where as when it is large, we need smaller sample.
- ***Standard of accuracy and acceptable confidence level:*** If the standard of accuracy or the level of precision is to be kept high, we shall require relatively larger sample. For doubling the accuracy for a fixed significance level, the sample size has to be increased fourfold.
- ***Power of the study:*** When we keep the power of the study low, we need lesser sample, whereas when we keep the power of the study high, we need large sample.
- ***Alternative hypothesis:*** When alternative hypothesis is one sided, we need small sample whereas if it is two sided, we may need, larger sample size.
- ***Effect size:*** To detect even smaller effect size, we need large sample whereas to detect large effect size, we need less sample. Effects are harder to detect in smaller samples. Increasing sample size is often the easiest way to boost the statistical power of a test.
- ***Availability of finance:*** In practice, size of the sample depends upon the amount of money available for the study purposes. This factor should be kept in view while determining the size of sample. Large samples result in increasing the cost of sampling estimates.
- ***Other considerations:*** Nature of units, size of the population, size of questionnaire, availability of trained investigators, the conditions under which the research is being conducted, the time available for completion of the study are a few other considerations to which a researcher must pay attention while selecting the size of the sample.

Estimation of Sample Size

Method 1: Calculation of Sample Size for a Ratio Level Variable

There is no simple rule to determine the appropriate sample size for a study. If someone says that the sample size should be 10% of the population, the advice may not be sound. Sample size determination depends on the number of factors. A general guideline is the larger the sample, the more accurate the findings. This is because a larger sample is more likely to be a representative of the population. A second guideline is the more heterogeneous the population, the larger the sample required. In a homogeneous population, the variability is very less so that one can go for lesser sample size. According to Gillis A and Jackson W (2002) the steps in calculation of sample size as follows:

Step 1: ***Decide on the confident level*** with which you want to prove or find something. In general we use the 95% confidence level. With this level, you can be confident that your sample mean will be within a given precision, 19 out of 20 times.

Step 2: ***Select the major variable to be measured.*** Normally the dependent variable is taken into consideration for the determination of sample size. Estimate the population standard deviation for this variable. This gives the idea about the homogeneity or heterogeneity of the population. Larger the standard deviation, more heterogeneous is the population. Smaller the standard deviation, homogenous is the population. Standard deviation gives idea about the variability of the population which helps us to consider to include the variability. The standard deviation of the particular variable can be found from the previous studies, surveys and at times common sense estimation will be of helpful.

Another suggestion for estimating an unknown population standard deviation is to approximate it by taking the range of values and dividing it by two (excluding the extreme values). At the same time one must understand that a study involving a larger number of variables, it is impossible to make claims with any certainty about the precision of all the variables.

Step 3: ***Determine the precision that would be acceptable.*** Suppose we can estimate the effectiveness within two percentage points of true value (effectiveness) or if we want to predict the weight of the children within a kg of true mean weight

Step 4: ***Compute the sample size. Ratio level measurement***

$$\text{Required sample size} = \left[\frac{(\text{Confidence limit})(\sigma_p)}{\text{Accuracy}}\right]^2$$

Example 2:

Suppose we want to estimate the sample size required to estimate the average weight of the newborn in Chennai. We fix 95% confidence level (Z = 1.96) and be within 0.2 kg of estimating the true weight. The estimated standard deviation of the population is 1.1 kg. The values can be substituted in the equation, as given below

$$\text{Required sample size} = \left[\frac{(\text{Confidence limit})(\sigma_p)}{\text{Accuracy}}\right]^2 = \left[\frac{(95\%)(1.1)}{0.2}\right]^2$$

$$= \left[\frac{1.96 \times 1.1}{0.2}\right]^2 = \left[\frac{2.156}{0.2}\right]^2 = (10.78)^2 = 116.2 = 116$$

Step 5: ***Compute the sampling fraction:*** The sampling fraction is the sample size in relation to the population.

Suppose if we have 10000 newborn population of newborn in a particular year and a sample of 116, the sampling fraction would be:

Sampling fraction = Sample size/Population = 116/10000 = 0.0116 = 1.16%

If the sampling fraction is less than 5% we have to question our self whether this sample size is adequate for complex statistical analysis especially when we go for cross tabulation. Whether each cell will have adequate frequency so as perform statistical analysis. In that case we should think of increasing the sample size.

If sampling fraction is more than 5% of the population, if $N = 1000$, we have to make an adjustment in our sample size. The required sample size may be reduced according to the following formula

$$\text{Adjusted sample size} = \frac{n}{\left(1+\frac{n}{N}\right)} = \frac{116}{\left(1+\frac{116}{1000}\right)} = \frac{116}{1+0.116} = \frac{116}{(1.116)}$$

$$= 103.9 = 104 \text{ samples.}$$

Gillis A and Jackson W (2002).

Method 2: **Calculation of Sample Size for a Nominal Level Variable**

Step 1: ***Decide on the confident level*** with which you want to prove or find something. In general we use the 95% confidence level. With this level, you can be confident that your sample mean will be within a given precision, 19 out of 20 times.

Step 2: ***Select the major variable to be measured***. The major variable may be to estimate the proportion of children attending integrated child development services (ICDS) program.

Step 3: ***Determine the precision that would be acceptable***. Suppose we can estimate the proportion of children attending the ICDS within 2% of its true percentage.

Step 4: ***Compute the sample size. Nominal level measurement***

$$\text{Required sample size} = \frac{(\text{Success})\times(\text{Failure})\times(\text{Confidence limit Z value})}{\text{Accuracy}^2}$$

Success = Proportion of children attending ICDS
Failure = 1 – p, i.e. proportion of children not attending ICDS
Confidence limit = Z score for 95%
Accuracy is the range within which we want the estimate to be.

Example 3:

Suppose we may predict that success (p) = 70%; failure = 30% and accuracy is 2%, the sample size can be calculated at 95% of confidence limit as follows:

$$\text{Required sample size} = \frac{(0.7)\times(0.3)\times(1.96)^2}{(0.02)^2} = \frac{(0.7)\times(0.3)\times 3.84}{0.0004} = \frac{0.8067}{0.0004} = 2016$$

Sample size = 2016.

Method 3:

Example 4:

A researcher is interested in determining the rate of milk usage per household in a city. She believes that yearly consumption per household is normally distributed with an unknown mean and a standard deviation of about 2 liters. How large a sample she should take in order to be 95% certain that the sample mean is within one half liter of the population mean? She would like to estimate with accuracy of one half liter difference between the sample and population mean.

The calculation of sample size is as follows:

$$\text{Allowable error} = e = z\frac{\sigma}{\sqrt{N}}$$

$$e = z\frac{\sigma}{\sqrt{N}} = (0.5) = \frac{1.96 \times 2}{\sqrt{N}}$$

$$(0.5)^2 = \frac{(3.92)^2}{N} = 0.25 = \frac{15.37}{N}$$

$$0.25\,N = 15.37$$

$$N = \frac{15.37}{0.25} = 61.48 = 62 \text{ households.}$$

Example 5:

A tooth paste manufacturer wants to know how much a resident of a hostel of a certain college spends annually on tooth paste. The company wants this estimate to be correct within plus or minus ₹ 2 of the real expenditure at 95% confidence. It is known that a student's annual expenditure on tooth paste is ₹ 120 and he bought a total of 6 numbers. How much sample does he requires to achieve an above end?

Standard deviation can be calculated as follows:

$$= \frac{120}{6} = 20$$

$$\text{Allowable error} = e = z\frac{\sigma}{\sqrt{N}}$$

$$e = z\frac{\sigma}{\sqrt{N}} = (2) = \frac{1.96 \times 20}{\sqrt{N}}$$

$$(2)^2 = \frac{(39.2)^2}{N} = 4 = \frac{1536.64}{N}$$

$$4N = 1536$$

$$N = \frac{1536}{4} = 384 \text{ students.}$$

Example 6:

On a casual inspection of a batch of students, we find 15% as anemic and so we wish to know the size of sample to determine p, the percentage of anemic students in the population within 5% of the true value with 95% degree of confidence.
If the quantity to be estimated is a binomial distribution, the allowable error, e, for any given confidence probability is?

$$e = z\sqrt{\frac{pq}{N}} = e^2 = (z)^2\frac{pq}{N}$$

$$e^2 = \frac{(z)^2 pq}{N}$$

$$N = \frac{(z)^2 pq}{e^2}$$

Applying the value in the above formula,

$$N = \frac{(1.96)^2 15\times 85}{5\times 5} = \frac{3.84\times 1275}{25} = \frac{4896}{25}$$

$$= 195.84 = 196 \text{ students}$$

POWER ANALYSIS

Power analysis is now integral to the health and behavioral sciences, and its use is steadily increasing whenever the empirical studies are performed. Power of the study, is the probability of detecting a predefined clinical significance. The ideal study is the one, which has high power. This means that the study has a high chance of detecting a difference between groups if it exists, consequently, if the study demonstrates no difference between the groups, the researcher can reasonably confident in concluding that none exists. The ideal power for any study is considered to be 80%.

The power of a statistical test is the probability that the test will reject the null hypothesis when the alternative hypothesis is true, i.e. the probability of not committing a Type II error. Statistical power is the probability of rejecting the null hypothesis when the null hypothesis is false. As the power increases, the chances of a Type II error occurring decrease and the power is equal to $1-\beta$. The power is also known as the sensitivity of the test. Although there are no formal standards for power (sometimes referred to as π), most researchers assess the power of their tests using $\pi = 0.80$ as a standard for adequacy (Table 6.1). This convention implies a four-to-one trade off between β-risk and α-risk. (β is the probability of a Type II error; α is the probability of a Type I error, 0.2 and 0.05 are conventional values for β and α).

Table 6.1: Statistical power

$Z_{1-\beta}$	Power
0.80	0.84
0.85	1.03
0.90	1.28
0.95	1.64
0.99	2.33

Why Should we do Power Analysis?

- It is used to calculate the minimum sample size required
- It can also be used to calculate the minimum effect size that is likely to be detected in a study using a given sample size
- It is used to make comparisons between different statistical testing procedures: for example, between a parametric and a non parametric test of the same hypothesis
- It is used to assess the probability of rejecting the null when the null is true.

When to do Power Analysis?

'Power analysis' can either be done before (*a priori* or prospective power analysis) or after (*post-hoc* or retrospective power analysis) data are collected.

- ***Priori power analysis:*** It is conducted prior to the research study, and is typically used in calculation of sample size to achieve adequate power. The prospective power analysis for experimental studies are universally accepted.
- ***Post-hoc power analysis:*** It is conducted after a study has been completed, and uses the obtained sample size and effect size to determine what the power was in the study, assuming the effect size in the sample is equal to the effect size in the population. There is a controversy in doing retrospective power analysis. The post-hoc power analysis occurs when the result turns out to be non-significant. In this case, statistical power is calculated to verify whether the non-significance result is due to lack of relationship between the groups or due to lack of statistical power.

Factors Influencing the Statistical Power

- Level of significance
- Effect size of the variable of interest in the population
- Sample size
- Precision
- Design of the study
- Outcome variable
- Variance or standard deviation

Level of Significance or Alpha

The definition of alpha is the probability of detecting a significant difference when the treatments are equally effective or risk of false positive findings. In general, we fix the level of significance as 0.05 (5%, 1 in 20), 0.01(1%, 1 in 100) and 0.001 (0.1%, 1 in 1000). We are sure that we may accept only 5% error that we reject null hypothesis when null hypothesis is true. Lower the alpha level, larger is the sample size. For example, a study with alpha level of 0.01 requires more subjects when compared to a study with alpha level of 0.05 for similar outcome variable. Lower alpha viz 0.01 or less is used when the decisions based on the research are critical and the errors may cause substantial, financial, or personal harm.

Look at the values given in table 6.2 below for various alpha level (Type I error).

Table 6.2: Z values for various alpha level

Alpha level	Z value (One tailed)	Z value (Two tailed test)
0.05	1.64	1.96
0.01	2.33	2.58
0.001	3.09	3.29

Effect Size or Minimum Detectable Difference

This is the expected difference or relationship between 2 independent samples, also known as the effect size. The obvious question is how to know the difference in a study, which is not conducted. If available, it may be useful to use the 'effect size' found from prior studies. Where no previous study exists, the effect size is determined from literature review, logical assertion and conjecture.

An effect size can be a direct estimate of the quantity of interest, or it can be a standardized measure that also accounts for the variability in the population. For example, in an analysis comparing outcomes in a treated and control population, the difference of outcome means $Y - X$ would be a direct measure of the effect size, whereas $(Y - X)/\sigma$ where σ is the common standard deviation of the outcomes in the treated and control groups, would be a standardized effect size. If constructed appropriately, a standardized effect size, along with the sample size, will completely determine the power. An unstandardized (direct) effect size will rarely be sufficient to determine the power, as it does not contain information about the variability in the measurements.

Sample Size

It is the number of samples to be included in a study. It determines the amount of sampling error inherent in a test result. Effects are harder to detect in smaller samples. Increasing sample size is often the easiest way to boost the statistical power of a test. Read the factors influencing the sample size estimation.

Precision

The precision with which the data are measured also influences statistical power. Consequently, power can often be improved by reducing the measurement error in the data.

Study Design

The design of an experiment or observational study often influences the power. For example, in a two-sample testing situation with a given total sample size *n*, it is optimal to have equal numbers of observations from the two populations being compared (as long as the variances in the two populations are the same). In regression analysis and ANOVA, there is an extensive strategies, for improving the power based on optimally setting the values of the independent variables in the model. Table 6.3 explains the sample size required for various research designs.

Table 6.3: Sample size for various research designs

Study design	Sample size	Reason
Descriptive studies	Larger sample size	To give acceptable confidence interval for smaller effects
Experimental studies	Lesser sample	Randomization and Control is exercised
Cross-over designs	One-quarter of the number required compared to a control group	Every subject gets the experimental treatment in cross-over study
Evaluation studies-One group pretest and post-test study	Half the number for a similar study with a control group	Control group aids in comparison which helps in assessing the true effect or chance occurrence
Study design with one-tailed hypothesis	20% lesser subjects compared to two-tailed studies	One tailed hypothesis is more directional and two tailed hypothesis is non directional
Non-randomized studies	20% more subjects compared to randomized studies	In order to accommodate confounding factors

Additional 10–20% subjects are required to allow adjustment of other factors such as withdrawals, missing data, lost to follow-up etc.

Outcome Variable

If the measurement of variable of interest is in nominal and ordinal level which will be usually expressed as percentages and rates, need larger sample size. They are usually of dichotomous (Yes/No; Male /Female) variable or categorical variable (blood group, religion, etc.). If the outcome variable is measured in interval or ratio scale, such as continuous variable (Weight, hemoglobin level, etc.) needs lesser sample size compared to dichotomous or categorical variable since they are expressed as mean and standard deviation.

Variance or Standard Deviation

The variance or standard deviation for sample size calculation is obtained either from previous studies or from pilot study. Larger the standard deviation, larger is the sample size required in a study.

Nature of Analysis

Complex multivariate statistics need larger samples than the simple univariate analysis.

Withdrawals, missing data and losses to follow-up: Sample size calculated is the total number of subjects who are required for the final study analysis. There are few practical issues, which need to be considered while calculating the number of subjects required. It is a fact that all eligible subjects may not be willing to take part and may be necessary to screen more subjects than the final number of subjects entering the study. In addition, even in well-designed and conducted studies, it is unusual to finish with a data set, which is complete for all the subjects recruited, in a usable format. The reason could be subject factor like-subjects may fail or refuse to give valid responses to particular questions, physical measurements may suffer from technical problems and in studies involving follow-up (e.g. Trials or cohort studies), there will be some degree of attrition. The reason could be technical and the procedural problem-like contamination, failure to get the assessment or test performed in time. It may, therefore, necessary to consider these issues before calculating the number of subjects to be recruited in a study in order to achieve the final desired sample size.

Example, say in a study, a total of N number of subjects are required in the end of the study with all the data being complete for analysis, but a proportion (q) are expected to refuse to participate or drop out before the study ends. In this case, the following total number of subjects (N^1) would have to be recruited to ensure that the final sample size (N) is achieved:

$$N^1 = \frac{N}{1-q}$$

where, q is the proportion of attrition and is generally 10%. The proportion of eligible subjects who will refuse to participate or provide the inadequate information will be unknown at the beginning of the study. Approximate estimates is often possible using information from similar studies in comparable populations or from an appropriate pilot study.

Sample size estimation for survey type of studies: The general rule relative to acceptable margins of error in survey research is 5–10%. The sample size can be estimated using the following formula,

$$N = \frac{Z^2 \times P \times (1-p) \times D}{E^2} \text{ where,}$$

P is the prevalence or proportion of event of interest for the study.

E is the Precision (or margin of error) with which a researcher want to measure something.

Generally, E will be 10% of P.

Z is normal deviate for two-tailed alternative hypothesis at a specified level of significance.

D is the design effect reflects the sampling design used in the survey type of study.

This is 1 for simple random sampling and higher values (usually 1–2) for other designs such as stratified, systematic, cluster random sampling etc. estimated to compensate for deviation from simple random sampling procedure. The design effect for cluster random sampling is taken as 1.5 to 2. For the purposive sampling, convenience or judgment sampling, D will cross 10. Higher the D, the more will be sample size required for a study. Simple random sampling is unlikely to be the sampling method in an actual filed survey. If another sampling method such as systematic, stratified, cluster sampling, etc. is used, a larger sample size is likely to be needed because of the 'design effect'. In case of impact study, P may be estimated at 50% to reflect the assumption that an impact is expected in 50% of the population. A P of 50% is also a conservative estimate.

Example 7:

A researcher is interested to know the sample size for conducting a survey for measuring the prevalence of malnutrition in certain community. Previous literature gives the estimate of malnutrition at 40% in the population to be surveyed, and assuming 95% confidence interval or 5% level of significance and 10% margin of error, the sample size can be calculated as follow as:

$$N = \frac{(1.96)^2 \times 0.4 \times (1-0.4) \times 2}{(0.1 \times 0.4)^2} = \frac{3.84 \times 0.4 \times 0.6 \times 2}{(0.04)^2} = \frac{1.84}{0.0016} = 1150 \text{ for cluster}$$

random sampling. Hence, sample size of 1150 is required to conduct community-based survey to estimate the prevalence of malnutrition. **Note** E is the margin of error, in the present example; it is 10% of the P (prevalence or proportion of event of interest for the study; P = 40%; E = 0.4/10 = 0.04).

To find the final adjusted sample size, allowing non-response rate of 10% in the above example, the adjusted sample size will be 1150/(1 – 0.10) = 1150/0.90 = 1277.77 = 1280.

Sample size estimation with single group mean: If a researcher is conducting a study in single group of students who were exposed to a structured learning strategies and the primary outcome is a continuous variable such as knowledge for which the mean and standard deviation are expression of results or estimates of population, the sample size can be estimated using the following formula,

$$N = \frac{Z^2 \times s^2}{d^2}$$

where, s is the standard deviation obtained from previous study or pilot study and d is the accuracy of estimate or how close to the true mean. $Z_{\alpha/2}$ is normal deviate for two-tailed alternative hypothesis at a level of significance. Research studies with one tailed hypothesis, the above formula can be rewritten as:

$N = (Z_\alpha)^2\ s^2/d^2$, the Z_α values are 1.64 and 2.33 for 5% and 1% level of significance.

Example 8:

In a study for estimating the hemoglobin of population and wants the error of estimation to be less than 0.5 g/dL of true mean (that is expected difference of hemoglobin to be 0.5 g/dL), the sample standard deviation was 2 and with a probability of 95%, and (that is) at an error rate of 5%, the sample size estimated as;

$$N = \frac{Z^2 \times s^2}{d^2} = \frac{(1.96)^2 \times (2)^2}{(0.5)^2} = \frac{3.84 \times 4}{0.25} = \frac{15.36}{0.25} = 61.44$$

gives the sample of 62 subjects, if the allowance of 10% for missing, losses to follow-up, withdrawals is assumed, then the corrected sample will be 62/0.9 = 68.88 subjects. Corrected sample size thus obtained is 70 and for 20% allowances, the corrected sample size will be 62/0.8 = 78 samples.

Problems in Sampling

Sampling bias: In statistics, sampling bias is a bias in which a sample is collected in such a way that some members of the intended population are less likely to be included than others. It results in a biased sample, a non-random sample of a population (or non-human factors) in which all individuals, or instances, were not equally likely to have been selected. If this is not accounted for, results can be erroneously attributed to the phenomenon under study rather than to the method of sampling.

Causes of Sampling Bias

- ***Selection of geographical area:*** If we want to study the quality of sleep of elderly, if we select samples only from the hospital which leads to bias because it does not include the elderly people residing at community area. Suppose if we want to assess the prevalence of child abuse, if we rely upon only reported case of child abuse in police station, that will not make true prevalence since there may be many unreported cases too.
- ***Over representation and under representation of the sample:*** Suppose our population is all women in the age group of 50–60 years and if we are selecting a women who come to religious places, we may miss out the samples who are ill and not having religious faith. And there are women, who may not come out of the home because of their cultural practice.
- ***Self-selection:*** This bias, which is possible whenever the group of people being studied has any form of control over whether to participate. Participants' decision to participate may be correlated with traits that affect the study, making the participants a non-representative sample. For example, people who have strong opinions or substantial knowledge may be more willing to spend time answering a survey than those who do not.
- ***Exclusion*** bias results from exclusion of particular groups from the sample, e.g. exclusion of subjects who have recently migrated as well as who have recently left the place. Exclusion of samples who are residing in the remote areas will also cause sampling bias.
- ***Under matching:*** Sometimes, it is possible that the population and sample may not match in many respects. For example, the study

population is likely healthier than the general population, e.g. workers (i.e. someone in ill-health is unlikely to have a job as manual laborer).

- ***Over matching:*** Sampling bias results due to overmatching when the control group becomes more similar to the cases in regard to exposure than the general population.

Probability and Sampling Error

Probability of Committing a Type I and Type II Error

Statistics derives its power from random sampling. The argument is that random sampling will average out the differences between sample and populations. But in practical, it is not so easy. There is little chance that one will pick random samples that result in significantly same populations. Even if they are the same populations, we can not be sure whether the results that we are seeing are just one time (or rare) events or actually significant (regularly occurring) events.

Hypothesis testing is based on the concept of normal distribution and sampling distribution. A researcher formulates null hypothesis for his research and tests the same based on the data obtained from the sample. Ultimately testing of null hypothesis depends on the data collected from the samples. If the samples selected are true representative of the population and data are accurately collected which will lead to correct decision making in the testing of null hypothesis.

In fact, there are four possible situations which may arise in testing of hypothesis. The researcher may make a correct decision by (a) accepting the null hypothesis when it is true or by (b) rejecting the null hypothesis when it is false. The researcher may also make a wrong decision by a (a) rejecting the null hypothesis when it is true or by (b) accepting the null hypothesis when it is false. The former of these two wrong decisions is known as the Type I error or the 'rejection error' and the latter is known as the Type II error or the 'acceptance error'. All these four situations are shown in a tabular form thus:

Null hypothesis is actually	**Null hypothesis is**	
	Accepted	Rejected
True	Correct decision (No error)	Wrong decision (Type I error)
False	Wrong decision (Type II error)	Correct decision (No error)

By rewriting
Reject the null hypothesis when it is true = Type I error = α
Accept the null hypothesis when it is false = Type II error = β
Accept the null hypothesis when it is true = Correct decision
Reject the null hypothesis when it is false = Correct decision

A level of significance represents the probability of committing Type I error. This probability is denoted by the Greek letter α (alpha). It is obvious that every researcher wants this probability to be small. Conventionally, this probability is fixed at 5% before a test is made, and more rarely at 1%. Five percent level of significance gives a value which has a rare chance of coming up only once in 20 trails. Similarly, 1% level of significance gives a value which has the chance of coming up only once in 100 trials. Hence none of these values can be considered by the researcher as substantially supporting his null hypothesis. So, when these values appear he rejects the hypothesis. This is why a level of significance is also called the region of rejection or the critical region. Needless to say, that a researcher feels more confident in rejecting H_0 at 1% level of significance than at 5% level of significance because in the former case the probability of his making a wrong decision (of rejecting the null hypothesis when it is actually true) is only one in a hundred (or 0.01). One can express this error thus:

Type I error or α = Probability (Rejecting H_0/H_0 is true)

The researcher can also fix the probability of committing the Type II error, i.e. accepting the null hypothesis when it is false. This probability which is denoted by the Greek letter β (beta) can be expressed thus:

Type II error or β = Probability (Accepting H_0/H_0 is false)

Every researcher likes β to be as small as possible. Alternatively, he likes $1-\beta$, i.e. the probability of rejecting the null hypothesis when it is false, to be as large as possible or to be as close to unity as possible. Thus, $(1-\beta)$ becomes the measure of how well the test is functioning or what is technically described as the power of the test.

Sampling Error

This is the difference between the values of sample and the population with regard to some phenomenon. It is the sample-to-sample variability in a statistic. In general we do not know the population parameters that we are interested in. Instead, we have to draw conclusions about them based on sample statistics usually from a single sample. We already know that such sample statistics are (probably) not going to match the corresponding population parameters exactly, so we have a problem.

The term for communicating that chance produced an unrepresentative sample is to say that the sample reflects sampling error. Sampling error results when chance produces a sample statistic such as mean, that is not equal to the population parameter it represents. Because of the luck of the draw, the sample is in error to some degree in representing the population. Sampling error is the reason researchers perform inferential statistics. There is always the possibility of sampling error in any sample. Whenever a sample mean is different from a particular population mean, it may be that the sample poorly represents that population of scores due to sampling error and the difference is not due to sampling error but the sample represents some other population.

Sample surveys do imply the study of a small portion of the population and as such there would naturally be a certain amount of inaccuracy in the information collected. This inaccuracy may be termed as sampling error or error variance. In other words, sampling errors are those errors which arise on account of sampling and they generally happen to be random variations (in case of random sampling) in the sample estimates around the true population values.

Sampling error = Frame error + Chance error + Response error

(If we add measurement error or the non-sampling error to sampling error, we get total error).

Sampling errors occur randomly and are equally likely to be in either direction. The magnitude of the sampling error depends upon the nature of the universe; the more homogeneous the universe, the smaller the sampling error. Sampling error is inversely related to the size of the sample, i.e. sampling error decreases as the sample size increases and vice-versa. A measure of the random sampling error can be calculated for a given sample design and size and this measure is often called the precision of the sampling plan. Sampling error is usually worked out as the product of the critical value at a certain level of significance and the standard error.

To deal with the possibility of sampling error, we apply inferential statistics. Inferential statistics are procedures for deciding whether sample data represent a relationship in the population. We decide whether the samples are likely to represent the populations that form a particular relationship or whether they are likely to represent population that do not form the relationship. The inferential procedure we use in a given research situation depends on the research design and the scale of measurement used when measuring the dependent variable. We use parametric and non parametric test to test the sampling error.

As opposed to sampling errors, we may have non-sampling errors which may creep in during the process of collecting actual information and such errors occur in all survey whether census or sample. We have no way to measure non-sampling errors.

Reasons for Sampling Error

- ***Population specification error:*** The sampling error creeps in when a researcher does not define the population of the study accurately. If the population is not specified properly, they may not form the representative of the population. Sampling frame error occurs when wrong subpopulation is used to select a sample.
- ***Selection error:*** Some of the bias is introduced by the use of defective sampling technique for the selection of a sample, e.g. purposive or judgment sampling in which the investigator deliberately selects a representative sample to obtain certain results.
- ***Substitution:*** If difficulties arise in enumerating a particular sampling unit included in the random sample, the investigators usually substitute a convenient member of the population.
- ***Faulty demarcation of sampling units:*** Bias due to defective demarcation of sampling units is particularly significant in area surveys such as agricultural experiments in the field or crop cutting surveys, etc.
- ***Error due to bias in the estimation method:*** Sampling method consists in estimating the parameters of the population by appropriate

statistics computed from the sample. Improper choice of the estimation techniques might introduce the error.

- ***Non-response error:*** This occur when respondents are different than those who do not respond. This may occur because either the potential respondent was not contacted or they refuse to respond.
- ***Non-sampling errors:*** These errors arise due to factors other than the inductive process of inferring about the population from a sample. Some factors which give rise to these errors are as under:
  - Defective frame and faulty sampling
  - Inappropriate methods of data collection, coding, tabulation, etc.
  - Untrained investigators
  - Inadequate inspection and supervision
  - Incomplete coverage.

All sampling errors are random and compensatory whereas all non-sampling errors are systematic and cumulative. Sampling error can be reduced by increasing the size of the sample whereas non-sampling errors can be reduced by suitably improving the collection and compiling techniques and streamlining the training and supervision of field staff. In a research, a researcher must try to reduce the sampling and non-sampling error. A researcher may not try to reduce any single error because to reduce sampling error if he increases the sample size, it may lead to increased non-sampling error. Hence the gain achieved in one direction may be more than offset by the loss suffered in the other direction.

SUMMARY

- An aggregate of objects or individuals under study is called population. A population comprises all the possible cases (persons, objects, events) that constitute a known whole. The number of units constituting the population is called the size of population.
- A population containing a finite number of units, individuals, or member is called a finite population. A population containing infinite number of units, individuals or members is called infinite population.
- The population of concrete individuals, is called as existent population and the collection of all possible ways in which an event can materialize is referred to as the hypothetical population.
- Target population refers to the entire group of individuals or objects to which researchers are interested in generalizing the conclusions. The target population usually has varying characteristics and it is also known as the theoretical population.
- The accessible population is the population in research to which the researchers can apply their conclusions. This population is a subset of the target population and is also known as the study population. It is from the accessible population that researchers draw their samples.
- A sample is a part of the population from which it was drawn. Sampling is the process of selecting a group of subjects for a study in such a way that the individuals represent the larger group from which they were selected.
- Sampling is the process of selection of samples from a population.

- Sampling frame is a list of all elements of the population and it is the list from which we draw a sample. A sample design is a definite plan for obtaining a sample from the sampling frame. It refers to the technique or the procedure the researcher would adopt in selecting some sampling units from which inferences about the population is drawn.
- In probability sampling, every item has equal chance of being included in the sample. Simple random sampling, systemic sampling, stratified sampling, cluster and area sampling and multistage sampling are examples of probability sampling techniques.
- Non-probability sampling does not afford any basis for estimating the probability that each item in the population has been included in the sample. Deliberate sampling, purposive sampling, quota and judgment sampling are non-probability sampling methods.
- Power of the study, is the probability of detecting a predefined clinical significance. The ideal study is the one, which has high power. This means that the study has a high chance of detecting a difference between groups if it exists, consequently, if the study demonstrates no difference between the groups, the researcher can reasonably confident in concluding that none exists. The ideal power for any study is considered to be 80%.
- Statistical power is the probability of rejecting the null hypothesis when the null hypothesis is false. As the power increases, the chances of a Type II error occurring decrease and the power is equal to $1-\beta$. The power is also known as the sensitivity of the test.
- Sampling error is the difference between the values of sample and the population with regard to some phenomenon. It is the sample-to-sample variability in a statistic.
- Sampling errors are those errors which arise on account of sampling whereas non-sampling errors may creep in during the process of collecting actual information and such errors occur in all survey whether census or sample. We have no way to measure non-sampling errors.

EXERCISE

- Mention the type of population
  - All mothers of under-five children residing at Chennai
  - All mothers of under-five children attending Pediatric OPD of Hospital X
  - All adolescent girls in Tamil Nadu
  - All adolescent girls studying in selected 10 schools in Chennai
  - All women who deliver twin baby in the forthcoming year.
- Calculate the size of sample to be selected from each strata.

Q. No.	Total population	Sample size required	Strata 1	Strata 2	Strata 3	Strata 4	Strata 5
1.	22500	500	50000	3000	2500	5000	7000
2.	12000	100	3600	5400	3000	—	—
3.	50000	1000	8000	10000	12000	13000	7000
4.	8000	82	1600	2400	2800	1200	—

  - In a population under study, there are 2000 women and 8000 men. If we have to select a sample of 250 individuals from this population, how many should be women to make our sample considered strictly representative?

  - You are interested in estimating per capita consumption of rice of adults living in Chennai. You want to state with 95% confidence that the population mean will lie within an allowable interval computed above the sample mean. Allowable error is 0.5 kg. Estimated standard deviation of the population using a pilot study is 3 kg per year. Determine the sample size for the research.
  - A random sample of houses is to be taken to estimate the percentage of houses that are not having toilet facilities in rural areas. The estimate is desired to be correct within plus or minus 1% with 95% confidence. One advance estimate is that the percentage of houses without toilet facilities will be about 6%. What size of samples are required?
- Reason out:
  - Why sample is selected from the population?
  - Why probability sampling technique is superior than non-probability sampling technique?
  - Why judgment sampling is used in qualitative studies?
  - What is the difference between the quota sampling and systematic sampling?
  - Why should we fix confidence level before undertaking a research?
  - Why priori power analysis is more useful than post-hoc power analysis?
- Identify the research setting where you could use the following types of sampling.
  - Simple random sampling
  - Quota sampling
  - Convenience sampling
  - Cluster sampling
  - Area sampling
  - Multistage sampling.

7

Data Collection

OBJECTIVES

After reading this chapter, you will be able to:

- State the meaning and definition of data and data collection
- Classify data collection methods and tools used in data collection
- Explain the methods of data collection
- Explain the tools used in data collection
- List the factors to be considered in selection of methods and tools of data.

INTRODUCTION

Data collection is an important aspect of any type of research study. Inaccurate data collection can impact the results of a study and ultimately lead to invalid results. Collection of data is the first step in the statistical treatment of a problem. Data may be primary and secondary. Primary data are original in character and it is collected for the first time. Secondary data refer to those, which have been collected already by previous researchers and have gone through the process of standardization. The researcher has to decide about the data that should be collected during his investigation. A researcher may have to collect primary data or secondary data or both based on the requirement of his research.

Definition of Data

Data can be defined as factual information (e.g. measurements or statistics) used as a basis for reasoning, discussion, or calculation. Data collection is the activity of acquiring and compiling information from different sources.

The word data is a plural form of the word datum which means information that is systematically collected in the course of the study. The data for a research is collected through various methods using appropriate tool.

Primary Data

Primary data are obtained by specifically designed methods to fulfill the data needs of the problem at hand. The primary data are those which are collected afresh and for the first time and thus happen to be original in character. For example, data obtained in a population census by the office of Registrar General and Census Commissioner are primary data.

Primary Source

A primary source is one that itself collects the data. A primary source has more detailed information on the procedure followed in collecting and compiling the data.

Advantages

It is advantageous to use the primary source for collecting the data for the following reasons:

- Primary source shows data in greater detail
- It frequently includes definitions of terms and units used
- It often includes a copy of schedule and description of procedure used in selecting the sample and in collecting the data
- The secondary source may contain mistakes due to errors in transcription made when the figures were copied from the primary source.

Secondary Data

The data which are not originally collected but rather obtained from published or unpublished sources are called secondary data. For example, for the office of Registrar General, the census data are primary whereas for all others, who use such data, they are secondary. The secondary data constitutes the chief material on the basis of which statistical work is carried out in many investigations.

Secondary Source

Usually the secondary data are available in following:

- Various publication of central, state and local government
- Various publications of foreign Government or international bodies and their subsidiary organization
- Technical and trade journals
- Books, magazines and newspapers
- Reports and publications of various associations connected with business and industries, banks, stock exchange etc.
- Reports prepared by research scholars, universities, economists, etc in different fields
- Public records and statistics, historical documents
- Diaries, letters, unpublished biographies and autobiographies, public/private individuals, etc.

Advantages

- If secondary data are available, they are much quicker to obtain than primary data
- It may be available on some subjects, where it would be impossible to collect primary data. For example, census data cannot be collected by individuals in research organization but can only be obtained from government publications

- It is highly convenient to use information which someone else has complied. There is no need for printing data collection forms, hiring numerators, editing and tabulating the results, etc.
- It is most economic and we can readily get it
- It saves time and effort of the researcher
- The findings based on primary data can easily be verified by the use of secondary data.

Disadvantages

- There is a problem in finding the data which are sufficiently accurate
- It is difficult to find data which exactly fit the need of the present project
- It may not be most suitable
- It may not be time and context specific
- It may not be very accurate and reliable
- It may not be up-to-date
- It may not be complete
- It may be biased.

Characteristics of Data

A researcher must see that the secondary data posses following characteristic:

- ***Reliability of data:*** The reliability can be tested by finding out such things about said data; Who collected the data? What were the sources of data? Were they collected by using proper methods? At what time were they collected? Was there any bias of compiler? What level of accuracy was desired?
- ***Suitability of data:*** The researcher must carefully scrutinize the definition of various terms and units of data collection used at the time of collecting the data from the primary sources because the data that are suitable for one enquiry may not necessarily be found suitable in another inquiry.
- ***Adequacy of data:*** If the level of accuracy achieved in data is found inadequate for the purpose of the present inquiry, they will be considered as inadequate and should not be used by the researcher. The data will be considered inadequate, if they are related to an area which may be either narrower or wider than the area of present inquiry.

Selection of Methods

Keeping in the view of following factors, the researcher should select the methods:

- ***Nature, scope and object of inquiry:*** This constitutes the most important factor affecting the choice of a particular method. The method selected should be such that it suits the type of inquiry that is to be conducted by the researcher. This factor is also important in deciding whether the data already available are to be used or the data not yet available are to be collected.

- ***Availability of funds:*** It determines to a large extent the method to be used for the collection of data. When the funds at the disposal of researcher are very limited, he will have to select a comparatively cheaper method which may not be as efficient and effective as some other costly method.
- ***Time factor:*** Availability of time has also to be taken into account in deciding a particular method of data collection. Some methods take relatively more time, whereas with others the data can be collected in a comparatively shorter duration.
- ***Precision required:*** Precision required is yet another important factor to be considered at the time of selecting method of collection of data.

Methods of Data Collection

There are three major methods of data collection. They are (Fig. 7.1):

1. Self-report
2. Observation
3. Biophysiological measurements.

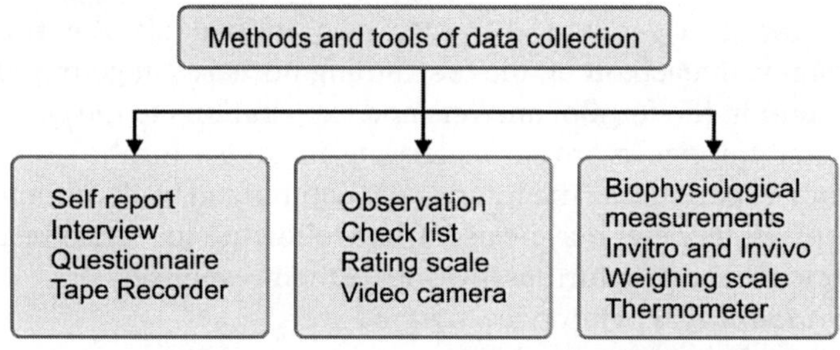

Fig. 7.1: Methods and tools of data collection

SELF-REPORT AS A METHOD OF DATA COLLECTION

The self-report method is strong with respect to its directness and versatility. If we want to know what people think, feel or believe, the most direct means of gathering the information is to ask them about it. Self-reports are also versatile with respect to content coverage. Self-reports are obtained by conducting interview or collection of information through personal contacts with individual respondents or by written questionnaire. Interview schedule and questionnaire is used to enhance interview. An equally common method of data collection that is used especially with educated respondents located over a wide geographical area is the questionnaire. During the interview, the participants are observed (Fig. 7.2).

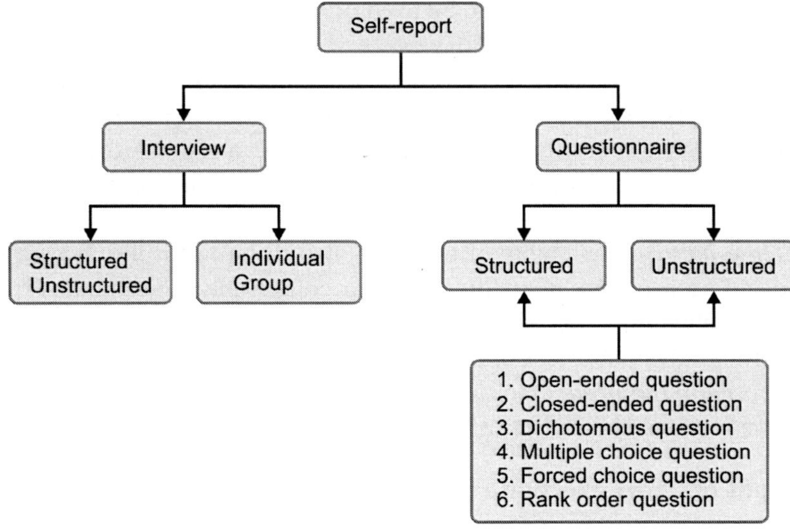

Fig. 7.2: Classification of methods of obtaining self-report

Interview Method

Introduction

The interview is a method in which two individuals are involved in conversation with each other, the first aiming primarily at getting responses from the other in the form of answers and explanations to the questions put by the former. Interviews are particularly useful for getting the story behind a participant's experiences. The interviewer can pursue in-depth information about a topic. Interviews may be useful as a follow-up to certain respondents to questionnaires, e.g. to further investigate their responses.

The main ***advantages*** of interview method are:

- It has a high degree of flexibility
- It can be used with both literate and non literates
- It provides for high returns in responses
- It can be used extensively in a wide variety of studies
- Supplementary data can also be collected
- It is thorough
- It permits exhaustive exploration and probing
- Its validity can be appraised
- It can observe reactions which enable the creation of a right atmosphere for interviewing
- In-depth information can be collected
- More accurate information can be collected
- More control can be exercised
- More information and too in greater depth can be obtained
- Interviewer by his own skill can overcome the resistance, if any, of the respondent

- Personal information can be obtained easily under this method
- The language of interview can be adapted to the ability or educational level of the person interviewed
- The interviewer can collect supplementary information about the respondent's personal character and environment which is often of great value in interpreting results.

The primary ***disadvantages*** of the interview method are:

- It is a very expensive procedure
- It requires trained investigators who know the language of the respondents
- It requires the active cooperation and participation of respondents
- It depends on the availability of respondents as it can be done only at their convenience
- It gives an interviewee a tendency to rationalize her actions
- The respondent may have memory lapses
- The respondents may evade answering some types of questions
- The interview method presumes the competence of the respondent to answer all questions
- It is time consuming especially when the sample is large and recalls upon the respondents are necessary
- Tend to be subjective
- Certain information cannot be obtained in face-to-face interview
- There remains the possibility of the bias of interviewer as well as that of the respondents
- The presence of the interviewer on the spot may over-stimulate the respondent, sometimes even to the extent that he may give imaginary information just to make the interview interesting.
- Under the interview method the organization required for selecting, training, and supervising the field staff is more complex with formidable problem
- Interview at times may also introduce systemic errors.

Preparation for Interview

- Choose a setting with little distraction. Avoid loud lights or noises, ensure the interviewee is comfortable, etc. Often, they may feel more comfortable at their own places of work or homes
- Explain the purpose of the interview
- Address terms of confidentiality. Note any terms of confidentiality. Explain who will get access to their answers and how their answers will be analyzed. If their comments are to be used as quotes, get their written permission to do so
- Explain the format of the interview. Explain the type of interview conducted and its nature
- Indicate how long the interview usually takes

- Tell them how to get in touch with the interviewer later if they want to
- Ask them if they have any questions before the interview begins.
- Do not count on memory to recall their answers. Ask for permission to record the interview or bring along someone to take notes.

Types of Interviews

- ***Informal, conversational interview:*** No predetermined questions are asked, in order to remain as open and adaptable as possible to the interviewee's nature and priorities; during the interview, the interviewer goes with the flow.
- ***General interview guide approach:*** The guide approach is intended to ensure that the same general areas of information are collected from each interviewee; this provides more focus than the conversational approach, but still allows a degree of freedom and adaptability in getting information from the interviewee.
- ***Standardized, open-ended interview:*** Here, the same open-ended questions are asked to all interviewees (an open-ended question is where respondents are free to choose how to answer the question, i.e. they do not select yes or no or provide a numeric rating, etc.); this approach facilitates faster interviews that can be more easily analyzed and compared.
- ***Closed, fixed-response interview:*** Where all interviewees are asked the same questions and asked to choose answers from among the same set of alternatives. This format is useful for those not practiced in interviewing.

Personal Interview

In this method of data collection, there is a face-to-face contact with persons from whom the information is to be obtained. The interviewer asks them questions pertaining to the survey and collects the desired information. The information thus obtained is original in character.

Techniques: There are various techniques of personal interviews:

Structured and unstructured: Structured interview involves the use of a set of predetermined questions and of highly standardized techniques of recording. The term 'structured' refers to the extent to which the questions are predetermined and degree of flexibility or rigorousness in the interviewing process. A schedule will include only those questions, which are essential and relevant to the study. In order that this takes place, not only should the questions be properly framed, but the responses should also be appropriate to the questions. The interviewer follows a rigid procedure laid down, asking questions in a form and prescribed order. It is used in descriptive studies. Unstructured interviews are characterized by a flexibility of approach of questioning. It does not follow a system of predetermined questions and standardized techniques of recording. The interviewer has greater freedom. This method is used in exploratory or formulative studies.

Focused Interview

It is to focus attention on the given experience of the respondents and its effects. The interviewer has freedom to decide the manner and sequence of the questions. These are generally used in the development of hypothesis and constitute a major type of unstructured interviews. Focus group discussion is another method of eliciting information from the participant in qualitative research. It is a carefully planned discussion designed to obtain perceptions on a defined area of interest in a non-threatening environment. It is an interview conducted by a trained moderator in a non-structured manner and natural manner with a small group of respondents. For this, a group of 6–12 people with similar characteristics are gathered to discuss a focused topic of interest. A moderator guides the discussion. A note taker records the nonverbal aspects of the group. Tape recorded notes are combined with the nonverbal notes and transcribed for analysis.

It helps in obtaining a range of perceptions, opinions or beliefs about an issue and to explore controversial topics. The data collected from this helps in generating hypotheses for further research. The ***advantages*** of focused group discussion are many. It is cost-effective. Quality data can be collected. Focus group tends to be enjoyable to participants. The ***disadvantages*** are the number questions are restricted; time consuming; sensitive and highly personal topic cannot be explored and confidentiality cannot be assured.

Clinical Interviews

It is concerned with broad underlying feelings or motivation or with the course of individual's life experience.

Nondirective Interviews

In this, the interviewer's function is simply to encourage the respondent to talk about the given topic with a bare minimum of direct questioning.

Types of Topics in Questions

Patton notes six kinds of questions. One can ask questions about:

1. ***Behaviors:*** What a person has done or is doing
2. ***Opinions/values:*** What a person thinks about a topic
3. ***Feelings:*** The respondents sometimes respond with I think
4. ***Knowledge:*** To get facts about a topic
5. ***Sensory:*** What people have seen, touched, heard, tasted or smelled
6. ***Background/demographics:*** Standard background questions, such as age, education, etc.

   The above questions can be asked in terms of past, present or future.

Prerequisites and basic Tenets of Interview

For successful implementation of interview method:

- Interviewer should be carefully selected, trained and briefed
- They should be honest, hard-working, sincere and impartial and must possess the technical competence and necessary practical experience

- Occasional field checks should be made to ensure that interviewer are neither cheating nor deviating from instructions given to them for performing their job efficiently
- Some provision should be made in advance so that appropriate action may be taken, if some of the selected respondents refuse to cooperate or not available when an interviewer calls upon them
- In fact, interviewing is an art governed by certain scientific principles. The interviewer's approach must be friendly, courteous, conversational and unbiased.

Sequence of Questions

- Get the respondents involved in the interview as soon as possible
- Before asking about controversial matters (such as feelings and conclusions), first ask about some facts. With this approach, respondents can more easily engage in the interview before warming up to more personal matters
- Intersperse fact-based questions throughout the interview to avoid long lists of fact-based questions, which tends to leave respondents disengaged
- Ask questions about the present before questions about the past or future. It is usually easier for them to talk about the present and then work into the past or future
- The last question might be to allow respondents to provide any other information they prefer to add and their impressions of the interview.

Wording of Questions

- Wording can be open-ended. Respondents should be able to choose their own terms when answering questions
- Questions should be as neutral as possible. Avoid wording that might influence answers, e.g. evocative, judgmental wording
- Questions should be asked one at a time
- Questions should be worded clearly. This includes knowing any terms particular to the program or the respondents' culture
- Be careful asking 'why' questions. This type of question infers a cause-effect relationship that may not truly exist. These questions may also cause respondents to feel defensive, e.g. they have to justify their response, which may inhibit their responses to this and future questions.

Conducting Interview

- Occasionally verify the tape recorder (if used) is working
- Ask one question at a time
- Attempt to remain as neutral as possible. That is, do not show strong emotional reactions to their responses. Patton suggests to act as if 'you have heard it all before'

- Encourage responses with occasional nods of the head, 'uh huhs', etc.
- Be careful about the appearance when note taking. That is, if you jump to take a note, it may appear as if you are surprised or very pleased about an answer, which may influence answers to future questions
- Provide transition between major topics, e.g. 'we have been talking about (some topic) and now I would like to move on to (another topic)'.
- Do not lose control of the interview. This can occur when respondents stray to another topic, take so long to answer a question or even begin asking questions to the interviewer.

Immediately after Interview

- Verify if the tape recorder, if used, worked throughout the interview
- Make any notes on your written notes, e.g. to clarify any scratching, ensure pages are numbered; fill out any notes that do not make senses, etc.
- Write down any observations made during the interview. For example, where did the interview occur and when, was the respondent particularly nervous at any time? Were there any surprises during the interview? Did the tape recorder break?

Principles in the Construction of Interview Schedule

The general principles in the formulation of a schedule are:

- The questions asked should have a bearing on the objectives and hypothesis of the study. That is to say, while one may be tempted to include interesting questions, only relevant ones should be framed. Relevance is determined by whether or not the item or items have already been listed in the first place
- Only those questions which cannot be elicited by any other method or technique should be included in a schedule
- The form should be as short as possible and take into consideration the time factor. Where long-winded schedules are used, not only will the interviewer find it difficult to retain the attention of the respondent, but it is also possible that the, latter may not be cooperative
- The questions included should be such as can' be answered by the respondents.
- Questions which are definitely known to bring in unreliable answers must also be avoided
- The question included should as far as possible, be short and to the point. The exception to this is when schedules are used in concealed studies, i.e. where a conscious attempt is made to hide from the respondent the actual purpose of the study. When the respondent knows the purpose of the study, there is a likelihood of biased answers
- Objective, factual and simple questions should precede subjective and complex questions
- Each question should include only one idea and elicit only one answer.

Telephone Interview

This method of collecting information consists in contacting respondents on telephone itself. It is not a very widely used method, but plays important part in industrial surveys, particularly in developed regions.

Merits

The chief merits of such systems are:

- It is more flexible in comparison to mailing method
- It is faster than other methods
- It is cheaper than personal interviewing method
- Recall is easy, callback are simple and economical
- There is a higher rate of response than what we have in mailing method
- Replies can be recorded without causing embarrassment to the respondents
- Interviewer can explain requirements more easily
- No field staff is required
- Representative and wider distribution of sample is possible
- At times access can be gained to respondents who otherwise cannot be contacted.

Demerits

It is not free from demerits:

- Little time is given to respondents for considered answers; interview period is not likely to exceed five minutes in most cases
- Surveys are restricted to respondents who have telephone facilities
- Extensive geographical coverage may get restricted by cost consideration
- It is not suitable for intensive surveys where comprehensive answers are required to various questions
- Possibility of bias of the interviewer is relatively more
- Questions have to be short and to the point, probes are difficult to handle.

Questionnaire Method

Questionnaires are an inexpensive way to gather data from a potentially large number of respondents. Often they are the only feasible way to reach a number of reviewers large enough to allow statistical analysis of the results. A well-designed questionnaire that is used effectively, can gather information on both the overall performance of the test system as well as information on specific components of the system. If the questionnaire includes demographic questions on the participants, they can be used to correlate performance and satisfaction with the test system among different groups of users.

It is important to remember that a questionnaire should be viewed as a multi-stage process beginning with definition of the aspects to be examined and ending with interpretation of the results. Every step needs to be designed carefully because the final results are only as good as the weakest link in the questionnaire process. Although questionnaires may be cheap to administer compared to other data collection methods, they are every bit as expensive in terms of design time and interpretation.

In this method a list of questions pertaining to the survey is prepared and sent to the various informants by post. The questionnaire contains questions and provides space for answers. A request is made to the informants through a covering letter to fill up the questionnaire and send it back within a specified time. This method is adapted by private individuals, research workers, private and public organizations and even by government. In questionnaire method, the researcher has to articulate clearly what problem or need is to be addressed using the information to be gathered by the questions and review the need for doing the evaluation and what is expected to accomplish by it. This helps the researcher to focus on the information needed and, ultimately, on what questions should be used.

There are three basic types of questionnaire:

1. Closed-ended
2. Open-ended
3. Combination of both.

- ***Closed-ended questionnaire:***
  - Closed-ended questions include all possible answers/prewritten response categories and respondents are asked to choose among them, e.g. multiple choice questions, scale questions
  - Type of questions used to generate statistics in quantitative research
  - As these follow a set format and most responses can be entered easily into a computer for ease of analysis, greater numbers can be distributed
  - This asks the respondent to rank the responses according to some criteria such as most favorable to least favorable or most important to less important.
- ***Open-ended questionnaire:***
  - Open-ended questions allow respondents to answer in their own words
  - Questionnaire does not contain boxes to tick but instead leaves a blank section for the respondent to write an answer
  - Open-ended questionnaires might be used to find out what people think about a service
  - As there are no standard answers to these questions, data analysis is more complex
  - As it is opinions which are sought rather than numbers, fewer questionnaires need to be distributed.
- ***Combination of both:***
  - This way it is possible to find out how many people use a service and what they think of the service in the same form

- Begins with a series of closed-ended questions, with boxes to tick or scales to rank, and then finish with a section of open-ended questions or more detailed response.

Requirement of a good questionnaire: The following general principles/ requirements are useful in framing questionnaire:

- ***Covering letter:*** The person conducting the survey must introduce himself and state the objectives of the survey. A short letter stating the purpose of survey should be enclosed along with the questionnaire.
- ***Number of questions:*** The number of questions to be included in the questionnaire would strictly depend upon the objective and the scope of the investigation and number of the questions should be as small as possible. Because if the questionnaire is lengthy, the rate of response will be lower.
- ***Should be arranged logically:*** The question should be arranged logically so that a natural and spontaneous reply to each is induced. For example it is illogical to ask a person about his income before asking him whether he is employed or not.
- ***Short and simple:*** The question should be short and simple to understand and technical terms should be avoided.
- ***Personal questions:*** Personal questions should be avoided such as income, income tax is paid, etc.
- ***Necessary instructions:*** The instructions about the unit of measurement or the time within which questionnaire should be sent back, etc. should be provided.
- ***Objective answers:*** The descriptive questions should be avoided while framing the questionnaire. As far as the question should be of such nature that can be answered easily in 'yes' or 'no'.
- ***Calculation:*** Question requiring calculation should be avoided. If calculation is included, informant may not answer the questions.
- ***Attractive:*** The quality of paper used and printing should be of high quality. Sufficient space should be given for answering.

The steps required to design and administer a questionnaire include:

- Defining the objectives of the survey
- Determining the sampling group
- Writing the questionnaire
- Administering the questionnaire
- Interpretation of the results.

Directions to respondents

- Include a brief explanation of the purpose of the questionnaire
- Include clear explanation of how to complete the questionnaire
- Include directions about where to provide the completed questionnaire
- Note conditions of confidentiality, e.g. who will have access to the information, if the investigator is going to attempt to keep their answers private and only accessed by the investigator and/or someone who will

collate answers. However, the investigator can assure that he/she will make every reasonable attempt to protect access to their answers.

Content of Questions

The question asked should be related and relevant to the problem and objectives. The below mentioned questions help in self evaluation of the researcher in asking questions with regard to content of the question.

- Ask about what need to known, i.e. get information in regard to the goals or ultimate questions to be addressed by the evaluation.
- Think whether the respondent be able to answer the question, i.e. do they know the answer?
- Is it too private or silly?
- Is it really necessary to gather information? Is it beyond the study objectives?

Wording of Questions

- Will the respondent understand the wording, i.e. are you using any slang, cultural-specific or technical words?
- Are any words so strong that they might influence the respondent to answer in a certain way? Attempt to be made to avoid use of strong adjectives with nouns in the questions, e.g. 'highly effective government', 'prompt and reliable', etc.
- To ensure that one question is asked at a time, avoid use of the word 'and' in the question.
- Avoid using 'not' in the questions if the respondents have to answer 'yes' or 'no' to a question. Use of 'not' can lead to double negatives and cause confusion.
- If multiple choice questions are used, be sure that choices are mutually exclusive and encompass the total range of answers. Respondents should not be confused about whether two or more alternatives appear to mean the same thing. Respondents also should not have a clearly preferred answer that is not among the alternative choices of an answer to the question.

Order of Questions

- Be careful not to include so many questions that potential respondents are dissuaded from responding.
- Attempt to get respondents' motivation to complete the questionnaire. Start with fact-based questions and then go on to opinion-based questions, e.g. ask people for demographic information about themselves and then go on to questions about their opinions and perspectives. This gets respondents engaged in the questionnaire and warmed up before more challenging and reflective questions about their opinions. (Consider if they can complete the questionnaire anonymously; if so, indicate this on the form where you ask for their name.)

- Attempt to get respondents' commentary in addition to their ratings, e.g. if the questionnaire ask respondents to choose an answer by circling an answer or provide a rating, ask them to provide commentary that explains their choices.
- Include a question to get respondents' impressions of the questionnaire itself. For example, ask them if the questionnaire was straightforward to complete ('yes' or 'no'), and if not, to provide suggestions about how to improve the questionnaire.
- Pilot or test your questionnaire on a small group of clients or fellow staff. Ask them if the form and questions seemed straightforward. Carefully review the answers on the questionnaires. Does the information answer the evaluation questions or provide what you want to know about the program or its specific services? What else would you like to know?
- Finalize the questionnaire according to results of the pilot. Put a date on the form so you can keep track of all future versions.

What can questionnaires measure?

Questionnaires are quite flexible in what they can measure, however, they are not equally suited to measuring all types of data. We can classify data in two ways, ***Subjective vs. Objective*** and ***Quantitative vs. Qualitative***.

When a questionnaire is administered, the researchers control over the environment will be somewhat limited. This is why questionnaires are inexpensive to administer. This loss of control means the validity of the results are more reliant on the honesty of the respondent. Consequently, it is more difficult to claim complete objectivity with questionnaire data than with results of a tightly controlled lab test. For example, if a group of participants are asked on a questionnaire how long it took them to learn a particular function on a piece of software, it is likely that they will be biased towards themselves and answer, on average, with a lower than actual time. A more objective usability test of the same function with a similar group of participants may return a significantly higher learning time. More elaborate questionnaire design or administration may provide slightly better objective data, but the cost of such a questionnaire can be much higher and offset their economic advantage. In general, questionnaires are better suited to gathering reliable subjective measures, such as user satisfaction of the system or interface in question.

Questions may be designed to gather either qualitative or quantitative data. By their very nature, quantitative questions are more exact than qualitative. For example, the word 'easy' and 'difficult' can mean radically different things to different people. Any question must be carefully crafted, but in particular questions that assess a qualitative measure must be phrased to avoid ambiguity. Qualitative questions may also require more thought on the part of the participant and may cause them to become bored with the questionnaire sooner. In general, we can say that questionnaires can measure both qualitative and quantitative data well, but that qualitative questions require more care in design, administration and interpretation.

When to use a questionnaire?

There is no all encompassing rule for when to use a questionnaire. The choice will be made based on a variety of factors including the type of information to be gathered and the available resources for the experiment. A questionnaire should be considered in the following circumstances.

- When resources and money are limited. A questionnaire can be quite inexpensive to administer. Although preparation may be costly, any data collection scheme will have similar preparation expenses. The administration cost per person of a questionnaire can be as low as postage and a few photocopies. Time is also an important resource that questionnaires can maximize. If a questionnaire is self-administering, such as an e-mail questionnaire, potentially several thousand people could respond in a few days. It would be impossible to get a similar number of usability tests completed in the same short time.
- When it is necessary to protect the privacy of the participants. Questionnaires are easy to administer confidentially. Often confidentiality is the necessary to ensure participants will respond honestly if at all. Examples of such cases would include studies that need to ask embarrassing questions about private or personal behavior.
- When corroborating other findings. In studies that have resources to pursue other data collection strategies, questionnaires can be a useful confirmation tools. More costly schemes may turn up interesting trends, but occasionally there will not be resources to run other tests on large participant groups to make the results statistically significant. A follow-up large scale questionnaire may be necessary to corroborate these earlier results.
- The construction of a research instrument or tool for data collection is the most important aspect of a research project because anything said by way of findings or conclusions is based upon the type of information collected. The data collected is entirely dependent upon the questions that are asked to the respondents. The famous saying about computers—'garbage in garbage out'—is also applicable for data collection. The research tool provides the input into a study and therefore the quality and validity of the output (the findings), are solely dependent on it.

How to construct questionnaires?

- ***Deciding which questionnaire to use:*** 'Closed or open ended' or 'self or interviewer administered.'
- ***Wording and structure of questions:***
  - Questions should be kept short
  - Avoid negative questions as it is confusing for respondent to agree or disagree
  - Question should not contain prestige bias–causing embarrassment or forcing the respondent to give false answer in order to look good. Questions about educational qualification or income might elicit this type of response

- Use indirect questions for sensitive issues—in indirect questions respondents can relate their answer to other people
- Using closed-ended questions—try to make sure that all possible answers are covered so that respondents are not constrained in their answer. 'Do not know' category also needs to be added.

- ***Avoiding leading questions:*** Do not lead the respondent to answer in a certain way, e.g. 'how often do you wash your car?' assumes that respondent has a car and he washes his car. Instead, ask a filter question to find if he has a car, and then, 'If you wash your car, how many times a year'?
- ***Length and ordering of the questions:***
  - Keep the questionnaire as short as possible
  - Ask easy questions which respondents will enjoy answering
  - If combined questionnaire, keep open-ended questions for the end
  - Make questions as interesting as possible and easy to follow by varying type and length of question
  - Group the questions into specific topic as this makes it easier to understand and follow
  - Layout and spacing is important as cluttered questionnaire is less likely to be answered.
- ***Piloting the questionnaire:*** Once the questionnaire is constructed, the researcher must pilot it. This means that the researcher must test it out to see if it is obtaining the result he requires. This is done by asking people to read it through and see if there are any ambiguities which the researcher have not noticed. They should also be asked to comment about the length, structure and wording of the questionnaire and the questions should be altered accordingly.

Merits

This method is most extensively employed in various economic and business surveys. The main merits are as follows:

- There is low cost even when the universe is large and is widely spread geographically
- It is free from the bias of the interviewer; answers are in respondent's own words
- Respondents have adequate time to give well out answers
- Respondents who are not easily approachable can also be reached conveniently
- Large sample can be made use of and thus the results can be more dependable and reliable
- Little skill is required to administer it
- It can be self-administered
- It can be sent through mail
- It ensures uniformity from one measurement situation to another, e.g. no pressure of time on respondent is required.

Demerits

- Low rate of return of the duly filled in questionnaires, bias due to no-response is often indeterminate
- It can be used only when respondents are educated and cooperating
- There is inbuilt inflexibility because of the difficulty of amending the approach once questionnaires have been sent
- The control over questionnaire may be lost once it is sent
- There is also the possibility of ambiguous replies or omission of replies altogether to certain questions, interpretation of omission is difficult
- It is difficult to know whether willing respondents are truly representative.
- This method is likely to be the slowest of all
- The information obtained is limited to the written responses of subject to prearranged questions
- It is too narrow in scope as only limited questions are asked
- The validity of responses cannot be assessed
- It does not permit deep probing.

Schedule Method

This method of data collection is very much like questionnaire method, with a little difference which lies in the fact that schedules are being filled in by the numerators who are specially appointed for this purpose. These numerators along with schedules go to respondents put to them the questions from the performa in the order questions are listed and record the replies in the space provided. Numerators explain them the objective of the investigation and also remove the difficulties felt by the respondents. The numerators should be trained to perform their job well and the nature and scope of the investigation should be explained to them thoroughly. The numerators should be intelligent and must possess the capacity of cross examination in order to find out the truth. This method of data collection is very useful in extensive enquiries and can lead to fairly reliable results. It is, however, very expensive and is usually adopted in investigations conducted by governmental agencies or by some big organizations. Population census all over the world is conducted through this method.

Difference between questionnaire and schedule: Both methods are important. The points of difference are:

- ***Mode of sending:*** The questionnaire generally sent through mail to informants to be answered as specified in a covering letter without further assistant from the sender. The schedule is generally filled out by the research worker or the numerator.
- ***Cost-effective:*** To collect data through questionnaire is relatively cheap and economical, since we have to spend money only on preparing the questionnaire and in mailing to the respondents. Schedule is relatively more expensive since considerable amount of money has to be spent in appointing numerators.

- ***Rate of response:*** Non-response is usually high in case of questionnaire as many people do not respond and return the question without answering. It is very low in case of schedule method.
- ***Identity:*** In case of questionnaire, it is not always clear who replies, but in schedule the identity of respondent is known.
- ***Collection time:*** The questionnaire, method is likely to be very slow, but in case of schedules the information is collected well in time as these are filled by numerators.
- ***Contacts:*** Personal contact is generally not possible in case of questionnaire, but in case of schedules direct personal contacts are established with respondents.
- ***Literacy:*** Questionnaire method can be used only when respondents are literate and cooperative. But in schedules, information can be gathered even when the respondents happen to be illiterate.
- ***Area:*** Wider and more representative distribution of sample is possible under questionnaire method, but in schedules there usually remains the difficulty in sending numerators over a relatively wide area.
- ***Accuracy:*** Risk of collecting incomplete and wrong information is relatively more under the questionnaire method, but in schedules, information collected are complete and correct.
- ***Results:*** The success of questionnaire method depends upon the quality of questionnaire itself but in schedules it depends upon the honesty and competence of numerators.
- ***Attraction:*** In order to attract the attention of respondents, the physical appearance of questionnaire must be quite attractive, but this may not be so in case of schedules.
- ***Other methods:*** Along with schedules, observation method can also be used but such things are not possible in questionnaire method while collecting data.

SCALING TECHNIQUES

Scaling describes the procedures of assigning numbers to various degrees of opinion, attitude and other concepts. We not only try to assess opinions of the respondents but also measure the intensity of it. Scaling has been defined as a procedure for the assignment of numbers or other symbols to a property of objects in order to impart some of the characteristics or numbers to the properties in question. A scale is a continuum consisting of a set of statement, logically related to the concept under study. The continuum consist of the highest point and the lowest point along with several intermediate points between these two extreme points. The scales must satisfy the principles of measurements. It must satisfy the characteristics of homogeneity, linearity, validity and reliability.

The scaling procedures may be based on the purpose of categorizing or making comparisons. A categorical scale is a rating scale and ranking scale allows the subject to compare and relatively rank the item. The scales may be of unidimensional or multidimensional. Unidimensional scale measures only one dimension whereas multidimensional scale measures more than one dimension.

The rating scale and attitude scales have the objective of assigning individual to positions with different numerical values in order to make possible the distinctions of degree.

Number of scale points depends upon:

- The discriminative ability of the raters (their training and experience)
- The kind of characteristic to be judged
- The conditions under which ratings are to be made.

Attitude Scale

An attitude scale measures how the participant feels about a subject at the moment when he or she answers the question. Several popular types of attitude scales are used in nursing research.

Types of Attitude Scales

There are various types of attitude scales used in nursing research, they are:

- Differential scale (LL Thurstone scale)
- Summated (Likert) scale
- Semantic differential attitude scales.

Likert Scale

The Likert scale is an ordered, one-dimensional scale from which respondents choose one option that best aligns with their view. It is designed to determine the opinion or attitude of a subject and contains a number of declarative statements with a scale after each statement. The original version of the scale included five response categories. Each response category was assigned a value, with a value of 1 given to the most negative response and a value of 5 to the most positive response. It is a bipolar scaling method, measuring either positive or negative response to a statement. Sometimes a four-point scale is used; this is a forced choice method since the middle option of 'Neither agree nor disagree' is not available.

Why is this scale known as Likert scale?

The scale is named after its inventor, Psychologist Rensis Likert.

A Likert item is simply a statement which the respondent is asked to evaluate according to any kind of subjective or objective criteria; generally the level of agreement or disagreement is measured. Often five ordered response levels are used, although many psychometricians advocate using seven or nine levels. The format of a typical five-level Likert item is:

1. Strongly disagree
2. Disagree
3. Neither agree nor disagree
4. Agree
5. Strongly agree.

Response choices in a likert scale most commonly addresses agreements, evaluation or frequency. Agreement options may include statements such as strongly agree, uncertain, disagree and strongly disagree. Evaluation responses ask the respondent for an evaluative rating along a good/bad dimension, such as positive or negative or excellent to terrible. Frequency responses may include statements such as rarely, seldom, sometimes, occasionally and usually. The terms used are versatile and need to be selected for their appropriateness to the stem. Use of uncertain or neutral category is controversial because it allows the subject to avoid making a clear choice of positive or negative statements. Thus, sometimes only 4 or 6 options are offered, with the uncertain category omitted. This type of scale is referred to as a forced choice version (Table 7.1).

The likert scale is the sum of responses on several likert items. Because likert items are often accompanied by a visual analog scale (e.g. a horizontal line, on which a subject indicates his or her response by circling or checking tick-marks), the items are sometimes called scales themselves. This is the source of much confusion; it is better, therefore, to reserve the term likert scale to apply to the summated scale and likert item to refer to an individual item. The phrasing of item stems depends on the type of judgment that the respondent is being asked to make.

Agreement items are declarative statements such as 'I feel good about my work on the job'. Frequency items can be behaviors, events or circumstances which the respondent can indicate how often they occur. A frequency stem may be 'I read research articles in journals', 'I do exercises and yoga'. An evaluation stem could be 'The effectiveness of computer as an aid in promotion of students' learning'.

Likert scale usually consists of 10–20 items each addressing an element of the concept being measured. Halves the statements should be expressed positively and half negatively to avoid inserting bias into the responses.

Scale value of negatively expressed items must be reversed before analysis. Usually the values obtained from each item in the instrument are summed to obtain a single score for each subject. Although the values for each item are technically ordinal-level data, the summed score is often treated as interval level data, thus allowing more sophisticated statistical analyses.

Likert scales may be subject to distortion from several causes. Respondents may avoid using extreme response categories (central tendency bias); agree with statements as presented (acquiescence bias); or try to portray themselves or their organization in a more favorable light (social desirability bias). Designing a scale with balanced keying (an equal number of positive and negative statements) can obviate the problem of acquiescence bias, since acquiescence on positively keyed items will balance acquiescence on negatively keyed items, but central tendency and social desirability are somewhat more problematic.

Advantages

- Questions used are usually easy to understand and so lead to consistent answers
- Easy to use.

Disadvantages

- Only a few options are offered, with which respondents may not fully agree.
- People may become influenced by the way they have answered previous questions. For example, if they have agreed several times in a row, they may continue to agree
- They may also deliberately break the pattern, disagreeing with a statement with which they might otherwise have agreed.

Example of a Likert Scale to assess the attitude towards ragging among college students.

Table 7.1: Likert scale to assess the attitude towards ragging

S. No.	Items	SA	A	UC	D	SD
1.	Ragging gives me a sense of authority.					
2.	I do ragging to impress my peer group.					
3.	Formal introduction is not ragging.					
4.	Ragging is done to remove the fear of freshman.					
5.	Playing the fool is ragging.					
6.	All juniors must assist seniors in the hostel.					
7.	Ragging satisfies the sadistic pleasures.					
8.	I rag because I am being ragged.					
9.	Ragging is for fun and joy.					
10.	Ragging will affect the victim and victim's family.					
11.	Ragging helps to establish friendship.					
12.	Ragging affects the self esteem of the person who is being ragged.					
13.	Ragging should be punished.					
14.	Helping is misunderstood as ragging in many context.					

Keys: SA, Strongly Agree; A, Agree; UC, Uncertain; D, Disagree; SD, Strongly Disagree.

Johncy Prabha (2013) has prepared a Likert scale to assess the attitude towards safety behavior among adolescents.

Table 7.2 is a 5 point Likert scale which consisted of 10 items. In these, item no 1, 2 ,4, 5, 8 are positive statements and item no 3, 6, 7, 9, 10 are negative statements to assess the attitude towards safety behavior among adolescents. Scale legend includes strongly agree, agree, uncertain, disagree and strongly disagree.

Table 7.2: Likert scale to assess the attitude towards safety behavior among adolescents

Statement	Strongly disagree	Disagree	Uncertain	Agree	Strongly Agree
1. Safe behavior maintains positive health (+)	0	1	2	3	4
2. Eating balanced diet is good for health (+)	0	1	2	3	4

contd...

contd...

Statement	Strongly disagree	Disagree	Uncertain	Agree	Strongly Agree
3. Consumption of fast food provides adequate nutrients (–)	4	3	2	1	0
4. Attending family function will promote social health (+)	0	1	2	3	4
5. Give and take is a good policy (+)	0	1	2	3	4
6. Night sleep can be compensated by day sleep (–)	4	3	2	1	0
7. Fighting with friends is an acceptable behavior (–)	4	3	2	1	0
8. Regular exercise prevents over weight (+)	0	1	2	3	4
9. Being social is difficult (–)	4	3	2	1	0
10. Parents and teachers always control adolescents (–)	4	3	2	1	0

Semantic differentials: The semantic differential was developed by Osgood and colleagues (1957) measures attitudes or beliefs. It consists of two adjectives with a 7-point scale between them. The subject is to select one point on the scale that best describes his or her view of the concept being examined. In a semantic differential, values from 1–7 are assigned to each of these space, with 1 being the most negative response and 7 the most positive response. Placement of negative responses to the left or right of the scale should be randomly varied to avoid global responses (in which the subject places checks in the same column of each scale). Each line is considered one scale. The values for the scales are summed to obtain one score for each subject.

The Semantic Differential (SD) measures people's reactions to stimulus words and concepts in terms of ratings or bipolar scales defined with contrasting adjectives at each end. An example of an SD scale is:

Good _ _ _ _ _ _ _ Bad
3 2 1 0 1 2 3

or

Good _ _ _ _ _ _ _ Bad
7 6 5 4 3 2 1

Usually, the position marked 0 is labeled neutral, the 1 positions are labeled slightly, the 2 positions quite and the 3 positions extremely. A scale, like this one, measures directionality of a reaction (e.g. good versus bad) and also intensity (slight through extreme).

A number of basic considerations are involved in SD methodology:

- Bipolar adjective scales are a simple, economical means for obtaining data on sample's reactions. With adaptations, such scales can be used with adults or children, persons from all walks of life and persons from any culture.

- Ratings on bipolar adjective scales tend to be correlated and three basic dimensions of response account for most of the covariation in ratings. The three dimensions, which have been labeled as Evaluation, Potency and Activity (EPA), have been verified and replicated in an impressive variety of studies.
- Some adjective scales are almost pure measures of the EPA dimensions, e.g. good-bad for Evaluation, powerful-powerless for Potency and fast-slow for Activity. Using a few pure scales of this sort, one can obtain, with considerable economy, reliable measures of a person's overall response to something. Typically, a concept is rated on several pure scales associated with a single dimension and the results are averaged to provide a single factor score for each dimension. Measurements of a concept on the EPA dimensions are referred to as the concept's profile.
- EPA measurements are appropriate when one is interested in affective responses. The EPA system is notable for being a multivariate approach to affect measurement. It is also a generalized approach, applicable to any concept or stimulus and thus it permits comparisons of affective reactions on widely disparate things.
- The SD has been used as a measure of attitude in a wide variety of projects. Osgood, et al. (1957), report exploratory studies in which the SD was used to assess attitude change as a result of mass media programs.

Evaluation dimensions are:

- nice-awful
- good-bad
- sweet-sour
- helpful-unhelpful
- hot-cold
- pleasant-unpleasant
- beautiful-ugly.

Potency dimensions are:

- big-little
- powerful-powerless
- strong-weak
- deep-shallow.

Activity scales are:

- fast-slow
- alive-dead
- noisy-quiet
- young-old
- passive-active.

Thurstone scale: In psychology, the Thurstone scale was the first formal technique for measuring an attitude. It was developed by Louis Leon Thurstone in 1928, as a means of measuring attitudes towards religion. It is made up of statements about a particular issue and each statement has a numerical value indicating how favorable or unfavorable it is judged to be.

People check each of the statements to which they agree and a mean score is computed, indicating their attitude. Thurstone was one of the first and most productive scaling theorists. He actually invented three different methods for developing a unidimensional scale: the method of equal appearing intervals; the method of successive intervals; and the method of paired comparisons. The three methods differed in how the scale values for items were constructed, but in all three cases, the resulting scale was rated the same way by respondents.

Construction of Thurstone scale (Method of equal appearing intervals)

Developing the focus: First decide on the concept or theme to which the respondent has to rate. Define the focus for the scale and the purpose for which it has to be created. The description of this concept should be as clear as possible so that the person(s) who are going to create the statements have a clear idea of what will be measured.

Generating potential scale items: The next step is to create a large set of candidate statements (e.g. 80–100), because the final scale items are selected from this pool. All of the statements are worded similarly—that they do not differ in grammar or structure.

Rating the scale items: The next step is to have the participants (i.e. judges, i.e. approximately 50 or more) rate each statement on a 1–11 scale in terms of how much each statement indicates a favorable attitude towards a particular concept. It is not that the judges rating their attitudes towards a concept or whether they would agree or disagree with the statements towards a concept. It is to rate their favorableness of each statement in terms of an attitude towards a concept for, e.g. AIDS, where 1 = extremely unfavorable attitude towards people with AIDS and 11 = extremely favorable attitude towards people with AIDS.

Computing scale score values for each item: The next step is to analyze the rating data. For each statement, from 50 judges values, the median and the inter-quartile range is computed. The median is the value above and below which 50% of the ratings fall. The first quartile (Q1) is the value below which 25% of the cases fall and above which 75% of the cases fall—in other words, the 25th percentile. The median is the 50th percentile. The third quartile, Q3, is the 75th percentile. The inter-quartile range is the difference between third and first quartile, or Q3 - Q1. These values can be computed easily with any introductory statistics program or with most spreadsheet programs. To facilitate the final selection of items for the scale, sort the table of medians and inter-quartile range.

Select the final scale items: The statements that are selected should be at equal intervals across the range of medians. Within each value, the statement with smallest inter-quartile range is selected. This is the statement with the least amount of variability across judges. And also, look over the candidate statements at each level and select the statement that makes the most sense. If the best statistical choice is a confusing statement, the next best choice is selected.

Administering the scale: The final selected items make a single Thurstone scale to measure the attitude towards a concept. This is given to the samples to measure the attitude. The participants have to either agree or disagree with each statement. To get that person's total scale score, get the average value for the scores of all the items that person agreed with.

OBSERVATION

Observation is a technique for collecting data through occurrences that can be observed through senses with or without medical devices. Goode and Hatt have rightly said that science begins with observation. Observation becomes scientific when,

- It is planned deliberately
- It is serving a formulated research purpose
- It is systematically recorded
- It is subjected to checks and controls of validity and reliability.

Observation is way of gathering data by watching behavior, events, or noting physical characteristics in their natural setting. It is the most commonly used method especially in studies relating to behavioral science. In this method, information are sought by way of investigator's own direct observation without asking from the respondent. For instance, in a study relating to consumer behavior, the investigator instead of asking the brand of wrist watch used by the respondent may himself look at the watch. There are two parts, i.e. someone is observing or observer and there is something to observe or the observed.

Processes of Observation

Observation involves ***three processes*** such as sensation, attention and perception.

1. ***Sensation:*** Sensation is gained through the sense organs which depends on physical alertness of the observer.
2. ***Attention or concentration:*** This is the person's ability to concentrate on certain activity. This is largely a matter of will power and adequate training and experience.
3. ***Perception:*** It involves the interpretation of sensory inputs. Thus, sensation merely reports the facts as observed but perception enables the mind to attach meaning and to understand it.

Observation is a two-part process:

1. Someone is observing—observer
2. There is something to observe—observed.

Types of Observation

Non concealment and concealment refer to whether the observer takes his intentions known to the persons observed or not, whereas Participant and Non-participant refer to the role of observer, that is, whether the observer is a part of the social setting or makes the observation from periphery of a social setting.

Observations can be overt (everyone knows they are being observed) or covert (no one knows they are being observed and the observer is concealed). The benefit of covert observation is that people are more likely to behave naturally, if they do not know that they are being observed. However, the researcher will typically need to conduct overt observations because of ethical problems related to concealing his observation.

Observations can also be either direct or indirect. Direct observation is when the researcher watches interactions, processes, or behaviors as they occur. Indirect observations are when the researcher watches the results of interactions, processes, or behaviors; for example, measuring the amount of plate waste left by students in a school cafeteria to determine whether a new food is acceptable to them (Fig. 7.3).

The observer-observed relationship: The observer/researcher can interact with individuals in the observational setting to varying degrees. The two most important aspects of this issue are intervention and concealment.

Observational methods differ in the degree of structure that the researcher imposes on the task of recording and encoding the obtained information. Relatively unstructured methods generally involved in the collection of extensive amounts of descriptive information, which is analyzed in a qualitative rather than quantitative fashion. Unstructured methods of recording observation are more commonly used in studies in which the observer is not concealed.

There are three types of observations:

1. ***Structured and unstructured observations:*** The observations which are characterized by a careful definition of the units to be observed, the style of recording the observed information, standardized conditions of observation and selection of pertinent data of observation are called 'structured observations'. These observations are considered appropriate in descriptive studies. When the observation is to take place without these characteristics to be thought of in advance, it is termed as 'unstructured observation'. Theses observations are most likely in exploratory studies.

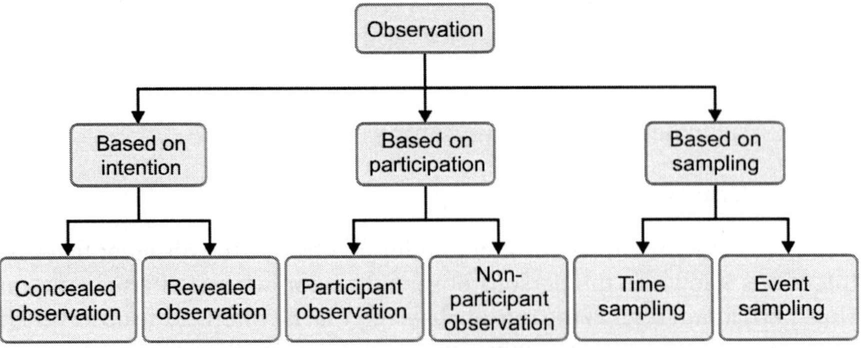

Fig. 7.3: Classification of methods of observation

2. ***Participant and Non-participant observations:*** These observations are used in social science. If the observer observes by making himself, more or less, a member of the group he is observing so that he can experience what the members of the group experience, the observation is called participant. But when that observer observes as detached emissary without any attempt on his part to experience through participation what others feel, the observation is termed as non-participant.
3. ***Controlled and uncontrolled observations:*** If the observation takes place in natural settings it may be termed as 'uncontrolled observation'. The major aim of this type of observation is to get a spontaneous picture of life and person. But when observation takes place according to definite pre arranged plans, involving experimental procedures, the same is then termed as controlled observation. Such observations has a tendency to supply formalized data upon which generalization can be built with some degree of accuracy (Fig. 7.3).

Participant Observation

Participant observation is a technique where in a researcher participates in the functioning of the social group that is under investigation. The aim of this approach is to secure insights and sources of information, which probably would be unattainable in other ways. Proponents of the participant observation approach claim that it represents both a sources of data and basis for understanding what the data mean. The most common forms of recordkeeping in participant observation studies are logs and field notes. A log is a record of events and conversations and usually maintained on a daily basis by field workers. Field notes may include the daily log but tend to be much broader, more analytic and more interpretive than a simple listing of occurrences.

Instruments and Tools used in Observation

Field notes may include daily log but tend to be much broader, more analytic and include more interpretation than more listing of occurrences.

Anecdotes' focus on behavior of particular interest. Anecdote typically selects specific kinds of events and behavior of observation before hand. The observer objectively, accurately records the observation.

'Check list' is a tool used for structured observation where phenomena are recorded by putting a tally against a particular behavior, events or characteristic depending upon its presence or absence. When developing a check list, the researcher must list all the expected behaviors related to the variable being measured. So that, all relevant behaviors in the subjects will correctly be identified.

Rating scales: Structured observation can also be rated in terms of qualitative points along a descriptive continuum. The rating usually is quantified during the subsequent analysis of the observation data. Here the observer is required to make ratings of behavior or events at frequent intervals throughout the observational period or he may make use of rating scale to summarize an entire events or transaction after the observation is completed where a more descriptive method have been used for maintaining observational record.

Field notes normally consist of records concerning the following elements of a social situation.

- The 'actors' or subjects, their roles and status and their characteristics and interrelationships
- The setting, its structure and appearance, and its atmosphere
- The timing of events, the season and time of day and the weather and other relevant environmental attributes
- The purpose or occasion for events
- The behavior and activities of the actors and the correlations, movements; non verbal communications
- The frequency and duration of events and behaviors.

Anecdotes: Anecdotes occasionally, can be scientific value, particularly if they are used in an illustrative fashion to add richness and vitality to what might otherwise be a dull and sterile statistical report. Anecdotal methods are considerably more focused on behavior of particular interest.

Observation Sampling Technique

Since it is usually possible to observe behaviors for extended period of time because of fatigue and boredom one must plan when to make the observation. The most commonly used techniques are:

- ***Time sampling method:*** This procedure involves the selection of time periods during which the observation will take place. One decides the day into units that are appropriate for observation. The time frame may be systematically selected.
- ***Event sampling:*** It is done when we want to observe an entire event in order to give the subject the opportunity to perform all of the expected behaviors. The observer selects integral behavior or event of a prespecified type of observation. Researcher either requires to know the occurrence of event or be in a position to wait for their occurrence.

Steps in developing observation schedule: The first step is to select the aspect of behavior to be observed. We cannot notice everything that happens and record everything we notice, so to carry out systematic observation, we must select certain aspects of categories of behavior to be observed.

- The investigator lists the categories of behaviors that may or may not be manifested by the subjects. The observer watches for the behaviors given on the list and put a check off beside the appropriate behavior when it occurs. The observer does not classify all the behaviors or characteristics of the individuals being observed but rather identifies the occurrence and frequency of particular behavior.

- The most common method used in structured observation is construction of category system to which observed behaviors or characteristics can be assigned. In category system, an attempt is made to designate in a systematic or quantitative fashion the qualitative behavior and events transpiring within the observation setting.
- ***Quantifying observation:*** When the behaviors specified have to provide certain measurement then some form of quantification is required. The quantification usually takes the form of counting.
- ***Developing procedure to facilitate recording:*** In order to have adequate account of what was observed during the observation, some procedure for recording should be followed, either during the observation or soon after the observation is completed.
- Observation of human beings involve some important ethical implications in terms of their rights, willingness to be observed.

When should the researcher use observation for evaluation?

- When the researcher is trying to understand an ongoing process or situation
- When the researcher wants to gather data on individual behaviors or interactions between people
- When the researcher needs to know about a physical setting
- When data collection from individuals is not a realistic option. If respondents are unwilling or unable to provide data through questionnaires or interviews, observation is a method of choice.

How do you plan for observations?

- Determine the focus
- Design a system for data collection
- Select the sites
- Select the observers
- Train the observers
- Time your observations appropriately.

Observation technique requires skill in administration

- Determine the observer observed relationship, i.e. participant or non-participant and concealment or no concealment
- Record responses exactly
- ***Training observer:*** Observational methods are more vulnerable to perceptual errors than any other data collection. To minimize the biases and maximize the accuracy, an objectivity of the observation and training of observer is essential.

Advantages of Observation

- To study human behavior
- All subjects are potential respondents
- Subjects are usually available
- It lends itself to the use of recording instruments

- Instrument is simple
- Subjective bias is eliminated, if observation is done correctly
- It can be stopped or started at anytime
- Recording eliminates bias because of the ability to recall
- One can make use of assistants to carry out observations
- Provides depth and variety of information
- The information obtained under this method relates to what is currently happening, it is not complicated by either the past behavior or future intentions or attitudes.

  This method is independent of respondent's willingness to respond and as such is relatively less demanding of active cooperation on the part of respondents as happen to be the case in the interview or the questionnaire method. This method is particularly suitable in studies which deal with subject, i.e. respondents who are not capable of giving verbal report of their feelings for one reason or the other.

Disadvantages of Observation

- Accurate prediction of situation is not possible. So we may miss key elements
- It is an expensive method
- It requires attention, perception and concentration
- Lack of consent
- Information provided by this method is very limited
- Presence of the observer leads to bias
- Data is vulnerable to many distortions and biases
- Subjectivity
- Recording devices are expensive
- Errors of leniency and halo effects are possible
- Sometimes unforeseen factors may interfere with the observational task. At times, the fact that some people are rarely accessible to direct observation creates obstacles for this method to collect data effectively.
- Does not rely on people's willingness or ability to provide information
- Susceptible to the 'Hawthorne effect,' that is, people usually perform better when they know they are being observed, although indirect observation may decrease this problem
- Can be expensive and time-consuming compared to other data collection methods.

CHECKLISTS

Checklists are lists of items or performance indicators requiring dichotomous responses such as satisfactory or unsatisfactory, pass or fail, yes or no, present or absent, etc. Gronlund (2005) describes a checklist as an inventory of measurable performance dimension of products with a place to record a simple yes or no judgment.

A checklist is a grouping of items by which something may be confirmed or verified. It can be called as a behavioral inventory. It is basically a method of recording whether a particular attribute is present or absent or whether an action had or had not taken place. It consists of a listing of steps, activities or behavior which the observer records when an incident occurs. The objectives of the research should be kept in mind when preparing and using a checklist.

Construction of Checklists

While constructing or preparing checklists, following points to be kept in mind:

- Express each item in clear, simple language
- Avoid lifting statements verbatim from the text
- Avoid negative statements wherever possible
- Review the items independently.

Utilization of Checklists

- Use checklist only when you are interested in ascertaining whether a particular trait or characteristics is present or absent
- Use only a carefully prepared checklist for more complex kind of trait
- Observe only one sample at a time and confine your observation to the points specified in the checklists
- Have separate checklists for each sample
- The observer must be trained, how to observe, what to observe and how to record the observed behavior. To make a valid judgment he should omit recording those behaviors for which he has insufficient information
- Checklists require the observer to judge whether certain behavior of sample has taken place. They can be used most effectively when components of clinical performance can be specified. It is possible for the observer to simply note whether the prescribed behavior has taken place or not. The actual physical, psychomotor skills involved can be jointly precisely stated.

Merits of Checklists

- Short and easy to assess and record
- Useful for evaluation of specific well-defined behaviors and are commonly used in the clinical and simulated laboratory setting
- They can be used for both process and procedure evaluation
- They are adaptable to most subject matter areas
- They allow inter individual comparisons to be made on a common set of traits or characteristics.

The checking process implies that standards and criteria are available for gauging items. The inspection procedure requires scrutiny of behavior under investigation. Checklists are most useful for determining the status of tangible items, such as inventory and maintenance of equipment and supplies.

They have the advantage that items to be observed can be determined in advance and will be the same criteria used in each situation. But there is no guarantee however, that the observed behavior is a persistent one and that the procedure will provide a representative picture of the individual being evaluated. It is recommended that only significant behaviors essential for a successful performance be included on the checklist.

Limitations

Does not indicate the quality of performance. Only a limited component can be assessed.

RATING SCALE

Rating means the judgment of one person by another. A rating scale is a method by which we systematize the expression of opinion concerning a trait. It is a common evaluation tool used in describing observed skills and performance. More than noting the presence or absence of a behavior, the rating scales locate the behavior to a point on a continuum and also involves judgments regarding quantitative and qualitative abilities. In simple words, it consists of a set of characteristics or qualities to be judged and a scale for indicating the degree up to which the particular attribute is present.

It can be defined as 'a standardized method of recording, interpretation of behavior, which is totally based on observation, strictly in line with the objectives'. It is a device used to evaluate situations or characteristics that can occur or be present in varying degrees, rather than merely be present or absent. The instrument is so designed as to facilitate appraisal of a number of traits or characteristics by reference to a common quantitative scale of values.

Rating scales resemble checklists but are used when finer discriminations are required. Instead of merely indicating the presence or absence of a trait or characteristic, it enables us to indicate the degree to which a trait is present. Rating scale provides systematic procedure for obtaining, recording and reporting the observer's judgment. That may be filled out while the observation is made, immediately after the observation is made or as often in the case, long after the observation.

Rating scales consist of a set of characteristics or qualities to be judged and some type of scale for indicating the degree to which an attribute is present.

Types of Rating Scales

Various types of rating scales that are commonly used are:

- Descriptive rating scales
- Graphic rating scales
- Numerical rating scales
- Behaviorally Anchored Rating Scales (BARS).

Descriptive Rating Scales

These types of rating scales use descriptive phrases to identify the points on a graphic scale (Fig. 7.4). The descriptions are brief details that convey in behavioral terms for each trait (how samples behave at different steps along the scale). The rater selects the one most applicable to the person. A space for comment is also frequently provided to enable the rater to clarify the rating or to record behavioral incidents pertinent to the rating. For example, observation of working hours can have scale legends as usually late, sometimes late and usually on time; Completion of work assignments can have scale legends such as usually late, sometimes late and usually on time (Table 7.3).

The descriptions may take the form of:

- ***Abstract labels:*** Such as A, B, C, D and E
- ***Frequency labels:*** Such as always, usually, frequently, sometimes, never.
- ***Qualitative labels:*** Superior, above average, average, below average.

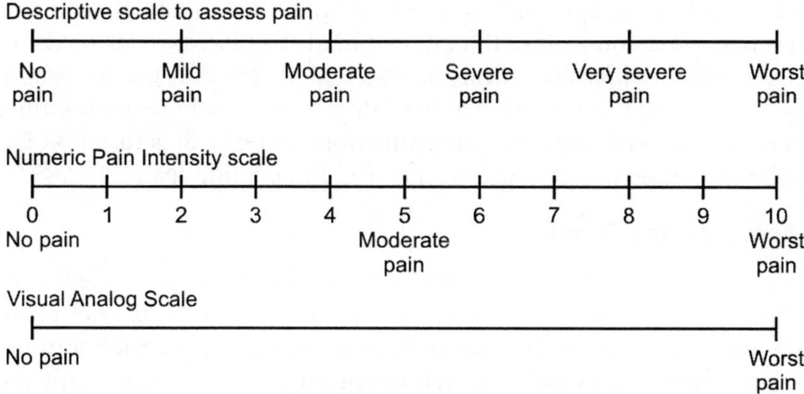

Fig. 7.4: Various rating scales

Table 7.3: Rating scale to assess the mental health of the students

S.No.	Items	None	Sometimes	Often	Almost always
1.	Able to concentrate				
2.	Losing much sleep over worry				
3.	Feeling mentally alert				
4.	Feeling full of energy				
5.	Having restless nights				
6.	Managing to keep busy				
7.	Getting out of the hostel				
8.	Managing as well as most people would				
9.	Doing things well				

Contd...

Contd...

S.No.	Items	None	Sometimes	Often	Almost always
10.	Feeling warmth and affection				
11.	Getting on with other people				
12.	Feeling that playing a useful part				
13.	Not capable of making decisions				
14.	Feeling constantly under stain				
15.	Not capable to overcome				
16.	Finding life a struggle all the time				
17.	Enjoying day-to-day activities				
18.	Taking things hard				
19.	Getting scared or panicky				

Graphic Rating Scales

The rater indicates the performer's standing in respect to each trait by placing a check mark at an appropriate point along the line. In this, each line is followed by a horizontal line. The rating is made by placing a tick on the line. A set of categories identify specific positions along the line, but the rater can also click between these points. Here the degree of each character is arranged so that the rater can make as fine distinctions as he wishes to make. Faces scale for pain assessment is an example of graphic rating scale.

Numerical Rating Scales

In this, the extent or degree to which a particular attribute is present in an individual is indicated by numbers (Fig. 7.4). The observer puts a tick or circle on the number to which the sample possess that attribute. Each number is given a verbal description that remains constant for a particular character.

It includes numbers against which a list of behaviors is evaluated. This is not a very reliable tool because of the inconsistent value attributed to the number. It can be partially overcome by adding a few quantitative terms. For example,

Ability to get along with others	1	2	3	4	5
Punctuality	1	2	3	4	5
Clinical performance	1	2	3	4	5
Communication skill	1	2	3	4	5

1 = Never 2 = Sometimes 3 = About half the time
4 = Usually 5 = Always Or
5 = Outstanding 4 = Above average 3 = Average
2 = Below average 1 = Dissatisfactory

The numerical rating scale is useful when the characteristics or qualities to be rated can be classified into a limited number of categories and when there is a general agreement concerning the category represented by each number.

Behaviorally Anchored Rating Scales

BARS is an acronym for Behaviorally Anchored Rating Scales, sometimes known as BES, Behavioral Expectation Scales. It evaluates behavior relevant to specific demands of the job and provides examples of specific job behaviors corresponding to good, average and poor performances. This reduces the amount of personal judgment needed by the rater. Separate BARS are needed for each job. BOS as an acronym for Behavioral Observation Scales. This system capitalizes on some of the strengths of BARS while avoiding some of the disadvantages. The evaluator lists a number of critical incidents for each performance dimension and rates the extent to which the behavior has been observed on a five point scale ranging from almost never to almost always.

Punctual	Almost never	1	2	3	4	5	Almost always
Gets along well with others	Almost never	1	2	3	4	5	Almost always

Principles in Preparing Rating Scales

- Rating scales should directly relate to objectives of the research
- They need to be confined to performance areas that can be observed
- Three to seven rating positions may need to be provided
- The scale may be made more objective, valid and reliable by getting a pooled rating from more than one observer
- All raters should be oriented to the specific scale as well as the process of rating in general
- As errors are common due to subjective judgment made by the observer, rater should be conscious enough to avoid them
- A rating scale provides the instructor with a convenient form on which to record judgments indicating the degree of sample's performance. This differs from a checklist in that it allows for more discrimination in judging behaviors as compared with dichotomous yes or no options.

Advantages of Rating Scales

- Rating scales are easy to administer and score
- They can be used for large number of samples
- They have a wide range of application
- They are used to evaluate skills, product outcomes, activities, interests, attitudes and personal characteristics
- It is used to observe and record qualitative and quantitative judgments about observed performance
- They tend to be adaptable and flexible
- They are efficient and economical in the use of time
- They can help to reduce the subjectivity and unreliability that are usually associated with the observation method
- It will direct observation towards specific aspects of behavior

- It will provide a common frame of reference for comparing all samples on the same set of characteristics
- It will provide a convenient method for recording the observer's judgments.

Disadvantages of Rating Scales

However, be careful, a degree of subjectivity is inevitable while using the rating scales.

Example of a rating scale to assess the mental health of the students

BIOPHYSICAL MEASUREMENTS

Nurses are involved in collection and measurement of biophysiological measures in clinical oriented research. Physiologic measurements can be classified in one of two major categories. Physiological measurement can be classified as *in vivo* and *in vitro* (Fig. 7.5). *In vivo* includes measurement of those which are performed directly with in or on living organisms themselves, such as blood flow determination through radiography, intravenous pyelogram (IVP), cholecystography. An *In vitro* measurement by contrast is performed outside the organism's body, such as blood glucose, blood urea, serum Na^+, K^+.

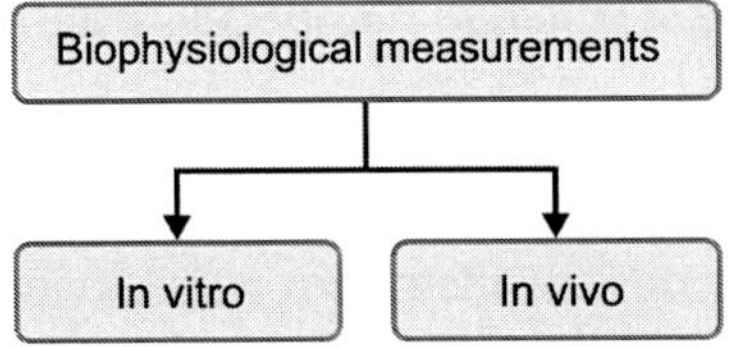

Fig. 7.5: Types of biophysiological measurements

Physiological measurements can also be classified as listed below:

- Physical measurement, e.g. temperature, volume, pressure, electrical measures
- Chemical measurement, e.g. hormnone levels, sugar, urea, Hb%, potassium level, etc.
- Microbiological measurement, e.g. bacterial counts and identification
- Anatomical and cytological measurements, e.g. X-rays, tissue biopsies, demography CAT scan etc.

PSYCHOLOGICAL AND SOCIOLOGICAL MEASUREMENT

Psychological measurement mainly makes use of psychological test and inventories. Psychological test is an instrument designed to measure only a certain aspect of human behavior, these tests yield objective and standardized descriptions of behavior, quantified by numerical scores. These tools attempt to quantify the feelings, attitudes, opinion of individuals, etc. for example, measurement of attitude, personality and intelligence achievements.

Sociological measurement attempts to measure groups or individuals in relation to a social set-up. For example, social distance scale which attempts to measure to what degree an individual or group is distanced from others. Socioeconomic status scale such as SES scale by B. Kuppuswamy and SES scale (Rural) Udai Pareek, G Trivedi measures the socioeconomic status of the samples.

Characteristics of Tools/Measuring Scales

- ***Initial acceptance:*** The tool we use to collect data must be acceptable to the researcher himself and samples. Unacceptable questions in the tool should be rejected and not be used in data collection activities. Instruments which are used to measure some biophysiological data must be acceptable by the both.
- ***Practicability/Feasibility:*** At the next level, practicability is of concern. If the gathering of data is onerous and time-consuming, conducting enough measurements to establish stability or reliability will be difficult and perhaps impossible.

  Validity cannot exist in the absence of reliability and a method of measurement that has no potential for valid use is worthless. Hence, acceptability and practicability are both necessary, but not sufficient requirements of sources of evaluation data. Factors to be considered in deciding feasibility are time and resources required, availability of an equivalent form of the test for measuring reliability and ease of administration, scoring and interpretation.

  The tool should be simple, easy to use, reliable and valid. In case of questionnaire as a tool, if the words in the questions are complex, ambiguous and difficult to understand, we cannot collect the relevant data. The tool may not be valid and reliable. If the instruments are used, it should be simple to operate, read and interpret the score. The instrument should not involve complex mechanisms, not too costly and easy to carry and use.
- ***Reliability:*** Reliability is the degree to which measurements are consistent and do not contain measurement error. Reliability was defined as the extent to which on repeated measures, an instrument yields similar results. Measurements should be stable over time and across situations. For example, if we use a weighing scale to measure the weight of a group of adults, then the weighing scale should show the similar results when it is used to measure the weight for the same adults in different time periods or when it is used by the different investigator for the same adults. When the three attributes of acceptability, practicability and reliability have been established, validity can be investigated. In simple terms, any tool or instrument should be stable, that is on

repeated usage or administration it should produce the similar findings or no variation between administration. Terms such as dependability, consistency, stability and accuracy are often used interchangeably to refer to reliability. The first three terms refer to the instrument's ability to produce the same results on repeated measures. The fourth term, accuracy, reflects a different dimension of reliability, the measurement tool's ability to reflect the true value being measured. Reliability is the term used to deal with accuracy.

True value is the value that would be obtained if the measurement tools were perfect. In other words, the true value is free of random measurement error.

A scale measurement is considered reliable if it measures that what it is supposed to measure. Further refining of the term reliable is that, when a test is repeated by the same researcher, i.e. with a different group representing the original group, the same results should be obtained.

Reliability refers to the stability or consistency of the measurement. Reliability is a measure of reproducibility of the test. In other words, if the same or an equivalent test is given to the students, the scores obtained by individual students and the group as a whole would be similar. Reliability refers to the results of the test, not to the instrument itself. A reliable test does not indicate a valid one since the test can consistently measure something but not necessarily what is intended to be measured.

Reliability is a relative term. It exists in degrees and is usually expressed as a form of correlation coefficient, with 1.00 indicates perfect reliability and 0.00 indicating an absence of reliability. Nunnally (1978) suggests that reliability coefficients of 0.70 or above for new instruments and 0.80 or above for established instruments are acceptable.

- ***Stability:*** Stability is concerned with the consistency of the results with repeated measures. Perhaps the easiest way to assess stability is to repeat a question that been posed. The idea of test retest is whether the respondent is able to understand the question on both occasions on identical terms and have and infer similar meaning. So that the variable measured would be the same on two occasions. This type of reliability is most important in repeated measures design, specially the one with the pretest and post-test design of single and two groups.
- ***Internal consistency:*** It refers to the ability of the items in an instrument to measure the same variable. Homogeneity is often used to refer to the internal consistency of an instrument. A homogenous instrument means which contains items that are strongly correlated with each other. The higher the correlations among the items, the greater the internal consistency of the instrument. Homogenous instruments are unidimensional, i.e. the items taken together measure one construct. Because all the items reflect the same underlying construct, the researcher can sum the individual item scores to get total score that

reflects the construct. Methods available to test the internal consistency of a measure include the Kuder-Richardson coefficient, item total correlations, split half reliability and Cronbach's alpha.

In split half method the items in a tool are randomly divided into two groups and correlation coefficient is calculated for the resulting two scores. The advantage of this method is that it allows the researchers to assess the test retest reliability without administering the instrument twice. The Spearman-Brown correlation is usually used in this procedure.

Another procedure to assess homogeneity is to compare an individual item's correlation with the total index score. If an item is consistent with the total score, it will correlate with it. This technique is known as the internal consistency approach to reliability.

The item total correlations represent a group of correlations between each item and total score for instrument. Item total correlations are useful in instrument development. They are helpful in deciding which items to retain and which ones to discard in creating a final index. The item total correlations should be high enough to indicate internal consistency but low enough that they are not redundant. Nunnally (1978) suggests that uncorrected item total correlations above 0.25 and below 0.70 are typically acceptable for item retention when developing a new index.

The most common method used by nurse researchers for assessing internal consistency is Cronbach's alpha. This test is based on the strength of the inter correlations of all the items in the instrument as well as the number of items used. The alpha value ranges from 0–1, with '1' indicating perfect internal consistency and '0' no internal consistency.

Equivalence refers to the degree of agreement among two or more different observers using the same measurement tool or the agreement between two or more alternate forms of an instrument.

Reliability can be measured by ***Test-Retest method*** and ***Split Half method***.

- ***Test-retest method:*** Two observations (measurements) are made using same instrument (either on different time period or by different persons) and calculating the correlations coefficient (r) is a method of establishing reliability. Value closer to 1 indicates the high reliability and low value indicates the low reliability.
- ***Split-half method:*** The values of the odd number and even number questions can be computed for each sample and with the resultant values the correlation coefficient can be calculated. Or else, the values of the first half and the second half of the questions can be computed for each individual and with the values the correlation coefficient value can be calculated.

Measures to improve reliability: Reliability can be increased by increasing length of a test or questionnaire to optimum level, ensure objectivity of scoring and ensuring validity of the instrument used. There are two general approaches to increasing the reliability of data especially in experimental desings: Practice trails and multiple trials.

- ***Practice trials:*** A participant's score may be unrepresentative because he or she has not 'warmed up' on the measurement task. When this is a possibility, we provide practice trials. We test participants as in the real study, but we ignore their scores from these trials when analyzing the results.
- ***Multiple trials:*** A major component of reliability is the number of real trials a participant performs in a condition. A score that is based on only one trial may reflect all sorts of extraneous factors: A participant may be momentarily distracted or may guess well. The trial may be easy or difficult, or some other aspect of the situation may make the trial peculiar. In such a case, the response and score are not representative of a subjects typical response and score. To avoid bias from one unique trial, we observe each participant several times in a condition, observing multiple trials. Providing practice trials and testing multiple trials tends to increase the reliability of data.

Multiple trials produce a new extraneous variable called 'order effects'. Order effects are the influence on a particular trial that arises from its position in the sequence of trials. Order effects have two components. Practice effects and carry over effects. Practice effects are the influence on performance that arises from practicing a task. Even after practice trials, participants may perform initial trials poorly because they are not warmed up. After more trials, performance may increase, at the same time, performance may decrease again because subjects become fatigued or bored.

The other component is carry over effects, the influence that a particular trial has on performance of subsequent trials. Carry over effects may arise first from simply experiencing a trial. Carry over effects also arise from a response set which is a bias toward responding in a particular way because of previous responses made. This occurs whenever responding becomes more of a habit than a natural reaction to the stimulus. This can be taken care by counterbalancing the order effects.

Counterbalancing order effects: Balancing order effects is called counter balancing. It is systematically changing the order of trials for different subjects in a balanced way to counter the biasing influence of any one order.

Validity: Validity on the other hand is concerned with the soundness and the effectiveness of the measuring instrument (Leedy 1993). Validity is the accuracy with which a test measures whatever it is intended to/supposed to measure. Validity is regarded as the absolutely indispensable property of any measuring instrument. Without validity, the instrument has no value. Validity is concerned with the general question: To what extent will this assessment information help us make an appropriate decision? It is a matter of degree; it does not exist on an all or nothing basis. It should be considered in terms of categories—highly valid, moderately valid, and invalid (Table 7.4).

Table 7.4: Types and its procedure of validity and reliability

Criteria	Types	Procedure
Reliability	Test-retest	Test and retest is conducted. Each subjects ratings on same tool on two occasions positively correlated.
	Split half	Subjects score from half of the item positively correlated with their scores from the other half.
	Inter rater	Ratings obtained by two raters are positively correlated.
Validity	Face	Procedure/items appears to be valid.
	Convergent	Procedure correlates with other accepted measures.
	Discriminant	Procedure does not correlate with other unintended measures.
	Predictive	Procedure correlates with a future behavior.

Types of Validity

- ***Face validity:*** A measure has face validity to the extent that it appears to measure what it sets out to measure. A measure may only appear to be a valid index of some characteristic under study but may really lack it. Conversely, a measure may lack face validity but be an excellent index of some characteristic.
- ***Content validity:*** Face validity of a measure is the most superficial type. A more systematic type is content validity. Content validity refers to whether we actually and only measure an intended variable. Content validity deals with the accuracy with which an instrument measures the factors or content of the course or situations, under study. It refers to the content in the tool whether does it measure whatever it is intended to measure?. Whether the content is appropriate to measure what is supposed to measure. A measure has content validity to the extent that it is representative of the subject matter or topic being measured. Content validity suffers when the measure contains items which measure subject matter or topic outside the domain of interest. For example, a tool which intends to measure the knowledge of the samples on prevention and management of anemia in adolescent girls supposed to measure the knowledge on anemia only. It should include the questions relevant to prevention and management of anemia in adolescent girls. Content validity suffers when the items in a measure under represent the relevant domain. Content validation is basically a judgmental. The content validity of the tool is ensured by showing the content of the tool to the experts in the field and getting approval for its appropriateness and relevance etc. Their suggestions and recommendations for improvising and modification of the tool can be taken for improving content validity.
- ***Criterion validity:*** The question of criterion related validity arises when the scores obtained by an individual on one measure (called predictor) are used to infer his standing on some other variable (called criterion). The criterion may be either a behavior or attitude. Criterion related validity is a measure of how well the test performance reflects either

concurrent performance of the same behavior based on some other measuring instrument or future performance obtained by another test given at some future time. Comparison of test scores with other scores obtained by other measuring instruments at the same time is called concurrent validity and comparison with subsequent scores obtained in future is called predictive validity (Table 7.4).

Criterion related validity may be of three different types depending upon when the predictor and criterion variables are measured:

- ***Predictive validity:*** When the predictor variable is measured at one point in time and the criterion at some future point, it is known as 'predictive validity.'
- ***Construct validity:*** Construct validity refers to whether a variable actually and only reflects the intended hypothetical construct. Abstract variables which cannot be directly observed (e.g. motivation, morale, beauty etc) are known as constructs. The values of such variables cannot be directly observed but can only be inferred from other observable variables. These other observable variables then become our operational definitions of these constructs. By construct validity of a measure it meant the appropriateness of the operational definition of the construct. Construct validity is interested in the degree to which the construct is actually measured. Construct validity is really a comparison of the test scores with scores obtained by other measuring instruments which measures a related ability.
- ***Internal validity:*** Internal validity is the degree to which the mathematical relationship we observe between subjects' scores actually and only reflects the relationship between the variables of interest. Internal validity is the degree to which we can draw the correct inferences about the relationship occurring within a study.
- ***External validity:*** External validity is the degree to which the results accurately generalize to other individuals and other situations. In other words, external validity is the question of whether the study provides a good example of the relationship that occurs in a situations 'external' to our study. External validity is the degree to which we can draw the correct inferences when generalizing beyond a study.
- ***Ecological validity:*** Ecological validity is the extent to which research can be generalized to common behaviors and natural situations. This issue is most important in highly controlled laboratory experiments. Ecological validity is the extent to which the situation and behaviors in a study are those found in the natural environment.

Threats to validity and reliability can be minimized by controlling extraneous variables. This is possible by eliminating extraneous variables, keeping extraneous variables constant and balancing extraneous variables.

Other than these criteria, certain other qualities are also used to select tools that include:

- ***Objectivity:*** A test is objective, when the scorer's personal judgment does not affect the scoring.

- ***Relevance:*** To what extent the items in the tool conform to the objectives of the measuring instrument.
- ***Specificity:*** The items in a tool should be specific to the objectives.
- ***Length:*** The number of items in the tool should depend upon the objectives of the research.
- ***Comprehensiveness:*** The total content and objectives has to be kept in mind while preparing items for the tool.
- ***Adequacy:*** A measuring instrument should be adequate on itself.
- ***Precise and clear:*** Items contained in the test should be clear and precise.
- ***Economic:*** Administration of the tool be cost efficient.

Factors to be Considered in Measurement of Variables

When designing a study a researcher observes the participants in a specific environment and applies a measurement procedure. The researcher must consider:

- ***Subject variables:*** The personal characteristics and experiences of participants that may influence their responses.
- ***Researcher variables:*** The behaviors and characteristics of the researcher that may influence the reactions of the subjects.
- ***Environmental variables:*** The aspects of the environment that can influence scores.
- ***Measurement variables:*** The aspect of the stimuli that can influence the measurement procedure employed may influence scores.
- ***Statistical error vs. systematic error:*** Researchers recognize two different sorts of error:
    - ***Statistical error:*** The difference between a computed, estimated, or measured value and the true, specified, or theoretically correct value that is caused by random and inherently unpredictable fluctuations in the measurement apparatus.
    - ***Systematic error:*** The difference between a computed, estimated, or measured value and the true, specified, or theoretically correct value that is caused by non-random fluctuations from an unknown source and which, once identified, can usually be eliminated.

SUMMARY

- Data can be defined as factual information (e.g. measurements or statistics) used as a basis for reasoning, discussion, or calculation. Data collection is the activity of acquiring and compiling information from different sources.
- The word data is a plural for the word datum which means information that is systematically collected in the course of the study. The data for a research is collected through various methods using appropriate tool.
- Primary data are obtained by specifically designed methods to fulfill the data needs of the problem at hand. The primary data are those which are collected afresh and

for the first time and thus happen to be original in character. For example, data obtained in a population census by the office of Registrar General and Census Commissioner are primary data.

- A primary source is one that itself collects the data. A primary source has more detailed information on the procedure followed in collecting and compiling the data.
- The data which are not originally collected but rather obtained from published or unpublished sources are called secondary data.
- The three major methods of data collection are self report, observation and bio-physiological measurements.
- Self reports are obtained by conducting interview or collection of information through personal contacts with individual respondents or by written questionnaire.
- The interview is a method in which two individuals are involved in conversation with each other, the first aiming primarily at getting responses from the other in the form of answers and explanations to the questions put by the former.
- Telephone interview is a method of collecting information consists in contacting respondents on telephone itself. It is not a very widely used method, but plays important part in industrial surveys, particularly in developed regions.
- Questionnaires are an inexpensive way to gather data from a potentially large number of respondents. Often they are the only feasible way to reach a number of reviewers large enough to allow statistical analysis of the results.
- There are three basic types of questionnaire: closed-ended, open-ended and the combination of both.
- An attitude scale measures how the participant feels about a subject at the moment when he or she answers the question.
- Likert scale is designed to determine the opinion or attitude of a subject and contains a number of declarative statements with a scale after each statement.
- The semantic differential was developed by Osgood and colleagues (1957) measures attitudes or beliefs. It consists of two adjectives with a 7-point scale between them. The subject is to select one point on the scale that best describes his or her view of the concept being examined.
- In psychology, the Thurstone scale was the first formal technique for measuring an attitude. It was developed by Louis Leon Thurstone in 1928, as a means of measuring attitudes towards religion. It is made up of statements about a particular issue and each statement has a numerical value indicating how favorable or unfavorable it is judged to be.
- Observation is a way of gathering data by watching behavior, events, or noting physical characteristics in their natural setting. It is the most commonly used method especially in studies relating to behavioral science.
- Checklists are lists of items or performance indicators requiring dichotomous responses such as satisfactory or unsatisfactory, pass or fail, yes or no, present or absent, etc.
- Rating means the judgment of one person by another. A rating scale is a method by which we systematize the expression of opinion concerning a trait. Rating scale is a common evaluation tool used in describing observed skills and performance.
- Physiological measurement can be classified as *in vivo* and *in vitro*. *In vivo* includes measurement of those which are performed directly with in or on living organisms themselves, such as blood flow determination through radiography, IVP, cholecystography. An *in vitro* measurement by contrast is performed outside the organism's body, such as blood glucose, blood urea, serum Na^+, K^+.
- Psychological measurement mainly makes use of psychological test and inventories. Psychological test is an instrument designed to measure only a certain aspect of human behavior, these tests yield objective and standardized descriptions of behavior, quantified by numerical scores.

- Sociological measurement attempts to measure groups or individuals in relation to a social set up. For example, social distance scale which attempts to measure to what degree an individual or group is distanced from others. Socioeconomic Status Scale such as SES scale by B Kuppuswamy and SES scale (Rural) Udai Pareek, G Trivedi measures the socioeconomic status of the samples.
- Measurements should be stable over time and across situations. Reliability refers to the stability or consistency of the measurement. Reliability is a measure of reproducibility of the test. Validity is the accuracy with which a test measures whatever it is intended to/supposed to measure. Validity is regarded as the absolutely indispensable property of any measuring instrument.

EXERCISE

- Calculate the reliability for the data given below.

Sample No.	Test	Retest
1	76	80
2	84	78
3	68	70
4	57	64
5	48	52
6	50	48
7	72	70
8	64	66
9	80	78
10	91	86

Sample No.	Rater 1	Rater 2
1	48	40
2	36	40
3	44	36
4	26	28
5	32	30
6	46	46
7	32	34
8	30	32
9	28	30
10	20	24

- Select a topic of interest and construct various types of questions.
- Select a standardized tool and critique.
- Select an appropriate topic and prepare the below mentioned tool:
  - Likert scale
  - Rating scale
  - Semantic differential scale
  - Checklist.

8 Pilot Study

OBJECTIVES

After reading this chapter, you will be able to:

- State the meaning and definition of pilot study
- Explain the importance of conducting pilot study
- Determine the samples for pilot study
- List the advantages of pilot study.

INTRODUCTION

Pilot study is the study carried out at the end of the planning phase of research, in order to explore and test the research elements. It is a small scale study that proceeds as if it were the actual study, except for the fact that subjects who will participate in the actual study are not used. However, they may be selected at this point. The primary objective of the pilot study is to test as many elements of the research proposal as possible, in order to correct any part that does not work well. For example, the pilot study tests whether the variable defined by operational definition are actually observable and measurable. Pretesting of instrument also carried in the pilot study.

Meaning and Definition of Pilot Study

A pilot experiment, also called a 'pilot study', is a small scale preliminary study conducted in order to evaluate feasibility, time, cost, adverse events and effect size (statistical variability) in an attempt to predict an appropriate sample size and improve upon the study design prior to performance of a full-scale research project. It is a smaller version of a larger study that is conducted to prepare for that study. A pilot study is an initial investigation to give information that will be necessary when designing a future trial or study. A pilot, or feasibility study, is a small experiment designed to test logistics and gather information prior to a larger study, in order to improve the latter's quality and efficiency. A pilot study can reveal deficiencies in the design of a proposed experiment or procedure and these can then be addressed before time and resources are expended on large scale studies. There should be an outline of the future study for which the pilot is being used to gather information. As the sample size of a pilot study is seldom sufficient to draw reliable conclusions, the pilot should not be an end in itself.

Pretesting is the process of measuring the effectiveness of the instrument used to gather data. After the research tool is completed it must be tested on subjects who met the criterion for the study sample. This is called 'pretesting'. Instruments and scales are likewise tested to determine if each actually measures what the researcher intends it to measure. It is important that all steps in a pilot study be carried through because it is only by completing the full procedures that weaknesses can be identified. Poorly worded items, ambiguous answers and any other corrections can be done before we proceed into main study. The time and effort to conduct a pilot study is well worth it. Pitfalls and errors that may prove costly in the actual study may be identified and avoided.

Reasons for Conducting Pilot Study

- A pilot study can involve pretesting a research tool, like a new data collection method. It can also be used to test an idea or hypothesis. Pilot studies can also be used in clinical trials, in order to test different doses, routes of administration, dosing schedules and possible barriers to adherence before a large-scale multicenter drug study is launched.
- Pilot studies are used as feasibility studies, to ensure that the ideas or methods behind a research are sound, as well as to 'work out the kinks' in a study protocol before launching a larger study.
- Pilot experiments are frequently carried out before large-scale quantitative research, in an attempt to avoid time and money being wasted on an inadequately designed project. A pilot study is usually carried out on members of the relevant population, but not on those who will form part of the final sample. This is because it may influence the later behavior of research subjects if they have already been involved in the research.
- A pilot experiment/study is often used to test the design of the full-scale experiment which then can be adjusted. It is a potentially valuable insight and should anything be missing in the pilot study it can be added to the full-scale (and more expensive) experiment to improve the chances of a clear outcome.
- The pilot study may, however, provide vital information on the severity of proposed procedures or treatments.
- Good pilot studies increase the likelihood of success in the main study. Pilot studies should warn of possible project failures, deviations from protocols, or problems with proposed methods or instruments and, it is hoped, uncover local politics or problems that may affect the research.
- The pilot study is a small preliminary investigation of the same general character as the major study, which is designed to acquaint the researcher

with problems that can be corrected in preparation for the larger research projects or is done to provide the researcher with an opportunity to try out the procedures for collecting data.

- A pilot study may address a number of logistical issues. As part of the research strategy, the following factors can be resolved prior to the main study:
  - Check that the instructions given to investigators (e.g. randomization procedures) are comprehensible
  - Check that investigators and technicians are sufficiently skilled in the procedures
  - Check the correct operation of equipment
  - Check the reliability and validity of results
  - Detect a floor or ceiling effect (e.g. if a task is too difficult or too easy there will be skewed results)
  - Assess whether the level of intervention is appropriate (e.g. the dose of a drug)
  - Identify adverse effects (pain, suffering, distress or lasting harm) caused by the procedure and the effectiveness of actions to reduce them (e.g. analgesia dose rate and schedule).

Samples for Pilot Study

The purpose of pilot study is two fold. Firstly, to make improvements in the research project and secondly to detect problems that must be eradicated before major study is attempted. The pilot study should be only large enough to be representative of the sample, which might in some cases be 10% anticipated sample size. This number would give some indication of the major problems that will arise in the research study. It is very important that information discussed during the pilot study should be kept confidential. Any publication of the purpose, nature or methods of pilot study may bias the major study.

The major advantages of pilot study are as follows:

- It tells about the completeness, accuracy and convenience of the sampling frame from which it is proposed to select the sample
- It unfolds the variability within the population to be surveyed or studied.
- It helps the researcher to determine the sample size
- It helps in checking the adequacy of the tool in eliciting the desired response. It helps to check about the content coverage
- It helps to check the difficulties experienced in administration and understanding by the researcher
- It allays interviewers' fears about overtly sensitive questions and builds their self-confidence
- It tests the efficiency of the survey organization in the field, including the type of supervision and instructions required while conducting the main study

- It helps in identifying the need for different kinds of equipment and vehicles which are necessary during the project
- It provides data for making estimates of time and costs for completing various phases of the project
- It helps the researcher to gain experience with methodology and instrument
- It helps to identify potential problems with data collection
- It helps to develop and refine protocol for the implementation of treatment.

Limitations

A pilot study is normally small in comparison with the main experiment and therefore can provide only limited information on the sources and magnitude of variation of response measures.

It may be necessary to carry-out a second pilot study to assess the revised main study or in some cases the main study may have to be abandoned.

SUMMARY

- Pilot study is the study carried out at the end of the planning phase of research, in order to explore and test the research elements. A pilot study is an initial investigation to give information that will be necessary when designing a future trial or study.
- Pretesting is the process of measuring the effectiveness of the instrument used to gather data. After the research tool is completed it must be tested on subjects who met the criterion for the study sample. This is called pretesting.
- Pilot study can also be used to test an idea or hypothesis. Pilot studies can also be used in clinical trials, in order to test different doses, routes of administration, dosing schedules and possible barriers to adherence before a large-scale multicenter drug study is launched.
- A pilot study is usually carried out on members of the relevant population, but not on those who will form part of the final sample.
- A pilot experiment/study is often used to test the design of the full-scale experiment which then can be adjusted. Good pilot studies increase the likelihood of success in the main study. The pilot study should be only large enough to be representative of the sample, which might in some cases be ten percent anticipated sample size.

9 Research Ethics

OBJECTIVES

After reading this chapter, you will be able to:

- Understand the history of evolution of research ethics
- Explain the universal declaration of human rights
- Explain the principles of ethics
- Enumerate the functions of Institutional Ethics Committee
- Understand the Informed consent process
- List the responsibilities of the researcher in maintaining research ethics.

INTRODUCTION

Research ethics involves the application of fundamental ethical principles to a variety of topics involving scientific research. These include the design and implementation of research involving human experimentation and animal experimentation. Research ethics is most developed as a concept in medical research. All research makes demands on others and is likely to involve some invasion of privacy. Because of the trust and intimacy inherent in the nurse-patient relationship nurses have privileged access to all kinds of information. Hence, the need for ethical guidelines. Almost all research involving human beings is intrusive. Research is done for the benefit of humanity. In all human research, some amount of data is collected. The data which we collect from the samples must be used only for the research purpose without any hidden agenda and intention other than the research. The samples should be given the top priority than the purpose of research itself. Nursing research relies on collaboration and partnerships based on mutual trust. When that trust is breached, the damage is irreversible. Honesty, openness, respect and sensitivity to others provide the cornerstones for ethical research. It is important that all nursing research is undertaken from a clear ethical stance, with ethical concerns.

History of Evolution of Research Ethics

The trial by the German medical practitioners during the post Second World War (1939–45) was shocking and they were accused of conducting experiments on human participants without their consent and exposing them to grave risk of death or permanent impairment of their faculties. This raised grave concern about subjecting human subjects to medical research.

Thus, the first International Statement on the ethics of medical research using human subjects namely, the Nuremberg Code was formulated in 1947. Although informed consent for participation in research was recorded in 1900, the Nuremberg Code highlighted the essentiality of voluntariness of this consent. In 1948, Universal Declaration of Human Rights (adopted by the General Assembly of the United Nations) expressed concern about rights of human beings being subjected to involuntary maltreatment. In 1966, the International Covenant on Civil and Political Rights specifically stated, 'No one shall be subjected to torture or to cruel, in human or degrading treatment or punishment. In particular, no one shall be subjected without his consent to medical or scientific treatment.' Based on the preliminary efforts of the Council for International Organization of Medical Sciences (CIOMS) in 1964 at Helsinki, Finland the World Medical Association formulated general principles and specific guidelines on use of human subjects in medical research, known as the Helsinki Declaration, which was revised from time to time. In February 1980, the Indian Council of Medical Research (ICMR) released 'Policy Statement on Ethical Considerations involved in Research on Human Subjects' for the benefit of all those involved in clinical research in India. In 1982, the World Health Organization (WHO) and the CIOMS issued the 'Proposed International Guidelines for Biomedical Research involving Human Subjects.' Subsequently the CIOMS brought out the 'International Guidelines for Ethical Review in Epidemiological studies' in 1991 and 'International Ethical Guidelines for Biomedical Research involving Human Subjects' in 1993. The most recent documents on ethics are those of UNESCO's 'The Universal Declaration on Human Genome and Human Rights' (1997), 'The International Declaration on Human Gene Data' (2003) and 'Universal Declaration on Bioethics and Human Rights' (2005).

Universal Declaration of Human Rights

The Universal Declaration of Human Rights (UDHR) is a declaration adopted by the United Nations General Assembly on 10th December 1948 at Palais de Chaillot, Paris. The Declaration arose directly from the experience of the Second World War and represents the first global expression of rights to which all human beings are inherently entitled. The full text is published by the United Nations on its website.

It consists of 30 articles which have been elaborated in subsequent international treaties, regional human rights instruments, national constitutions and laws. The International Bill of Human Rights consists of the Universal Declaration of Human Rights the International Covenant on Economic, Social and Cultural Rights and the International Covenant on Civil and Political Rights and its two Optional Protocols. In 1966, the General Assembly adopted the two detailed Covenants, which complete the International Bill of Human Rights and in 1976, after the Covenants had been ratified by a sufficient number of individual nations, the Bill took on the force of international law.

Preamble

Whereas recognition of the inherent dignity and of the equal and inalienable rights of all members of the human family is the foundation of freedom, justice and peace in the world.

- Disregard and contempt for human rights have resulted in barbarous acts which have outraged the conscience of mankind, and the advent of a world in which human beings shall enjoy freedom of speech and belief and freedom from fear and want has been proclaimed as the highest aspiration of the common people.
- It is essential, if man is not to be compelled to have recourse, as a last resort, to rebellion against tyranny and oppression, that human rights should be protected by the rule of law.
- It is essential to promote the development of friendly relations between nations.
- The peoples of the United Nations have in the Charter reaffirmed their faith in fundamental human rights, in the dignity and worth of the human person and in the equal rights of men and women and have determined to promote social progress and better standards of life in larger freedom.
- Member States have pledged themselves to achieve, in co-operation with the United Nations, the promotion of universal respect for and observance of human rights and fundamental freedoms.
- A common understanding of these rights and freedoms is of the greatest importance for the full realization of this pledge.

Now, therefore the General Assembly proclaims this UNIVERSAL DECLARATION OF HUMAN RIGHTS as a common standard of achievement for all peoples and all nations, to the end that every individual and every organ of society, keeping this Declaration constantly in mind, shall strive by teaching and education to promote respect for these rights and freedoms and by progressive measures, national and international, to secure their universal and effective recognition and observance, both among the peoples of Member States themselves and among the peoples of territories under their jurisdiction.

Article 1: All human beings are born free and equal in dignity and rights. They are endowed with reason and conscience and should act towards one another in a spirit of brotherhood.

Article 2: Everyone is entitled to all the rights and freedoms set forth in this Declaration, without distinction of any kind, such as race, color, sex, language, religion, political or other opinion, national or social origin, property, birth or other status. Furthermore, no distinction shall be made on the basis of the political, jurisdictional or international status of the country or territory to which a person belongs, whether it be independent, trust, non-self-governing or under any other limitation of sovereignty.

Article 3: Everyone has the right to life, liberty and security of person.

Article 4: No one shall be held in slavery or servitude; slavery and the slave trade shall be prohibited in all their forms.

Article 5: No one shall be subjected to torture or to cruel, inhuman or degrading treatment or punishment.

Article 6: Everyone has the right to recognition everywhere as a person before the law.

Article 7: All are equal before the law and are entitled without any discrimination to equal protection of the law. All are entitled to equal protection against any discrimination in violation of this Declaration and against any incitement to such discrimination.

Article 8: Everyone has the right to an effective remedy by the competent national tribunals for acts violating the fundamental rights granted him by the constitution or by law.

Article 9: No one shall be subjected to arbitrary arrest, detention or exile.

Article 10: Everyone is entitled in full equality to a fair and public hearing by an independent and impartial tribunal, in the determination of his rights and obligations and of any criminal charge against him.

Article 11: (1) Everyone charged with a penal offense has the right to be presumed innocent until proved guilty according to law in a public trial at which he has had all the guarantees necessary for his defense. (2) No one shall be held guilty of any penal offense on account of any act or omission which did not constitute a penal offense, under national or international law, at the time when it was committed. Nor shall a heavier penalty be imposed than the one that was applicable at the time the penal offense was committed.

Article 12: No one shall be subjected to arbitrary interference with his privacy, family, home or correspondence, nor to attacks upon his honor and reputation. Everyone has the right to the protection of the law against such interference or attacks.

Article 13: (1) Everyone has the right to freedom of movement and residence within the borders of each state. (2) Everyone has the right to leave any country, including his own and to return to his country.

Article 14: (1) Everyone has the right to seek and to enjoy in other countries asylum from persecution. (2) This right may not be invoked in the case of prosecutions genuinely arising from nonpolitical crimes or from acts contrary to the purposes and principles of the United Nations.

Article 15: (1) Everyone has the right to a nationality. (2) No one shall be arbitrarily deprived of his nationality nor denied the right to change his nationality.

Article 16: (1) Men and women of full age, without any limitation due to race, nationality or religion, have the right to marry and to find a family. They are entitled to equal rights as to marriage, during marriage and at its dissolution. (2) Marriage shall be entered into only with the free and full consent of the intending spouses. (3) The family is the natural and fundamental unit of society and is entitled to protection by society and the State.

Article 17: (1) Everyone has the right to own property alone as well as in association with others. (2) No one shall be arbitrarily deprived of his property.

Article 18: Everyone has the right to freedom of thought, conscience and religion; this right includes freedom to change his religion or belief, and freedom, either alone or in community with others and in public or private, to manifest his religion or belief in teaching, practice, worship and observance.

Article 19: Everyone has the right to freedom of opinion and expression; this right includes freedom to hold opinions without interference and to seek, receive and impart information and ideas through any media and regardless of frontiers.

Article 20: (1) Everyone has the right to freedom of peaceful assembly and association. (2) No one may be compelled to belong to an association.

Article 21: (1) Everyone has the right to take part in the government of his country, directly or through freely chosen representatives. (2) Everyone has the right of equal access to public service in his country. (3) The will of the people shall be the basis of the authority of government; this will shall be expressed in periodic and genuine elections which shall be by universal and equal suffrage and shall be held by secret vote or by equivalent free voting procedures.

Article 22: Everyone, as a member of society, has the right to social security and is entitled to realization, through national effort and international cooperation and in accordance with the organization and resources of each State, of the economic, social and cultural rights indispensable for his dignity and the free development of his personality.

Article 23: (1) Everyone has the right to work, to free choice of employment, to just and favorable conditions of work and to protection against unemployment. (2) Everyone, without any discrimination, has the right to equal pay for equal work. (3) Everyone who works has the right to just and favorable remuneration ensuring for himself and his family an existence worthy of human dignity and supplemented, if necessary, by other means of social protection. (4) Everyone has the right to form and to join trade unions for the protection of his interests.

Article 24: Everyone has the right to rest and leisure, including reasonable limitation of working hours and periodic holidays with pay.

Article 25: (1) Everyone has the right to a standard of living adequate for the health and well-being of himself and of his family, including food, clothing, housing and medical care and necessary social services, and the right to security in the event of unemployment, sickness, disability, widowhood, old age or other lack of livelihood in circumstances beyond his control. (2) Motherhood and childhood are entitled to special care and assistance. All children, whether born in or out of wedlock, shall enjoy the same social protection.

Article 26: (1) Everyone has the right to education. Education shall be free, at least in the elementary and fundamental stages. Elementary education shall be compulsory. Technical and professional education shall be made generally available and higher education shall be equally accessible to all on the basis of merit. (2) Education shall be directed to the full development of the human personality and to the strengthening of respect for human rights and fundamental freedoms. It shall promote understanding, tolerance and friendship among all nations, racial or religious groups, and shall further the activities of the United Nations for the maintenance of peace. (3) Parents have a prior right to choose the kind of education that shall be given to their children.

Article 27: (1) Everyone has the right freely to participate in the cultural life of the community, to enjoy the arts and to share in scientific advancement and its benefits. (2) Everyone has the right to the protection of the moral and material interests resulting from any scientific, literary or artistic production of which he is the author.

Article 28: Everyone is entitled to a social and international order in which the rights and freedoms set forth in this Declaration can be fully realized.

Article 29: (1) Everyone has duties to the community in which alone the free and full development of his personality is possible. (2) In the exercise of his rights and freedoms, everyone shall be subject only to such limitations as are determined by law solely for the purpose of securing due recognition and respect for the rights and freedoms of others and of meeting the just requirements of morality, public order and the general welfare in a democratic society. (3) These rights and freedoms may in no case be exercised contrary to the purposes and principles of the United Nations.

Article 30: Nothing in this Declaration may be interpreted as implying for any state, group or person any right to engage in any activity or to perform any act aimed at the destruction of any of the rights and freedoms set forth here in.

According to ICMR statement, the medical and related research using human beings as research participants must necessarily ensure that:

- The PURPOSE, of such research is that it should be directed towards the increase of knowledge about the human condition in relation to its social and natural environment, mindful that the human species is one of the many species in a planet in which the well-being of all species is under threat, no less from the human species as any other, and that such research is for the betterment of all, especially the least advantaged.
- Such research is CONDUCTED under conditions that no person or persons become a mere means for the betterment of others and that human beings who are subject to any medical research or scientific experimentation are dealt within a manner conducive to and consistent with their dignity and well-being, under conditions of professional fair treatment and transparency; and after ensuring that the participant is placed at no greater risk other than such risk commensurate with the well-being of the participant in question in the light of the object to the achieved.
- Such research must be subjected to a regime of EVALUATION at all stages of the proposal, i.e. research design and experimentation, declaration of results and use of the results thereof and that each such evaluation

shall bear in mind the objects to be achieved, the means by which they are sought to be achieved, the anticipated benefits and dangers, the potential uses and abuses of the experiment and its results and above all, the premium that civilized society places on saving and ensuring the safety of each human life as an end in itself.

Sources of Ethical Issues

- Ethical issues arise from the kinds of problems a nursing researcher investigates and the methods used to obtain valid and reliable data. They include:
    - ***The research problem itself:*** Problems based on genetic engineering, health practices, health habits, lifestyles, effect of treatment, etc.
    - ***Setting:*** Hospitals, health centers, prisons, public schools government agencies, communities, etc.
    - ***Procedures:*** Exposure of the experimental group to some intervention which may bring unwanted effect.
    - ***Method of data collection:*** Participants are observed based on concealed method.
    - ***Participants:*** The kind of persons serving as research participants, e.g. men, women, children People with HIV/AIDS, etc.
    - ***Data:*** Personal information on past and present health status, signs and symptoms, health habits, lifestyles, etc.

Principles of Ethics

The word ethics means moral principles. Ethical means morally correct. Ethics in Nursing research can be defined as 'the set of moral principles which the researcher has to follow while conducting nursing research to ensure the rights and welfare of persons and communities which are the subjects of his/her study.' The principles of ethics is as follows:

Beneficence or Nonmaleficence

Beneficence is a concept in research ethics which states that researchers should have the welfare of the research participant as a goal of any research activity. The antonym of this term, maleficence, describes a practice which opposes the welfare of any research participant. Beneficence refers to the ethical obligation to maximize benefits and to minimize harms. This principle gives rise to norms requiring that the risks of research be reasonable in the light of the expected benefits, that the research design be sound and that the investigators be competent both to conduct the research and to safeguard the welfare of the research subjects. Beneficence further proscribes the deliberate infliction of harm on persons; this aspect of beneficence is sometimes expressed as a separate principle, nonmaleficence (do not harm).

These four concepts often arise in discussions about beneficence:

1. One should not practice evil or do harm, often stated in Latin as Primum non nocere

2. One should prevent evil or harm
3. One should remove evil or harm
4. One should practice good.

The principle of beneficence includes:

- Freedom from harm
- Freedom from exploitation
- Benefits from research
- The risk/benefit ratio.

Justice

Justice is a concept in research ethics which refers to fair selection of research participants. Justice describes the ideal distribution of risks and benefits. The concept gives guidelines on how scientific objectives and not membership in either a privileged or vulnerable population should determine which members of which communities should meet inclusion criteria to participate in research in order to most equitably share the risks and benefits of the research. Study participants have the right to fair and equitable treatment in all phases of research. Fair treatment includes the fair and non discriminatory selection of participants, nonprejudicial treatment of individuals, the honoring of all agreements between the researcher and the participants, debriefing and respectful and courteous treatment at all times. Justice refers to the ethical obligation to treat each person in accordance with what is morally right and proper, to give each person what is due to him or her. In the ethics of research involving human subjects the principle refers primarily to distributive justice, which requires the equitable distribution of both the burdens and the benefits of participation in research. Differences in distribution of burdens and benefits are justifiable only if they are based on morally relevant distinctions between persons; one such distinction is vulnerability. 'Vulnerability' refers to a substantial incapacity to protect one's own interests owing to such impediments as lack of capability to give informed consent, lack of alternative means of obtaining medical care or other expensive necessities, or being a junior or subordinate member of a hierarchical group. Accordingly, special provision must be made for the protection of the rights and welfare of vulnerable persons.

Respect for Persons

Respect for persons incorporates at least two fundamental ethical considerations, namely:

- Respect for autonomy, which requires that those who are capable of deliberation about their personal choices should be treated with respect for their capacity for self-determination
- Protection of persons with impaired or diminished autonomy, which requires that those who are dependent or vulnerable be afforded security against harm or abuse.

Respect for persons is the concept that all people should be given the right to fully exercise their autonomy. An autonomous person is defined as an individual who is capable of self-legislation and is able to make judgments and actions based on his/her particular set of values, preferences and beliefs. Respecting a person's autonomy thus involves considering his/her choices and decisions without deliberate obstruction. It also requires that subjects be treated in a non-degrading manner out of respect for their dignity. In practice, respect for persons is operationalized by obtaining Informed Consent from all individuals who are going to be research subjects.

The standard case for applying respect for persons is when the person receiving the health intervention is of sound mind, fit to make personal decisions, and empowered to choose from various options. Other cases involve showing respect to people who for whatever reason are not free to choose among the typical range of options when making a decision.

The word 'vulnerability' stems from the Latin vulnerare, 'to wound.' In medical research ethics, the term Vulnerable Populations generally refers to individuals whose situations do not allow them to protect their own interests. These include individuals who are minors, prisoners, pregnant, physically handicapped, mentally disabled, old, economically disadvantaged, educationally disadvantaged, or subordinates in hierarchical groups (e.g. a soldier). These individuals are entitled to protection, and additional ethical justification is needed to involve such populations in human subject studies. In such cases, a balance should be established between protecting subjects from exploitation and depriving these subjects of access to the potential benefits of research. Reasons justifying the participation of these subjects would include that some studies could not be carried out without a vulnerable population. Another justification would be that the aim of the study is to gain knowledge to improve diagnosis, prevention or treatment of diseases associated specifically with that population. The right to withdraw is a concept in clinical research ethics that a study participant in a clinical trial has a right to end participation in that trial at will. When children participate in clinical research their parents or guardians must give assent for them to participate, but ethics dictate that even in this case it is best to get the consent of the research subject. Studies have shown that children participating in research have little understanding of the right to withdraw when they are presented with the option.

Return of Results

Return of results is a concept in research ethics which describes the extent of the duty of a researcher to reveal and explain the results of research to a research participant.

Privacy

Privacy for research participants is a concept in research ethics which states that a person in human subject research has a right to privacy when participating in research. People decide to participate in research for any number of different reasons, such as a personal interest, a desire to promote research which benefits their community, or for other reasons. Various guidelines for human subject research protect study participants who choose to participate in research and the international consensus is that the rights of people who participate in studies are best protected when the study participant can trust that researchers will not connect the identities of study participants with their input into the study.

Many study participants have experienced problems when their privacy was not upheld after participating in research. Sometimes privacy is not kept because of insufficient study protection, but also sometimes it is because of unanticipated problems with the study design which inadvertently compromise privacy. The privacy of research participants is typically protected by the research organizer, but the institutional review board is a designated overseer which monitors the organizer to provide protection to study participants.

A privacy attack is the exploitation of an opportunity of someone to identify a study participant based on public research data. The way that this might work is that researchers collect data, including confidential identifying data, from study participants. This produces an identified dataset. Before the data is sent for research processing, it is 'de-identified,' which means that personally identifying data is removed from the dataset. Ideally this means that the dataset alone could not be used to identify a participant.

Institutional Ethics Committee

The basic responsibility of an Institutional Ethics Committee (IEC) is to ensure a competent review of all ethical aspects of the project proposals received by it in an objective manner. IECs should provide advice to the researchers on all aspects of the welfare and safety of the research participants after ensuring the scientific soundness of the proposed research through appropriate Scientific Review Committee. In institutions where this is lacking, the IEC may take up the dual responsibility of review of both, the scientific content and ethical aspects of the proposal. It is advisable to have separate Committees for each, taking care that the scientific review precedes the scrutiny for ethical issues. The scientific evaluation should ensure technical appropriateness of the proposed study. The IECs should specify in writing the authority under which the Committee is established.

Special Situations

Small institutions could form alliance with other IECs or approach registered IEC (ind). Large institutions/Universities with large number of proposals can have more than one suitably constituted IECs for different research areas for which large number of research proposals are submitted. However, the institutional policy should be same for all these IECs to safeguard the research participant's rights. A sub-committee of the main IEC may review proposals submitted by undergraduate or postgraduate students or if necessary, a committee may be separately constituted for the purpose, which will review proposals in the same manner as described above. The responsibilities of an IEC can be defined as follows:

- To protect the dignity, rights and well-being of the potential research participants.
- To ensure that universal ethical values and international scientific standards are expressed in terms of local community values and customs.
- To assist in the development and the education of a research community responsive to local health care requirements.

Composition

The IECs should be multidisciplinary and multisectorial in composition. Independence and competence are the two hallmarks of an IEC. The number of persons in an ethics committee should be kept fairly small (8 –12 members). It is generally accepted that a minimum of five persons is required to form the quorum without which a decision regarding the research should not be taken. The IEC should appoint from among its members a Chairman who should be from outside the Institution and not head of the same Institution to maintain the independence of the Committee. The Member Secretary should be from the same Institution and should conduct the business of the Committee. Other members should be a mix of medical/non-medical, scientific and non-scientific persons including lay persons to represent the differed points of view.

The composition may be as follows:

- Chairperson
- One-two persons from basic medical science area
- One-two clinicians from various Institutes
- One legal expert or retired judge
- One social scientist/representative of non-governmental voluntary agency
- One philosopher/ethicist/theologian
- One lay person from the community
- Member Secretary.

As per revised Schedule Y of Drugs & Cosmetics Act, 1940, amended in 2005, the ethics committee approving drug trials should have in the quorum at least one representative from the following groups:

- One basic medical scientist (preferably one pharmacologist)
- One clinician
- One legal expert or retired judge
- One social scientist/representative of non-governmental organization/ philosopher/ethicist/theologian or a similar person
- One lay person from the community

The Ethics Committee (EC) can have as its members, individuals from other institutions or communities with adequate representation of age and gender to safeguard the interests and welfare of all sections of the community/society. If required, subject experts could be invited to offer their views, for instance, a pediatrician for pediatric conditions, a cardiologist for cardiac disorders, etc. Similarly, based on the requirement of research area, for example HIV, genetic disorders, etc. it is desirable to include a member from specific patient groups in the Committee.

Informed Consent Process

Informed consent of participants: Diener and Crandall (1978) defined informed consent as the procedure in which individuals choose whether to participate in an investigation after being informed of the facts that would be likely to influence their decisions. The informed consent involves four elements that is competence, voluntarism, full information and comprehension.

Competence is any decision made by a responsible mature individual who is given the relevant information, will be the correct decision. In general persons are incapable of providing consent if they have impaired mental capacity or a questionable ability to exercise self-determination, e.g. young children, comatose patients and patients with psychiatric illnesses. The guardian, parents and others responsible for such incompetent individuals are asked to make decisions for them. By ***voluntarism***, the researcher ensures freedom to participants to choose whether or not to take part in a research project and guarantees that exposure to known risks is undertaken voluntarily. The researcher might give ***full information*** to the participants about the study. At the same time, the researcher may not be aware of the consequence of the research activity as they are in the process of finding out. Therefore, reasonably informed consent must be adopted which includes the explanation of the procedure to be followed and their purposes, a description of participants' discomfort and risks to be expected, an offer to answer to any queries concerning the procedure an instruction that the person is free to withdraw at anytime without prejudice to the participant. ***Comprehension*** refers to the confidence that the participant has gained by knowing the details of the research. It can be ensured by selecting educated participants, availability of consultant to discuss the study with the participant, the time lag between the request for participation and the decision to take part in the study.

For all biomedical research involving human participants, the investigator must obtain the informed consent of the prospective participant or in the case of an individual who is not capable of giving informed consent, the consent of a legal guardian. Informed consent protects the individual's freedom of choice and respect for individual's autonomy and is given voluntarily to participate in research or not. Adequate information about the research is given in a simple and easily understandable unambiguous language in a document known as the Informed Consent Form with Participant/Patient Information Sheet. The latter should have following components as may be applicable:

- Nature and purpose of study stating it as research
- Duration of participation with number of participants
- Procedures to be followed
- Investigations, if any, to be performed
- Foreseeable risks and discomforts adequately described and whether project involves more than minimal risk
- Benefits to participant, community or medical profession as may be applicable
- Policy on compensation
- Availability of medical treatment for such injuries or risk management
- Alternative treatments if available
- Steps taken for ensuring confidentiality
- No loss of benefits on withdrawal
- Benefit sharing in the event of commercialization
- Contact details of principal investigator (PI) or local PI/Co-PI in multicentric studies for asking more information related to the research or in case of injury
- Contact details of Chairman of the IEC for appeal against violation of rights
- Voluntary participation
- If test for genetics and HIV is to be done, counseling for consent for testing must be given as per national guidelines
- Storage period of biological sample and related data with choice offered to participant regarding future use of sample, refusal for storage and receipt of its results.

A copy of the participant/patient information sheet should be given to the participant for her/his record. The informed consent should be brief in content highlighting that it is given of free will or voluntarily after understanding the implications of risks and benefits and she/he could withdraw without loss of routine care benefits.

Assurance is given that confidentiality would be maintained and all the investigations/interventions would be carried out only after consent is obtained.

When the written consent as signature or thumb impression is not possible due to sensitive nature of the project or the participant is unable to write, then verbal consent can be taken after ensuring its documentation by an unrelated witness. In some cases ombudsman, a third party, can ensure total accountability for the process of obtaining the consent. Audiovisual methods could be adopted with prior consent and adequate precaution to ensure confidentiality, but approval of EC is required for such procedures. For drug trials, if the volunteer can give only thumb impression then another thumb impression by the relative or legal custodian cannot be accepted and an unrelated witness to the project should then sign.

Fresh or re-consent is taken in following conditions:

- Availability of new information which would necessitate deviation of protocol

- When a research participant regains consciousness from unconscious state or is mentally competent to understand the study. If such an event is expected then procedures to address it should be spelt out in the informed consent form
- When long term follow-up or study extension is planned later
- When there is change in treatment modality, procedures, site visits
- Before publication if there is possibility of disclosure of identity through data presentation or photographs (which should be camouflaged adequately).

Waiver of Consent

Voluntary informed consent is always a requirement for every research proposal. However, this can be waived if it is justified that the research involves not more than minimal risk or when the participant and the researcher do not come into contact or when it is necessitated in emergency situations. If such studies have protections in place for both privacy and confidentiality, and do not violate the rights of the participants then IECs may waive off the requirement for informed consent in following instances:

- When it is impractical to conduct research since confidentiality of personally identifiable information has to be maintained throughout research as may be required by the sensitivity of the research objective, e.g. study on disease burden of HIV/AIDS.
- Research on publicly available information, documents, records, works, performances, reviews, quality assurance studies, archival materials or third party interviews, service programs for benefit of public having a bearing on public health programs, and consumer acceptance studies.
- Research on anonymized biological samples from deceased individuals, left over samples after clinical investigation, cell lines or cell free derivatives like viral isolates, DNA or RNA from recognized institutions or qualified investigators, samples or data from repositories or registries, etc.
- In emergency situations when no surrogate consent can be taken.

Obligations of investigators regarding informed consent: The investigator has the duty to:

- Communicate to prospective participants all the information necessary for informed consent. Any restriction on participant's right to ask any questions related to the study will undermine the validity of informed consent.
- Exclude the possibility of unjustified deception, undue influence and intimidation. Although deception is not permissible, if sometimes such information would jeopardize the validity of research it can be withheld till the completion of the project, for instance, study on abortion practices.
- Seek consent only after the prospective participant is adequately informed. The investigator should not give any unjustifiable assurances to prospective participant, which may influence the her/his decision to participate.

- Obtain from each prospective participant a signed form as an evidence of informed consent (written informed consent) preferably witnessed by a person not related to the trial, and in case the participant is not competent to do so, a legal guardian or other duly authorized representative.
- Take verbal consent when the participant refuses to sign or give thumb impression or cannot do so. This can then be documented through audio or video means.
- Take surrogate consent from the authorized relative or legal custodian or the institutional head in the case of abandoned institutionalized individuals or wards under judicial custody.
- Renew or take fresh informed consent of each participant under circumstances described earlier in this chapter.
- If participant loses consciousness or competence to consent during the research period as in Alzeimer or psychiatric conditions, surrogate consent may be taken from the authorized person or legal custodian.
- The investigator must assure prospective participants that their decision to participate or not will not affect the patient-clinician relationship or any other benefits to which they are entitled.

Essential information for prospective research participants: Before requesting an individual's consent to participate in research, the investigator must provide the individual with the following information in the language she or he is able to understand which should not only be scientifically accurate but should also be sensitive/adaptive to their social and cultural context:

- The aims and methods of the research
- The expected duration of the participation
- The benefits that might reasonably be expected as an outcome of research to the participant or community or to others
- Any alternative procedures or courses of treatment that might be as advantageous to the participant as the procedure or treatment to which she/he is being subjected
- Any foreseeable risk or discomfort to the participant resulting from participation in the study
- Right to prevent use of her/his biological sample (DNA, cell-line, etc.) at anytime during the conduct of the research
- The extent to which confidentiality of records could be maintained, i.e. the limits to which the investigator would be able to safeguard confidentiality and the anticipated consequences of breach of confidentiality
- Responsibility of investigators
- Free treatment for research related injury by the investigator and/ institution and sponsor(s)
- Compensation of participants for disability or death resulting from such injury
- Insurance coverage if any, for research related or other AEs
- Freedom of individual/family to participate and to withdraw from research anytime without penalty or loss of benefits which the participant

would otherwise be entitled to the identity of the research teams and contact persons with address and phone numbers
- Foreseeable extent of information on possible current and future uses of the biological material and of the data to be generated from the research and if the material is likely to be used for secondary purposes or would be shared with others, clear mention of the same
- Risk of discovery of biologically sensitive information and provision to safeguard confidentiality
- Publication, if any, including photographs and pedigree charts.

The quality of the consent of certain social and marginalized groups requires careful consideration as their agreement to volunteer may be unduly influenced by the Investigator.

Compensation for Participation

Participants may be paid for the inconvenience and time spent, and should be reimbursed for expenses incurred, in connection with their participation in research. They may also receive free medical services. When this is reasonable then it cannot be termed as benefit. During the period of research if the participant requires treatment for complaints other than the one being studied necessary free ancillary care or appropriate referrals may be provided. However, payments should not be so large or the medical services so extensive as to make prospective participants consent readily to enroll in research against their better judgment, which would then be treated as undue inducement. All payments, reimbursement and medical services to be provided to research participants should be approved by the IEC. Care should be taken:
- When a guardian is asked to give consent on behalf of an incompetent person, no remuneration should be offered except a refund of out of pocket expenses.
- When a participant is withdrawn from research for medical reasons related to the study, the participant should get the benefit for full participation.
- When a participant withdraws for any other reasons she/he should be paid an amount proportionate to the amount of participation.

Ethical Responsibilities of the Researcher

- Researcher is responsible for all decisions regarding procedural matters and ethical issues related to research project
- Researcher has to ensure that all activities carried out must be consistent with the ethical standards of the home and host community
- She should consider the ethical issues from the perspectives of the participant's society
- She has to obtain assistance or necessary guidance from the colleagues and superiors when unresolved or difficult dilemmas arise
- Research should be conducted not for the sake of conducting research, but for the benefit of humanity. Participant's benefit is the prime importance

- The researcher has to ensure that all research personnel are qualified to use any procedures employed in the project
- Researcher has to eliminate any bias in the design, conduct or reporting of the research
- Researcher must seek informed consent from the participant. Official permission form the settings must be obtained
- The researcher has to protect dignity, privacy and interest of the research participants and welfare of the participants should take priority over all other concerns
- The researcher has to terminate the research if danger to the participants arise
- She has to keep all research data confidential and maintain the anonymity of the participants
- She has to give appropriate credit to all parties contribution to the research.

The rights of all persons to life, esteem, self-determination, privacy, and protection from all forms of injury and manipulation are values which must govern researchers in their conduct towards those whom they involve as participants/subjects and co-researchers.

Informed Consent

The provision of information on which consent is to be based has to be nicely judged so that it does not overwhelm or confuse those whom it is intended to inform. Valid consent to participate in research is dependent on full understanding and freedom from coercion and deception. Usually the information to prospective participants/subjects needs to be presented both orally and in written form and should cover:

- The nature and extent of involvement expected of them
- The purpose of the research, particularly any benefits which are anticipated for the participants directly and for the public more generally through increased knowledge
- The right to refuse and to withdraw at any point without prejudice to their care or welfare
- Ongoing opportunities for further discussion or clarification of any aspect of the study
- Their rights with respect to any publication which comes out of the research
- Any actual or potential risks.

Group consent does not replace individual consent. Generally no person can give consent for another except for those mentally incapable of giving consent for themselves, in which case a guardian may make the decision.

Consent should be written or recorded, and reconfirmed from time to time if the study extends over a long period, and there is doubt about a participant's memory. Nurse researchers need to be particularly careful that captive populations, such as students and patients are not exploited. Consent is not open ended and refers only to the current project. Qualitative research presents a major challenge to the principle of informed consent because the study may evolve in ways that could not be foreseen at the outset.

Confidentiality

Confidentiality refers to what happens to the data. It is an extension of the concept of privacy. Having consented to an initial invasion of privacy by supplying information, research participants have the right to maintain control over any further release of those data. Participants/subjects should be able to trust that strict confidentiality will be maintained during the collection, storage and use of the data. They should know who, if anyone other than the researcher, will have access to the data, and for what purposes. Use of photographs should be specifically negotiated. Anonymity refers to the protection given to individuals or organizations from being identifiable in the data and the report.

Protection from Risk and Injury

Researchers have a responsibility to ensure that their participants/subjects are not directly or indirectly harmed in the course of the research. Safety must encompass physical and nonphysical well-being (psychological, cultural, social, financial and spiritual). Normally, the risk of harm must be no greater than in ordinary life, i.e. participants should not be exposed to risks greater than or additional to those encountered in their normal lifestyles.

Where research may involve behavior or experiences that participants may regard as personal and private the participants must be protected from stress by all appropriate measures, including the assurance that answers to personal questions need not be given. There should be no concealment or deception when seeking information that might encroach on privacy. In research involving children, great caution should be exercised when discussing the results with parents.

Qualitative research requires very careful monitoring in the respect. Because the scope of open ended interviewing is not definable in advance, the researcher is unable to predict what painful experiences or memories may be triggered by the questioning? When questioning in sensitive areas, the researcher must set the limits for what is ethical? Possible strategies for debriefing and providing additional support for participants should be rehearsed in case they are needed. In clinical settings, it should be the concern of caregivers, as well as the researcher, to ensure that services to nonparticipants are not diminished in anyway because of the demands of the research.

Debriefing

In studies where the participants are aware that they have taken part in an investigation, when the data have been collected, the investigator should provide the participants with any necessary information to complete their understanding of the nature of the research. The investigator should discuss with the participants their experience of the research in order to monitor any unforeseen negative effects or misconceptions.

Debriefing does not provide a justification for unethical aspects of any investigation. Some effects which may be produced by an experiment will not be negated by a verbal description following the research. Investigators have a responsibility to ensure that participants receive any necessary debriefing in the form of active intervention before they leave the research setting.

Withdrawal from the Investigation

At the onset of the investigation, investigators should make plain to participants their right to withdraw from the research at anytime, irrespective of whether or not payment or other inducement has been offered. It is recognized that this may be difficult in certain observational or organizational settings, but nevertheless the investigator must attempt to ensure that participants (including children) know of their right to withdraw.

Observational Research

Studies based upon observation must respect the privacy and psychological well-being of the individuals studied. Unless those observed give their consent to being observed, observational research is only acceptable in situations where those observed would expect to be observed by strangers. Additionally, particular account should be taken of local cultural values and of the possibility of intruding upon the privacy of individuals who, even while in a normally public space, may believe they are unobserved.

Implementation of Poorly Planned or Designed Research is Unethical

Where possible beginning researchers should work as part of a team. In team research, the principal researcher has responsibility for ensuring that others in the team are competent, and have the information they need in order to act in an ethical manner. There should be inbuilt checks and balances. Researchers who have to work alone should establish informal mentorship or supervision. Even more experienced researchers should still use peer review regularly.

Publication and Dissemination of Findings

This last phase of the research process also has ethical aspects. First and foremost is the need for honesty in reporting. The researcher has an obligation to publish both the process and the findings, so that the former can be subjected to peer scrutiny and the latter will add to the pool of nursing knowledge. Prior to publication participants/subjects should be given an opportunity to confirm that they are faithfully represented in what is being published and, if anonymity has been promised, that this has been retained? The required qualities of the researcher in fulfilling ethics:

- Honesty
- Objectivity

- Integrity
- Carefulness
- Openness
- Respect for intellectual property
- Confidentiality
- Responsible publication
- Responsible mentoring
- Respect for colleagues
- Social responsibility
- Non-discrimination
- Competence
- Legality
- Human subjects protection.

SUMMARY

- The trial by the German medical practitioners during the post Second World War (1939–45) was shocking and they were accused of conducting experiments on human participants without their consent and exposing them to grave risk of death or permanent impairment of their faculties. This raised grave concern about subjecting human subjects to medical research.
- The first International Statement on the ethics of medical research using human subjects namely, the Nuremberg Code was formulated in 1947. In 1948, Universal Declaration of Human Rights (adopted by the General Assembly of the United Nations) expressed concern about rights of human beings being subjected to involuntary maltreatment.
- Based on the preliminary efforts of the Council for International Organization of Medical Sciences (CIOMS) in 1964 at Helsinki, Finland, the World Medical Association formulated general principles and specific guidelines on use of human subjects in medical research, known as the Helsinki Declaration, which was revised from time to time.
- The most recent documents on ethics are those of UNESCO's 'The Universal Declaration on Human Genome and Human Rights' (1997), 'The International Declaration on Human Gene Data' (2003) and 'Universal Declaration on Bioethics and Human Rights' (2005).
- Beneficence refers to the ethical obligation to maximize benefits and to minimize harms. The principle of beneficence includes freedom from harm, freedom from exploitation, benefits from research and the Risk /Benefit Ratio.
- Justice refers to the ethical obligation to treat each person in accordance with what is morally right and proper, to give each person what is due to him or her.
- Respect for persons is the concept that all people should be given the right to fully exercise their autonomy. An autonomous person is defined as an individual who is capable of self-legislation and is able to make judgments and actions based on his/her particular set of values, preferences and beliefs.
- Return of results is a concept in research ethics which describes the extent of the duty of a researcher to reveal and explain the results of research to a research participant.
- Privacy for research participants is a concept in research ethics which states that a person in human subject research has a right to privacy when participating in research.

- The basic responsibility of an Institutional Ethics Committee (IEC) is to ensure a competent review of all ethical aspects of the project proposals received by it in an objective manner.
- For all biomedical research involving human participants, the investigator must obtain the informed consent of the prospective participant or in the case of an individual who is not capable of giving informed consent, the consent of a legal guardian. Informed consent protects the individual's freedom of choice and respect for individual's autonomy and is given voluntarily to participate in research or not.

10 Interpretation, Communication and Utilization of Research Findings

OBJECTIVES

After reading this chapter, you will be able to:
- Interpret the findings of the research
- State the ways of communicating research findings
- Explain the method of writing research report for various purposes
- State the meaning of research utilization
- List the importance of research utilization
- Explain the steps involved in research utilization
- Explain the steps of critiquing the research
- Explain the steps of writing a research proposal.

INTRODUCTION

After collecting and analyzing the data, the researcher has to accomplish the task of drawing inferences followed by report writing. This has to be done very carefully, otherwise misleading conclusions may be drawn and the whole purpose of doing research may get vitiated. In case of studies aimed at hypothesis testing, the researcher either rejects or accepts the hypothesis. But in studies without hypothesis, the researcher tries to explain the findings of his study based on some theories. All this findings must be well communicated. The purpose of research is to be of use—to change current practice, or to confirm it. Yet the process of moving new understandings and new products from research to practice is long and cumbersome. For many innovations, the timeline involves decades, even generations. The task of dissemination is precisely to bridge that gap. The nurse researchers should understand this and develop strategies for effective utilization.

INTERPRETATION OF RESEARCH FINDINGS

Interpretation refers to the task of drawing inferences from the collected facts after analysis. In fact, it is a search for broader meaning of research findings. Interpretation helps in establishment of some explanatory concepts. After analysis of data we want to draw conclusions for the population. Drawing conclusion involves generalization of the findings for the population. Interpretation is essential for the simple reason that the usefulness and utility of research findings lie in proper interpretation. Through interpretation, the researcher can link his findings with that of others. The interpretation of the findings of exploratory research study often results into hypotheses for experimental research and as such interpretation is involved in the transition from exploratory to experimental research. Since an exploratory study does not have a hypothesis to start with, the findings of such study have to be interpreted on a post factum basis in which case the interpretation is technically described as 'post factum' interpretation.

One should remember that post factum interpretation is different from hypothesis testing. In hypothesis testing, the investigator begins with a specific interpretation and determines whether or not the data are consistent with it. But in the post factum interpretation, the analyst begins with the data and seeks an interpretation consistent with it. Post factum interpretations have generally low evidential value compared with hypothesis testing. This is because they suffer from three distinctive limitations, viz.,

1. They are flexible
2. They are not nullifiable
3. They are not dependent on external confirmation.

Excessive flexibility is one of the most conspicuous limitations of post factum interpretations. In principle, one is free to choose or change one's interpretation at will. If, for example, one finds that unmarried nurses are punctual with less absenteeism than the married staff nurses for duty, one can bring out a number of possible interpretations of this result. On the other hand if it is reverse, one could have come up with equally satisfactory explanations.

The second limitations is that post factum interpretations are not nullifiable. If one finds that working class people are more radical, one might interpret this finding to be due to their resentment at their economic exploitation. But, as it stands, there is no way to prove this interpretation wrong. In hypothesis testing, on the other hand, the theory presumably generates the data examination and the data are thus capable of nullifying the hypothesis and the theory underpinning it.

The third limitation is that post factum interpretations are not dependent on external confirmation. If an interpretation is offered after the data are in, there is no confirmation that the interpretation is correct. One cannot refer back to the data for confirmation, the strength of the interpretation resides soley in the logical system in which it is imbedded. In hypothesis testing, on the other hand, the data came after the hypothesis has been formulated and thus represent external confirmation of one's line of reasoning.

Correct interpretation requires a high degree of critical thinking, knowledge, skill, care, judgment and objectivity on the part of the researcher. Statistics are the most dangerous tools in the hands of the inapt. One can misinterpret data easily if a person is not well versed in the science of statistics.

Misinterpretation can be avoided by the following:

Making appropriate comparisons: A researcher cannot compare apples and oranges. When he wants to compare two groups, he has to define the variable of interest in the group properly. He could compare the outcome of one group with the similar outcome of the other group. For example, a research wants to compare the per capital income of the two countries, say example, India and Japan, then the per capita income should be defined properly in the study. Definitely the per capita income in both countries are not same. There are various factors influencing the per capita income in a country. All those factors must be considered in defining a variable and then the data can be compared.

If we want to compare the performance of nurses working in multi-speciality hospitals with that of nurses working in small clinic. The two groups may not stand similar. A researcher has to see whether the two groups are equal on certain factors before comparisons are made or else the measurement should be very specific so that other confounding variables may not influence the outcome of the research.

Adequacy of data: Inadequate data leads to misinterpretation. For example, if we conclude that 80 percentage of those who are obese developed diabetes mellitus in the middle age, we may infer that obesity leads to diabetes. This is not a valid interpretation. Since we do not know the percentage of non obese developing diabetes at middle age. The results can be generalized based on the comparison of obese and nonobese persons developing diabetes. Similarly comparison of the mortality of patients admitted in critical care unit and general medical ward does not sound good since the nature of health problem for which the patients admitted to these areas are not the same.

Proper sample selection: The samples selected should be a good representative of the population. Proper definition, appropriate sampling technique, adequacy of sample size are mandatory for generalization of the data for population. For example, job satisfaction of nurses working in private hospitals may not be generalized for nurses working in government sector. Similarly studies on job turnover of nurses working in private setting should not be generalized for nurses working in government sectors.

Avoiding errors in statistical analysis: Use of absolute numbers instead of percentages make a difference in interpretation.

Look at the below mentioned data.

Staff Turnover	2013	2014
Nurses	100	122
Doctors	24	30

Suppose if a researcher states that the turnover of nurses is increased when compared to the doctors, it may not be a right interpretation. Since they are absolute numbers, they may not give the correct information to us. Calculation percentages for these two groups to compare the turnover, gives correct information.

In the above example, if the total number of staff nurses working in the hospital is 650 and the doctors are 80 then the percentage is;

Nurses	15.4	18.8
Doctors	30	37.5

But if percentages are compared we can see the difference. Actually the turnover is increased in doctors when compared to the nurses.

On the other hand if the researcher uses the percentage instead of absolute number at inappropriate context he may misinterpret data.

Suppose a researcher reports that 33.3% of the students admitted to the MSc (N) program is male. This looks like a considerable number of male candidates are joining MSc (N). But if only 2 girls and one male candidate is admitted to MSc (N) that gives wrong interpretation. If a finding says that 75% of the students of PG in Nursing stays in hostel, we may think that majority is staying in the hostel. But if only 4 students are enrolled and 3 of them are staying in the hostel, could give wrong interpretation.

Appropriate use of correlation: A linear correlation between any two variables may exist only within limits. For example, one may get a negative correlation between the fees to be paid for admission of students to a course and the number of admission. That does not mean that if fees are very less more students will enroll or if fees are very high less students only will enroll to a course. We have a curvilinear correlation with a positive relationship up to a certain point and then a negative relationship setting in after that point and vice versa. If fees are less many students will join the course up to certain limit then there may be a declining trend in admission. Because of low fees, institution may comprise its quality which will affect the admission.

In a study among nursing students, an investigator reported that Post graduate students learn faster the skill than the undergraduates. This does not mean that educational program is the cause of skill learning. The explanation is that PG students may have faster skill learning because they have the good foundation of working experience and the undergraduate education.

In a longitudinal study where an investigator reported that those who performed better in college had earned less monthly income than those who scored less in the college studies. This does not mean that good students earn less. The students who scored better in academics might be in teaching than those who scored less. Obviously the number of faculty in college is less in number than who are working in the hospitals.

In a city, the average number of vehicles a family use was collected among a sample of working men and women. This showed a comparatively large figure. This may be due to the fact that all or majority of working people may possess one or more vehicle than others and if both gender is included, two samples belonging to a same family may respond for the same question which will increase the number.

Heterogeneity of the sample: If study says that the average age at enrollment of students for Post Basic BSc (N) program is 35 years, it may not be sounding good. This may be due to the heterogeneity of the sample that if one sample with age of 50 is enrolled that it will affect the average.

Consultation with the experts: It is advisable that before arriving at final conclusion, to consult with the experts who is frank and honest and will not hesitate to point out omissions and errors in logical augmentation. Such consultation will result in correct interpretation and will enhance the utility of research results.

COMMUNICATION OF RESEARCH FINDINGS

Research study is complete only when the findings have been shared with others. It is of no value unless the research finding is disseminated to the people. It is the researcher's responsibility to ensure that the research study, and its findings/recommendations are disseminated to as wide an audience as possible. Scientific communication takes place in many ways, including archival publication in scholarly journals and informal communication among groups of scientists, known as invisible colleges. For this, a report of entire study should be written by the researcher. The writing of research report necessitates specific methods which depends on the purpose for which it is to be written and skill on the part of the researcher to write a report on one's own work. The purpose of writing research report is to document the research findings, to share the results with other interested groups and apply the results in practice. It is a challenging job and requires imagination, creativity, and resourcefulness. The research report aims at telling the readers the problem identified, investigated and methods adopted, the results found and the conclusion reached. Research outcome needs to be shared with other professionals, regardless of the study's outcome.

There are many ways of communicating one's research findings. They are:

- Writing dissertation
- Writing for publication in scholarly journals/books/newspapers
- Writing and presenting at conferences
- Writing for funding agencies
- Preparing and doing poster presentation
- Verbal report/presentation at meetings
- Presentation at journal clubs and
- Presentation at continuing nursing education programs.

Guidelines for Writing the Research Report

The research task is not completed until the report has been written. A research report is the ultimate output of the research process. As a matter of fact even the most brilliant hypothesis, highly well designed and conducted research study and the most striking generalizations and findings are of little value unless they are effectively communicated to others. The purpose of research is not well served unless the findings are made known to others. Writing of report is the last step in a research study and requires a set of skills which are as follows:

Have good critical thinking: Research is not merely the accumulation, evaluation and assimilation of facts, it is the process of rebuilding facts into a meaningful whole. This requires deep understanding, comprehension and background knowledge by the researcher.

Use appropriate tense and voice: In general the report is written in past tense since it is the report of completed work. Past tense cannot be used in all segments of research report. For example, the studies' implication and its utilization has to be written in present tense.

Appropriate use of language: When the report is written for the professional people, one should use standard language using all technical terms. When the report is prepared for the general public one should use simple, easy to understand language. Technical words should be avoided.

Appropriate use of diagrams and tables: Use of diagrams and tables whenever and wherever appropriate, should be used to illustrate the principal findings of the study.

Objectivity: The report should be unbiased and objective and it should contain only facts. As a general rule, long excerpts from works of others should be avoided. Too many quotations or references of other writers either create an impression of showmanship or that the researcher has done very little work of his own. Inclusion of all works of others should be properly acknowledged in the foot notes.

Confidentiality of the data: This is not an issue when the samples have voluntarily provided the data with full awareness that these will be revealed to others. But where the researcher has promised to the respondents to protect their anonymity, the same should be fulfilled at the time of writing the report. This implies that the report should be written in such a way as to preclude the possibility of respondents' identification.

Revise and rewrite: Revising is part of writing. Novice writers should read many times after completion of the report for any omission or corrections. An experienced researcher can do the job better on the first try even for him a second reading will reveal newer information. The common changes that requires are restructuring of faulty sentences, shortening of concepts or simplifying complex concepts, rearrangement of content, change of tense and voice, numbering of tables, correction of spelling mistakes, etc. This should not dishearten the writer. He should understand that these are common occurrences in all writings and among the best writers.

The report should normally go through three drafts. The first draft should aim at making the report as comprehensive and full of facts as possible. The second should aim at improving the language, form and style of the report and final draft should aim at making the report authoritative by checking its foot notes, references and bibliography, etc.

Revision of the first draft should be done after some time gap. This will increase the objectivity towards one's own work. If the gap is less he cannot detach himself and have a third person look at the article for its completeness. If the gap is too long he may tend to forget the major ideas.

Writing Research Report for Various Purposes

Dissertations: Dissertations are written for the submission to the universities for requirement of partial fulfillment of the award of a degree. Each and every discipline will have a standard rule for writing dissertations. The dissertation in nursing is expected to be written by following specific methods which are as follows:

Front pages: It usually consists of the title, candidate and the supervisors information and signature, acknowledgement, information on chapters, main and subheading with its page numbers, list of tables and figures.

Chapters: The entire research report is organized under 6 chapters so as to present in a sequential manner.

Chapter I: It gives information on planning phase of the research study and it includes:

- Introduction
- Background of the study
- Need for the study
- Statement of the problem
- Research objectives
- Hypothesis
- Operational definition
- Assumptions and delimitations
- Projected outcome.

Chapter II: It gives information on the work of others on the same topic and it includes:

- Review of literature
- Conceptual framework.

Chapter III: It details on the research methodology used and it includes:

- Research approach
- Research design
- Major variables of the study
- Setting
- Population
- Sample and sample size
- Sampling technique
- Inclusion criteria
- Exclusion criteria
- Tool for data collection
- Data collection procedure
- Ethical considerations
- Pilot study
- Modification after the pilot study
- Validity and reliability of the tool
- Main study data collection
- Plan for data analysis.

Chapter IV: It details on the analysis and interpretation of the data in tables and figures and it includes:

- Tables and figures on demographic data and data about the study variables and its interpretation.

Chapter V: This chapter, on discussion gives details on:

- The major findings of the study
- Discussion on the demographic variables
- Discussion on the variables of the study based on the objectives
- Discussion on the acceptance or rejection of hypothesis and note on assumption.

Chapter VI: This chapter on summary and recommendations gives details on:
- Summary of the findings
- Implications for nursing
- Suggestions and recommendations
- Limitations.

Bibliography and Reference: It includes:
- Books
- Journals
- Online reference.

Appendix: It includes:
- Tool
- Permission letters from the settings
- Informed consent form
- Any other relevant information which cannot be accommodated in the chapters.

Writing research report for journal publication/conferences: While dissertation is the elaborate report of the research work, the research report for the journal or conference publication is the exclusive, concise but complete report. The editorial board gives the clear directions of how a research should be reported. A researcher need not to write in detail as it is required for the dissertation. In general, the parts of a paper are:
- ***Title:*** The title should convey the main idea of the paper in a few words.
- ***Authors and their affiliations:*** The authors of the paper are listed in the order of the importance of their contributions and the details of their affiliation is also given.
- ***Abstract:*** The abstract is a brief summary of the paper and includes elements from the introduction, method, results and discussion sections.
- ***Introduction:*** The introduction states the general problem the paper deals with, discusses the relevant literature and the need for the study, research objectives/questions, hypothesis, definition of terms, assumptions and delimitations and states what the paper will contribute to the understanding of the problem.
- ***Method:*** It includes the details on the research approach, design, setting, population, sample, sampling technique, tool for data collection and the methods of data collection.
- ***Results and discussion:*** The results section describes the results and their statistical analysis. Graphs and tables are described here. The discussion section interprets the results and relates them to the literature. It states the contributions that the study makes to the understanding of the problem posed in the introduction. A list of suggestions, recommendations and implications to nursing is also given. It also reports limitation of the study.
- The other elements are:
    - References
    - Footnotes
    - Tables
    - Figure captions
    - Figures.

APA Style of Writing Research Report

American Psychological Association (APA) has given a standard format for writing scientific and scholarly article. There are many specific rules for preparing a research article, so refer to the Publication Manual for complete instructions. Some general rules for preparing a research article that conforms to APA style:

- A report should be written in past tense since it describes a completed study. The exception is to state in the present tense any conclusions that apply to present or future situations.
- To distinguish your study from other studies, refer to it as 'this study' or 'present study'. Use accepted psychological terminology as much as possible. Avoid abbreviations.
- Use words for numbers between zero and nine, and digits for numbers that are 10 and larger. However use digits for any size of number if you are writing a series of numbers in which at least one is 10 or larger or the number contains a decimal or refers to a statistical result or to a precise measurement. Also never begin a sentence with a number expressed in digits.
- The manuscript is written as 12 font size, Times New Roman font with double line space. Indent the first line of every paragraph one-half inch. Align the text to the left hand margin.
- Quotations fewer than 40 words are incorporated into the text using quote marks. Cite the specific page of the quote. If a quotation is 40 or more words, start a new line, using a block quotation; indent as if a new paragraph, double space and do not use quotation marks. Do not include references to personal communications, such as letters, e-mails, interviews, telephone conversations on the reference page as they are not recoverable. You may however, cite them in-text. What you cite should have scholarly relevance.
- APA style uses five level headings.
- Proper citation should be given for the quotation of others work.

Reducing bias in language: The information should be specific. Any risk is mentioned means, it should specify the risk they are at and if age is mentioned, it should specify for example it can be written as 18 to 35 years instead of writing as above 18 years. When we write about the roles of individuals in an experiment, it should be written as active participants rather than passive recipients of the intervention. It should be written as 'the samples completed the procedure/activity' instead of the procedure/activity was completed by the samples.

APA style is used for:

- Empirical studies
- Research reports
- Literature reviews
- Theoretical articles
- Methodological articles
- Case studies.

The whole content is organized as follows:

- Title
- Abstract
- Introduction
- Methods
- Results
- Discussion
- References
- Appendices.

Title page: It is the first page. Short title of the paper in all caps in each page is given as running head. The title is typed as sentence case and aligned as centre and positioned in the upper half of the page. It should be no longer than 12 words. The author and the institutional affiliation is given below the title. Each page is numbered starting with the title page.

Title should attract the readers and motivate them to read further. It should communicate the variables and relationship being studied. Title also often begin with the phrase 'Effect of' or 'Assessment of' or 'Evaluation of'. This running head will be printed at the top of each page in the published article. So, if any pages become separated the publisher can identify them as belonging to a particular manuscript. This is another reason for all researchers not to use titles beginning 'A study of'.

Abstract page: It is the second page. An abstract is a brief comprehensive summary of the paper between 150 and 250 words. It provides the reader with a brief overview of the article. Abstract is typed in block format, one paragraph, no indentations and double spaced. Key words are given. The abstract describes the specific variables used, important subject characteristics, a brief description of the overall design and the key general statistical relationship obtained. One should remember that the title describes the relationship under investigation whereas the abstract summarizes the report.

Body of the paper: Page 3 begins the body of the paper. It contains introduction, method, results and discussion. One inch margin is given on all sides. Title is centered on the paper on this page. Title should not be bold or underlined.

Introduction: It should explain the concepts which helps you to derive the objectives and hypotheses of the study. It should provide the empirical evidence that supports the hypothesis. The introduction presents all information that will be used to interpret the results: The conceptual and theoretical logic of the study, relevant past research and the predictions of the study.

Method: The method section contains the information needed to understand, critique and literally replicate the data collection procedures. To collect data we need participants, testing materials and equipment and a specific testing procedure and design. APA style requires that these categories be presented in three separate subsections, in this order: (1) Participants, (2) Materials and (3) Procedure.

Participants: This should give details about the subject characteristics and specification of any criteria used to select the subjects as samples. It also includes the details on the sample size, methods of selecting them and the ethical principles followed in recruitment of samples.

Materials or apparatus: This mainly deals with the instruments or tools used to measure the variables.

Procedure: This section describes about the procedure of data collection. This elaborates on obtaining permission from the setting, selection of samples, data collection procedure, etc.

Results: It reports the statistical procedure performed and the statistical outcomes obtained. However, the results are not interpreted here. The analysis then involves first computing the descriptive statistics that summarize the scores and relationship and then the inferential statistics. Remember that for any inferential procedure, one result cannot be 'more significant' than another and there is no such thing as a 'very significant' or 'highly significant' result. Also do not attribute human actions to statistical procedures, saying such things as 'according to the ANOVA...' or 'the t gave significance'. Instead it can be stated as 'there was a significant differences between the means of two groups'.

Discussion: In this section, the results are interpreted and conclusions are drawn. Discussion on hypothesis testing and post factum interpretations are carried out. While interpreting one should think of internal and external validity. The discussion section answers the questions posed by the study, interpreting the results in terms of what is now known about the underlying behavior or variables.

References: Arrange entries in alphabetical order by the author's last name, or if no author, by the 1st word in the citation. All citations should be listed in the reference list except for personal communications and classical work. References are written in authors' surname. Entire reference should be double spaced. References should contain the following information:

- Authors name
- Publication data
- Title of the work
- Publication details.

References should begin on a new page after the last page of text. Each table begins on a new page after the references. Each figure begins on a new page after the tables. Each appendix begins on a new page. The publication manual provides specific rules for referencing books, book chapters, journals, magazines and so on.

Figures and tables: Every figure and table need to be numbered and titled. The figures and tables are placed after the references at the end of the manuscript starting at a separate page. There are many specific rules to prepare the figures. Check the publication manual for details. In general, the Y-axis should be about 60–75% of the length of the X-axis. Label each axis and use legends or keys to describe. Each figure should have figure number and figure caption.

Do's and Don'ts of Writing a Research Report

Do's

- Read the instruction carefully before preparing a research report. The reporting will vary based on the purpose. Look for any standard instruction and format to be used. If it is given, better to adhere to it.
- Organize and limit your content based on the number of pages. There is usually limitation placed on the number of pages. Too many pages and too less pages may not be effective. Too many pages beyond limitation conveys the inefficiency of the researcher to organize his/her content and too less pages conveys the inadequacy of the content.
- References wherever appropriate should be cited in the text by author name and year.
- Always proofread your work for typos. For example, the spell checker will not alert you to 'trials' being incorrectly spelled as 'trails'.
- Look for sequence and continuity of the content. There should be a continuity from chapter to chapter.
- The language should be based on the purpose of the reader. If the expected readers are professionals/colleagues and the educated group, use standard research language. If the target readers are the general public better use simple language and not the technical terms and jargons.
- Tables and diagrams are to be numbered and referred within the text.
- Remember that the work is yours and you are the best person to present it in a best possible way. Copying and imitating the style and presentation from others may not do justice. Think critically and analytically, comprehend and then present the content.

Don'ts

- ***Use of personal pronouns (we, I, our, me, etc.):*** Use of personal pronouns as far as possible, should be avoided. Avoid contradicting words (don't, can't, couldn't, etc.)
- ***The word 'data' is plural.*** For example, write: 'the data were collected', not 'the data was collected'
- Avoid using unnecessary figures and diagrams in the report
- Avoid repeating the same information in the form table and diagram
- Avoid selecting dark colors for the diagram
- Avoid using variety of graphs and diagrams in the report. The use of diagrams and graphs is to present the content well. It is not to prove the researcher's knowledge and efficiency in using this. There should be an appropriate selection of the diagrams and graphs based on the need
- Avoid using unnecessary background and filling in the diagram or graph. Sometimes it may not look like a professional work
- ***Use of tenses:*** Tenses can be very difficult to use correctly. The research proposal can be written using future tense since it is a plan for future action whereas a research report should be written in past tense since

it is a report of the work already done especially the methodology and the results. Basically, anything that is history should be written in the past tense. At the same time, the theories and models that were derived from the results and conclusions still make predictions today and their predictions thus should be described using the present tense. The conclusions of previous workers are history, however, the present project is still current and should be described in the present tense.

Thus, for a previous piece of work that a researcher wants to describe: 'Sudha, et al. (2012) found that... they concluded that...and developed the ABC model. This predicts that...'

In order to discuss the findings: 'It was found that... and thus we conclude that.... the ABC model predicts that...'

Oral Presentation

Preparation of report for oral presentation needs a different approach. First the researcher should think of the audience to whom he is going to present. The preparation should start from this thought of audience and their level of background. The purpose of presentation should be identified. It may be to sell, persuade, inform, entertain or solicit support. The introduction and conclusion are the most important part of any oral presentation. The introduction should attract the audience and should create curiosity. It is very important to spice these parts with relevant stories, anecdotes, analogies, examples and visuals. In between the presentation, there should a self-posed questions that do not really expect answers but their use in the report focuses listeners, sets their mind to thinking and enhances their sense of well being and makes them feel a part of what is taking place.

Techniques of Good Oral Presentation

- ***Spontaneous presentation:*** Presentation should be free flowing, it should come off as spontaneous speech even though it is a carefully prepared speech.
- ***Conversational:*** A presentation attracts the audience when it is presented in a conversational style rather than a formal one.
- ***Tone of voice:*** An excellent presenter takes advantage of the rich range of vocal resources available to increase interest, impact and persuasive power.
- ***Involvement through gesture:*** An excellent presenter involves listeners through the skillful use of gestures. Gestures provide a visual narrative that goes along with the verbal one. They are displayed thinking.
- ***Creativity:*** An excellent presenter shows imagination and resourcefulness by drawing on a variety of verbal tools to enliven presentations and renew enthusiasm.
- ***Relevancy:*** A presentation related to the topic and audience will relate to the listeners in a personal way.
- ***Clarity:*** A good presenter has the ability to present his concepts very clearly which results in giving everyone the same message.

- ***AV aids:*** A power point preparation and using over head projector will facilitate the presentation. One should not overly dependent on the AV aids.

CRITIQUING OF RESEARCH REPORT

Evidence-based practice, is the use of the best clinical evidence in making patient care decisions and such evidence typically comes from research conducted by nurses and other health care professionals. Research is systematic inquiry that uses disciplined methods to answer questions or solve problems. Nursing research has experienced remarkable growth in the past three decades, providing nurses with an increasingly sound evidence base to practice. The authenticity of the research findings, need to be assessed by careful critical analysis as to broaden the understanding, determine evidence for use in practice and provide a background for conducting further study. All nurses should possess skills to evaluate relevant research reports since all published studies are not sound and all information available on internet are not reliable.

A research critique is a careful appraisal of the strengths and weaknesses of the study. An intellectual research critique is a careful, complete examination of a study to judge its strengths, weaknesses, logical links, meaning and significance. It is the process of objectively and critically evaluating a research report's content for scientific merit and application to practice, theory or education.

In common a research critique is a appraisal of—

- Strengths and limitations of a study
- Adequacies, inadequacies, virtues as well as faults
- Merits and demerits.

Need for critiquing a research:

- To learn the process of critiquing
- To identify a valid research
- To find evidence for research utilization
- To accept a study for publication in journal.

Prerequisites for a research critique

- A person who makes a critique should have a knowledge on research concepts
- He should read the entire content of the research
- It is not finding fault in others work
- It is not proving one's talent in critiquing
- He cannot be hypercritical
- He should be very specific in critiquing
- He cannot be so general
- It should not be a review or summary
- Be open in critiquing and should not be prejudiced or biased
- Identify both strengths and weakness of a study
- Read thoroughly and critique the entire study
- Examine the organization and presentation of the research report

- Check for the logic in presentation and use of excessive jargon
- Examine the significance of the problem studied for nursing practice
- Be objective and realistic in identifying the study's strength and weaknesses
- Provide a rationale for the critique
- Suggest modifications for future studies
- Discuss the usefulness of the findings for practice.

Critiquing a research article: A research can be critiqued on various dimensions such as theoretical dimensions, methodological dimensions, ethical dimensions, interpretive dimensions and presentation dimensions. Both quantitative and qualitative studies can be critiqued on these dimensions.

Theoretical dimension: It mainly assesses for formulation of research problem, objectives, hypothesis and the variables or concepts and its relationships. It mainly checks whether a problem formulated is based on theory, formulation and derivation of hypothesis, whether the hypothesis formulated from existing theory or based on sound review of literature and also checks for the proper statement of need.

Methodological dimension: It mainly deals with the research approaches and design, sampling methods, sampling size, data sources, setting, recruitment of participants and measurement tools. It also checks for data analysis, reliability and validity of the tool.

Ethical dimensions: In this, a research report should be critiqued for protection of human rights of participants and checks whether ethical principles are followed in the conduction of study.

Interpretive dimension: This mainly deals with the interpretation of the data and generalization. This also ensures the implications for nursing, suggestions and recommendations.

Presentation dimension: It assesses the language, organization of the content, logic in presentation, appropriate use of figures and diagrams.

The questions on each heading will help for critiquing the research report.

Title:

- Is the title attractive?
- Does it include key variables and the study population?
- Is it appropriately worded neither too lengthy nor too small?

Abstract:

- Does the abstract clearly and concisely summarize the main features? (problem, methods, research conclusions)
- Is it too lengthy or too short?

Introduction:

- Is the introduction well written?
- Does it explains the concepts and variables of the study?
- Does it introduce the topic logically and clearly?
- Is the introduction relevant?

Problem statement:

- What is the study problem? Is it easy to locate?
- Is the problem stated clearly and unambiguously? Is it easy to identify?
- Is the problem researchable one?
- Is the problem formulated based on sound review of literature?
- Does the problem includes all elements such as variables, population and setting?
- Has the research problem been substantiated with adequate experiential and scientific background material?
- Does the problem stated, expresses a relationship between two or more variables or at least between dependent and independent variable, implying empirical testability?
- Does the problem specify the nature of the population being studied?
- Does the problem have significance and relevance to nursing?
- Is there a match between the research problem and paradigm and methods used?
- Is the problem sufficiently narrow in scope without being trivial?
- Was this study feasible to conduct in terms of money commitment; the researcher's expertize; availability of subjects, facility, equipment; ethical considerations?
- Has the research problem been placed within the context of an appropriate theoretical framework?

Purpose:

- What is the study purpose?
- Does the purpose narrow and clarify the focus or aim of the study and identify the research variables, population and setting?
- Is it worded appropriately?
- Are verbs used appropriately to suggest the nature of the inquiry and or the research tradition?

Objectives:

- Are the objectives adequate in number?
- Was the objectives formally stated? Clearly and concisely stated?
- Is it logically linked to purpose?
- Is it linked to concepts and relationships from the framework?
- Is the objectives measurable or potentially measurable and achievable?
- Do they clearly identify the variables and population studied?

Hypotheses:

- Is hypothesis present or absent?
- If present, how many in number?
- Are they properly worded?
- Are they stated objectively without value laden words?
- Does it state the relationship between variables?
- Is it directional or nondirectional?
- Is it testable?
- Is it a research or null hypothesis?
- Is it a simple or complex, causal or associative?

- Is it formulated based on theory?
- Is it formulated based on sound literature review?
- Does it include all other elements such as setting, population, level of significance?
- Is the hypothesis linked to the research problem and purpose?
- Is the hypothesis linked to concepts, relationships from the framework and literature review?
- Is the hypothesis directs the research study?
- If hypothesis absent, is their absence justifiable?

Conceptual framework:

- Is it a content or process framework?
- Is the study framework identified?
- Is a particular theory or model identified as a framework for the study?
- Is the framework appropriate?
- Does the concepts fit into the theory?
- Is the relationship stated clearly?
- Is the directions between the variables clear?
- Does the framework describe and define the concepts of interest or major features of the theory/model?
- Is a map or model of the framework provided for clarity?
- If there was an intervention, was there a cogent theoretical basis or rationale for the intervention?
- Is the theory or model used as the basis for generating hypothesis that were tested or is it used as an organizational or interpretive framework? Was this appropriate?
- Are deductions from theory are logical?
- Is the framework presented with clarity?
- Are the concepts adequately defined in way that is consistent with the theory? If there is an intervention, are intervention components consistent with the theory?
- Do the problem and hypothesis naturally flow from the framework? Or is the link contrived?
- Is the framework related to nursing's body of knowledge? Is it based on a conceptual model of nursing or a model developed by nurses? Is it borrowed from another discipline, is there adequate justification for its use?
- Is the framework linked to the research purpose?
- Is there a link between the framework, concepts being studied and the methods of measurement
- If the proposition from a theory is to be tested, is the proposition clearly identified and linked to the study hypotheses?
- Did the framework guide the study methods?
- Does the researcher tie the findings of the study back to the framework at the end of the report?
- How do the findings support or undermine the framework? Are the findings interpreted within the context of the framework?

Variables:

- Do the variables reflect the concepts identified in the framework?
- Are the variables clearly defined (conceptually and operationally) based on previous research and or theories?
- Is the conceptual definition of a variable consistent with the operational definition?
- Are the variables measurable?
- Do the theoretical definitions correspond to the conceptual definitions?
- What attribute or demographic variables are examined in the study?
- Were the extraneous variables identified and controlled as necessary in the study?
- Is the potential impact of these variables on the findings discussed?

Review of literature:

- Is the literature review presented? Does it reflect critical thinking?
- Is the review adequate?
- Is the recent articles reviewed?
- Are all relevant concepts and variables included in the review?
- Are relevant theories and models identified and described?
- Are the references current? Examine the number of sources in the last five and ten years in the reference list.
- Does it identify/uncover the gaps or inconsistencies in literature?
- Is it based on primary sources? Are secondary sources cited?
- Does it provide solid basis for the new study? Does the summary of the current empirical and theoretical knowledge provide a basis for the study?
- Are the studies critiqued by the author?
- Is a summary of the current knowledge provided? This summary needs to include what is known and not known about the research problem.
- Is the review well organized, flow logically, written concisely? Is the development of ideas clear to demonstrate the progressive development of ideas through previous research?
- Is the review objective?
- Is there use of appropriate language?
- Is a theoretical knowledge base developed for the problem and purpose? Does it follow the purposes of the study?
- Is there a written summary synthesis of the reviewed scholarly literature?

Research design:

- Is the research approach and design appropriate and clearly addressed?
- Is the selection of research design appropriate for the problem and hypothesis?
- Does the researcher use the various concepts of control that are consistent with the type of design chosen?
- What elements are controlled? What elements could have been controlled to improve the design?
- What elements of the design were manipulated and how were they manipulated?

- How adequate was the manipulation? What elements should have been manipulated to improve the validity of findings?
- What are the threats to internal and external validity?
- What are the controls for the threats of internal and external validity?
- Does the study include a treatment or intervention? If so is the treatment clearly defined conceptually and operationally? Clearly described and consistently implemented?
- Was the control of comparison condition adequately explained? What justification from the literature provided for development of the experimental intervention?
- Who implemented the treatment? If more than one person, were they trained to ensure consistency in the delivery of the treatment?
- Was there a protocol developed to ensure consistent or reliable implementation of the treatment with each subject throughout the study?
- Were randomization procedures adequately explained?
- Is there adequate justification for failure to randomize subjects to treatment conditions?
- If the study was non experimental, was the study inherently non experimental? What was the design used?
- If the study has more than one group, how were the subjects assigned to groups?
- What type of comparisons are specified in the design (before-after, between groups)?
- Was the study longitudinal? Was the timing of the collection of data appropriate?
- Was the number of data collection points reasonable?
- Was masking and blinding used at all? If yes who was blinded and was this adequate? If not, was there an adequate rationale for failure to mask?
- Did the design minimize biases and threats to the internal and external validity of the study?
- Are the extraneous variables identified and controlled?
- Were pilot study findings used to design the major study?
- Is the design logically linked to the sampling method and statistical analyses?

Setting:

- Is the setting appropriate and adequate?
- Whether adequate sample is obtained from the setting?
- Is the proper permission obtained from the setting?

Population and sample:

- Was the population identified and described?
- Was the sample described in sufficient detail?
- Is the target population to which the findings will be generalized defined?
- Was the best possible sampling design was used to enhance sample's representativeness?
- Were sample biases minimized?
- Is the sampling method adequate to produce a sample that is representative of the study population?

- Is the sample representative of accessible and target population?
- Was the sample size adequate?
- Are the sample selection procedures clearly delineated?
- Did the researchers identify the sampling frame for the study?
- What type of sampling plan was used?
- Are key characteristics of the sample described (female or male percentage, mean age, etc.)?
- Is the inclusion and exclusion criteria clearly stated? Are they acceptable?

Instrument/Tools:

- Are all of the measurement strategies/instruments identified and described?
- Identify the author of each measurement strategy. Identify the type of each measurement strategy (Likert, visual analogue, physiological measurement, questionnaire, interview, observation).
- Is there rationale for their selection given?
- Is the method used appropriate to the problem being studied?
- Are they similar for all subjects?
- Is there a discussion on the reliability and validity of each instrument?
- What was the precision and accuracy of the physiological measurement methods used in a study?
- Were the set of data collection instruments adequately pretested?
- Do the instruments adequately measure the study variables? Determine whether the type of measurement is direct or indirect?
- Are the specific instruments adequately described in terms of reading level of questions, length of time to complete it, number of modules included and so on? Were they good choices, given the study purpose and study population?
- Was the mode of obtaining data appropriate? (in personal interview, mailed questionnaire, internet questioning)
- Were self-report data gathered in a manner that promoted high quality and unbiased responses (e.g. Privacy, efforts to put respondents at ease)?
- If observational data were used did the report adequately describe what specific constructs were observed? What was the unit of observation – was the approach molar or molecular?
- Are the instruments sufficiently sensitive to detect differences between subjects?
- If validity and reliability is reported, which method of validity and reliability appraisal have been used? Was it appropriate?
- Is the reliability sufficiently high or the validity appear adequate? Should another method have been used?
- Are the instruments clearly described? Described well enough to know whether it covers the subject?
- Are techniques to administer, complete and score instruments provided?
- If the instrument was developed for the study, is the instrument process development described?
- Is there a clear indication that the subjects understood the questionnaire?

- Is there evidence that subjects were able to perform the task?
- Are the accuracy, precision, selectivity, sensitivity, error of the physiological instruments discussed?
- Are the methods for recording data from the physiological measures clearly described?
- Are the records used appropriate to the problem being studied?
- Are the data examined in such a way as to provide new information and not summarize the records?
- Has the author addressed questions of internal and external criticism?
- Is there any indication of selection bias in the available records?

Ethical considerations:

- Are the rights of human subjects protected?
- Were appropriate procedures used to safeguard the rights of study participants used?
- Was the study subjected to an external review? Was the study approved and monitored by an institutional review board, research ethics board or other similar ethics review committee?
- Was the study designed to minimize risks and maximize benefits to participants?
- Did the benefits outweigh any potential risks or actual discomfort they experienced?
- Did the benefits to society outweigh the costs to participants?
- Did they have the right to refuse to participate or to withdraw without penalty?
- Were the study participants subjected to any physical harm, discomfort or psychological distress?
- Were participants deceived in anyway?
- Were they fully aware of participating in a study and did they understand the purpose and nature of research?
- Were the subjects informed about the purpose and nature of the study?
- Were appropriate informed consent procedures used with all subjects?
- Was the information essential for the consent provided?
- Were the subjects capable of comprehending the information, competent to give consent?
- Were adequate steps taken to safeguard the privacy of the participants?
- How data was kept anonymous or confidential? Was a certificate of confidentiality obtained?
- Were vulnerable groups involved in the research? If yes, were special precautions instituted because of their vulnerable status?

Data Collection:

- Did the researcher make the right decision about collecting new data versus existing data for the study?
- Did the researcher make good data collection decisions with regard to structure, quantification, researcher obtrusiveness and objectivity?
- Were the right methods used to collect the data?

- Was triangulation of methods used appropriately—were multiple methods used sensibly? Are the data collection procedures were same for all subjects?
- Was the right amount of data collected? Were data collected to address the varied needs of the study?
- Did the researcher use good instruments, in terms of congruence with underlying constructs, data quality, reputation, efficiency and so on?
- Were new instruments developed unnecessarily?
- Did the report provide adequate information about data collectors and data collection procedure?
- Is the data collection process clearly described?
- Is the data collection process conducted in a consistent manner?
- Are the data collection methods ethical?
- Do the data collected address the research objectives, questions or hypotheses?
- Who collected the data?
- Was the training of data collectors described? Was the training adequate?
- Was the setting for data collection appropriate?
- Were data collected in a manner that minimized bias?
- What methods were used to sample observational units? Was the sampling approach good one?
- To what degree were observer biases controlled or minimized?
- Were biophysiologic measures used in the study and was this appropriate?
- Were appropriate methods used to measure the variables of interest?
- Did the researcher appear to have the skills necessary for proper interpretation of biophysiologic measures?

Data analysis:

- Are data analysis procedures clearly described?
- What statistical analyses are included in the research report?
- Do data analyses address each objective, question or hypothesis?
- Are data analyses procedures appropriate to the type of data collected?
- Are the results presented in an understandable way?
- Are tables and figures used to synthesize and emphasize certain findings?
- Were the tables, graphs, pictures clear, with a good title, carefully labeled headings?
- Were appropriate descriptive statistics used?
- What level of measurement is used to measure each of the major variables?
- Was the most powerful analytic method was used? Were type I and II errors avoided or minimized?
- Does the level of measurement and sample size permit the use of parametric statistics?
- Are the statistics used appropriate to the problem, the hypothesis, the method, the sample and the level of measurement?
- If nonparametric tests were used was a rationale provided and does the rationale seem sound?
- Are the results for each of the hypotheses presented appropriately?

- Do the findings support the study framework?
- Are the results clearly and completely stated? Are the results presented objectively?
- Was the level of significance or alpha identified?
- Are significant and nonsignificant findings explained?
- Are the analyses interpreted appropriately? Does the interpretation of findings appear biased?
- What conclusions did the researcher identify based on this study and previous research?
- Are any generalizations made, how did the researcher generalize the findings?
- Are the generalizations within the scope of the findings or beyond the findings?
- Are the findings adequately summarized?

Discussion:

- What is the researcher's interpretation of findings?
- Are all important results discussed?
- Did the researcher identify and discuss important study limitations and their effects on the results?
- Are the findings consistent with the results and with study's limitations?
- Are all major findings interpreted and discussed within the context of prior research and or the study's conceptual framework?
- Are the findings consistent with previous research findings?
- Does the report address the issue of the generalizability of the findings?
- Do the researchers discuss the study's implications for clinical practice, nursing education, nursing administration, nursing theory or make specific recommendations?
- What implications do the findings have for nursing practice? Are they reasonable and complete?
- What suggestions/recommendations are made for further studies?
- What are the missing elements of the study? Is the description of the study sufficiently clear to allow replication?

Application and utilization:

- Do the study appear valid?
- Are the findings related to the framework?
- Are the findings linked to those of previous studies? To what populations can the findings be generalized?
- What research questions emerge from the findings? Are these questions identified by the researcher?
- What is the overall quality of the study when strengths and weaknesses are summarized?
- Do the findings have potential for use in nursing practice? What risk/benefit are involved for patients if the research findings would be used in practice?
- Can the study be replicated by other researchers? Are the findings credible?

- Is direct application of the research findings feasible in terms of time, effort money and legal and ethical crisis?
- How and under what circumstances are the findings applicable to nursing practice?

Researcher credibility and presentation:

- Does the researchers' clinical, substantive or methodological qualifications and experience enhance confidence in the findings and their interpretation?
- Is the report well written, well organized and sufficiently detailed for critical analysis? Is the report placed logical sequence and useful location?
- Was it written in a manner that makes the findings accessible to practicing nurses?

RESEARCH UTILIZATION

It refers to the use of some aspect of a scientific investigation in an application unrelated to the original research. The research findings are utilized by the investigator herself or any other who is interested in utilizing the findings.

The need for utilization:

- Nursing research contributes to improving the patient outcome and ultimately to the health care system.
- Research utilization facilitates an innovative change in practice or the verification of existing practice protocols.
- Knowledge about published materials and what other people have tried is vital when exploring solutions to a problem.
- Research utilization helps in improving nursing practice by providing answers to clinical questions, evaluating effectiveness of the nursing actions, testing theories relevant to nursing practice and expanding nursing knowledge (Lanuza,1999).
- Research utilization facilitates evidence based practice thus improves autonomy and professionalism.
- It ultimately leads to development of the profession.

Dissemination and Utilization

Dissemination is the important item on most people's agendas. How to get research results to intended audiences in the most effective, cost-efficient manner. But utilization is a critical element in increasing the effective reach of research outcomes. Dissemination speaks primarily to the process of knowledge transfer—the who, what, when and how of moving ideas and information from the source(s) to intended recipient(s). ***Utilization*** speaks primarily to purpose and to impact—why we want people to get the research outcomes we are putting forth, what use we want people to make of the ideas, information, or products, and how people are actually using them (Table 10.1).

The phenomenon of 'utilization' varies from person to person. In order to change pre-existing understandings, groups or individuals first must recognize a certain 'need.' A reason has to be perceived in order to make a shift in thinking. Or, People and organizations develop the energy to change when faced with real pain. When old ways do not seem to be working as well as they should, when current explanations cannot account for a new circumstance, when the status quo is no longer comfortable, these are times when real change in understanding and behavior are possible.

Knowledge Transfer

It is the process and tools by which researchers disseminate evidence or new knowledge. (Centre for knowledge transfer)

It is the exchange, synthesis and ethically sound application of knowledge within a complex system of relationships among researchers and users. (Jacobson, et al. 2004).

Those involved in utilization efforts must not underestimate the complexities of the dissemination/utilization process. A successful utilization model must rely on effective and well-defined interactions between basic process elements of the potential user, the content of the message, the context required to obtain the message, the medium of the message and the source of the message/research result(s).

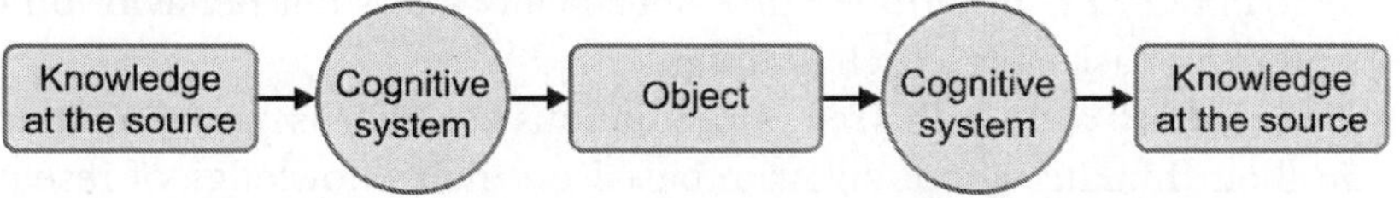

The researcher is the source of knowledge. For the knowledge transfer to be effective, the object has primarily to fit the cognitive characteristics of the recipient. As a consequence, even a simple set of data can represent an important source of knowledge for people who can interpret those data and get benefits from them. This perspective also stresses the fundamental action of the cognitive processes which includes codification and interpretation.

Codification is the process by which knowledge is represented in various forms (codes) that can be leveraged and transferred (Ruggles, 1997). The knowledge code can vary in a wide range, including natural language, numbers, analytical models, images. Consequently, the means used for the transfer can be different, including face-to-face communication, telephone, fax, e-mail. In codification, the selection and organization of information seem the fundamental processes, which are necessarily affected by the cognitive characteristics of the subject who performs codification. It is interesting to note that adopting the 'object' perspective makes the distinction between codification and interpretation clear. In particular, this is typical in those cases where the interaction between individuals is mediated by technology, which enables creating, transferring and storing knowledge objects. However, the two processes are also recognizable in knowledge transfer without the support of technology, as in teaching, where the code is often the natural language and in apprenticeship, where codification is reduced to showing things at work and the interpretation is left to the observation capability.

Table 10.1: Difference between dissemination and utilization

S. No.	Dissemination	Utilization
1.	A process of getting research results to intended audience in the most effective manner	A process of using findings from conducting research to guide practice. The process by which scientifically produced knowledge is transferred to practice
2.	It requires preparation of research report, identification of means of dissemination and actual dissemination	Research utilization refers to the review and critique of scientific research, and then the application of the findings to clinical practice
3.	It focuses on communicating the findings	It focuses on improving the outcome of the practice
4.	It is the process of knowledge transfer—who, what, when, where and how a research is conducted	It focuses on application of the findings in actual practice.

Terms Related to Research Utilization

- ***Instrumental utilization:*** Nurse specifically alters her behavior on the empirical basis of research findings.
- ***Conceptualization:*** This refers to situations in which users are influenced in their thinking about an issue based on their knowledge of research studies but do not put this knowledge to any specific documentable use. Knowledge creep refers to an evolving percolation of research ideas and findings. Decision accretion refers to the manner in which momentum for a decision builds over time based on accumulated information gained through readings, informal discussions, meetings and so on.
- ***Indirect research utilization:*** This involves changes in nurses' thinking and therefore analogous to conceptual utilization.
- ***Direct research utilization:*** It involves the direct use of findings in giving patient care and therefore analogous to instrumental utilization.
- ***Persuasive utilization:*** It involves the use of findings to persuade others (typically those in decision making positions) to make changes in policies or practices relevant to nursing care.

Elements of Research Utilization

To develop the knowledge transfer base that underlies utilization, there are five common core elements that are keys to success. These core elements strongly influence whether utilization efforts will be effective:

- ***Source:*** It is the source of research information from where where the research information can be obtained.
- ***Content:*** It is the information on the specific problem or questions to be answered or issue of clinical importance, etc.

- ***Context:*** It is relating the research information to existing knowledge or products. It is the way of linking the new information with the existing.
- ***Medium:*** It is the method of obtaining research information. It may be by attending the journal club, reading journals, etc.
- ***User:*** It is the person who wants to utilize the findings or the beneficiary.

A nurse who wants to utilize or shows interest in research utilization undergoes the continuum ranging from receiving information without internalization to application of received information.

Stage 1: A nurse receives information but no internalization occurs.

Stage 2: A nurse receives information and internalization occurs but rejected or ignored to apply.

Stage 3: A nurse receives information, internalizes and partially applies or rejects.

Stage 4: A nurse receives information, internalizes and fully replicates.

Stage 5: A nurse receives information, internalizes and fully adapts for application.

Utilization Continuum, identifies some examples of outcomes that may represent utilization. Intended use and effective use are not always synonymous. Sometimes consumers make adaptations or find effective uses never considered by researchers; sometimes cultural differences between researchers and consumers shift the assumptions as to what constitutes effective use. Utilization measurement is made complex by the nature of use.

Steps in Research Utilization

Research utilization refers to the use of some aspect of a scientific investigation in an application unrelated to the original research. The Dissemination (Knowledge transfer) is the step prior to the Utilization which also varies from person to person. The nurse researcher's duty not only rest with conducting research. It also includes promotion for effective utilization otherwise their research work is meaningless. By recognizing the difference between the dissemination and utilization, she can prepare model for utilization by which one can encourage effective utilization. Evidence- Based Practice (EBP) involves making clinical decisions on the basis of the best possible evidence. Usually the best evidence comes from rigorous research, but EBP also uses other sources of credible information. The major steps involved in research utilization are as follows:

- ***Identification of need or problem:*** The nurse must experience a need to solve a problem or face a burning problem for which she is in need of a solution.
- ***Identification of sources and looking for evidence:*** The nurse has to search and analyze various resources of research for seeking solution for her problem. In the process of doing this, she may either come across with lot of research findings or there may be inadequate or little information related to her clinical problem. The nurse who seeks for evidence should have keen interest and attitude in utilizing research in practice. There are many factors facilitating and hindering research utilization.

- ***Analyzing and identification of appropriate solution:*** When she searches for the data, she may either obtain lot of information and may be confused with the information to select and apply for her practice. She should analyze the credibility, validity and reliability of the findings. She should critique the research whether it is properly conducted. The number of researchers supporting one particular evidence and the reason for supporting it and also the number of researchers opposing the same findings and its reason can be analyzed. She should evaluate the findings for its application in the patient care. Finally she should arrive at conclusion on which evidence can be applied and tested to solve the problem.
- ***Utilization:*** She can apply the identified evidence on patient care and evaluate whether the problem is solved. She could try this solution in many patients and properly document the response of the patient. Before utilizing the evidence, she can consult with the peers and experts.
- ***Evaluation:*** Once tested on reasonable number of patients while providing care she can evaluate the outcome of a particular intervention that is the evidence. In doing this, she can compare the new practice with the existing practice. She can see how far a new practice has improved patient care than the existing practice.
- ***Recommendation:*** Once proved that the new practice is effective in improving patient care, she can disseminate this to many others for its wider utilization and promoting independent nursing actions.

If no satisfied results or solution found for a clinical problem, that is the area for a nurse to undertake a research. She can plan and conduct a research for identification of solution to a problem.

Barriers in utilization of research in nursing practice:

- Research related barriers
- Nurse related
- Organizational
- Barriers related to nursing profession.

Research related barriers: For many practical nursing problems, the studies are scarce or are not conducted. There are many unexplored areas. Studies are many times replicated. Studies based on clinical problems are very less. Studies for clinical utilization is not carried out. Lack of research knowledge pose barriers to knowledge diffusion to most practicing nurses.

Strategies to improve:

- High quality research should be conducted
- Establish a research utilization group in the hospital or working area
- Collaborate with clinicians for conducting research
- Communicate clearly
- Write clearly about the clinical problems which needs solution
- Collaborate with academic nurses for conduction of research
- Suggest clinical implications
- Disseminate broadly
- Prepare integrative research reviews.

Nurse related barriers: The knowledge and attitude of nurses towards research and research utilization is lacking. There is a resistance to change the age old practice. There is a lack of interest in learning new things and identification of evidences. They may not have knowledge in computer skills.

Strategies to improve:

- Read widely and critically
- Learn and update the concepts
- Attend professional conferences
- Be connected with the researchers
- Look for evidences
- Become involved in journal club
- Participate in research activities
- Write, communicate and disseminate clearly.

Organizational barrier: The organization especially hospital, may not have the climate of research utilization. They do not motivate or reward nurses for their research effort. The nurses may not have time during working hours to seek, do literature reviews and read research articles. Organizations may be reluctant to allocate resources. There may not be adequate journals, computer and internet facilities, time to discuss with peers and colleagues, etc. There may not be any fund to try this out.

Strategies:

- Foster a climate of intellectual curiosity
- Offer emotional or moral support
- Allocate specific time in their working schedule for research utilization
- Offer financial resource
- Reward efforts for using research
- Provide facilities
- Seek opportunities for research utilization projects.

Barriers related to the nursing profession: Nurse clinicians and nurse researchers do not collaborate. They work separately. Practicing nurses may not perceive themselves as independent professionals capable or recommending changes based on research results. Nurse educators teach research, but undertaking research which solves clinical problems is less.

Strategies:

- Incorporate research findings into the curriculum
- Encourage research and research use
- Place demands on researchers
- Bridge the gap between theory and practice.

RESEARCH PROPOSAL

Before an attempt is made to start with a research project, a research proposal should be compiled. For the beginner researcher, this is usually the most difficult part. It is, however, the most important aspect of the research project and should be considered carefully by the researcher. This does not only require subject knowledge, but also insight into the problem that is going to be investigated, so as to give logic and structure to research envisaged.

Meaning of Research Proposal

The research proposal can be envisaged as the process (step by step guidelines) to plan and to give structure to the prospective research with the final aim of increasing the validity of the research. It is therefore a written submission to spell out in a logic format the nature of the design and the means and strategies that are going to be used.

The sections of the proposal:

- ***Title:*** The title should be attractive, short in length and should give clue to the reader.
- ***Introduction:*** Prospective researchers can search within their own subject field for suitable problems. The introduction should introduce the problem with sufficient background information. It should be crisp, not too exhaustive and provide relevant information.
- ***Need for the study:*** The prospective researcher should think on what caused the need to do the research. The proposed researcher should state clearly the reason why he wants to conduct the research on particular topic by elaborating with the evidence. He can detail what is already done and what information is lacking and justify his interest and how it would be beneficial. The researcher should indicate and defend why it is necessary to undertake the research. A thorough review of literature will be helpful.
- ***Problem statement:*** The problem should be stated with all elements and it should arise from the need of the study. The research problem should always be formulated grammatically correct and as completely as possible.
- ***Research objectives/questions and hypothesis:*** Based on the problem statement, either research objectives or research question should be formulated. Formulation of hypotheses give structure and direction to research. Hypotheses can only be formulated after the researcher has gained enough knowledge regarding the nature, extent and intensity of the problem.
- ***Operational definition:*** This involves defining the key words in the problem statement based on how it will be operated in the study.
- ***Assumptions and Delimitations:*** In this, a precise indication is given of the scope of the research with indication of the assumptions made, limitations and delimitations of the research before the research is started.
- ***Research approach and research design:*** This is indicating the approach and design used for the study.
- ***Major variables:*** It is indicating the independent and dependent variables in the experimental study or in descriptive study which aims to correlate or find cause and effect relationship. In other studies, the major variable will be indicated.
- ***Setting:*** It is the proposed setting where the researcher will have access to the samples and the feasibility of obtaining permission is also mentioned.
- ***Population and sample:*** The proposed investigator should clearly state the target and accessible population, sampling method and sample

size. Empirical research almost always depends upon a sample which is assumed to accurately represent a population. Therefore, the techniques by which the samples will be chosen are vital to a discussion.

- ***Criteria for sample selection:*** It is the inclusion and exclusion criteria for the selection and exclusion of sample in the research study.
- ***Data collection methods and tool:*** It includes the description of the method of data collection and the type of tool to be used. It also should give details on the scoring and interpretation of the tool and the method of administration.
- When particular measurement instruments are used, it is often important to explain how those instruments are developed, where they have previously been used (if at all) and to what effect.
- ***Plan for data analysis:*** It is the plan for the descriptive analysis and inferential analysis.
- ***Projected outcome:*** This indicates of what the researcher expects to get out of the research. It is projected based on the possible outcome of the study and its significance to theory and practice. The benefits that will result from the research and to whom it will be beneficial should be indicated.
- ***Ethical principles:*** A note of how ethical principles will be fulfilled in the study helps to check for ethical agreement or any violation.
- ***Budget:*** A detailed indication of the funds needed to undertake the research. This is necessary where the researcher intends to apply for funding from the funding agency.
- ***Duration of the research project:*** A detailed proposed time schedule is supplied.
- ***Bibliography:*** This is the list of the relevant works. The reference list contains an entry for each work cited in the text and no others. The list of resources used will only include resources referred to in the research proposal. Use the APA style.
- ***Profile of the researcher:*** A list of all the qualification the researcher obtained up to date is indicated. This is must in case if the investigator applies for fund or scholarship.

Do's of writing a research proposal: Many people assume that any literate person can write a research proposal. This is not automatically true. Writing is a difficult skill to master and one that requires practice and some dedication.

- Read everything you can find in your area of interest. Take notes and talk to your advisor or expert about the topic.
- Write about the topic a lot. Later you can re-think and re-type and you can edit.
- Generate the research question, critical observation, interpretations of the possible outcomes and the expected results. These are the core of the project and will help focus your reading and thinking. Modify them as needed as your understanding increases.
- Use some systematic way of recording notes and bibliographic information from the very beginning.

- Make sure that you find a proposal structure that suits the needs of your research. If you are submitting to different organizations, make sure that you find out what those organizations' requirements are. Some institutions have very rigid formats and often proposals are disadvantaged because they do not conform to the requirements laid down.
- Apart from the sections outlined above, many organizations demand other sections as well.
- Know what you want to say before trying to write it.
- Every sentence must contain one idea only. Each sentence must follow logically from the one before. A well written text is a 'chain of ideas.'

Technical Editing of the Research Proposal

Although the research proposal is considered as the preliminary planning of a research problem, it should comply with the following requirements:

- It should preferably be typed in double spacing on size A4 paper
- 12, font size in Times New Roman
- A margin of 1 inch in all sides would give neat appearance
- Produce a professional looking proposal
- Be interesting and informative
- Use clear headings and subheadings
- Be concise and precise
- Use simple language wherever possible
- Check the spelling and grammar
- Give reference using an acceptable format
- Do not use words when you are not absolutely certain of their meaning
- Before submitting, make sure you have completed each of the following steps:
  - ❒ Proofread your work carefully
  - ❒ Ask a friend or relative to read your proposal
  - ❒ Ask an experienced researcher or your supervisor to read your proposal

The following should also accompany the research proposal:

- A front page
- The name and address of the researcher
- Research proposal prepared for a project with the details of the title.

What should however be emphasized is the fact that the research proposal forms part of the research project, and is not merely a means to acquire funding. A well prepared research proposal is characterized by an orderly logical outline. It should be emphasized that various disciplines and different research types, requires different approaches and methods.

SUMMARY

- Interpretation refers to the task of drawing inferences from the collected facts after analysis. In fact, it is a search for broader meaning of research findings. It is of two types such as hypothesis testing and post factum interpretation.

- The post factum interpretation is different from hypothesis testing. In hypothesis testing the investigator begins with a specific interpretation and determines whether or not the data are consistent with it. But in the post factum interpretation, the analyst begins with the data and seeks an interpretation consistent with it.
- Research study is complete only when the findings have been shared with others. It is of no value unless the research finding is disseminated to the people. It is the researcher's responsibility to ensure that the research study and its findings/ recommendations are disseminated to as wide an audience as possible.
- Scientific communication takes place in many ways, including archival publication in scholarly journals and informal communication among groups of scientists, known as invisible colleges.
- American Psychological Association (APA) has given a standard format for writing scientific and scholarly article.
- Research critique is a careful appraisal of the strengths and weaknesses of the study. A research can be critiqued on various dimensions such as theoretical dimensions, methodological dimensions, ethical dimensions, interpretive dimensions and presentation dimensions. Both quantitative and qualitative studies can be critiqued on these dimensions.
- Research utilization refers to the use of some aspect of a scientific investigation in an application unrelated to the original research. The research findings are utilized by the investigator herself or any other who is interested in utilizing the findings.
- The research proposal can be envisaged as the process (step by step guidelines) to plan and to give structure to the prospective research with the final aim of increasing the validity of the research. It is therefore a written submission to spell out in a logic format the nature of the design and the means and strategies that are going to be used.

EXERCISE

- Write a proposal for a research.
- Write research report for communication.
- Write an article for publication in journal.
- Write an article following APA style.
- Select one quantitative and qualitative study and critique.

Section 2

Biostatistics

11. Introduction to Statistics
12. Presentation of Data
13. Measures of Central Tendency (Averages)
14. Measures of Dispersion
15. Measures of Skewness and Kurtosis
16. Measures of Relationship—Correlation Coefficient
17. Measures of Relationship—Regression Analysis
18. Probability Distribution
19. Estimation of Parameters
20. Hypothesis Testing
21. Research Designs and its Statistical Application
22. Z Distribution
23. t Distribution
24. F Distribution
25. Chi Square Distribution
26. Nonparametric Tests
27. Application of Statistics in Psychology and Education
28. Vital Health Statistics

11 Introduction to Statistics

OBJECTIVES

After reading this chapter, you will be able to:

- Define terms
- List the importance of data analysis
- Explain the steps in processing of data analysis
- Explain the levels of measurement
- Formulate frequency distribution
- Classify methods of data analysis.

INTRODUCTION

The word 'statistics' seems to have been derived from the Latin word 'status' or Italian word 'statista' or the German word 'statistik', each of which means a political state, originally meant information useful to the state, for example, information about the sizes of populations and armed forces. But this word has now acquired different meanings. Almost all fields, like medicine, nursing, education, agriculture, economics, sociology, business management, etc. are now using statistical methods. The word 'statistics' is used in two different senses–Plural and Singular. When used as a plural, statistics means numerical set of data and when used in singular sense, it means the science of statistical methods embodying the theory and techniques used for collecting, analyzing and drawing inferences from the numerical data.

The word 'statistics' can be used to denote (1) data; (2) the science of statistics; and (3) sample measures. A census data is a data about the population statistics. We also heard about the statistics of birth and death, road accidents, statistics of crimes, statistics of enrollment into educational institutions, admission rates and ratio, pass percentage, etc. In all these examples, the word 'statistics' denotes a set of numerical data in the respected fields. The science of statistics includes the principles and methods for the collection, presentation, analysis and interpretation of numerical data of different kinds. Also any calculated value of the samples is also known as 'statistics'. Data are collected either as part of a normal routine or for specific investigation. The raw material of statistics is called 'data'. Depending on the nature of the problem, the data may be related to the individual, family, community or any program. The data collected from these are known as observations. The individual subject or object upon whom the data are collected are known as statistical units. The items or characteristics on which the observations are made, known as 'variables'.

Data may be quantitative or qualitative. A quantitative raw data cannot explain anything and, in order to understand and draw inference, it is subjected to analysis. Raw data are mere numbers with which one cannot interpret anything. A qualitative data is not subjected to statistical analysis since the data is about the variables of qualitative nature, such as emotions, feelings and perceptions of the human beings.

The statistical analysis are of two types. They are ***descriptive*** and ***inferential statistics***. The descriptive statistics are used to describe the data whereas the inferential statistics is used to draw conclusions for the population. Suppose if we want to prove that a specific nursing intervention/ protocol is effective in reducing pain while administering intramuscular injection among children, we test this protocol on a sample of children and test its effectiveness. Based on the measures on the sample, we can draw conclusion for the population. Practically, it is not possible to study the entire subject and prove something is effective. A mother cooks biryani at home. In order to check whether it is cooked well or tastes good, she takes a sample of biryani (a spoon or two) and checks it and makes inference for the whole biryani. It is not needed or meaningless as well as not practically possible to eat the entire biryani and check for the taste. At the same time, before tasting, if it is not mixed well, the mother may end up in wrong conclusion. The sample should be a good representative of a population so that it facilitates drawing of accurate inferences.

DEFINITION OF TERMS

Statistics

'Statistics' is the study of how to collect, organize, analyze and interpret numerical information from the data.

According to Bowley, 'statistics are numerical statements of facts in any department of enquiry placed in relation to each other'.

According to BusinessDictionary.com, 'statistics' is a branch of mathematics concerned with collection, classification, analysis and interpretation of numerical facts for drawing inferences on the basis of their quantifiable likelihood (probability).

Biostatistics

The concept and techniques of statistics are employed in many fields—education, psychology, economics, medicine and nursing, etc. When the concepts of statistics are used in biological sciences, it is termed as 'biostatistics'. It is the branch of statistics that deals with data relating to living organisms. It is the application of statistics to biological and medical data.

It is a branch of biology that studies biological phenomena and observations by means of statistical analysis.

Biostatistics is the application of statistical methods to health sciences. The basic task of biostatistics is to describe the data and to draw inferences for the underlying population.

IMPORTANCE OF STATISTICAL ANALYSIS

Statistical analysis of data is done to:

- Understand about the data
- Give meaning to the data
- Describe about the sample
- Simplify complex nature of data
- Reduce the data
- Measure the variable(s)—association or relationship
- Test hypothesis
- Draw conclusions for the population
- Make predictions or estimate for the future
- Facilitate communication to others
- Make comparisons easier
- Make others also understand in a similar way
- Determine the success or failure of a program
- Plan and promote for policy-making and implementation.

PROCESSING OF DATA FOR ANALYSIS

- ***Data—the basic unit of statistical analysis:*** Research as a scientific enquiry involves lot of observation, which means collection of data. Data collection is the precise, systematic gathering of information relevant to the research purpose or the specific objectives, questions or hypothesis of a study. Data is the basis of any statistical work or calculation. The raw material of statistics is data. In our everyday life, we collect a lot of data. Nurses collect data from patients. During admission of a candidate to BSc (N) program, data is collected about the candidate. Data are collected intentionally or unintentionally. We are now living in information-rich world. The importance of data in this technological world cannot be ignored.
- ***Quantitative data vs Qualitative data:*** Data may be used to arrive at conclusions or generate interpretations. For example, a nurse collects data from a patient to identify his or her problem. A doctor collects information from a patient which will lead to a diagnosis. However, if data are to be treated statistically, or if we want to analyze data, it should be in numerical form. They must be quantitative or measurable. The pulse rate, temperature, respiration, oxygen saturation, etc. are in numerical form. Height expressed in centimeters, weight expressed in kilograms or pounds, knowledge on subject expressed as scores, etc. all are measurements and are quantitative in nature. This kind of data is known as 'quantitative data'.

  Some phenomena or information cannot be translated into numbers. Information on gender cannot be quantified. Data on religion, educational status, occupation, etc. cannot be quantified. This kind of data is known as 'qualitative data'. We collect both quantitative as well as qualitative data in research. In general, we collect and use two kinds of numbers in statistics. One kind of number comes as a result of measurement and the other arises as a result of counting. The example of measurement is temperature, height and weight. Measurement is assignment of numbers to objects or events according to a set of rules. The examples for numbers arising as a result of counting are pulse rate, respiration rate, number of patients admitted, number of students passing the final-year exam, number of male and female children in a class, etc.

- ***Primary data vs secondary data:*** 'Primary data' is the one collected by a particular person or organization for his own use from the primary source. Primary data can be collected by direct personal observation, using questionnaires, using enumerators to collect data and by personal investigation. It is the collection of original data for the first time (Table 11.1).

  'Secondary data' is the data collected by some other person or organization for his/her own use but the investigator also gets it for his own use. Secondary data can be collected from newspapers, periodicals, information obtained from the publications by university, special agencies, etc. and official publications of state, central and the local governments, etc.

Table 11.1: Distinction between primary data and secondary data

S. No.	Primary data	Secondary data
1.	It is collection of original data for the first time	It is a compilation of existing data
2.	It is collected by the researcher or by the trained persons appointed by him	It is compiled by persons other than who collected it
3.	Its collection is relatively more costly	Its collection is relatively less costly
4.	It is collected based on the purpose of investigation	Secondary data may not be related to the purpose of enquiry
5.	It is directly used	It may require some modification before using
6.	There is a chance for subjectivity	There is no possibility of subjectivity since the data is already collected
7.	There may be less error	There is a chance of error since it was not collected by the person other than the present researcher
8.	There is a possibility of verification and rechecking of data	There is less possibility of rechecking
9.	More reliable	There is a chance of less reliablity
10.	The data is time-specific and context-specific	The data may not suit to the present situation.

Variables

Variables are anything which vary from person to person or object to object. When we collect data or make observation, we can find that the values, measurements or characteristics vary from individual to individual. Height, weight, place of residence, intelligence score, etc. are different in individuals.

These are known as 'variables' which is classified as quantitative and qualitative (Fig. 11.1). Variables are quantitative when these are measurable, whereas these are qualitative when we cannot measure them. Quantitative variables are either continuous or discontinuous. Numerical random variables yield numerical responses, such as height and weight. Continuous variables are measured in decimal numbers. Continuous random variables produce numerical responses that arise from a measuring process. Weight is an example of a continuous random variable because the response takes on any value within a continuum or interval, depending on the precision of the measuring instrument. For example, height of 155.5 cm, weight of 50.8 kg, etc. Discontinuous variables are measured in whole numbers, for example, number of patients admitted in a ward, number of births in a hospital on a specific date, etc. Some data can only be categorized. For example, gender—male vs female, religion—hindu, christian, muslim, place of residence-urban vs rural are examples of qualitative variables. Discrete random variables produce numerical responses that arise from a counting process. For example, number of children in a family. Measurements made on quantitative variables give information regarding amount whereas measurement (counting) made on qualitative variables gives information regarding an attribute. Simply having data for large numbers may not make any sense. Statistical methods are used to analyze these data in order to make sense of the data.

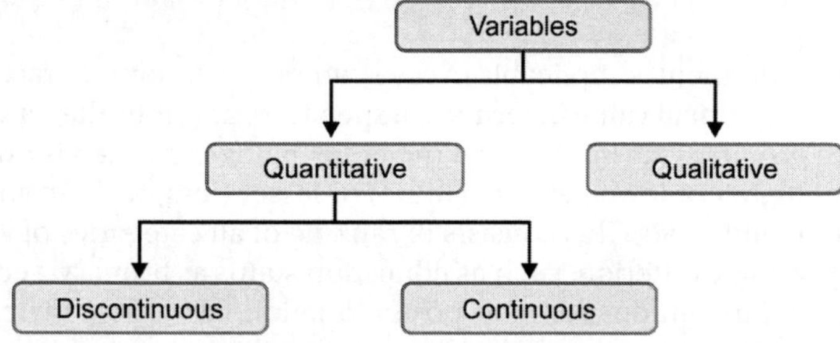

Fig. 11.1: Types of variables

The data, after collection, has to be processed and analyzed in accordance with the outline laid down for the purpose at the time of developing the research plan. This is essential for a scientific study and we can ensure that we have all relevant data for making comparisons and analysis. Processing of data implies editing, coding, classification and tabulation of collected data so that they are amenable to analysis. The term 'analysis' refers to the computation of certain measures along with searching for patterns of relationship that exist among data-groups. The data are measured at four levels. Understanding of these levels of measurement helps us to process the data for analysis.

LEVELS OF MEASUREMENT

We collect data in research. The data we collect will belong to any one category of the level or scales of measurement. The types or levels of measurement were originally developed by the psychologist Stanley Smith Stevens. He claimed that all measurements in science were conducted using four different types of scales that he called 'nominal', 'ordinal', 'interval' and 'ratio'.

Nominal

In this, the observations are placed in a broad category which may be denoted by a symbol or label or name. For example, observations based on gender, male or female; or place of residents, urban or rural; or based on religion, hindu, christian, muslim, etc. The data may be dichotomous or non-dichotomous. Nominal measurement includes the awarding of a numeral value to a specific characteristic. This type of measurement is the most basic form of measurement. In this measurement, a male can be assigned '1' and a female can be assigned '2'. Urban can be assigned '1' and rural can be assigned '2'. The numerical value '1' does not mean half of '2'. It merely indicates a difference. This scale of measurement is used mainly for the compiling of frequency tables.

With a nominal scale, each score does not actually indicate an amount; rather it is used simply for identification, as a name. In research, a nominal scale is used to identify the categories of a qualitative or classification variable. Numbers assigned to a variable in a nominal scale do not have the mathematical properties normally associated with the numbers.

Ordinal

Ordinal measurement is applicable in cases where a criterion/characteristic is awarded to numerical value in terms of a specific order (thus the name of the scale). The ordinal scale implies that the entity being measured is quantified in terms of higher or lower, greater (more) or lesser (less) without specifying the size of the intervals. This consists of ranking of all categories of variables according to some criterion, such as education status as primary, secondary, higher secondary, graduation and postgraduation, also categorizing based on the socioeconomic status. In this measurement, each category is in a unique position in relation to other categories but the distance between these categories is not known.

When a variable is measured using ordinal scale, the scores indicate rank order. The score of '1' means the most or least of the variable, '2' means the second most or least and so on. Each score indicates an amount of sorts, but it is a relative amount.

Interval

The interval scale of measurement is characterized by two features, namely equal units of measurement (equal intervals), and a zero point which has been established arbitrarily (Leedy 1993). The latter indicates that there is not an absolute zero point. For example, an individual's intelligence score is 110 whilst that of another is 100. The difference between these scores is exactly 10. It should also be remembered that intelligence measurement has no zero point. A second example of interval measurement is the Likert attitude scale.

When a variable is measured using an interval scale, each score indicates an actual amount, and there is an equal unit of measurement separating any two scores: The difference between 2 and 3 is the same as the difference between 3 and 4.

Ratio

This is considered the highest order of measurement that exists, because of the fixed proportions (ratio) between the number (numerical) and the amount of the characteristic that it represents. There is a fixed (absolute) zero point. Ratio level of measurement thus enables researchers to determine whether aspects possess something of a characteristic or not. The following can serve as an example of ratio level of measurement—the average weight of an adolescent girl is 45 kilograms. On the other hand, the average weight of an adolescent boy is 50 kilograms. Kilograms are expressed in constant units, and a zero point does exist, because 'no weight' can be determined. Because scores on this type of measuring scale possess absolute values, any type of arithmetical calculations is allowed.

Only with a ratio scale do the scores reflect the true amount of a variable that present, because the scores measure an actual amount. There is an equal unit of measurement and '0' truly means that zero amount of the variable is present. Therefore, ratio scales do not allow negative numbers.

A continuous scale allows for fractional amounts. It continues between the whole-number amounts. With a continuous scale, decimals make sense. Age is a continuous variable. On the other hand, a discrete scale can be measured only in whole number amounts. Here, decimals do not make sense. Usually, nominal and ordinal variables are discrete. In addition, some interval and ratio variables are discrete. For example, the number of children someone has is a discrete ratio variable. There is a type of discrete variable. When there can be only two amounts or categories of the variable, it is a dichotomous variable—pass/fail, male/female and married/unmarried are examples of dichotomous variable.

EDITING

Editing of data is a process of examining the collected raw data (specially in surveys) to detect errors and omissions and to correct these when possible. Editing involves a careful scrutiny of the completed questionnaires and/or schedules. The possible errors while collecting data are wrong entry of data, missing data and collection of unrelated data. These errors are committed when the investigator depends on his memory for entering data after data collection. It is always good to proceed data collection in a systematic and organized way so as to ensure for complete data collection. Data should be entered in the tool as soon as it is collected and one question must be completed before proceeding to the next question in case if the interview schedule is used. In case of questionnaire, there is a possibility that the samples may omit few questions without answering and, if possible, the investigator has to collect it immediately after it is received from the samples. Editing is done to assure that the data are accurate, consistent with other facts gathered, uniformly entered, as completed as possible and have been well arranged to facilitate coding and tabulation.

The data may be collected by the investigator herself or by an appointed person in case if it is a large-scale study. Field editing consists in the review of the reporting forms by the principal investigator for completing (translating or rewriting) what the later has written in abbreviated and/or in illegible form at the time of recording the respondents' responses. This type of editing is necessary in view of the fact that individual writing styles often can be difficult for others to decipher. This sort of editing should be done as soon as possible after the interview, preferably on the very day or on the next day. While doing field editing, the investigator must restrain himself and must not correct errors of omission by simply guessing what the informant would have said if the question had been asked.

In a large-scale study, where many research assistants are employed to collect data, central editing is mandatory. It should take place when all forms or schedules have been completed and returned to the office. This type of editing implies that all forms should get a thorough editing by a single editor in a small study and by a team of editors in case of a large inquiry. Editor(s) may correct the obvious errors, such as an entry in the wrong place, entry recorded in months when it should have been recorded in weeks, and the like. In case of inappropriate or missing replies, the editor can sometimes determine the proper answer by reviewing the other information in the schedule. At times, the respondent can be contacted for clarification. All the wrong replies, which are quite obvious, must be dropped from the final results, especially in the context of mail surveys.

Editors should be familiar with instructions given to the interviewers and coders as well as with the editing instructions supplied to them for the purpose. Once editing is over, the forms can be numbered and arranged in bundles so as to make entry easy and, if necessary, the same can be retrieved for further clarification in future.

CODING

Coding refers to the process of assigning numerals or other symbols to answers so that responses can be put into a limited number of categories or classes. Such classes should be appropriate to the research problem under consideration. They must also possess the characteristic of exhaustiveness (i.e. there must be a class for every data item) and also that of mutual exclusiveness which means that a specific answer can be placed in one and only one cell in a given category set. Another rule to be observed is that of unidimensionality which is meant that every class is defined in terms of only one concept. For example, assigning '1' for male gender and '2' for female gender is an example of coding gender information. In 'yes' or 'no' question, assigning '1' for the 'yes' response and '0' for the 'no' response is also coding. While coding, we should remember that there should be only one code number for information on single variable. Code no. 1 for a female should be used consistently.

Coding is necessary for efficient analysis and through it several replies may be reduced to a small number of classes which contain the critical information required for analysis. By coding, the data can be subjected to statistical analysis, especially when it is done by the computers. Coding decisions should usually be taken at the designing stage of the questionnaire.

TRANSFORMATION

A transformation is a mathematical procedure for systematically converting a set of scores into a different set of scores. One reason to transform data is to make different kinds of scores comparable. However, by transforming each score to a percent of total, we are no longer comparing apples to oranges. Second, we transform data because it makes scores easier to work with. For example, if the scores each contain on one decimal place, multiplying every score by 10 eliminates the decimals.

CLASSIFICATION

Classification is the process of arranging the available data into various homogenous classes and sub-classes according to some common characteristic or attribute or objective of investigation. According to Secrist, 'Classification is the process of arranging data into sequences and groups according to their common characteristics or separating them into different but related parts.'

Most research studies result in a large volume of raw data which must be reduced into homogenous groups if we are to get meaningful relationships. This fact necessitates classification of data which happens to be the process of arranging data in groups or classes on the basis of common characteristics. Data having a common characteristic are placed in one class and, in this way the entire data get divided into a number of groups or classes. Classification is the process of arranging things in the groups according to their resemblances, similarity, or identity.

Need for Classification of Data

- To reduce large volume of data
- To facilitate presentation of data
- To compare data
- To identify the relationship between the data
- To facilitate statistical analysis

- To communicate findings
- To facilitate easy interpretation
- To eliminate unnecessary details.

Types of Classification

The four types of classification are:

1. ***Chronological or temporal classification:*** It requires the arrangement of data according to the order of time expressed in years, months, weeks, etc. The data are generally classified in ascending order of time.

Example 1:

The estimates of pass percentage of 1 year BSc Nursing students in an organization during 2001–2010 are:

Year:	2001	2002	2003	2004	2005	2006	2007	2008	2009	2010
Pass percentage:	88.4	92	96.2	80.8	88.2	88	90.1	78.7	76.6	78.3

2. ***Geographical or spatial classification:*** It requires the data to be classified according to geographical region or place.

Example 2:

Number of deaths due to diarrhea in under-five children per year in different states in India.

1. When names of the countries are in alphabetical order:

States:	Andhra	Assam	Bihar	Gujarat	Haryana	Kerala	Manipur	Nagaland
Deaths:	120	100	90	68	40	20	60	70

2. When the observations are in descending order:

States:	Andhra	Assam	Bihar	Nagaland	Gujarat	Manipur	Haryana	Kerala
Deaths:	120	100	90	70	68	60	40	20

3. ***Qualitative classification:*** In this type of classification, data are classified on the basis of some attributes or qualities, like sex, literacy , religion, employment, etc.
   Types:
   - ***Simple or dichotomous classification:*** The data are classified with respect to one attribute, which is dichotomous in nature. For example, number of patients attended outpatient department of a hospital—male and female.
   - ***Manifold classification:*** In which the data are classified based on two or more attributes and several classes are formed.
4. ***Quantitative classification:*** In quantitative classification, the collected data are grouped with reference to the characteristics, which can be measured and numerically described, such as height, weight, sales, age, income, etc. Qualitative and quantitative classification are explained in detail.

TABULATION

Tabulation or classification is the process by which data of long series of observation are systematically organized and recorded so as to enable analysis and interpretation. In order to classify data, a set of categories are formed. The essential requirement of any such categories is that these categories should be selected in such a way that each one of the observations falls into one and only one of these categories and all that observation falls into any one of these categories. The lowest value of the observation falls into the first category and the highest value of the observation falls into the last category. The interval or width of the category must be same for all categories. Minimum of five categories are ideal. Tabulation is discussed in detail in the second chapter.

STATISTICAL SERIES

Statistical series are prepared to present the collected data in a properly arranged way. A series of data are some measurements arranged in a logical order. One way of arranging data is arranging them in an ascending or descending order of its magnitude. It is called an 'array'. But it does not reduce the volume of data.

Classification can be one of the following two types, depending upon the nature of the phenomenon involved:

1. ***Classification according to characteristics or attributes:*** Data are classified on the basis of common characteristics which can either be descriptive (such as gender, education status, occupation, religion, etc.) or numerical (such as weight, height, income, etc.) Descriptive characteristics refer to qualitative phenomenon which cannot be measured quantitatively; only their presence or absence in an individual item can be noticed. Data obtained this way on the basis of certain attributes are known as statistics of attributes.
2. ***Classification according to class-intervals:*** Unlike descriptive characteristics, the numerical characteristics refer to quantitative phenomenon which can be measured through some statistical units. Data relating to age, income, weight, height, hemoglobin level, etc. fall under this category. Such data are known as statistics of variables and are classified on the basis of class intervals.
   - ***Classes:*** Classes are the range which has specific lower and upper values. For example, 10–20, 20–30, 30–40 are the example of classes.
   - ***Class limits:*** The class limits are the smallest or the lowest and the largest or the highest values in the class. For example, in the class of 10–20, the lowest value is 10 and the highest value is 20. The two boundaries of the class are known as the lower limit and upper limit of the class. Class limit is also known as 'class boundaries'.
   - ***Class interval:*** Each group of class-interval, thus, has an upper limit as well as a lower limit which are known as class limits. The difference between the two class limits is known as class interval or class

magnitude. For example, in a class of 10–20, the class interval or class magnitude is (20 – 10 = 10) 10. We may have classes with equal class magnitudes or with unequal class magnitudes.

- ***Frequency:*** The number of items which fall in a given class is known as the 'frequency of the given class.'
- ***Frequency distribution:*** All the classes or groups, with their respective frequencies taken together and put in the form of a table, are described as group frequency distribution or simply frequency distribution.

  Erricker states frequency distribution is 'a classification according to the number possessing the same values of the variables'. It is simply a table in which the data are grouped into classes and the number of cases which fall in each class is recorded.

  One can formulate frequency distribution with class intervals and without class intervals. The frequency distribution can be formulated without class interval as follows:

Frequency distribution of children admitted in pediatric medical ward

Diagnosis	Tally marks	Frequency
Fever	~~IIII~~ ~~IIII~~ I	11
Common cold	~~IIII~~ ~~IIII~~ IIII	14
Acute diarrhea	~~IIII~~ ~~IIII~~ III	13
Urinary tract infection	II	02
Bronchopneumonia	~~IIII~~	05
Anemia	II	02
Typhoid	III	03
	Total	50

In setting up a frequency distribution with class intervals, one must first decide how many intervals to use and how wide the intervals will be. If the class intervals are fewer and wider, there would be information loss. At the same time, if the intervals are narrow and more, it would not convey the proper information and is less comprehensible. In addition, the number of intervals 'n' should be small enough so that the average interval frequency (N/n) is greater than 5. The researcher needs skill and experience in deciding the number of class intervals. It is ideal to have 5–15 classes. It is good to have equal width to the extent possible, but, in some cases, unequal width or magnitudes may result in better classification. Hence, the researcher's objective judgment plays an important role in this connection. Multiples of 2, 5 and 10 are generally preferred while determining class magnitudes.

Some statisticians adopt the following formula, suggested by HA Sturges, in determining the number and width of class interval:

- ***Formula to calculate the number of classes:***

$K = 1 + 3.32 * \log N$
K = No. of classes
N = No. of observations
For example, if the total number of observations is 100, number of classes would be:
$K = 1 + 3.32 * \log 100$
$K = 1 + 3.32 * 2$
$K = 1 + 6.64 = 7.64 = 8$ (fractions are always rounded up).
For example, if the total number of observations is 1,000, number of classes would be:
$K = 1 + 3.32 * \log 1000$
$K = 1 + 3.32 * 3$
$K = 1 + 9.96 = 10.96 = 11$ (fractions are always rounded up).

- ***Formula to calculate the magnitude of class interval:***

$W = R/K$ or
$W = R/(1 + 3.3 \log N)$
W = Width of the class interval
R = Range
K = No. of class intervals.
Range can be calculated by computing the difference between the largest value and smallest value among the given observations. $R = L - S$
For example, if the marks of 10 students are varied between 30 and 80 and if we want to form 5 classes, the class interval would be:

$$L = 80; S = 30; K = 5$$

$$W = \frac{80 - 30}{5} = \frac{50}{5} = 10$$

Therefore, 5 classes can be formulated with the class-interval of 10 as follows: 30–40, 40–50, 50–60, 60–70 and 70–80.

It should also be kept in mind that in case one or two or very few items have very high or very low values, one may use what are known as open-ended intervals in the overall frequency distribution. Such interval may be expressed like under ₹ 1,000 or ₹ 1,0001 and over. Such intervals are generally not desirable, but often cannot be avoided.

While choosing class-limits, the researcher must take into consideration the criterion that the mid-point (calculated by adding the value of upper limit and lower limit of a class and then dividing this sum by 2) of a class-interval and the actual average of items of that class-interval should remain as close to each other as possible. Consistent with this, the class-limits should be located at multiples of 2, 5, 10, 20, 100 and such other figures. Class-limits may generally be stated in any of the following forms:

- ***Exclusive type class intervals (overlapping):*** In this method, the upper limit of one class-interval is the lower limit of the next class-interval. They are usually stated as follows:
  10–20
  20–30
  30–40
  40–50
  The above intervals should be read as under:
  10 and under 20
  20 and under 30
  30 and under 40
  40 and under 50.
  Thus, under the exclusive type class-intervals, the items whose values are equal to the upper limit of a class are grouped in the next higher class. For example, an item whose value is exactly 30 would be put in 30–40 class interval and not in 20–30 class interval. In simple words, we can say that under exclusive type class-intervals, the upper limit of a class-interval is excluded and items with values less than the upper limit (but not less than the lower limit) are put in the given class-interval. It ensures continuity of data. A student whose marks are between 30 and 39.9 would be included in 30–40 class whereas these with 40–49.9 would be included in a class of 40–50.
- ***Inclusive type class intervals:*** They are usually stated as follows:
  11 - 20
  21 - 30
  31 - 40
  41 - 50
  In inclusive type class-intervals, the upper limit of a class-interval is also included in the concerned class-interval. Thus, an item whose value is 20 will be put in 11–20 class-interval. The stated upper limit of the class-interval, 11–20 is 20 but the real limit is 20.99999 and, as such, 11–20 class-interval really means 11 under 21.
  When the phenomenon under consideration happens to be a discrete one (i.e. can be measured and stated only in integers), we adopt inclusive type classification. But when the phenomenon happens to be a continuous one capable of being measured in fractions as well, we can use exclusive type class intervals.
- ***How to determine the frequency of each class?***
  This can be done either by tally sheets or by mechanical aids. Under the technique of tally sheet, the class-groups are written on a sheet of paper (commonly known as the 'tally sheet') and for each item, a stroke (usually a small vertical line) is marked against the class-group in which it falls. The general practice is that after every four small vertical lines in a class-group, the fifth line for the item falling in the same group is indicated as horizontal line through the said four lines and the resulting flower (||||) represents five items.

Example 3:

The scores on aggression inventory for 100 adolescent children who played violent video games were given below. Develop a frequency distribution table.

27.0	78.0	84.0	53.0	76.0	71.0	56.0	56.0	71.0	75.0	36.0	31.0	73.0
88.0	80.0	89.0	77.0	60.0	77.0	67.0	26.0	50.0	82.0	40.0	62.0	26.0
71.0	66.0	60.0	60.0	89.0	67.0	71.0	73.0	35.0	44.0	28.0	50.0	35.0
75.0	51.0	73.0	48.0	51.0	46.0	62.0	33.0	40.0	31.0	24.0	69.0	45.0
76.0	84.0	44.0	26.0	33.0	44.0	82.0	62.0	51.0	38.0	52.0	49.0	49.0
54.0	27.0	49.0	56.0	56.0	27.0	53.0	38.0	65.0	34.0	54.0	25.0	29.0
33.0	54.0	47.0	53.0	53.0	51.0	34.0	54.0	63.0	67.0	60.0	27.0	62.0
51.0	69.0	56.0	68.0	78.0	81.0	56.0	67.0	78.0				

Formula to calculate the number of classes:

K = 1 + 3.32*log N
K = No. of class-intervals
N = No. of observations
K = 1 + 3.328 log 100
K = 1 + 3.32*2 (log 100 = 2)
K = 1 + 6.64
K = 7.64 = 8
Range = Largest number – Smallest number
Formula to calculate the width/magnitude of class-interval:
W = R/K or
W = R/(1 + 3.3 log N)
W = Width of the class-interval
R = Range
K = No. of class-intervals.

Range can be calculated by computing the difference between the largest value and smallest value among the given observations.

Range = 89 – 24 = 65
Width = 65/7.64 = 8.5

Class-interval	Tally marks	Frequency
21–30	~~||||~~ ~~||||~~ |	11
31–40	~~||||~~ ~~||||~~ ||||	14
41–50	~~||||~~ ~~||||~~ ||	12
51–60	~~||||~~ ~~||||~~ ~~||||~~ ~~||||~~ ||||	24
61–70	~~||||~~ ~~||||~~ ||||	14
71–80	~~||||~~ ~~||||~~ ~~||||~~ ||	17
81–90	~~||||~~ |||	8

Class-interval	Frequency
21–30	11
31–40	14
41–50	12
51–60	24
61–70	14
71–80	17
81–90	8

Example 4:

The pulse rate for 100 adolescent children who played violent video games are given as follows. Develop a frequency distribution table.

77	72	68	86	82	88	78	68	78	70	90	76	75
80	70	72	88	88	88	88	76	88	78	88	74	66
74	110	85	81	90	88	82	96	86	84	72	74	82
80	68	88	84	72	82	78	78	82	70	80	82	86
76	76	80	86	90	98	86	90	98	86	80	90	86
76	82	90	88	96	81	76	80	80	80	84	70	72
108	76	78	80	82	82	80	74	104	78	76	86	86
90	84	82	78	80	82	82	76	78				

Formula to calculate the number of class interval (K):
$K = 1 + 3.32 \times \log N$
K = No. of class-intervals
N = No. of observations
$K = 1 + 3.328 \log 100$
$K = 1 + 3.32*2$ ($\log 100 = 2$)
$K = 1 + 6.64$
$K = 7.64$
Range = Largest number – Smallest number
Formula to calculate the width/magnitude of class-interval:
$W = R/K$ or
$W = R/(1 + 3.3 \log N)$
W = Width of the class-intervals
R = Range
K = No. of class-intervals

Range can be calculated by computing the difference between the largest value and smallest value among the given observations.

Range = 110 – 66 = 44
Width = 44/7.64 = 5.8

Class-interval	Tally marks	Frequency
65–71	~~IIII~~ III	08
72–78	~~IIII~~ ~~IIII~~ ~~IIII~~ ~~IIII~~ ~~IIII~~ III	28
79–85	~~IIII~~ ~~IIII~~ ~~IIII~~ ~~IIII~~ ~~IIII~~ ~~IIII~~ IIII	34
86–92	~~IIII~~ ~~IIII~~ ~~IIII~~ ~~IIII~~ III	23
93–99	IIII	04
100–106	I	01
107–113	II	02

Class-interval	Frequency
65–71	08
72–78	28
79–85	34
86–92	23
93–99	04
100–106	01
107–113	02

To Recapitulate

A frequency distribution is a tool for organizing data. We use it to group data into categories and show the number of observations in each category. Some guidelines for constructing a frequency distribution are as follows:

- Each value should fit into a category. The classes should be mutually exhaustive.
- No value should fit into more than one category. The classes should be mutually exclusive; there should be no overlapping of classes.
- If possible, make the classes of equal size. This makes it easier to compare the frequency in one class to another.
- Open-ended classes such as '75 and over' can be avoided if possible.
- Too less and too many number of classes should be avoided. Preferably, 5–15 classes are ideal. If the number of classes are less than 5, it indicates that the data are not organized, whereas if the number of classes are more than 20, this may probably be an information overflow.
- It is usually convenient to use class sizes of 5 or 10; in other words, to have each class containing 5 or 10 possible values.
- It is usually convenient to make the lower limit of the first category a multiple of the class size.

The first two rules are mandatory. The rest of the rules are merely suggestions. Sometimes, it may be required to violate some of these suggestions but, as far as possible, all these rules can be followed.

Example 5:

The weight of 50 adolescent children are given below. Develop a frequency distribution table.

52.0	44.0	38.0	57.0	65.0	52.0	44.0	46.0	47.0	35.0	45.0	55.0	45.0
50.0	48.0	65.0	50.0	75.0	36.0	32.0	51.0	34.0	51.0	59.0	64.0	38.0
70.0	62.0	68.0	58.0	74.0	70.0	42.0	65.0	35.0	32.0	57.0	35.0	46.0
37.0	45.0	66.0	68.0	32.0	68.0	55.0	40.0	54.0	40.0	37.0		

Log 50 = 1.7
Formula to calculate the number of class-intervals:
K = 1 + 3.32 × log N
K = No. of class-intervals

N = No. of observations
K = 1 + 3.328 log 50
K = 1 + 3.32*1.7
K= 1 + 5.64
K = 6.64
Range = Largest number – Smallest number
Formulá to calculate the width/magnitude of class-intervals:
W = R/K or
W = R/(1 + 3.3 log N)
W = Width of the class-intervals
R = Range
K = No. of class-intervals

Range can be calculated by computing the difference between the largest value and smallest value among the given observations.

Range = 75 – 32 = 43
Width = 43/6.64 = 6.5 can be rounded off as 10.

Class-interval	Tally marks	Frequency
31–40	~~IIII~~ ~~IIII~~ IIII	14
41–50	~~IIII~~ ~~IIII~~ II	12
51–60	~~IIII~~ ~~IIII~~ I	11
61–70	~~IIII~~ ~~IIII~~ I	11
71–80	II	02

Class-interval	Frequency
31–40	14
41–50	12
51–60	11
61–70	11
71–80	02

CLASSIFICATION OF METHODS OF ANALYSIS

If someone asks you to describe about your classmates, think of the possible answers you would give. You may tell them about the number of classmates and how many of them are male and female; also you may tell them how many of them are hostellers and day scholars. You may tell them based on certain characteristics, such as their performance, speciality chosen, etc. and you may also express what is the average weight, height, marks of the students, etc. It is also interesting and easy to name the tallest and shortest; overweight and thin; a good performer and a poor performer in the class. One can be compared with the good performer too. It is also very difficult to tell all the characteristics of each and every individual if a group size is big, which may not be necessary and may also be time-consuming.
From the above example, it is inferred that the total number of classmates is the sample size (N); gender, place of residence, speciality chosen, height and weight are the variables which vary from one student to other student. The average height and weight is the good measure of the group (classmates) and at the same time the extreme values (tallest vs shortest; good performer vs poor performer) is also a measure. The difference between the first and the later though both are measures first one takes the account of all students whereas the later takes the account of extreme cases. All these are few examples of descriptive statistics.

Data can be analyzed using descriptive and inferential statistical methods. There are various methods of descriptive statistics which are used for different purposes. Inferential statistics are used to estimate population parameters and hypothesis testing. Refer to Fig. 11.2 for classification of data analysis.

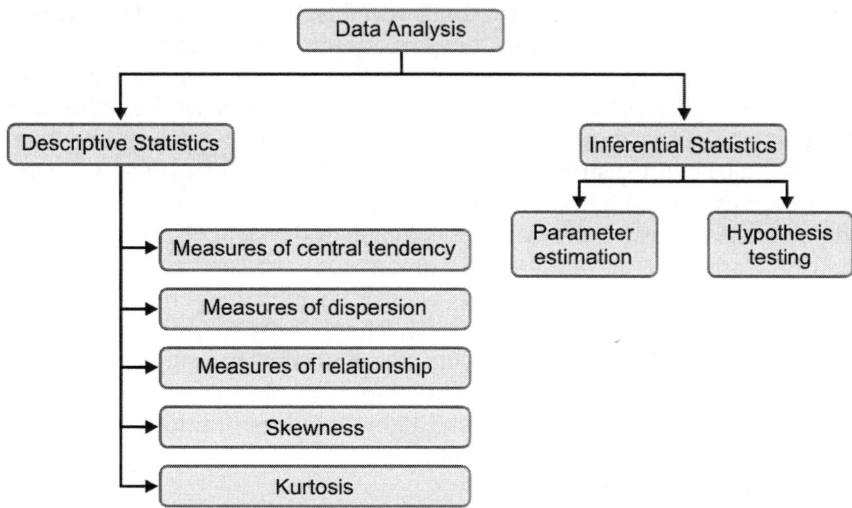

Fig. 11.2: Classification of data analysis

Descriptive Statistics

Smit (1983) sees descriptive statistics as the formulation of rules and procedures, according to which data can be placed in useful and significant order. Landman (1988) states that descriptive statistics deals with the central tendency, variability (variation) and relationships (correlations) in data that are readily available at hand.

All statistical tests or measures which are used to describe the data are known as descriptive statistics. These descriptive statistics are used to analyze single variables (univariate analysis), two variables (bivariate analysis) and more than two variables (multivariate analysis). Refer to Fig. 11.3 for classification of descriptive analysis.

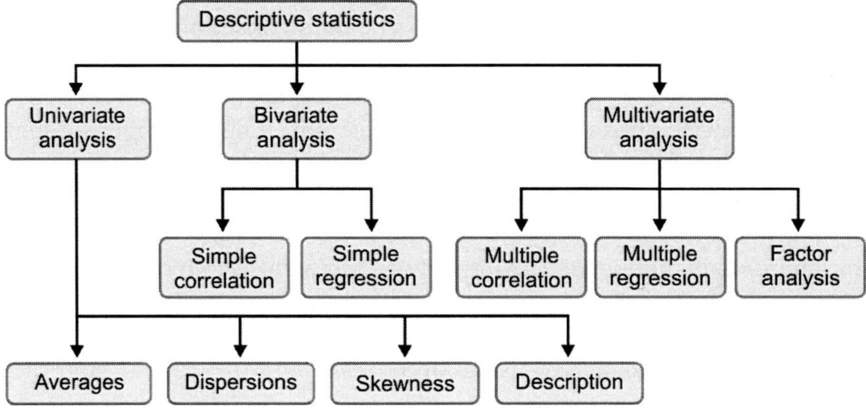

Fig. 11.3: Classification of descriptive statistics

Univariate Analysis

In many situations, we measure a single variable. For example, if we measure Hb level of 100 adolescent girls, they are often presented either in the form of frequency table or in series. Every distribution of a variable has certain characteristics. These characteristics account for differences in distributions. If we take height as a variable of a sample size of 100 adolescent boys in a school, this height distribution has certain characteristics. For the same samples, if we take weight as a variable, the weight distribution has got certain characteristics. These characteristics of height and weight distribution can be measured and in terms of these measures, data is analyzed and interpreted.

The long series of any data are reduced by forming frequency distribution. The next step is the calculation of certain characteristics which may be used to describe the characteristic of that distribution. The values will enable comparisons to be made between one series of observation and another. There are four major characteristics of a frequency distribution. These are:

1. The Measures of Central Tendency
2. The Measures of Dispersion
3. The extent of symmetry in the shape of the distribution
4. The flatness or peakedness of the distribution.

Bivariate Analysis

There are circumstances where we want to measure two variables and the kind of relationship between these two. For example, we may be interested to know the relationship between the childrens' intelligence and their academic performance. Naturally, there are some relationships existing between two variables. In general, there is a positive relationship between body temperature and pulse rate. As the body temperature increases, the pulse rate of a person increases. There is a negative relationship between the age and the pulse rate. As age increases, the pulse rate of a person decreases. The study of two variables is known as bivariate analysis in which we can study the correlation and the regression. Correlation deals with the relationship between the variables, whereas regression analysis deals with the effect of one variable on the other.

Multivariate Analysis

If we want to study about the relationship between more than two variables, the multiple correlation technique is of good use, whereas the effect of more than two independent variables on the dependent variable is analyzed through the multiple regression analysis. Factor analysis is also a technique where we can study about more than two variables.

Inferential Statistics

The purpose of any research is to benefit humanity. Though research is conducted for various purposes, like description, identification, explanation, exploration, prediction and control, ultimately the findings are utilized for the welfare of human beings. Apart from descriptive statistics that deal with central tendencies and measures of variation, there are statistical methods which enable researchers to go from the known to the unknown data. From the research findings, one can draw inference for the population. Practically, we cannot conduct research on population and it is not feasible too. So, we take samples who are representative of the population for the study. The statistics we calculate from the samples are utilized to draw inference for the population. This is to say to make deductions or statements regarding the broad population as the samples from which the 'known' data are drawn. These methods, according to literature, are called 'inferential' or 'inductive statistics.'

Statistical inference may be of two types: parameter estimation and hypothesis testing. Refer to figure 11.4 for classification of inferential statistics. In parameter estimation, we use some formula in which we substitute the observations of the sample in order to obtain a numerical estimate of the population parameters. In hypothesis testing, we formulate assumption or hypothesis about the population. In order to test the hypothesis, data are collected from the samples and statistics are computed to accept or reject hypothesis. Hypothesis testing is concerned with passing a judgment on some assumption which we make (on the basis of some theory or information) about the true value of a population parameter. Both types of statistical inferences utilize the information of a sample for drawing some conclusions about the population. In parameter estimation, we use some formula in which we substitute the observations of the sample in order to obtain a numerical estimate of the population parameters. In hypothesis testing, we begin with some assumption about the true value of the population parameter and then we use the information of the sample to compute a certain test statistic with which we will decide whether to accept or reject the assumption (hypothesis), which we made about the true population parameter.

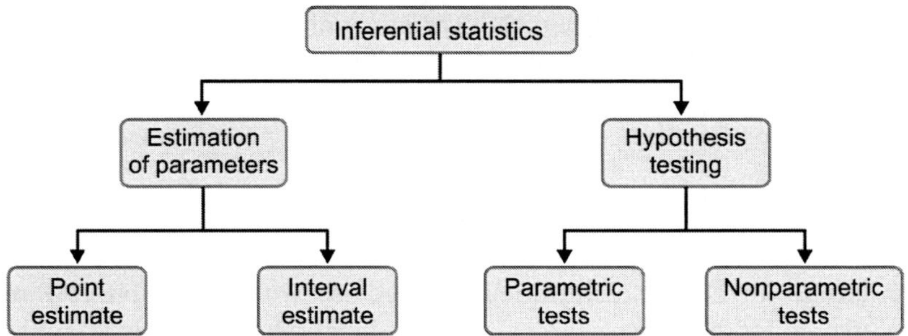

Fig. 11.4: Classification of inferential statistics

USES OF COMPUTERS IN RESEARCH AND STATISTICS

Computers are a modern-world tool, which is one of the important gadgets in everyone's life. Computer, because of its speed, accuracy, memory, storage and retrieval, becomes one of the important elements in all fields and disciplines. Computers are the wonderful tool of mankind. The uses of computer in day-to-day life as well as in the field of medicine, engineering, education, research and others are many. The uses of computers in research and statistics are as follows:

Uses of a Computer in Research

- ***Review of literature:*** There are a variety of databases which provide lots of research articles. One can have access to abstracts as well as full-text articles. Simultaneously, you can review literature from more than one database. Within seconds, the computer can list down the number of articles on a particular topic. The advanced search option in the PubMed helps us search better. The filter option in the databases helps us to focus on the selected topics. Computer helps to prepare the report after the review. The information can be downloaded faster and modified easily. It is easy to perform corrections in the report of literature review without discarding the previous one.
- ***Getting background information:*** Books and journals can give only limited information and are time-oriented. The updated data can be obtained from various websites managed by the government as well as

private organizations. The computer and the specific websites can give data on any topic. The local, national and international data can be obtained within a minute for comparison. The trend and the differences in the problem can be assessed based on the data. Comparison of data on a specific topic is possible. Context-specific, cultural-specific and time-oriented data can be accessed.

- ***Preparation of report:*** Computer helps in preparation of research report. Corrections can be made very easily. The document can be communicated easily. At any point of time, at any part of the world, one can retrieve the information as well as data. Referencing is very easy. There are options like inserting footnotes, inserting citations and adopting particular style of preparing the research article and references. These are built in bibliography in software which makes the researcher's work easy. Reports can be mailed to many people for easy reach and access.
- ***Preparation of research proposal:*** Like preparation of research report, a proposal can also be prepared and submitted to many reviewers simultaneously. Mailing reduces the cost and time of delivery. It saves time and energy of the researcher.
- ***Presentation of report:*** Computer helps in oral presentation of research report as well as proposal presentation. Powerpoint presentation enhances the delivery of the content. It makes presentation more attractive; tables and figures help to promote understanding and comparison of data. Posters can be designed using computers.
- ***Development of conceptual framework:*** Conceptual framework can be designed and developed using computers. There are built-in options and one can modify using shapes and diagrams.
- ***Communication/dissemination:*** It facilitates easy communication, retrieval of data, and dissemination of data. It is time-saving since delay in other modes of delivery can be avoided. Sharing of information is easy through computers. You can share information with anybody in any part of the world.
- ***Tool preparation:*** Computers helps in preparation of tools. Questionnaires, rating scales, observation checklists, etc. can be prepared very easily. It facilitates us to prepare a simple as well as complex tool for data collection.
- ***Preparation of tables and diagrams:*** Software available in computer helps in drawing various diagrams and tables. Within no minute, if data are given, the required diagram can be developed. One can easily change the color, background and do editing of the diagram. Simple as well as complex tables can be prepared very easily.
- ***Editing:*** Computer makes the work of editing easy. It is a paperless work. Any number of times, the information can be corrected, modified and improved.
- ***Storage and retrieval:*** Large volume of data and information can be stored and retrieved immediately. It is also easy to organize and store the data, which makes retrieval easy.

Uses of Computer in Statistics

- ***Data management:*** Computers are useful in effective data management. Large volume of data are collected during any research. Especially in longitudinal study and census enumeration, large volume of data are collected and handled. It is easy to handle any portion of data for part analysis.
- ***Analysis of data:*** Computers help in the task of data analysis. There are softwares available in the computers, such as Excel which facilitate us to perform descriptive and inferential statistics.

  Besides this, there are special software packages available to perform simple as well as advanced statistics. Statistical packages are statistical softwares, which are specialized computer programs for statistical analysis. There are free as well as paid statistical softwares. Examples of some of the statistical packages are as follows:

Epi Info

Epi Info is a public domain statistical software developed by Centers for Disease Control and Prevention (CDC) in Atlanta, Georgia(USA). Epi Info has been in existence for over 20 years and is currently available for Microsoft windows. The software is in the public domain, free, and can be downloaded from http://www.cdc.gov/epiinfo.

Utilities of Epi Info

The program allows for:
- Development of a questionnaire and customization of the data entry process.
- Quick entry of data into that questionnaire, and then analyzing of the data.
- Electronic survey creation, data entry and analysis.
- Analysis of data using t-tests, ANOVA, nonparametric statistics.
- Cross-tabulations and stratification with estimates of odds ratios, risk ratios and risk differences.
- Performance of logistic regression, survival analysis, and analysis of complex survey data.
- Saving considerable amounts of time versus using paper surveys.

Modules in Epi Info

- ***Designer modules:*** Electronic questionnaires are created in the designer module.
- ***Classic analysis:*** It is used to analyze the data. Many advanced statistical routines are provided, such as t-tests, ANOVA, nonparametric statistics, cross-tabulations and stratification with estimates of odds ratios, risk ratios and risk differences, logistic regression (conditional and unconditional), survival analysis (Kaplan Meier and Cox proportional hazard) and analysis of complex survey data.

- ***Map module:*** With the help of map module, data can be displayed either by geographic reference or by GPS coordinates.
- ***Report module:*** This allows the user to edit and format output from various Epi Info tools and modules. The resulting HTML document can then be printed or emailed to others.
- ***Menu module:*** It allows for the editing and re-arranging of the basic Epi Info menu structure.

Open Epi is a free, web-based, open source, operating system-independent series of programs for use in epidemiology, biostatistics, public health and medicine, providing a number of epidemiologic and statistical tools for summary data. It helps in hypothesis testing and analysis of data using various parametric tests and epidemiological investigation including randomized controlled trials. Because Open Epi is easy to use, requires no programming experience, and can be run on the internet, students can use the program and focus on the interpretation of results.

CSPro, short for the ***Census and Survey Processing System,*** is a public domain statistical package developed by the US Census Bureau and ICF International. The software can be used for entering, editing, tabulating, mapping, and disseminating census and survey data. This package is widely used by statistical agencies in developing countries. As of version 5, Unicode data entry is supported.

CSPro was designed and implemented through a joint effort by the developers of two software packages that were previously used to process census and survey data on DOS machines: the Integrated Microcomputer Processing System (IMPS) and the Integrated System for Survey Analysis (ISSA). The public domain distribution is binary-only, running exclusively on the Microsoft Windows family of operating systems.

Statistical Packages for Social Sciences (SPSS) is one of the most widely used statistical package for data analysis. It helps in data management, coding, editing, preparation of tables and diagrams, performance of descriptive and inferential statistics, various parametric and non parametric tests, assessing the reliability of the tool, etc. It makes the transfer of data easy and transformation of data can be done easily. It is easy-to-learn-and-use software and trial versions are available which can be downloaded for short period of time for learning purpose.

SUMMARY

- The word 'statistics' can be used to denote data, the science of statistics and sample measures. The science of statistics includes the principles and methods for the collection, presentation, analysis and interpretation of numerical data of different kinds.
- Statistics is the study of how to collect, organize, analyze, and interpret numerical information from data.
- Biostatistics is the branch of statistics that deals with data relating to living organisms. It is the application of statistical methods to health sciences. The basic

task of biostatistics is to describe the data and to draw inferences for the underlying population.

- The statistical analysis are of two types. They are descriptive and inferential statistics. The descriptive statistics is used to describe the data whereas the inferential statistics is used to draw conclusions for the population.
- There are four levels of measurement. They are nominal, ordinal, interval and ratio level. Among these four, the ratio level measurement is considered as the highest order of measurement.
- Editing of data is a process of examining the collected raw data (specially in surveys) to detect for errors and omissions and also to make corrections whenever possible. Editing involves a careful scrutiny of the completed questionnaires and/or schedules.
- Coding refers to the process of assigning numerals or other symbols to answers so that responses can be put into a limited number of categories or classes.
- Tabulation or classification is the process by which data of long series of observation are systematically organized and recorded so as to enable analysis and interpretation. In order to classify data, a set of categories are formed.
- Data are classified on the basis of common characteristics which can either be descriptive (such as gender, education status, occupation, religion, etc.) or numerical (such as weight, height, income, etc.)
- Descriptive characteristics refer to qualitative phenomenon which cannot be measured quantitatively; only their presence or absence in an individual item can be noticed. Data obtained this way on the basis of certain attributes are known as statistics of attributes. Unlike descriptive characteristics, the numerical characteristics refer to quantitative phenomenon which can be measured through some statistical units. Data relating to age, income, weight, height, hemoglobin level, etc. fall under this category. Such data are known as statistics of variables and are classified on the basis of class intervals.
- All statistical tests or measures which are used to describe the data are known as descriptive statistics. These descriptive statistics are used to analyze single variables (univariate analysis), two variables (bivariate analysis) and more than two variables (multivariate analysis).
- There are statistical methods which enable researchers to go from the known to the unknown data. From the research findings, one can draw inference for the population. Statistical inference may be of two types: parameter estimation and hypothesis testing.
- Computers are most useful in research and statistics. They are useful in data management and analysis of data.

EXERCISES

- Classify whether the following are quantitative or qualitative data:
  - Pulse
  - Admissions to a hospital on a specific day
  - Experience
  - Pain perception
  - Oxygen saturation
  - No. of staff nurses on duty on a day
  - No. of deaths on a day
  - No. of child births on a day
  - Serum pottasium level
  - Hemoglobin level

- Emotions
- Gender
- Feelings
- Score on stress inventory
- Stress
- Marital status
- Dietary pattern
- Age
- Urine output
- Satisfaction.

• Which one of the following are measurable or countable? Write 'M' for measurable and 'C' for countable:
  - Students in a classroom
  - Size of the classroom
  - Amount of syrup to be taken
  - Tablets to be taken
  - Pulse
  - Temperature
  - Height
  - Weight
  - Age
  - Knowledge
  - Patients admitted in a ward
  - Head circumference
  - Platelet
  - White blood cells
  - Blood glucose
  - Urine output
  - Abdominal circumference
  - Respiration
  - Serum calcium level
  - Birth of baby in a hospital.

• Write the level of measurement against each variable:
  - Intelligence score
  - Test score
  - Temperature
  - Pulse
  - Respiration
  - Income status
  - Educational status
  - Religion
  - Gender
  - Pain level
  - Grading of muscle strength
  - Place of residence
  - Attitude score
  - Dietary pattern
  - Weight
  - Urine output
  - Chest circumference
  - Platelet count
  - Pus cells in urine
  - Occupation.

- State which one of the following are inclusive-or exclusive- type class-intervals:

  20–30
  30–40
  40–50
  21–30
  31–40
  41–50
  05–15
  15–25
  25–35
  5–15
  16–25
  26–35
- State which of the following are descriptive or inferential statistics:
  - Testing of hypothesis
  - Correlation analysis
  - Standard deviation
  - Average
  - Range.
- Prepare the frequency distribution for the data given below:

36	40	22	33	42	54	24	33	42	46	48	24	30
38	20	32	36	28	40	25	36	28	23	24	27	31
50	52	48	46	36	42	44	30	32	36	42	40	30
40	32	34	36	28	46	48	41	32	33	37		

The hemoglobin level of 30 adolescents are given below. Prepare a frequency distribution.

10	10.5	10.8	10.3	11	11.2	10.4	10.8	11.6	12	11.3	11.4	11
12	11.8	12.2	10.8	10	12.1	11.6	12.4	11.8	11	12.6	10.9	12
11	11.6	10.5	10.6									

- The systolic blood pressures of 40 adults are given below. Prepare a frequency distribution.

100	110	112	120	124	128	130	110	100	150	164	170	200
130	120	110	100	132	134	164	170	180	190	110	100	100
126	126	112	140	142	136	138	138	120	120	110	112	110
100												

12 Presentation of Data

OBJECTIVES

After reading this chapter, you will be able to:

- Explain the tabulation of data
- Explain the diagrammatic presentation of data
- Explain the graphical representation of data
- Formulate table, diagrammatic and graphical presentation of data.

INTRODUCTION

In research, we collect large volumes of data. The data which we collect has to be presented for various purposes. Data can be presented as text, in tables, or pictorially as graphs and charts. Presentation of data is a task which requires thinking, logical reasoning about the classification and grouping of data. Meaningful classification of data is mandatory for any statistical analysis and for the purpose of communication. Tables and diagrammatic representations are the most important forms of presentation of data. Tables help us to present the data in a reduced form where as figures help us to present about the specific characteristics. Tables and graphs are attractive and uses only less space. Both make the comparisons easier. Tables are usually the best way of showing structured numeric information, whereas graphs and charts are better for showing relationships, making comparisons and indicating trends. Even where a graph or chart is used, it is usual to include a table to show the data from which it was drawn.

TABULATION OF DATA

Tabulation is a scientific process used in setting out the collected data in an understandable form. Tables are commonly used in collecting and organizing raw data during a research and also for representing final data to be included in a paper or report. When a mass of data has been assembled, it becomes necessary for the researcher to arrange the same in some kind of concise and logical order. This procedure is referred to as tabulation. Thus, tabulation is the process of summarizing raw data and displaying the same in compact form (i.e. in the form of statistical tables) for further analysis. In a broader sense, tabulation is an orderly arrangement of data in columns and rows. Rows are horizontal arrangements whereas columns are vertical arrangements. The representation of data in a table is formally referred to as 'tabular presentation'. Tabular presentation of data allows data to be organized for further analysis, allows large amounts of raw data to be sorted and reorganized in a neat format, and allows the inclusion of only the most important or relevant data. Good tables should be easy to read across rows and down columns, easy to understand, and easy to refer to in the text of the report. They should also include only relevant data.

Tabulation may be defined as logical and systematic arrangement of statistical data in rows and columns. It is designed to simplify the presentation of data for the purposes of analysis and statistical inferences. According to Gregory D and Ward H, tabulation is the process of condensing classified data in the form of a table so that it may be more easily understood and so that any comparison involved may be more readily made.

Objectives of Tabulation

The objectives of tabulation are stated below:

- ***To reduce large volume of data:*** When large volumes of data are collected, tabulation enables the data to be arranged sequentially following principles. When data are arranged systematically in a table, such data become more meaningful and can be easily understood.
- ***To facilitate comparison:*** Tabulation facilitates comparison when different sets are presented. Two way and cross tabulation enables comparison.
- ***To conserve the space:*** A statistical table furnishes maximum information relating to a study in minimum space.
- ***To provide basis for statistical analysis:*** Tabulation facilitates computation of statistics such as measures of central tendency and measures of dispersion and then interpretation of data. When we tabulate data, errors and omissions can be detected.
- ***To provide reference:*** Tabulation enables us to give reference whenever and wherever the data in a table are discussed.
- ***To provide meaning to the data:*** Data simply written cannot give any meaning to the reader. When it is organized, it conveys meaning to the reader.
- ***To facilitate presentation of the data:*** Data once collected to be presented. There are various methods by which the data can be presented to the readers. Tabulation is one such method.

Parts of a Table

- ***Table Number:*** A table should be numbered for easy reference and identification. This is usually written just before the title.
- ***Title of the table:*** An appropriate title should be given to the table. The title should be simple, clear and short in length. The title should be placed centrally on the top of a table.
- ***Head note:*** It is placed below the title of the table.

- ***Caption or column headings:*** Captions are the brief, self explanatory headings of vertical columns. It may have heading and sub headings as well. It is preferable to mention the unit of data given for each column. For example, if some data are given as percentage then under the main heading % or percentage is given.
- ***Stubs or row designations:*** Stubs are brief self explanatory headings of horizontal rows.
- ***Body:*** The body of the table contains the numerical information of frequency of observations in the different cells. This arrangement of data is according to the description of captions and stubs. The actual data should be arranged in such a manner that any figure may be readily located.
- ***Unit of measurements:*** The unit of measurement should always be stated along with the title, if this is uniform throughout. If different units have been adopted, then they should be stated along the stubs or captions.
- ***Dividers:*** Dividers are lines that frame the top and bottom of the table and, or mark the different parts of a table. They are often used for division within the body of a table.
- ***Source notes:*** A note at the bottom of the table should always be given to indicate the primary source as well as the secondary source from where the data has been taken, particularly when there is more than one source.
- ***Footnotes:*** Footnotes are given at the foot of the table for explanation of any fact or information included in the table which needs some explanation. Thus, they are meant for explaining or providing further details about the data that have not been covered in title, captions and stubs.

Types of Table

On the basis of the number of characteristics, tables may be classified as follows:

- ***Simple or one-way table:*** A simple or one-way table is the simplest table which contains data of one characteristic only. A simple table is easy to construct and simple to follow (Table 12.1).

Table. 12.1: Frequency and percentage distribution of the age of the children

Age of the children	Frequency	Percentage (%)
13 years	92	26.3
14 years	77	22.0
15 years	51	14.6
16 years	22	06.3
17 years	21	06.0
18 years	87	24.9
Total	350	100.0

- ***Two-way table:*** A table, which contains data on two characteristics, is called a two way table. In such case, therefore, either stub or caption is divided into two coordinate parts (Table 12.2).

Table 12.2: Frequency distribution of the children based on parent's education

Educational Status	Father's Education		Mother's Education	
	Frequency	Percentage	Frequency	Percentage
High school	97	27.7	111	31.7
Higher secondary	85	24.3	98	28.0
Graduate	109	31.1	92	26.3
Post graduate	59	16.9	49	14.0
Total	350	100.0	350	100.0

- ***Manifold table:*** A table, which has more than two characteristics of data, is considered as a manifold table. Manifold tables, though complex are good in practice as these enable full information to be incorporated and facilitate analysis of all related facts. Still, as a normal practice, not more than four characteristics should be represented in one table to avoid confusion. Other related tables may be formed to show the remaining characteristics (Table 12.3).

Table 12.3: Mean and standard deviation of physiological variables of children playing violent video games

Age group	Statistic	Pulse	Respiration	Systolic BP	Diastolic BP	Weight	Height
16 years	Mean	79.77	20.18	117.32	76.64	54.327	156.159
	N	22	22	22	22	22	22
	SD	6.094	1.053	11.765	8.080	12.8539	10.3479
17 years	Mean	83.57	20.86	116.10	76.57	55.476	155.229
	N	21	21	21	21	21	21
	SD	5.372	2.056	12.498	7.018	15.3505	11.8283
18 years	Mean	81.56	21.86	122.23	80.41	59.382	160.052
	N	87	87	87	87	87	87
	SD	5.720	4.713	12.805	9.150	10.4753	7.4227

On the basis of the content, tables may be classified as follows:

- ***Textual (Word) tables:*** When tables have only textual information in the body, it is known as ***textual tables***.
- ***Statistical tables:*** These tables can present descriptive or inferential statistics or both. Descriptive statistics are tabulations such as mean, standard deviation, mode, range, or frequency. Inferential statistics refers to statistical tests. In such tables, statistical test values are presented.
- ***Numerical tables:*** These are the most common types of data, which typically represent quantitative data, but sometimes may present a combination of quantitative and qualitative data. As its name suggests, most of the body of the table consists of specific number values.
- ***Mock or dummy tables:*** These are the tables without any content in the body. It is developed before the data collection and organization to facilitate thinking.

On the basis of objective (purpose), tables may be classified as follows:

- ***General purpose table:*** It is also known as ***informative table*** and provides information for general use; and usually in chronological order. The detailed table in the census reports are of this kind.

- ***Special purpose table:*** It is also called a ***summary table*** or analytical table or derived table. It presents the data for special purpose.

On the basis of Originality, tables may be classified as follows:

- ***Primary table:*** The primary table contains actual figures or data.
- ***Derived table:*** It consists of figures or numerical values that are derived from the primary data. It presents frequencies, percentages, ratios, mean, standard deviations, coefficient of correlations, etc.

Points to be Remembered in Preparing a Table

- Be certain that table is self explanatory.
- Let the table be supplementary to the text.
- Refer to all tables by numbers, e.g. Table 1, 2, 3.
- Always give units of measurement in table headings.
- Align decimal places.
- Round numbers as much as possible. Try to round to two decimal places unless more decimals are needed.
- Data in the body should be arranged logically. The arrangement of rows and columns also should be in a logical and systematic order. This arrangement may be an alphabetical; chronological or according to size
- Place the tables near the text that refers to them.
- Decide on a length of the table. Let the table not be too lengthy. Break the data in a meaningful way to organize additional table. Too many rows or columns could make it difficult for the reader to understand the data.
- The rows and columns are separated by single, double or thick lines to represent various classes and sub-classes used.
- Combine the tables when there are identical columns or rows of data in two or more tables.
- Provide column/row totals or other numerical summaries that can make it easier to understand the data.
- Align the data in the table to look neat and clear. For example, all numbers in the columns should line up with each other and with their headings.
- Highlight the information in the table by 'bold' or any other ways if necessary.
- Be consistent with the tabular presentation and formats.
- In case it is not possible to accommodate all the information in a single table, it is better to have two or more related tables.

DIAGRAMMATIC PRESENTATION OF THE DATA

In our day to day life, we come across various diagrams in newspapers, journals, magazines and advertisements. Diagrams are visual representation of data. Diagrams are advantageous than the tables for its attractiveness and it is easily understood by anybody with a single glance. Diagrams are used either alone or with the tables. According to MJ Moroney, 'diagrams register a meaningful impression almost before we think.'

Importance or Utility of Diagrams

- Diagrams give a clear picture of data. Anybody can understand diagram easily and in a short time.
- Diagrams make comparison easier without the use of any statistical technique.
- The scope of diagram is wider and it can be used in all fields.
- Diagrams are more attractive than the tables by visually appealing the audience.
- It is economical, saves time and energy.
- Diagrams promote understanding and critical thinking when compared to tabulation.
- Diagrams are easily remembered than tables.
- Data can be condensed with diagrams.
- Diagrams provide more information than the data in the table.

General Guidelines for Diagrammatic Presentation

- The diagram should be neat and properly drawn. The purpose should be considered before it is drawn.
- Various colors and symbols can be used to make the diagram more meaningful and appealing.
- Appropriate diagram must be chosen to present a set of figures.
- The diagrams should be drawn at an appropriate scale. Diagrams should neither be too big nor too small.
- A proportion between a height and width of the diagram should be maintained. The diagram may look ugly when the proportion is not maintained.
- The size of the diagram can be decided based on the size of the paper too.
- Footnote can be given wherever necessary for clarification of certain information.
- Diagrams should be self explanatory.
- Different colors and shades can be used to make the diagrams more attractive and easily understandable.
- It must be accurate as well as simple to understand.

Limitations of Diagrammatic Presentation

- Diagrams do not present the small differences properly.
- It is not an alternative to tabulation.
- Diagrams require skill.
- Diagrams are not useful in statistical analysis whereas tables are useful.
- Diagrams cannot show so many facts as a statistical table can do.
- Only a limited set of data can be presented in the form of diagram.
- Diagrams may present preliminary conclusions.

Parts of a Diagram

- ***Figure number:*** Each diagram should be numbered for easy identification and reference.
- ***Title:*** The diagram should be given appropriate title. It can be written at the bottom of the diagram and it should be short and self explanatory.
- ***Keys/index (labels):*** An index or labels illustrating the different types of lines or different shades, symbols, colors should be given to show that the reader can easily make out the meaning of the diagram.
- ***Footnote:*** Footnotes are given at the bottom of the diagram for clarification of any information included in the diagram which needs further explanation.
- ***Source note:*** Source note, wherever possible, should be appended at the bottom of the diagram. It is given to indicate the source from where the data have been taken.

Types of Diagrams

There are various types of diagram. One can choose the diagram based on the purpose.

- ***Line diagrams:*** It is the simplest of all diagrams. In line diagram only line is drawn to represent the data of a variable. These lines may be vertical or horizontal. The lines are drawn such that their length is the proportion to value of the terms or items so that comparison may be done easily (Fig. 12.1).

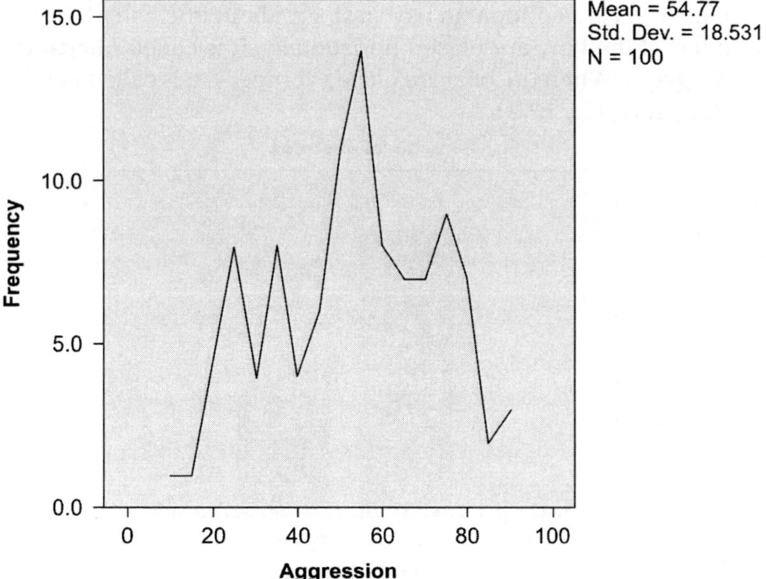

Fig. 12.1: Line diagram showing the frequencies of the aggression scores of the children

Example 1:

10 nursing students test mark is given. Draw a line graph for the data given below.

Student	1	2	3	4	5	6	7	8	9	10
Marks	50	60	70	70	80	80	85	85	75	65

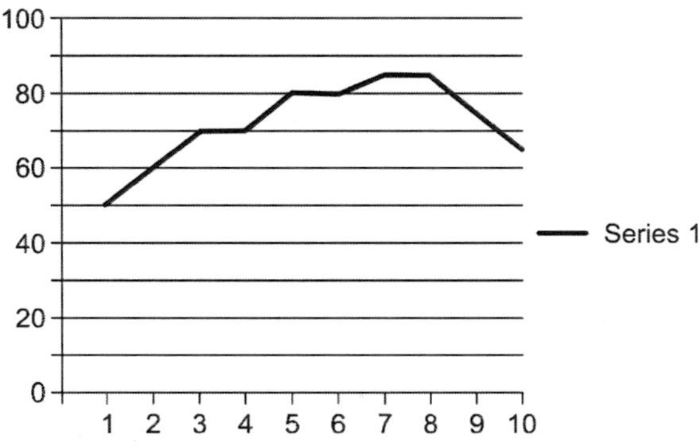

Fig. 12.2: Line graph showing test mark of nursing students.

Solution. Plot the points (1, 50), (2, 60), (3, 70), (4, 70), (5, 80), (6, 80), (7, 85), (8, 85), (9, 75) and (10, 65). Join them to get the line graph.

- ***Bar diagram***
  - ***Simple bar diagram:*** The simple bar diagram usually explains only one variable. The bars are erected on the horizontal axis and its height is equivalent to the percentage of occurrence which is exhibited on the vertical axis. It can even be drawn vertically. The width of bars is not governed by any set rules. Regarding the space between two bars, it is conventional to have a space about one half of the width of a bar. If the bars are placed horizontally, it is called ***horizontal bar diagram***. When the bars are placed vertically, it is called ***vertical bar diagram (Fig. 12.3)***.

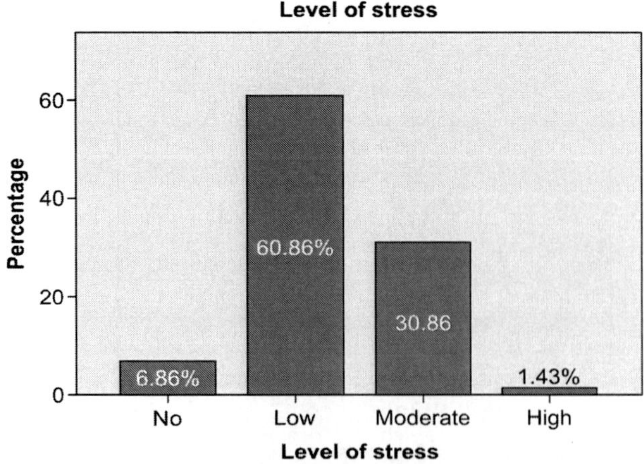

Fig. 12.3: Bar diagram showing the percentage distribution of the children based on level of stress

Example 2:

Draw a bar diagram for the data given below.

Year	2009	2010	2011	2012	2013
No. of deaths	60	50	60	70	40

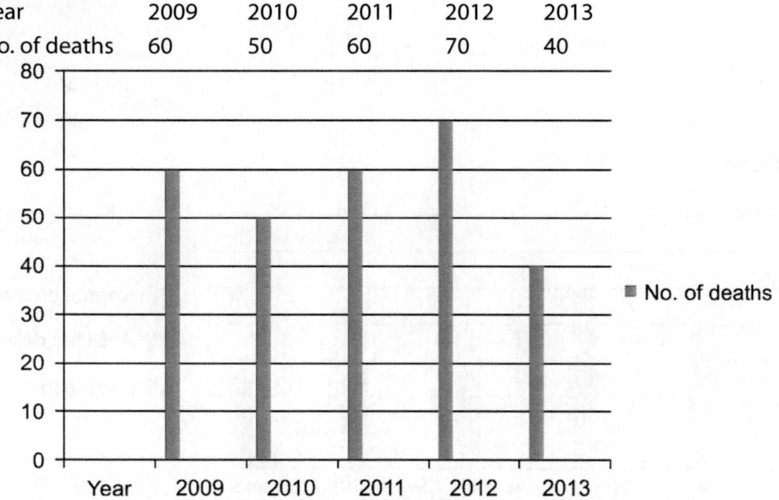

Fig. 12.4: Bar diagram showing number deaths in various years

- ***Multiple bar diagrams:*** The diagram is used, when we have to make comparison between more than two variables. The number of variables may be 2, 3 or 4 or more. In case of 2 variables, pair of bars is drawn. Similarly, in case of 3 variables, we draw triple bars. The bars are drawn on the same proportionate basis as in case of simple bars. The same shade is given to the same item. Distance between pairs is kept constant (Fig. 12.5).

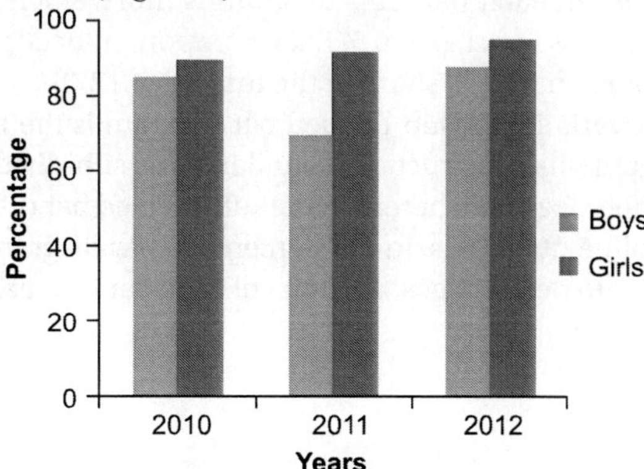

Fig. 12.5: Multiple bar diagram showing the pass percentage of boys and girls in three years.

Example 3:

Draw a suitable diagram for the data given below. In a hospital total number of deliveries were given for 5 months.

contd...

contd...

Month	Normal delivery	Assisted delivery (Forceps, etc.)	Cesarean delivery
June	50	10	40
July	40	15	50
August	60	18	35
September	70	10	45
October	50	10	25

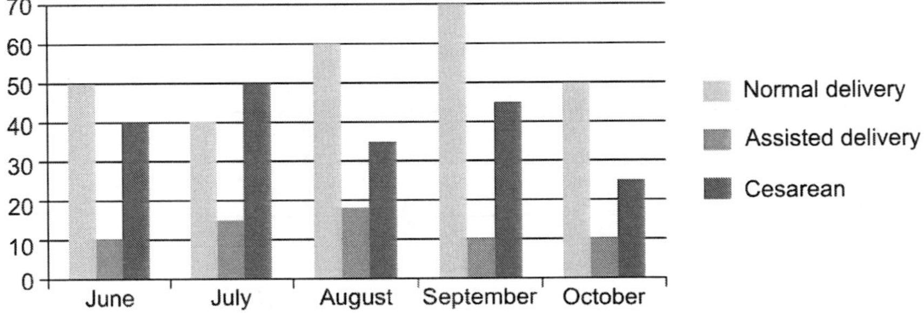

Fig. 12.6: Multiple bar diagram showing the types and number of deliveries in various months

- ***Sub-divided bar diagram:*** The sub-divided or component bar diagram is formed by dividing a single bar into several component parts. The data which is presented by multiple bar diagram can be presented by this diagram. In this case, we add different variables for a period and draw it on a single bar. The components must be kept in same order in each bar. This diagram is more efficient if number of components is less, i.e. 3 to 5. Each component occupies a part of the bar proportional to its share in the total (Fig. 12.7).

The another variation of sub-divided bar diagram is the percentage sub-divided bar diagram. Its construction is similar to the sub-divided bar diagram with the only difference that whereas in the sub-divided bar diagram segments are used in absolute quantities, in the percentage bar diagram the quantities are transformed into percentages. The total of each bar is equal to 100%.

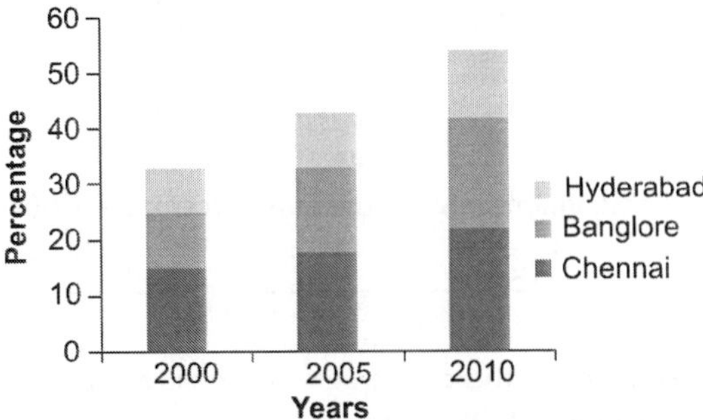

Fig. 12.7: Sub-divided bar diagram showing the rainfall in three cities

Example 4:

Represent the following data by sub-divided or component bar diagram. The admission of students for various program is given below.

Year	BSc (N)	PBBSc (N)	MSc (N)
2011	38	20	18
2012	40	15	11
2013	50	8	10

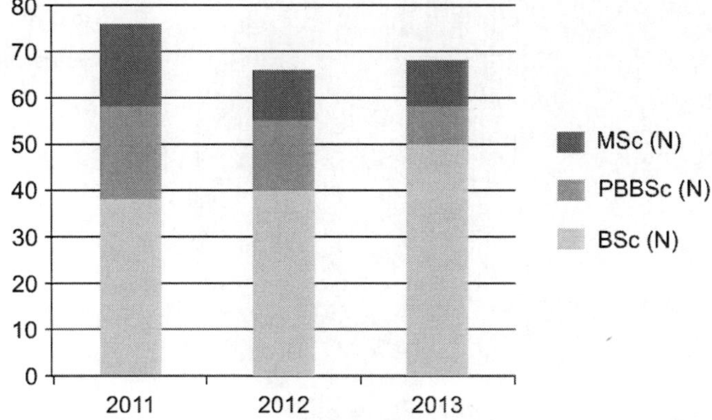

Fig. 12.8: Subdivided bar diagram showing the pass percentage of various nursing programs in various years

- ***Duo-directional bar diagram:*** In this case the diagram is on both the sides of base line, i.e. to left and right or to above or below sides.
- ***Broken bar diagram:*** This diagram is used when value of some variable is very high or low as compared to others. In this case the bars with bigger terms or items may be shown broken. A broken bar graph is used when one value, or a few values, goes up very high. Instead of scaling everything down, the abnormally high value is indicated with the broken bar graph (Fig. 12.9).

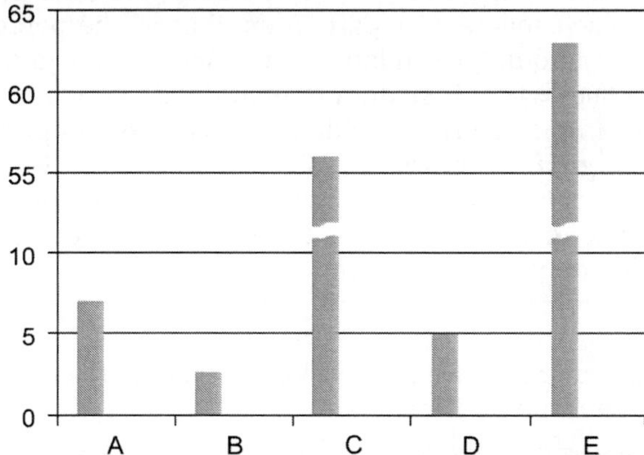

Fig. 12.9: Diagram showing the broken bar diagram

- ***Pie diagram or angular diagram:*** A pie diagram is a circular diagram divided into sectors, illustrating numerical proportion. In a pie chart, the arc length of each sector (and consequently its central angle and area), is proportional to the quantity it represents (Fig. 12.10).

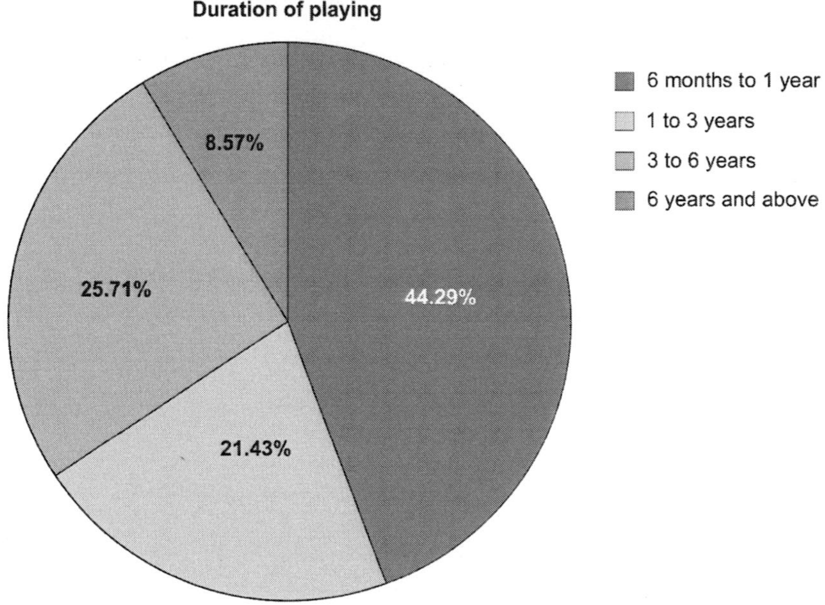

Fig. 12.10: Pie diagram showing the duration of playing violent video games by the adolescents

The area of the circle represents the total value and the different sectors of the circle represent the different parts. Every sector in the graph represents an item in the data that marches the fraction or percentage of the total data set. It is used to show visually the proportions of parts of something being studied. A pie chart shows data at one point in time, like a snapshot; it does not show change in data over time like a line chart does. To draw a pie chart, one should find the total value for the entire category being studied and calculate the percentage for each segment or part. Then convert the percentage values for each segment into degrees relative to the 360 degrees in the circle. (For example, 12% × 360° = 43°). Then draw a circle and divide it into appropriately sized segments. In pie diagram, the data are expressed as percentages. It is also known as ***angular diagram***.

The name pie diagram is given to a circle diagram because in determining the circumference of a circle we have to take into consideration a quantity known as ***pie*** (written as π).

Example 5:

The data on percentage of patients with various illnesses who had attended a clinic is given below. Draw a pie diagram.

Disease	Fever	Common cold	Hypertension	Diabetes	UTI	Others
Percentage	36	24	18	12	4	6

Solution

Disease	Percentage	Central angles (degrees)
Fever	36	$\frac{36}{100} \times 360 = 130°$
Common cold	24	$\frac{24}{100} \times 360 = 86°$
Hypertension	18	$\frac{18}{100} \times 360 = 65°$
Diabetes	12	$\frac{12}{100} \times 360 = 43°$
UTI	4	$\frac{4}{100} \times 360 = 14°$
Others	6	$\frac{6}{100} \times 360 = 22°$

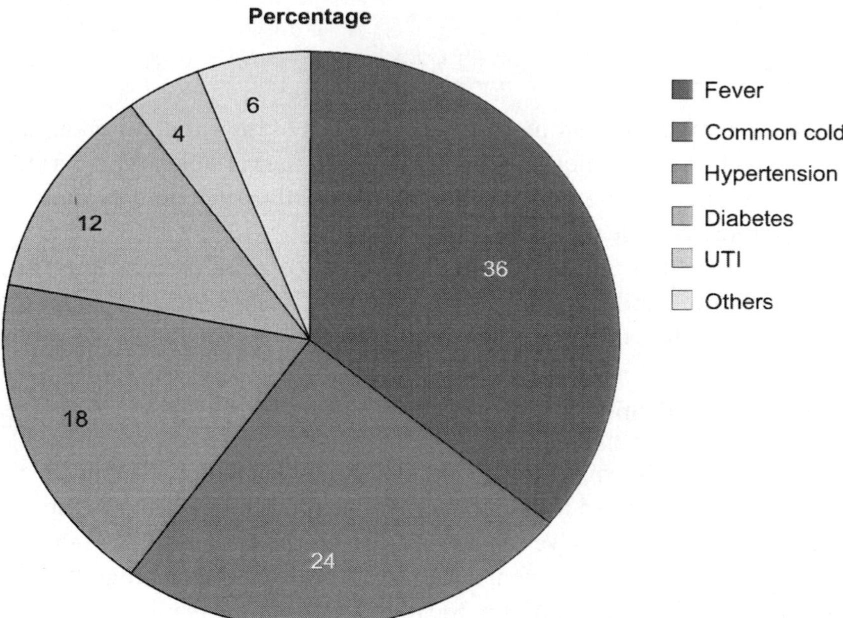

Fig. 12.11: Pie diagram showing the percentage of patients with various illness who had attended a clinic

- ***Pictogram:*** Pictogram is a device of representing statistical data in pictures. They are very attractive and are easily understood. For the purpose of propaganda, the pictorial presentations of facts are quite popular and extensively used by the government and private sector organizations.

Color	Number of smarties	Frequency
Green	●●●◖	7
Orange	●●●●	8
Blue	●●◖	5
Pink	●●●	6
Yellow	●●●●●◖	11
Red	●●●●	8
Purple	●●●◖	7
Brown	●◖	3
	Key ● = 2 smarties	

GRAPH

A graph refers to the plotting of different values of the variables on a graph paper which gives the movement or a change in the variable over a period of time. Diagrams can present the data in an attractive style but still there is a method more reliable than this.

According to AL Boddington, 'The wandering of a line is more powerful in its effect on the mind than a tabulated statement; it shows what is happening and what is likely to take place, just as quickly as the eye is capable of working'.

Advantages of Graphs

Think of a graph shown during the time of the cricket match. Usually the two team's score is depicted as a comparative line graph which shows the runs and the out of batsman gives a good picture for the audience. By seeing this one can understand which team is doing well and what is the progress and to some extent predictions can be made about the winning team.

- The data can be presented in an attractive and effective way
- It presents the complex data in a simple way
- Graphs can be used to compare and interpret the data
- Graphs facilitates the remembrance of the data and also help us to predict in a better way
- It not only provides information but helps in transmission of information.

Rules for the Construction of Graph

The following are the main rules to construct a graph:

- Every graph must have a suitable title.
- The graph must suit to the size of the paper.
- The scale of the graph should be in even numbers or in multiples.
- Footnotes should be given at the bottom to illustrate the main points about the graph.
- Graph should be as simple as possible.
- In order to show many items in a graph, index for identification should be given.
- A graph should be neat and clean.
- It should be appealing to the eyes.
- Every graph should be given with a table to ensure whether the data has been presented accurately or not.
- A good graph is the one which the observer can interpret it. Thus care should be taken in drawing the graph.

Limitations

Following are the main drawbacks/limitations of graphs.

- Graphic representation is useful for a common man but for an expert, its utility is limited.
- Graphs do not measure the magnitude of the data. They only depict the fluctuations in them.
- Graphs are subjective in character. Their interpretation varies from person to person.
- The person who has no knowledge can draw misleading conclusions from graphs.

How to Choose a Scale for a Graph

The scale indicates the unit of a variable that a fixed length of axis would represent. Scale may be different for both the axes. It should be taken in such a way so as to accommodate whole of the data on a given graph paper in a lucid and attractive style. Sometimes data to be presented does not have low values but with large terms.

Types of Graphs

There are two types of graphs:

1. ***Time Series Graph:*** Time series graphs may be of one variable, two variables or more variables graph. A time series graphs is a line graph where time is measured on the horizontal axis and the variable being observed is measured on the vertical axis (Fig. 12.12).

Inflation and short-term interest rate

Fig. 12.12: Time series graph showing the inflation and the short-term interest rate

2. ***Frequency Distribution Graphs:***

- ***Histogram:*** A histogram is a graphical representation showing a visual impression of the distribution of data. The histogram is a graphic representation of frequency distribution and is being used to represent simple frequency distribution. It is an estimate of the probability distribution of a continuous variable and was first introduced by Karl Pearson. It is a special kind of bar diagram used to present a frequency distribution of characteristics measured on a continuous scale (Fig. 12.13).

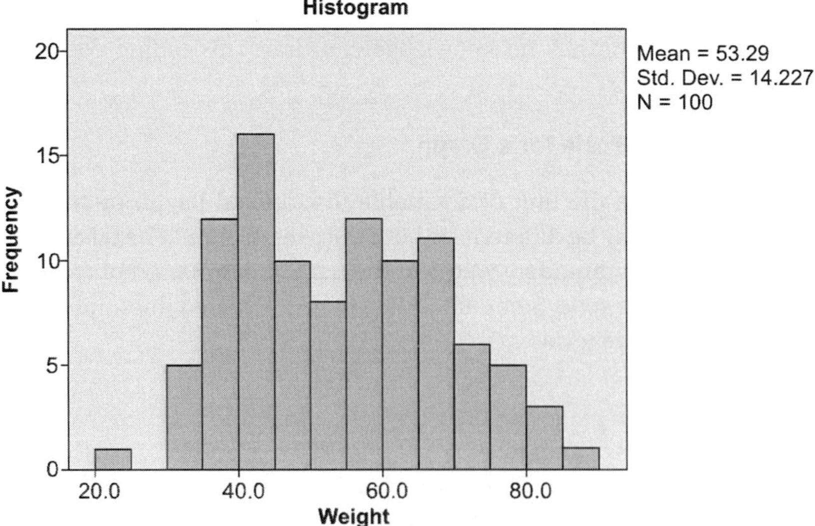

Fig. 12.13: Histogram showing the weight of the children

(Note the gap between the cells in the diagram which should be avoided)

A histogram is a graph containing a set of rectangles, each being constructed to represent the size of the class interval by its width and the frequency in each class-interval by its height. The area of each rectangle is proportional to the frequency in the respective class interval and the total area of the histogram is proportional to the total frequency. When we construct a histogram the values of the variable under consideration are represented by the horizontal axis, while the vertical axis has as its scale the frequency of occurrence. Rectangles (bar or cell) are erected on the horizontal axis, i.e. the class intervals to represent frequencies of the class intervals. In histogram the area of each rectangle represents frequency of the corresponding class interval. The cells of a histogram must be joined and to accomplish this we must take into account the true boundaries of the class intervals to prevent gaps from occurring between the cells of a graph. Histograms are used to plot density of data, and often for density estimation. The total area of a histogram used for probability density is always normalized to 1. If the lengths of the intervals on the x-axis are all 1, then a histogram is identical to a relative frequency plot (Fig. 12.14).

In histogram, the bars are placed continuously side by side with no gap between adjacent bars. That is, in histogram rectangles are erected on the class intervals of the distribution. The areas of the rectangle are proportional to the frequencies The difference between histogram and bar diagram is given in Table 12.4.

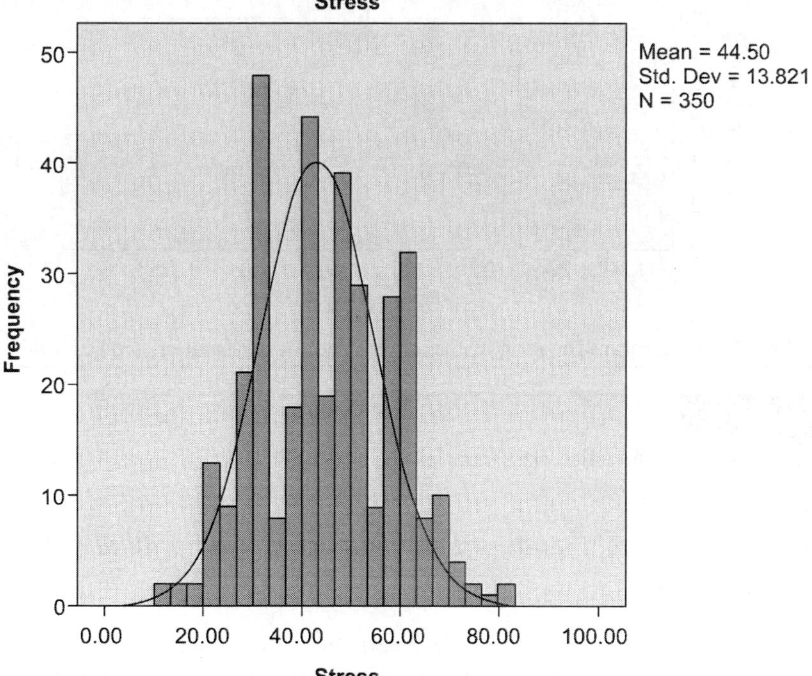

Fig. 12.14: Histogram with the normal curve showing the stress score of the children

Table 12.4: Difference between Histogram and Bar diagram

Histogram	Bar diagram
It can be drawn only for a continuous variable	It can be drawn for a continuous as well as discrete variable
It facilitates calculation of mode	It does not facilitate calculation of mode
Both width and height of the bar is important	Width is unimportant
There is no space between the bars	Space is left between two consecutive bars except in multiple (or component) bar diagram

Example 6:

Drawing a histogram for continuous frequency distribution.

Class-interval	0–10	10–20	20–30	30–40	40–50	50–60	60–70	70–80
Frequency	4	6	8	10	12	10	10	5

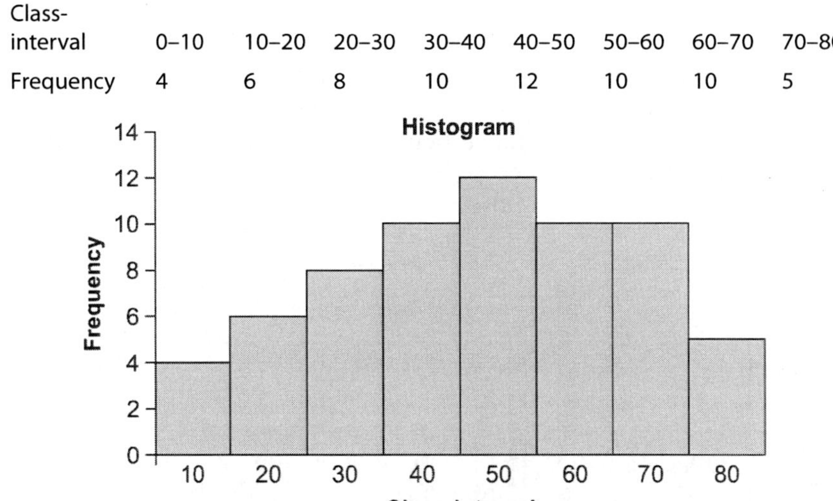

Fig. 12.15: Diagram showing histogram for continuous frequency distribution

Example 7:

Drawing a histogram when class intervals are not continuous.

Class-interval	16–20	21–25	26–30	31–35	36–40	41–45	46–50
Frequency	10	15	20	25	30	20	10

In this, the class intervals are discontinuous (inclusive form). If we draw histogram for this data, there will be a gap in between the class interval. This needs to be changed into a continuous form. For this we need an adjustment factor,

Adjustment factor = 1/2 [(lower limit of the second class) – (upper limit of the first class)]

= 1/2(21 – 20) =1/2 × 1 = 0.5

In the above class interval, we should subtract 0.5 from each lower limit and add 0.5 in each upper limit. Therefore, we rewrite the given table into the following table.

Class-interval	15.5–20.5	20.5–25.5	25.5–30.5	30.5–35.5	35.5–40.5	40.5–45.5	45.5–50.5
Frequency	10	15	20	25	30	20	10

For these values, the histogram can be drawn. Drawing a histogram when class-intervals are not continuous.

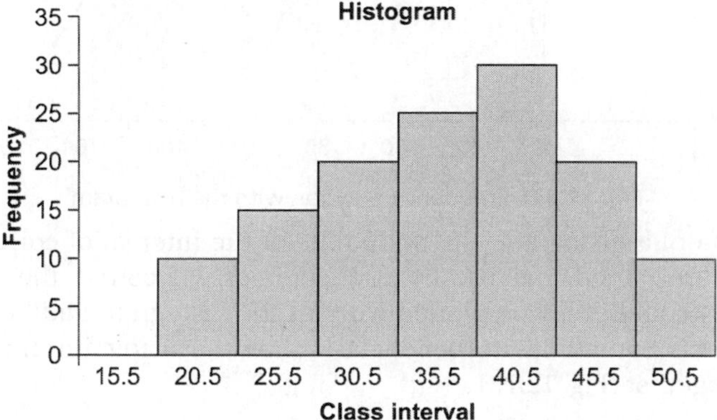

Fig. 12.16: Diagram showing histogram for discontinuous class intervals

- ***Frequency Polygon:*** Frequency polygon is another method of representing frequency distribution graphically. Draw a histogram for the given continuous data. Mark the middle points of the tops of adjacent rectangles. If we join these middle points successively by line segments, we get a polygon (Fig. 12.17). This polygon is called the ***frequency polygon***. It is customary to bring the ends of the polygon down to base level by assuming a lower class of frequency and highest class of a frequency. Frequency polygon can be constructed in two ways. (i) Using histogram and (ii) without using histogram.

It is a variation of histogram. To draw a frequency polygon we first place a dot above the midpoint of each class interval represented on the horizontal axis of a graph. The height of a given dot above the horizontal axis corresponds to the frequency of the relevant class interval. Connecting the dots by straight lines produces the frequency polygon. It gives a polygon, i.e. a figure with many angles. It is used when two or more sets of data are to be illustrated on the same diagram such as death rates in smokers and nonsmokers, birth and death rates of a population, etc.

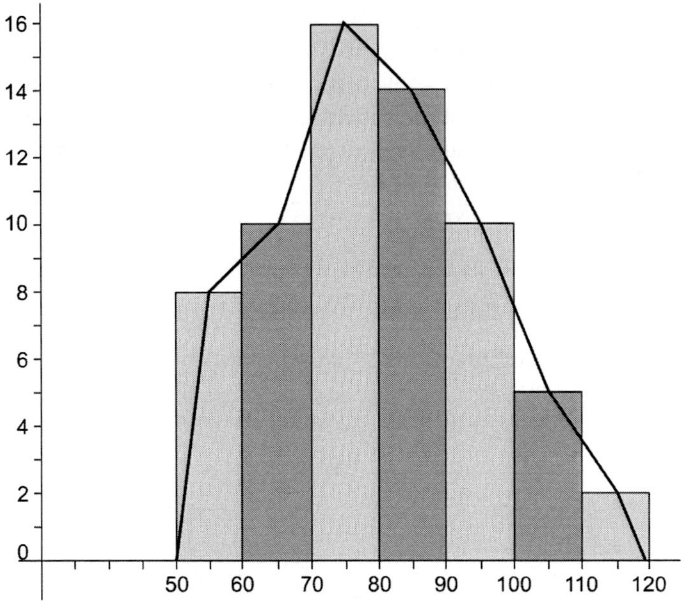

Fig. 12.17: Frequency polygon with the histogram

In case of a histogram, the midpoints of the interval of corresponding rectangle are joined together by straight lines. Of course the midpoints themselves could easily be plotted without the histogram and be joined by line segments. Sometimes it is beneficial to show the histogram and frequency polygon together (Fig. 12.18).

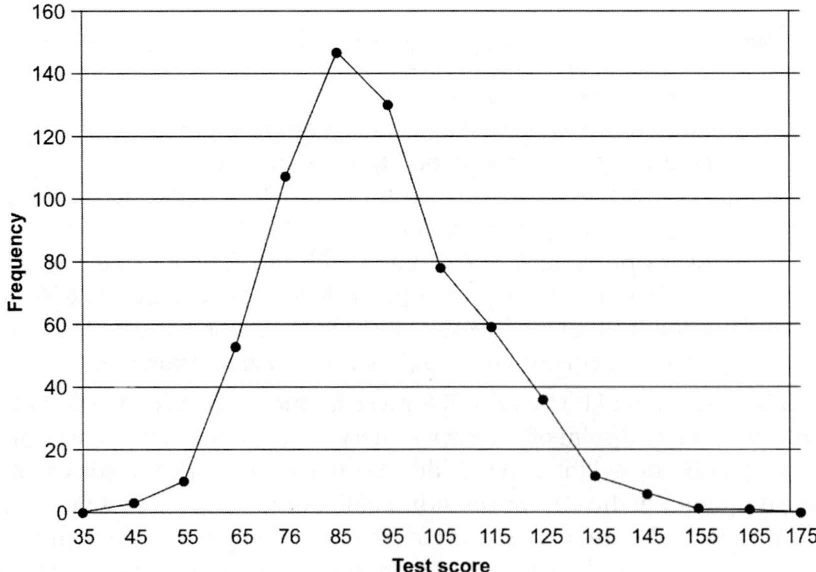

Fig. 12.18: Frequency polygon without histogram showing the test score of the children in test

Example 8:

Draw a frequency polygon imposed on the histogram for the following distribution.

Class-interval	10–20	20–30	30–40	40–50	50–60	60–70	70–80	80–90
Frequency	5	6	8	10	12	14	7	5

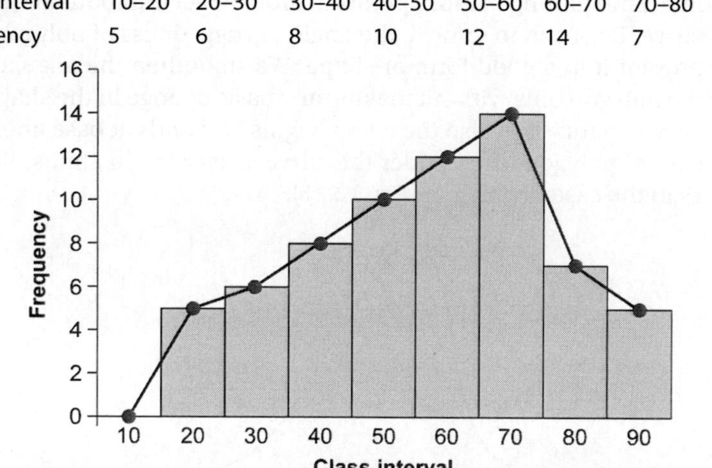

Fig. 12.19: Diagram showing the frequency polygon imposed on the histogram

Example 9:

Draw a frequency polygon without using histogram for the following distribution.

Class-interval	10–20	20–30	30–40	40–50	50–60	60–70	70–80	80–90
Frequency	5	6	8	10	12	14	7	5

Class-interval	10–20	20–30	30–40	40–50	50–60	60–70	70–80	80–90
Mid points	15	25	35	45	55	65	75	85
Frequency	5	6	8	10	12	14	7	5

Plot the points A(15, 5), B(25, 6), C(35, 8), D(45, 10), E(55, 12), F(65, 14), G(75, 7) and H(85, 5).

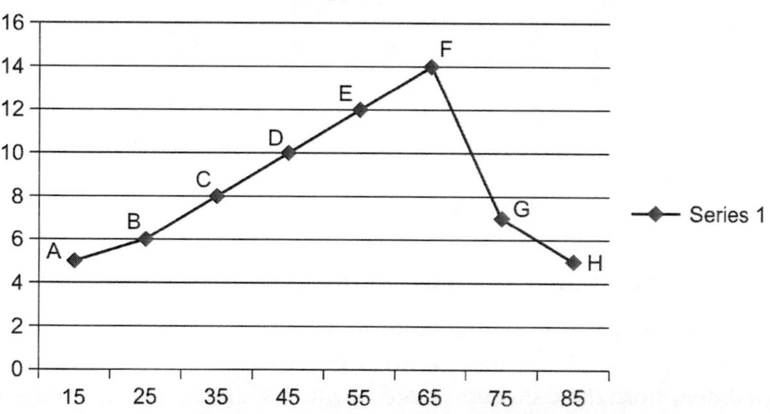

Fig. 12.20: Diagram showing frequency polygon without using histogram

- ***Frequency Curve:*** Frequency curve is obtained by joining the points of frequency polygon by a freehand smoothed curve. Unlike frequency polygon, where the points are joined by straight lines, we make use of free hand joining of those points in order to get a smoothed frequency curve. It is used to remove the angle or ruggedness of polygon and to present it in a good form or shape. We smoothen the angularities of the polygon only without making any basic change in the shape of the curve. In this case also the curve begins and ends at base line, as is in case of polygon. Area under the curve must remain almost the same as in the case of polygon (Fig. 12.21).

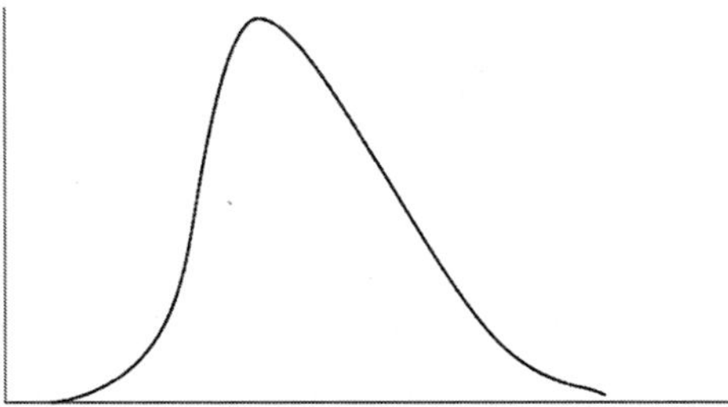

Fig. 12.21: Frequency curve

- ***Cumulative Frequency Polygon or Ogive:*** An Ogive (a cumulative line graph) is best used when we want to display the total at any given time. An Ogive is a graph that represents cumulative frequencies or cumulative relative frequencies (Fig. 12.22).

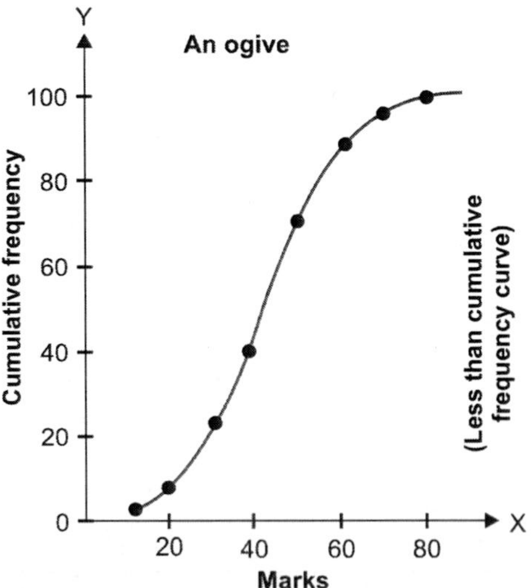

Fig. 12.22: An ogive showing the marks of the children

An ogive, when it is drawn, is in the form of a curve. The curve drawn from the data cumulated downward is known as ***less than ogive*** and the curve drawn from the data cumulated upward is known as ***more than ogive***. An ogive is used to find median, quartiles, deciles and percentiles, etc. A cumulative frequency curve or ogive is obtained by plotting the successive cumulative frequencies on the graph paper and joining them by a free hand. It represents the cumulative frequency distribution by plotting actual upper limits of the class intervals in the X axis and the cumulative frequency of these class intervals on the Y axis.

There are two types of ogive curve.

1. Less than ogive
2. More than ogive.

In drawing an ogive, if the cumulative frequencies are plotted at the upper limit of the class interval, it is a less than ogive. But in the case of more than ogive, the cumulative frequencies are plotted against the lower class boundaries of the respective class intervals.

Example 10:

Draw a less than and more than ogive for the following data.

IQ	70–80	80–90	90–100	100–110	110–120	120–130
No. of students	10	20	25	20	10	5

Ogive by less than method

Class interval	Frequency		Cumulative frequency	Plots to be plotted
70–80	10	Less than 80	10	(80, 10)
80–90	20	Less than 90	30	(90, 30)
90–100	25	Less than 100	55	(100, 55)
100–110	20	Less than 110	75	(110, 75)
110–120	10	Less than 120	85	(120, 85)
120–130	5	Less than 130	90	(130, 90)

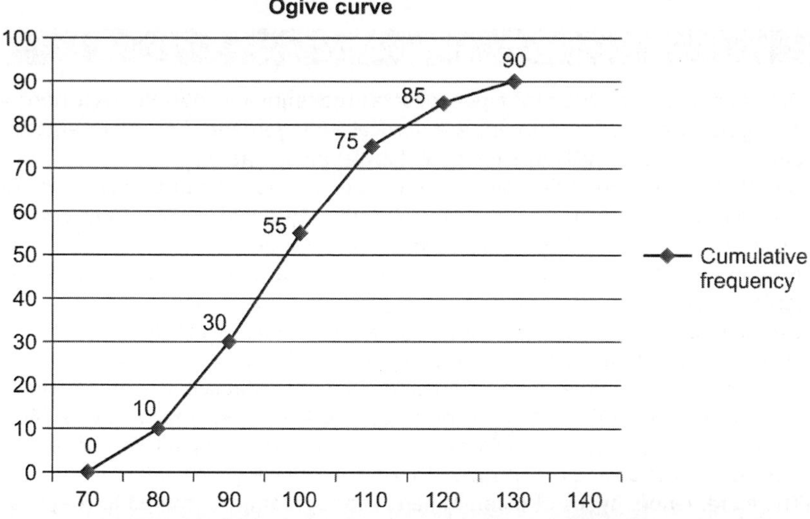

Fig. 12.23: Diagram showing Ogive by less than method

Ogive by more than method

Class interval	Frequency		Cumulative frequency	Plots to be plotted
70–80	10	More than 70	90	(70, 90)
80–90	20	More than 80	80	(80, 80)
90–100	25	More than 90	60	(90, 60)
100–110	20	More than 100	35	(100, 35)
110–120	10	More than 110	15	(110, 15)
120–130	5	More than 120	5	(120, 5)

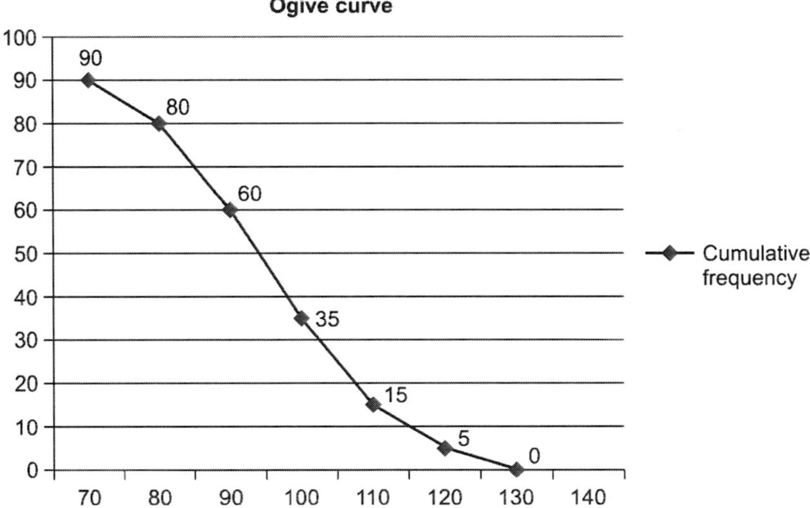

Fig. 12.24: Diagram showing Ogive by more than method

SUMMARY

- Tabulation is an orderly arrangement of data in columns and rows. Rows are horizontal arrangements whereas columns are vertical arrangements. The representation of data in a table is formally referred to as 'tabular presentation.'
- Tabular presentation of data allows data to be organized for further analysis, allows large amounts of raw data to be sorted and reorganized in a neat format, and allows the inclusion of only the most important or relevant data.
- A simple or one-way table contains data of one characteristic only. A simple table is easy to construct and simple to follow. A table, which contains data on two characteristics, is called a ***two way table***. A table, which has more than two characteristics of data is considered as a manifold table.
- Statistical tables can present descriptive or inferential statistics or both. When tables have only textual information in the body, it is known as ***textual tables***. Mock or dummy tables are the tables without any content in the body. It is developed before the data collection and organization to facilitate thinking.
- There are various types of diagrammatic representation of the data. They are line diagram, simple bar diagram, Multiple bar diagram, sub divided bar diagram, broken bar diagram, etc.

- A pie diagram is a circular diagram divided into sectors, illustrating numerical proportion. In a pie chart, the arc length of each sector (and consequently its central angle and area), is proportional to the quantity it represents. Every sector in the graph represents an item in the data that marches the fraction or percentage of the total data set.
- A graph refers to the plotting of different values of the variables on a graph paper which gives the movement or a change in the variable over a period of time.
- A histogram is a graphical representation showing a visual impression of the distribution of data. The histogram is a graphic representation of frequency distribution and is being used to represent simple frequency distribution.
- Frequency polygon is a variation of histogram. It is drawn by joining the midpoints of the interval of corresponding rectangle in a histogram. An ogive is a graph that represents cumulative frequencies or cumulative relative frequencies.

EXERCISE

- Draw a line diagram.

  a.

Marks scored	50	60	65	70	75	80
No. of students	4	10	25	15	10	5

  b.

Hb value	9.5	10	10.5	11.5	12.5	13.5	14.5
Frequency	10	12	20	25	15	10	5

- Draw a bar diagram.

  a. The population details of a village is given below:

Children	Adults	Old age	Antenatal mother
200	1000	200	50

  b. The number of students studying in various courses are given below:

DGNM	BSc (N)	PBBSc (N)	MSc (N)
62	140	60	30

- Draw a multiple bar diagram.

  a. The expenditure details of two students are given below.

Items of Expenditure	**Student A**	**Student B**
Food	1500	2000
Clothing	1000	1000
Travelling expenses	500	250
Stationary	750	500

  b.

Details	**BSc (N)**	**PBBSc (N)**
Admission	100%	50%
Pass	80%	70%
Discontinuation	5%	10%

- Draw a sub divided bar diagram.
  a. The income expenditure details of a College is given below:

Years	Income (in crores)	Expenditure (in crores)
2000	2.5	1.5
2011	3.5	1.6
2012	2.5	1.2
2013	2.0	1.5

- Draw a pie diagram.
  a. The university examination result of a college is as follows:

Result	Distinction	First class	Second class	Third class	Failed
Students(%)	10	30	40	15	5

  b. Nalini's mark in various subjects as follows:

Subject	Education	Management	Research	Statistics	Clinical specialty
Mark(%)	72	80	90	70	75

  c. There are 50 students in a class room. The details of the membership of various program as follows:

Programme	VBDC	YRC	RRC	NSS	Social club
No. of students	12	10	10	10	8

- Draw a histogram for the following data.
  a.

Marks	0–10	10–20	20–30	30–40	40–50	50–60	60–70
No. of students	5	10	20	10	5	10	5

  b.

Hb value	8.5–9.5	9.5–10.5	10.5–11.5	11.5–12.5	12.5–13.5
Frequency	10	20	25	15	10

  c.

Class-interval	10–19	20–29	30–39	40–49	50–59	60–69	70–79
Frequency	5	10	15	10	15	20	25

- Construct a frequency polygon for the following data using histogram.
  a.

IQ	70–80	80–90	90–100	100–110	110–120
No. of students	10	20	25	20	10

  b.

Hb value	8.5–9.5	9.5–10.5	10.5–11.5	11.5–12.5	12.5–13.5
Frequency	10	20	25	15	10

- Construct a frequency polygon without using histogram.

a.

Age in years	10–20	20–30	30–40	40–50	50–60	60–70
No. of patients	20	25	30	25	20	30

b.

Hb value	8.5–9.5	9.5–10.5	10.5–11.5	11.5–12.5	12.5–13.5
Frequency	10	20	25	15	10

- Draw less than and more than ogive for the following.

Marks	0–10	10–20	20–30	30–40	40–50	50–60	60–70
Frequency	2	5	10	20	15	10	8

13 Measures of Central Tendency (Averages)

OBJECTIVES

After reading this chapter, you will be able to:

- List the measures of central tendency
- Explain mean
- Explain median
- Describe mode
- Calculate measures of central tendency.

INTRODUCTION

In research, we collect large volume of data. Statistical analysis requires reduction of large volume of data. One such measure of data, known as measures of central tendency, known as averages represent the characteristics of entire data and also makes further statistical analysis possible. One common feature of any given statistical data is that there is a tendency to concentrate or cluster around some central value on observation which can be taken for some purposes as a representative for whole data. Measures of central tendency (or statistical averages) tell us the point about which items have a tendency to cluster. Such a measure is considered as the most representative figure for the entire mass of data. For example, the weight of the group of one year old infants may cluster around 9 kg. The height of a group of children aged 4 years may cluster around 100 cm. These central values such as 9 kg and 100 cm respectively around which the weight of the infants and height of the 4-year-old children cluster or locate is known as the measures of location or measures of central tendency of the two groups.

MEASURES OF CENTRAL TENDENCY

Measure of central tendency is also known as 'statistical average'. Average is a single figure, which represents the characteristic or general significance of the data. It is the point or location around which individual values of the data cluster. Mean, median and mode are the most popular averages. According to Murry R Speigal, 'Average is a value which is typical or representative of a set of data'. Clark and Sekkade defined, 'Average is an attempt to find one single figure to describe whole of figures'. There are three measures of central tendency (Fig. 13.1). They are mean, median and mode.

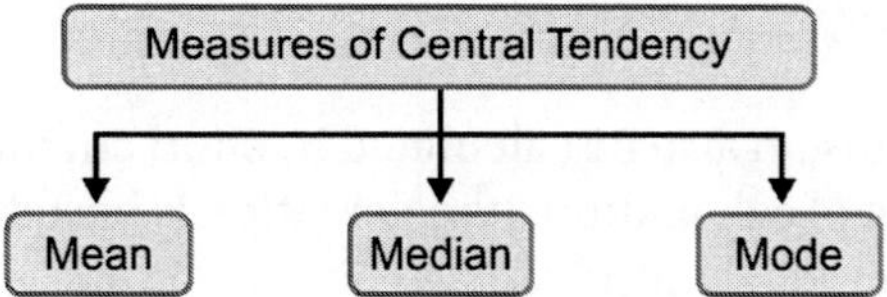

Fig. 13.1: Classification of measures of central tendency

Uses of Average

- Average by its calculation reduces large volume of data into a single value.
- Average gives idea about the entire mass of data since it represents the data.
- It is easy to remember.
- It facilitates comparison of groups and interpretation.
- It helps in estimating value for the population from the sample value.
- It forms the base for further mathematical analysis.

MEAN

We often use the term average in our day-to-day life. For example, the average number of patients attending out patient department, average rain fall in a year, average in patient census, average test performance in a particular subject, etc. The average as a single value is used in all areas to indicate something or to understand something. ***Mean***, also known as arithmetic average, is the most common measure of central tendency.

The 'mean', for a set of data is the sum of the elements in the set divided by the number of elements in the set.

Mean for Series or Ungrouped Data

In case of series of data (ungrouped data), mean is calculated by adding all values of the given observation and dividing by the number of observation. That means finding the sum of all data and dividing it by number of observation/data. We can work it out as under:

$$\text{Mean (or } \overline{X}) = \frac{\Sigma x_i}{n} = \frac{x_1 + x_2 + \ldots + x_n}{n}$$

Where $\overline{X}$ = The symbol we use for mean (pronounced as X bar)
Σ = Symbol for summation
X_i = Value of i item X, i = 1,2,...,n
n = total number of items

For example, the weight of 10 children are as follows:
20, 30, 35, 15, 25, 12, 48, 45, 15, 55
Sum of all observations = 20 + 30 + 35 +15 + 25 + 12 + 48 + 45 + 15 + 55 = 300
Number of children = 10

$$\text{Arithmetic mean} = \frac{\Sigma x_i}{n} = \frac{300}{10} = 30$$

Short Cut Method

The arithmetic mean can also be calculated by short cut method. This method reduces the amount of calculation. Its calculation is based on assumed mean.

For example, the weight of 10 children are as follows:

20, 30, 35, 15, 25 12, 48, 45, 15, 55

The mean can be calculated by the following formula,

$$\overline{X} = A + \frac{\Sigma d}{n}$$

where, A = Assumed mean

n = Number of items

Σd = Σ (X – A), i.e. the sum of deviation of each item from the assumed mean.

In the above example, let us take the assumed mean as 25.

X	X – A
20	20 – 25 = –5
30	30 – 25 = 5
35	35 – 25 = 10
15	15 – 25 = –10
25	25 – 25 = 0
12	12 – 25 = –13
48	48 – 25 = 23
45	45 – 25 = 20
15	15 – 25 = –10
55	55 – 25 = 30
Total =	88 – 38 = 50

$$\overline{X} = A + \frac{\Sigma d}{n} = \overline{X} = 25 + \frac{50}{10} = 25 + 5 = 30$$

Any value, whether existing in the data or not, can be taken as the assumed mean and the final answer would be the same. The answer is not affected by the value selected as the assumed mean. However, in order to simplify the calculations the mid-point of one, the centrally located classes in the given distribution should be selected as the assumed mean.

Calculation of Mean for Discrete Series

To find out the total of items in discrete series, the frequency of each value is multiplied with the respective number or size. The values are totalled up and divided by the number of frequencies to obtain the arithmetic mean.

For example,

Weight (X)	No. of children (f)	fX
15	3	45
16	8	128

Weight (X)	No. of children (f)	fX
17	10	170
18	6	108
19	8	152
20	5	100
Total	40	703

$$\overline{X} = \frac{\Sigma fX}{\Sigma f} = \frac{703}{40} = 17.58$$

Short cut method: Let us assume 17 as assumed mean.

Weight (X)	No. of children(f)	d = (X – A)	fd
15	3	-2	-6
16	8	-1	-8
17	10	0	0
18	6	1	6
19	8	2	16
20	5	3	15
Total	40		23

$$\overline{X} = A + \frac{\Sigma fd}{n} = \overline{X} = 17 + \frac{23}{40} = \overline{X} = 17 + 0.575 = 17.58$$

Mean for Grouped Data or Continuous Series

In case of grouped data (frequency distribution), arithmetic mean is calculated assuming that each observation in a class-interval is equal to the midpoint of the class-interval. It is calculated by the following formula:

$$\overline{X} = \frac{\Sigma f_i x_i}{\Sigma f_i} = \frac{f_1x_1 + f_2x_2 + ... f_nx_n}{f_1 + f_2 + ... + f_{n=n}}$$

or

$$= \frac{\Sigma fx}{\Sigma f}$$

f is the frequency and x is the midpoint of the given class-interval.

For example, the data on age and number of patients are given below. Calculate the mean.

Age of patients	0–10	10–20	20–30	30–40	40–50
Frequency	6	8	10	12	10

Age of patients	Frequency(f)	Mid-value(X)	fx
0 –10	6	5	30
10–20	8	15	120
20–30	10	25	250
30–40	12	35	420
40–50	10	45	450
Total	46		1270

$$\overline{X} = \frac{\Sigma fx}{\Sigma f} = \frac{1270}{46} = 27.6$$

Short cut method: The formula to calculate the mean value is as follows:

$$\overline{X} = A + \frac{\Sigma fd}{n}$$

A = Assumed mean

n = Sum of items

Σd = Σ(X – A), i.e. the sum of deviation of each item from the assumed mean.

In this, let us assume 25 as the assumed mean

Age of patients	Frequency(f)	Mid-value(X)	d = x – a	fd
0 -10	6	5	5 - 25 = -20	-120
10–20	8	15	15 – 25 = –10	-80
20–30	10	25	25 – 25 = 0	0
30–40	12	35	35 – 25 = 10	120
40–50	10	45	45 – 25 = 20	200
Total	46			120

$$\overline{x} = 25 + \frac{120}{46} = 25 + 2.6 = 27.6$$

Open End Classes

In certain cases, the lower limit of the first class-interval and upper limit of the last class-interval are not known and such intervals are termed as open end classes. In such circumstances mean cannot be calculated. If class-intervals are of equal magnitude, then the class should be made accordingly.

For example,

Less than 20

20–40

40–60

60–80

More than 80

Less than 20 can be made as 0–20 and more than 80 can be made as 80 -100.

Less than 15

15–20

20–25

25–30

More than 30

Less than 15 can be made as 10–15 and more than 30 can be made as 30–35.

If the magnitude of class-intervals increases gradually at an even rate, then the same pattern should be adopted.

For example,

Below 10

10–30

30–60
60–100
Above 100
Below 10 can be made as 0–10 and above 100 can be made as 100–150.

If there is no consistency in class-intervals then the first class-interval should be formed on the pattern of the second class-interval and last class-interval on the pattern of the preceeding class-interval.

Below 20
20–35
35–55
55–70
Above 70
Below 20 can be made as 5–20 and above 70 can be made as 70–85.

Merits and Demerits of Mean

Merits

- It is unique. For a given set of data there is only one arithmetic mean.
- It is the best measure to compare the two or more series.
- It is amenable to algebraic treatment and is used in further statistical calculations.
- It is a relatively stable measure of central tendency.
- It is easy to understand and calculate.
- Its calculation is based on all items in the series.
- It is least affected by fluctuations of sampling.
- Arithmetic mean of a group multiplied by the size of the group gives the aggregate value of the group.
- Its formula is rigidly defined and same value is obtained by people whoever calculates it for the given set of data.

Demerits

- It is unduly affected by extreme items.
- It may not coincide with the actual value of an item in a series.
- It may lead to wrong impressions, particularly when the item values are not given with the average.
- It cannot be computed unless all the items are known.
- It cannot be located by observation or the graphic method.
- Mean value cannot be calculated for qualitative data, such as beauty, honesty, etc.

MEDIAN

A more commonly used statistic is the median. As the name suggests, the median is the value in the middle of the distribution, by which we mean that there are equal number of observations above and below the median.

The 'median' is the middle number of a set of data when the numbers are arranged in numerical order.

Median may be defined as the value of that item which divides the series into two equal parts, one half containing values greater than it and the other half containing values less than it. Median is distinct from the arithmetic mean, which is calculated from the value of every item in the series, whereas median is known as a 'positional average'.

Median for Ungrouped Data

Median is the value of the middle item of series (ungrouped data) when it is arranged in ascending or descending order of magnitude in case if it is odd numbers. It divides the series into two halves; in one half all items are less than median, whereas in the other half all items have values higher than median. If the values of the items arranged in the ascending order are: 50, 55, 60,75, 80, 85, 90, 95,100, then the value of the 5th item viz., 80 is the value of median.

If N is odd, the median is the value in position.

Median (M) = Value of $\left(\frac{N+1}{2}\right)$ th item

In the above series, the N is 9. So the position of the median is $\frac{9+1}{2}=\frac{10}{2}=5$. So, the 5th observation of the series is 80 which is the median.

In case of even number of observations, the median is calculated by finding the average of the middle pair of the observation after arranging it in an ascending or descending order of magnitude.

If the values of the items arranged in the ascending order are: 20, 30, 40, 50, 60, 70, then the value of the median is calculated by $\left(\frac{N+1}{2}\right)=\frac{6+1}{2}=\frac{7}{2}\text{th}=3.5$ item which is the size of the average of the 3rd and 4th item which is $\frac{40+50}{2}=\frac{90}{2}$ = 45.

Other Method

If N is even, the median is the average of the values falling in positions, $\frac{N}{2}$ and $\frac{N}{2}+1$.

In the above series, N is 6. So, the position of the median is, $\frac{6}{2}$ and $\frac{6}{2}+1$ i.e. 3rd and 4th position. The values of the 3rd and 4th position are 40 and 50. So, the median is calculated as follows:

$$\frac{40+50}{2}=\frac{90}{2}=45$$

In general, we can use this $\left(\frac{N+1}{2}\right)$ irrespective of odd or even numbers.

In the above example, the median value is $\frac{6+1}{2}$ = 3.5 th item which is the size of the average of the 3rd and 4th item which is $\frac{40+50}{2}=\frac{90}{2}$ = 45.

One concept we must understand. The median value of 45 did not correspond to any observation or value of the series. When N is even the median can be an observed value only if the middle pair of the observations happen to be equal. If the middle pair of the values are unequal, it has to be calculated.

Median for Discrete Data

Calculation of median weight of children:

Weight (X)	No. of children (f)	Cumulative frequency
15	3	3
16	8	11
17	10	21
18	6	27
19	8	35
20	5	40

$$\text{Median} = \text{weight of} \left(\frac{N+1}{2}\right) \text{th child}$$

$$= \left(\frac{40+1}{2}\right) = \frac{41}{2} = 20.5 \text{ ; the weight of 21st child is 17}$$

The median weight of the child is 17 kg.

Median for Grouped Data

When data are grouped, the median is that value at or below which exactly 50% of the observations fall. In case of grouped data, the median is calculated by assuming that the observation in each class-interval are uniformly distributed over that class-interval. The formula for calculating the median for grouped data is:

$$\text{Median} = L + \frac{\frac{N}{2} - F}{f} \times c$$

L is the lower limit of the middle class,
N is the total of observation,
F is the number of observation up to the median class,
f is the frequency of the median class,
c is the interval of median class.

The class-interval that contain the median is called the median class. The median is in the class where the cumulative frequency reaches the sum of the absolute frequencies. That is to say, the median is within the class N/2.

For example,

Age of patients	Frequency (f)	Cumulative frequency
0–10	6	6
10–20	8	14
20–30	**10**	**24**
30–40	12	36
40–50	10	46
Total	46	

$$= \frac{N}{2} = \frac{46}{2} = 23$$

The median item lies in the 20–30.

$$\text{Median} = \frac{L + \frac{N}{2} - F}{f} \times c$$

L = 20; N = 46; F = 14; c = 10; f = 10

Applying the above values in the formula,

$$= 20 + \frac{23 - 14}{10} \times 10$$

$$= 20 + \frac{9}{10} \times 10 = 20 + 0.9 \times 10$$

$$= 20 + 9 = 29$$

$$\text{Median} = 29.$$

Merits and Demerits of Median

Merits

- It is easy to identify and calculate in series of data.
- It is quite rigidly defined.
- There is only one median for a given set of data. The median is always single valued.
- It eliminates the effect of extreme items since those values are not taken into consideration while calculating the median value except for arranging into ascending or descending order.
- The values of the middle items only required to calculate the median. It does not require all items of observation for the calculation of the median value.
- It can be found even for data which cannot be measured quantitatively. For example, if girls are arranged according to their height, the median height is the height of the middle girl.
- Its value generally lies in the distribution.

Demerits

- Median is a positional average. Median is not useful where items need to be assigned relative importance and weights.

- It may not be representative when the distribution is irregular that is the items vary greatly in magnitude. For example, if the runs score by the players of cricket team are 0, 2, 4, 8, 20, 22, 40, 60, 61, 68, 78 the median run score 22 is not the proper representative of the performance.
- It cannot be located with precision when the items are grouped. It can only be estimated and estimated value may not be found in the series.
- The aggregate value of the item cannot be obtained where the median and the number of items are known.
- It requires the data to be arranged first. This is an operation which involves considerable work if the number of item is large.
- It is not amenable to further statistical analysis except in non parametric tests.
- It is not frequently used in sampling statistics.

MODE

Mode is the most commonly or frequently occurring value in a series. The mode in a distribution is that item around which there is maximum concentration. The mode is the number that occurs most often in a set of data.

For example, in the series of data 4, 5, 6, 6, 6, 7, 8 the value 6 is the most commonly occurring or observed value and hence the mode is 6.

If we have a series of data such as 3, 4, 5, 6, 8, 9, 11 in which there is no value which is repeated. In this case, mode is calculated as using the formula

$$\text{Mode} = 3\text{ Median} - 2\text{ Mean}$$

For grouped data, the following formula is used,

$$\text{Mode} = L + \frac{d_1 \times c}{d_1 + d_2} \times 10$$

L is the lower limit of modal class

d_1 = Frequency in modal class - Frequency in the preceding class

d_2 = Frequency in the modal class - Frequency in the succeeding class

C = Class-interval of modal class

In general, mode is the size of the item which has the maximum frequency. Like median, mode is a positional average and is not affected by the values of extreme items. It is, therefore, useful in all situations where we want to eliminate the effect of extreme variations (Table 13.1).

For example:

Age of patients	Frequency (f)	Cumulative frequency
0–10	6	6
10–20	8	14
20–30	10	24
30–40	**12**	**36**
40–50	10	46

Find out the highest frequency in the given frequency distribution and the corresponding class-interval is the modal class-interval. In this highest frequency (12) lies in 30–40 which is the modal class.

$L = 30; d_1 = 12–10; d_2 = 12–10; C = 10$

$$\text{Mode} = L + \frac{d_1 \times c}{d_1 + d_2}$$

$$\text{Mode} = 30 + \frac{2 \times 10}{2 + 2} = 30 + \frac{20}{4} = 30 + 5 = 35$$

$$\text{Mode} = 35$$

If no number occurs more often than the other numbers, then a set of data has no mode. A set of data may have more than one mode. For a set in which there are two modes, it is said to be bimodal, a set of three modes, trimodal and so on.

Table 13.1: Comparison of mean, median and mode

S. No.		Mean	Median	Mode
1.	Average	Calculated	Positional	Positional
2.	Calculation	Includes all observations	Includes middle most observations	Includes most repeated items
3.	Arrangement of data	Not required	Required to be arranged in ascending or descending order	Required to be arranged in ascending or descending order
4.	Influence of extreme values	Affected by extreme values	Not affected by extreme values	Not affected by extreme values
5.	Number	Only one	Only one	One or more than one
6.	Reliability	More reliable	Less reliable	Less reliable
7.	Treatment	Capable of mathematical treatment	Not capable of mathematical treatment	Not capable of mathematical treatment
8.	Utility	Widely used	Not widely used	Not widely used

Merits and Demerits

Merits

- It is easily identifiable. Very often it can be identified by mere observation.
- It is easy to interpret.
- Only the values occurring with high frequency are required to be known for its determination and all values are not required to be known.
- It eliminates the effect of extreme values.
- The existence of more than one mode may give a good indication of the heterogeneity of a population.

Demerits

- It is not amenable to algebraic treatment.
- It is considered unsuitable in cases where we want to give relative importance to items under consideration.
- There may be sometimes more than one mode and then mode has hardly any equity as an average.
- Mode multiplied by the number of items does not yield the total value of the items.
- It is not based on all observation of a series.
- It may not fully representative of a group where the modal frequency occur near an extremity of the range of the variate.
- The mode tells us only the most popular value(s) in the distribution and considers neither the other values nor their frequencies.

SELECTION OF APPROPRIATE MEASURES OF CENTRAL TENDENCY

- If the data are symmetrically distributed or approximately symmetrical anyone of these measures, mean, median, mode may be used since the values are same in case of symmetrical distribution.
- When the distribution of observation is skewed, the arithmetic mean is usually not suitable. In a positively skewed series, the mean gives a higher value than the other two measures and for a negatively skewed series a lower value. It is preferable to use the median than mode.
- When calculation of these measures are required for further statistical analysis, the arithmetic mean has a definite advantage than the other two values.

To practice computation of measures of central tendency for ungrouped data

Find the Mean

To Recapitulate: The mean of a given data is defined as the sum of all the values of the data divided by the total number of values.

$$\text{Mean} = \frac{\text{Sum of all observations}}{\text{Total No. of observations}}$$

The arithmetic mean refers to a measure of central tendencies found by adding all scores and dividing them by the number of scores.

Example 1:

5 3 6 4 6 8 4

Sum of all observations = 36

Total number of observations (N) = 7

Mean = 36/7 = 5.140

Mean = 5.14

Example 2:

10 20 30 10 20 40 50

Sum of all observations = 180

Total number of observations (N) = 7

Mean = 180/7 = 25.71

Mean = 25.71

Example 3:

Compute the mean for the following distribution. The data represents the number of days stay in a hospital as follows:

Days	1	2	3	4	5	6
No.	20	40	50	40	30	20

x	**f**	**fx**
1	20	20
2	40	80
3	50	150
4	40	160
5	30	150
6	20	120

$$\bar{x} = \frac{\Sigma fx}{\Sigma f} = 680/200 = 3.4$$

Short cut method: Let us take assumed mean as 4

X	f	d = X – 4	fd
1	20	–3	–60
2	40	–2	–80
3	50	–1	–50
4	40	0	0
5	30	1	30
6	20	2	40
Total	200		–120

$$\bar{x} = A + \frac{\Sigma fd}{n}$$

$$\bar{x} = 4 + \frac{-120}{200}$$

$$\bar{x} = 4 - 0.6 = 3.4$$

Mean = 3.4

Example 4:

Calculate the mean for the following data. The data represents the number of days of absence/leave by the students for a course in a year.

Number of days Leave/Absent	1	2	3	4	5
Frequency	10	8	6	5	2

x	f	fx
1	10	10
2	08	16
3	06	18
4	05	20
5	02	10
Total	31	74

$$\bar{x} = \frac{\Sigma fx}{\Sigma f} = 74/31 = 2.39$$

Short cut method: Let us take assumed mean as 3

X	f	d = X – 3	fd
1	10	–2	–20
2	08	–1	–08
3	06	0	00
4	05	1	05
5	02	2	04
Total	31		–19

$$\bar{x} = A + \frac{\Sigma fd}{n}$$

$$\bar{x} = 3 + \frac{-19}{31}$$

$$\bar{x} = 3 - 0.61 = 2.39$$

Find the Median of the Following Data

To Recapitulate: The median indicates the middle value of a series of sequentially ordered scores. Because the median divides frequencies into two equal parts, it can also be described as being the fiftieth percentile.

Example 5:

2 5 4 7 4 8 9 5 3

Arrange the data in ascending or descending order as follows:

2 3 4 4 5 5 7 8 9

The median score is the fifth score that is $\left(\frac{N+1}{2}\right) = \frac{9+1}{2} = \frac{10}{2} = 5$. There are 4 counts on both sides of the numerical value 5.

Median = 5

Example 6:

13 14 10 25 19 22 25 15 18

Arrange the data in ascending or descending order as follows:

10 13 14 15 18 19 22 25 25

The median in the above-mentioned is the fifth score that is 18. There are 4 counts on both sides of the numerical value 18.

Median = 18

Example 7:

In cases where you have even numbers, for instance:

14 15 18 10 13 19 29 22 26 25

Arrange the data in ascending or descending order as follows

10 13 14 15 18 19 22 25 26 29

Median $= \frac{10+1}{2} = \frac{11}{2} = 5.5$ (So the average of 5th and 6th item is the median)

There are 2 numerical values indicating the median. By dividing the result by 2, the median can be determined. The fifth score with a numerical value of 18 and the sixth score with the numerical value of 19 are in the middle of the sequentially ordered scores. The median for the above mentioned scores is therefore (18 + 19)/ 2 = 18.5.

Median = 18.5

Example 8:

40 70 80 30 50 60

Arrange the data in ascending or descending order as follows

30 40 50 60 70 80

Median $= \frac{6+1}{2} = 3.5$ (The average of 3rd and 4th item is the median).

There are 2 numerical values indicating the median. By dividing the result by 2, the median can be determined. The third score with a numerical value of 50 and the fourth score with the numerical value of 60 are in the middle of the sequentially ordered scores. The median for the above mentioned scores is therefore (50 + 60)/ 2 = 55.

Median = 55

Example 9:

Find the median of the given data.

Income of the staff	4500	5000	5500	6000	6500	7000	8000
Number of staff	10	11	25	16	15	12	4

Solution:

Income of the staff	Number of staff	Cumulative Frequency
4500	10	10
5000	11	21
5500	25	46
6000	**16**	**62**
6500	15	77
7000	12	89
8000	4	93
Total	93	

Here, the number of observations (n) = 93

The median is $\left(\frac{N+1}{2}\right)$th observation where 'n' is the number of observations.

i.e. $\frac{93+1}{2} = 94/2 = 47$

So, the 47th observation is in 6000. This means 50% of the staffs received the income of less than ₹ 6000 and another 50% received more than ₹ 6000.

Example 10:

Compute the median for the following distribution. The data represents the number of days stay in a hospital as follows:

Days	1	2	3	4	5	6
No.	20	40	50	40	30	20

x	f	Cumulative frequency
1	20	20
2	40	60
3	**50**	**110**
4	40	150
5	30	180
6	20	200

N = 200

Median $= \frac{N+1}{2} = \frac{200+1}{2} = 100.5$, i.e. average of 100th and 101th observation or 100.5th value.

Here, the 100.5th value is in between 60 and 110 of cumulative frequency. So, we take higher cumulative frequency which is 110. The corresponding X value of cumulative frequency 110 is 3.

Therefore, median is 3. Median days stay in the hospital is 3 days.

Example 11:

Calculate the median for the following data. The data represents the number of days of absence/leave by the students for a course in a year.

Number of days Leave/Absent	1	2	3	4	5
Frequency	10	8	6	4	2

x	f	Cumulative frequency
1	10	10
2	**08**	**18**
3	06	24

x	f	Cumulative frequency
4	04	28
5	02	30
Total	30	

N = 30

Median = $\frac{N+1}{2} = \frac{30+1}{2}$ = 15.5, i.e. average of 15th and 16th observation is 15.5th value.

Here, the 15.5th value is in between 10 and 18 of cumulative frequency. So, we take higher cumulative frequency which is 18. The corresponding X value of cumulative frequency 18 is 2. Therefore, median is 2. Median days of leave or absence are 2 days.

Find the Mode

To Recapitulate: The mode is defined to be that number which occurs most frequently in a given data.

Example 12:

3 7 5 8 6 4 5 9 5

Arrange the data in ascending or descending order as follows:

3 4 5 5 5 6 7 8 9

From the above mentioned, the mode equal to 5 because 5 appears to be the most frequent score amongst all the numbers (occurred 3×).

Mode = 5

Example 13:

The weight of the 10 students in class are as follows in (kg):

33 32 35 33 40 33 36 34 39 40

Arrange the data in ascending or descending order as follows

32 33 33 33 34 35 36 39 40 40

Obviously, 33 occurs the most number of times. Hence, mode is 33kg.

Mode = 33 kg

Example 14:

Find the mode of the following data:

90 44 66 88 55 22 33

Arrange the data in ascending or descending order as follows:

22 33 44 55 66 88 90

This data does not possess any value occurring more than once. So, there are no frequently occurring values. Hence, this mode can be calculated by 3-median-2 mean.

$$\text{Mean} = \frac{\Sigma x}{n} = \frac{22+33+44+55+66+88+90}{7} = 56.86$$

$$\text{Median} = \frac{N+1}{2} = \frac{7+1}{2} = \text{4th item} = 55$$

Mode = 3 × 55 – 2 × 56.86

Mode = 165 – 113.72 = 51.28

Mode = 51.28

Example 15:

Compute the mode for the following distribution. The data represents the number of days stay in a hospital as follows:

Days	1	2	3	4	5	6
No.	20	40	50	40	30	20

The mode of a discrete distribution is the value of the variable which shows maximum frequency.
In the above data, 3 is the mode which shows the maximum frequency, 50.

Example 16:

Calculate the mode for the following data. The data represents the number of days of absence/leave by the students for a course in a year.

Number of days Leave/Absent	1	2	3	4	5
Frequency	10	8	6	5	2

The mode of a discrete distribution is the value of the variable which shows maximum frequency.

In the above data, 1 is the mode which shows the maximum frequency, 10.

Find the Measures of Central Tendency for the Grouped Data

Example 17:

Calculate the Mean, Median and Mode for the data given below:

Class-interval	Frequency
21–30	11
31–40	14
41–50	12
51–60	24
61–70	14
71–80	17
81–90	8

Calculation of the Mean: The formula to calculate the mean is $\frac{\Sigma fx}{\Sigma f}$ where f is the frequency and x is the midpoint of the given class-interval.

Class-interval	f	x	fx
21–30	11	25.5	280.5
31–40	14	35.5	497.0
41–50	12	45.5	546.0
51–60	24	55.5	1332.0
61–70	14	65.5	917.0
71–80	17	75.5	1283.5
81–90	8	85.5	684.0
	$\Sigma f = 100$		$\Sigma fx = 5540$

$$\bar{x} = \frac{\Sigma fx}{\Sigma f} = 5540/100 = 55.4$$

Mean = 55.4

Short cut method: The formula to calculate the mean value is as follows:

A = Assumed mean

n = Sum of items

$\Sigma fd = f(X - A)$, i.e. the sum of deviation of each item from the assumed mean.

Let us take assumed mean as 55.5.

Mid value (X)	f	d = X – 55.5	fd
25.5	11	–30	–330
35.5	14	–20	–280
45.5	12	–10	–120
55.5	24	0	0
65.5	14	10	140
75.5	17	20	340
85.5	08	30	240
Total	100		–10

$$\bar{x} = 55.5 + \frac{-10}{100} = 55.5 - 0.10 = 55.4$$

Calculation of the median:

Class-interval	f	Cumulative frequency
21–30	11	11
31–40	14	25
41–50	12	37
51–60	24	61
61–70	14	75
71–80	17	92
81–90	8	100
	$\Sigma f = 100$	

Median = $\frac{100+1}{2}$ = 50.5, i.e. average of 50th and 51th observation or 50.5th value.

Here, the 50.5th value is in between 37 and 61 of cumulative frequency. So, we take higher cumulative frequency which is 61. The corresponding class of cumulative frequency 61 is 51–60 which is the median class.

The formula for calculating the median for grouped data is $L + \frac{\left(\frac{N}{2} - F\right)}{f} \times c$

L is the lower limit of the median class,

N is the total number of observation

F is the number of observation upto the median class

f is the frequency of the median class

c is the class-interval of median class.

The class-interval that contain the median is called the median class. The median class is the one where the average of the lower limit of first class-interval and higher value of the last class-interval falls.

L = 51, N = 100, F = 37, f = 24, c = 10

$$\text{Median} = 51 + \frac{\left(\frac{100}{2} - 37\right)}{24} \times 10$$

$$= 51 + \frac{(50 - 37)}{24} \times 10$$

$$= 51 + \frac{13}{24} \times 10$$

$$= 51 + 130/24 = 51 + 5.4 = 56.4$$

Median = 56.4

Calculation of mode:

The formula to calculate the mode is:

$$\text{Mode} = L + \frac{d_1 \times c}{d_1 + d_2};$$

L is the lower limit of modal class

d_1 = Frequency in modal class-frequency in the preceding class

d_2 = Frequency in the modal class-frequency in the succeeding class

c = Class-interval of modal class

Find out the highest frequency in the given frequency distribution and the corresponding class-interval is the modal class-interval. The maximum frequency 24 lies in the class-interval of 51–60.

L = 51, $d_1 = 24 - 12 = 12$, $d_2 = 24 - 14 = 10$, c = 10

$$\text{Mode} = 51 + \frac{12 \times 10}{12 + 10}$$

$$\text{Mode} = 51 + \frac{120}{22} = 51 + 5.5 = 56.5$$

Mode = 56.5

Example 18:

Calculate the mean, median and mode for the following:

Class-interval	Frequency
65–71	08
72–78	28
79–85	34
86–92	23
93–99	04
100–106	01
107–113	02

Calculation of the mean: The formula to calculate the mean is $\bar{x} = \frac{\Sigma fx}{\Sigma f}$ where f is the frequency and x is the midpoint of the given class-interval.

Class-interval	f	x	fx
65–71	08	68	0544.0
72–78	28	75	2100.0
79–85	34	82	2788.0
86–92	23	89	2047.0
93–99	04	96	0384.0
100–106	01	103	0103.0
107–113	02	110	0220.0
	$\Sigma f = 100$		$\Sigma fx = 8186$

$$\bar{x} = \frac{\Sigma fx}{\Sigma f} = 8186/100 = 81.86$$

$$\text{Mean} = 81.9$$

Short cut method: The formula to calculate the mean value is as follows:

$$\bar{x} = A + \frac{\Sigma fd}{n}$$

A = Assumed mean

n = Sum of items

Σfd = f(X – A), i.e. the sum of deviation of each item from the assumed mean.

Let us take assumed mean as 89.

Midvalue (X)	f	d = X – 89	fd
68	08	–21	–168
75	28	–14	–392
82	34	–07	–238
89	23	0	0
96	04	07	028
103	01	14	014
110	02	21	042
Total	100		–714

$$\bar{x} = 89 + \frac{-714}{100} = 89 - 7.14 = 81.86 = 81.9$$

Calculation of the median

Class-interval	f	Cumulative frequency
65–71	08	08
72–78	28	36
79–85	**34**	**70**
86–92	23	93
93–99	04	97
100–106	01	98
107–113	02	100
	$\Sigma f = 100$	

The formula for calculating the median for grouped data is: $L + \dfrac{\left(\dfrac{N}{2} - F\right)}{f} \times c$

Median = $\dfrac{100 + 1}{2}$ = 50.5, i.e. average of 50th and 51th observation or 50.5th value which falls in the class-interval of 79–85.

L is the lower limit of the middle class

N is the total number of observation

F is the number of observation upto the median class

f is the frequency of the median class

c is the interval of median class.

The class-interval that contain the median is called the median class. The median class is the one where the average of the lower limit of first class-interval and higher value of the last class-interval falls.

L = 79, N = 100, F = 36, f = 34, c = 7.

$$\text{Median} = 79 + \frac{\left(\frac{100}{2} - 36\right)}{34} \times 7$$

$$= 79 + \frac{(50 - 36)}{34} \times 7$$

$$= 79 + \frac{14}{34} \times 7$$

$$= 79 + \frac{98}{34}$$

$$= 79 + 2.88 = 81.88$$

Median = 81.88

Calculation of mode: The formula to calculate the mode is

$$\text{Mode} = L + \frac{d_1 \times c}{d_1 + d_2}$$

L is the lower limit of modal class

d_1 = Frequency in modal class – Frequency in the preceding class

d_2 = Frequency in the modal class – Frequency in the succeeding class

c = Class-interval of modal class

Find out the highest frequency in the given frequency distribution and the corresponding class-interval is the modal class-interval. The highest frequency (34) lies in the class-interval of 79–85.

L = 79 d_1 = 34 – 28 = 6 d_2 = 34 – 23 = 11 c = 7

$$79 + \frac{6 \times 7}{6 + 11}$$

79 + 42/17

79 + 2.47 = 81.47

Mode = 81.47

Example 19:

Calculate mean, median and mode for the following;

No. of Beds	0–10	10–20	20–30	30–40	40–50
No. of Hospitals	10	4	5	3	2

Calculation of the mean

The formula to calculate the mean is $\bar{x} = \frac{\Sigma fx}{\Sigma f}$ where f is the frequency and x is the midpoint of the given class-interval.

Class-interval	f	x	fx
0–10	10	5	50
10–20	4	15	60
20–30	5	25	125
30–40	3	35	105
40–50	2	45	90
	$\Sigma f = 24$		$\Sigma fx = 430$

$$\bar{x} = \frac{\Sigma fx}{\Sigma f} = 430/24 = 17.91$$

Mean = 17.91

Shortcut method: The formula to calculate the mean value is as follows:

$$\bar{x} = A + \frac{\Sigma fd}{n}$$

A = Assumed mean

n = Sum of items

Σfd = f(X – A), i.e. the sum of deviation of each item from the assumed mean.

Let us take assumed mean as 25

Midvalue (X)	f	d = X - 25	fd
5	10	-20	-200
15	04	-10	-040
25	05	0	0
35	03	10	030
45	02	20	040
Total	24		-170

$$\bar{x} = 25 + \frac{-170}{24} = 25 - 7.08 = 17.92$$

Mean = 17.92

Calculation of the Median

Class-interval	f	Cumulative frequency
0–10	10	10
10–20	4	14
20–30	5	19
30–40	3	22
40–50	2	24

The formula for calculating the median for grouped data is: $L + \dfrac{\left(\dfrac{N}{2} - F\right)}{f} \times c$

Median= $\dfrac{24+1}{2}$ = 25/2 = 12.5 th item which is in the class-interval of 10–20.

L is the lower limit of the middle class
N is the total number of observation
F is the number of observation up to the median class
f is the frequency of the median class
c is the interval of median class.

The class-interval that contain the median is called the median class. The median class is the one where the average of the lower limit of first class-interval and higher value of the last class-interval falls.

L = 10, N = 24, F = 10, f = 4, c = 10.

$$\text{Median} = 10 + \frac{\left(\frac{24}{2} - 10\right)}{4} \times 10$$

$$= 10 + \frac{(12 - 10)}{4} \times 10$$

$$= 10 + \frac{2}{4} \times 10$$

$$= 10 + 20/4 = 10 + 5 = 15$$

Median = 15

Calculation of mode: The formula to calculate the mode is:

$$\text{Mode} = L + \frac{d_1 \times c}{d_1 + d_2}$$

L is the lower limit of modal class

d_1 = Frequency in modal class – Frequency in the preceding class

d_2 = Frequency in the modal class – Frequency in the succeeding class

c = class-interval of modal class

Find out the highest frequency in the given frequency distribution and the corresponding class-interval is the modal class-interval. The highest frequency (10) lies in the class-interval of 0–10.

$L = 0, \quad d_1 = 10 - 0 = 10, \quad d_2 = 10 - 4 = 6, \quad c = 10$

$$\text{Mode} = 0 + \frac{10 \times 10}{10 + 6}$$
$$= 0 + (100/16)$$
$$= 0 + 6.25 = 6.25$$
$$\text{Mode} = 6.25$$

Example 20:

Calculate the mean, median and mode.

Weight (x) = 53.9 69 43.8 61.8 55.3 69.6 60.3 59 56.4 66.2 58.8 49.7 54.6 58.8

$$\bar{x} = \frac{\Sigma X}{N} = \frac{817.2}{14} = 58.37$$

Median $= \left(\frac{n+1}{2}\right)$ th item $= \frac{14+1}{2} = \frac{15}{2} = 7.5$th item , the average of 7th and 8th item.

Arrange the data in ascending order.

43.8 49.7 53.9 54.6 55.3 56.4 58.8 58.8 59 60.3 61.8 66.2 69 69.6

$$\text{Median} = \frac{58.8 + 58.8}{2} = 58.8$$

Median = 58.8

Mode = 58.8 (Repeated twice)

Example 21:

Calculate the mean, median and mode.

Height (x) = 158 164 148 158 150 168 160 160 158 168 160 158 160 164

$$\bar{x} = \frac{\Sigma x}{N} = 2234/14 = 159.57$$

Median $= \left(\frac{n+1}{2}\right)$ the item $= \frac{14+1}{2} = 15/2$, the average of 7th and 8th item.

Arrange the data in ascending order.

148 150 158 158 158 158 160 160 160 160 164 164 168 168

$$\text{Median} = \frac{160 + 160}{2} = 160$$

Median = 160

Mode = 158, 160 (each repeated four times)

Example 22:

Calculate the mean, median and mode.

BMI(x) 21.2 20.4 22.8 22 23.4 24.5 25.2 23.6 20.6 22.2 21.6 21.9 22.5 22.8 23.4 23.4 22.8 23.1 24.1 22.9

contd...

contd...

$$\bar{x} = \frac{\Sigma x}{N} = 454.4/20 = 22.72$$

Median $= \left(\frac{n+1}{2}\right)$ th item $= \frac{20+1}{2} = 10.5$th item , the average of 10th and 11th item.

Arrange the data in ascending order.

20.4 20.6 21.2 21.6 21.9 22 22.2 22.5 22.8 22.8 22.8
22.9 23.1 23.4 23.4 23.4 23.6 24.1 24.5 25.2

Median = 22.8 (the 10th and 11th item is same, i.e. 22.8)

Mode = 22.8, 23.4 (each repeated three times)

Choosing the right measure of Central Tendency

When we select the appropriate measure of central tendency, we should keep two factors in mind.

- Nature of data
- Purpose for which the average is required.

The examples given below will explain the selection of right measure of central tendency.

1. Suppose we are given weights of 10 infants as (in kg):
   8.5, 9, 9.4, 10, 8.8, 9, 8.9, 9.8, 9.5, 9
   On observation of the given values, we can understand that there are no extreme values and the range, mode and mean can be used to represent the data correctly. The range is calculated by computing the difference between the highest value and the lowest value. The range is 10 – 8.5 = 1.5 and the mean is:
   $$\frac{8.5+9+9.4+10+8.8+9+8.9+9.8+9.5+9}{10} = \frac{91.9}{10} = 9.19$$
   Mean = 9.19
   Mode = 9
   Mode is usually used as a representative number if the given data has many identical values. One must remember that in similar age groups certain variables also more or less similar and the variation will be less. For example, the height of the two-year-old children will be more or less same as like that of the weight of the infants of 1-year-old. In that case, mode would be an appropriate value to represent a group. Shoe size, shirt size, etc. for similar age group of students can be chosen based on the mode value.
2. Suppose we are given the marks obtained by 9 students in a test are as: 50, 60, 58, 70, 68, 72, 73, 64, 55 and are asked to divide the students based on marks obtained into two groups for some purpose.
   Arrange the values either in ascending or descending order
   50 55 58 60 64 68 70 72 73
   Here, we can use median as the representative value of the group. Those getting less than 64 marks as one group of students and those getting more than 64 marks as the other group of students.

When to use median or when not to use mean: As already discussed, the mean takes into consideration of all the values whereas the median takes only the middle number(s) of observation for its calculation. The mean is susceptible to the influence of outliers or extreme values. In a series of observation, there are values which are unusual compared to the rest of the data set by being small or large in numerical value. For example, consider the salary of staff at a hospital given below:

Staff	1	2	3	4	5	6	7	8	9	10
Salary (in thousands)	10	12	10	12	15	12	16	14	50	50

The mean salary for these ten staff is ₹ 20,100.

The mean salary does not reflect the typical salary of a staff and most of the staffs have salaries in the range of 10–16 thousands. The mean is being skewed by the two large salaries. In this situation, the best measure of central tendency is the median. When the data is skewed, the median is preferred over the mean or mode, i.e. the frequency distribution for our data is skewed. In normal distribution, i.e. when the data is perfectly normal, the mean, median and mode are identical. Moreover, they all represent the most typical value in the data set. However, as the data becomes skewed the mean loses its ability to provide the best central location for the data because the skewed data is dragging it away from the typical value. However, the median best retains this position and is not as strongly influenced by the skewed values. The following table gives information regarding when to use mean/median/mode as a measure of central tendency.

Types of variable	Best measure of central tendency
Nominal	Mode
Ordinal	Median
Interval/Ratio (not skewed)	Mean
Interval/Ratio (skewed)	Median

Understanding of the measures of central tendency in a research

N = 220

Mean value of the physiological variables of children

Age in years	No of children	Pulse	Respiration	Systolic BP	Diastolic Bp	Weight in Kg	Height in cms
13	92	84.32	22.87	102.45	70.24	37.10	137.43
14	77	83.05	22.45	108.10	71.3	42.13	143.51
15	51	82.49	21.98	112.71	75.41	43.62	146.48

The above table shows the mean value of the children in the age group of 13–15 years in respect to their pulse, respiration, systolic and diastolic blood pressure, weight and height. The mean pulse rate was 84 (rounded of) in children in the age group of 13 years whereas it was 83 in 14 years. From this one should learn that out of 92 children for whom the pulse rate was measured the average is 84 which gives a single value which can be compared with the normal value which ranges from 55–85.

Regarding weight the mean value for 13 years was 37.1 kg whereas it was 43.62 for 15 years. The mean weight was calculated for 92 children for 13 years and for 15 years it was calculated from 51 children. This single value help us to compare with the normal values as well as with the other groups. As per Agarwal et al. (2009) in the weight statistics of Indian affluent percentiles, the mean weight (50th percentile) for 13-year-old boy was 39.4 kg, 14-year-old boy was 44.1 kg and 15-year-old boy was 48.6 kg. In this, the mean weight for the ages 13–15 was comparatively lesser.

SUMMARY

- Mean, median and mode are the three popular measures of central tendency. Mean, also known as arithmetic average, is the most common measure of central tendency. In case of series of data (ungrouped data), mean is calculated by adding all values of the given observation and dividing by the number of observation.
- Median is the value of the middle item of series (ungrouped data) when it is arranged in ascending or descending order of magnitude in case if it is odd numbers. It divides the series into two halves; in one half all items are less than median, whereas in the other half all items have values higher than median.
- Mode is the most commonly or frequently occurring value in a series. The mode in a distribution is that item around which there is maximum concentration.
- If the data are symmetrically distributed or approximately symmetrical anyone of these measures, mean, median, mode may be used since the values are same in case of symmetrical distribution.
- When the distribution of observation is skewed, the arithmetic mean is usually not suitable. In a positively skewed series, the mean gives a higher value than the other two measures and for a negatively skewed series a lower value. It is preferable to use the median than mode.
- When calculation of these measures are required for further statistical analysis, the arithmetic mean has a definite advantage than the other two values.

EXERCISES

- Find the Mean, Median and Mode for the following data.
  - 4, 6, 6, 9, 12, 5, 10
  - 7, 8, 13, 4, 7, 8
  - 3, 4, 6, 10, 5, 8, 15
  - 8, 7, 9, 9, 11, 9, 9, 8
  - 300, 24, 36, 40, 50, 60
  - 23, 23, 12, 12, 32, 32
- Find the Mean, Median and Mode for the following data.
  -
Class-interval	Frequency
0 – 10	21
10–20	14
20–30	25
30–40	13
40–50	22
  -
Class-interval	Frequency
100–110	8
110–120	6

120–130	10
130–140	04
140–150	2

-

Age	Frequency
05–10	3
10–15	6
15–20	8
20–25	7
25–30	10

-

Weight in kg	Frequency
45–50	02
50–55	11
55–60	12
60–65	04
65–70	03

- Solve the problems given below:
  - The price list for various nursing books are ₹ 400/-, ₹ 350/-, ₹ 500/-, ₹ 250/- and ₹ 525/-. Find the median price.
  - Find the mode for the following data.
    The common health reasons quoted by the nursing students in their leave application.

Reasons	**Frequency**
Common cold	42
Fever	58
Dysmenorrhea	22
Abdominal pain	14
Diarrhea	26
Vomiting	12
Giddiness	4

  - Find out the median income group from the following data.

No income	Low income	Middle income	Upper income
12	38	88	22

  - The following table represents the marks obtained by a batch of 9 students in a class tests in research and statistics.

S. No.	1	2	3	4	5	6	7	8	9
Research	63	54	50	48	60	46	28	25	48
Statistics	55	58	48	49	30	32	26	20	38

    Indicate in which subject, is the level of achievement higher?

- Answer the following questions
  - Which measure of central tendency is greatest when data is normally distributed?
  - What is the best measure of central tendency when a distribution is skewed?
  - Does all data have all measures of central tendency?
  - When the mean is the ideal measure of central tendency?
  - What measure of central tendency to be used when data has outliers?
  - Which measure of central tendency has more than one value?
  - What is the only measure of central tendency in case of nominal data?

14 Measures of Dispersion

OBJECTIVES

After reading this chapter, you will be able to:
- List the measures of dispersion
- Explain Range
- Explain mean deviation
- Describe inter quartile deviation
- Explain standard deviation

INTRODUCTION

In measures of central tendency, we understood that one of the characteristics of a group of data is to cluster or concentrate around a particular value of the observations. Besides this, the another characteristic is the scatter or dispersion of the data. A group of data can be described on the basis of how the data are scattered and how each value of the series differ from each other and also from the arithmetic mean. This is otherwise known as the measures of dispersion or variability.

MEASURES OF DISPERSION

A measure of dispersion conveys information regarding the amount of variability present in a set of data. If all the values are same, there is no dispersion. The amount of dispersion may be small, when the values, though different are close together. Variation, spread and scatter are synonyms for the word variation. If the values are widely scattered, the dispersion is greater.

According to AL Bowley, dispersion is the measure of the variation of the items. According to Spiegal, dispersion is the degree to which numerical data tend to spread about an average value is called the variation of dispersion of the data. Dispersion is a measure of extent to which the individual items vary said by Connor, LR. Figure 14.1 gives various measures of dispersion.

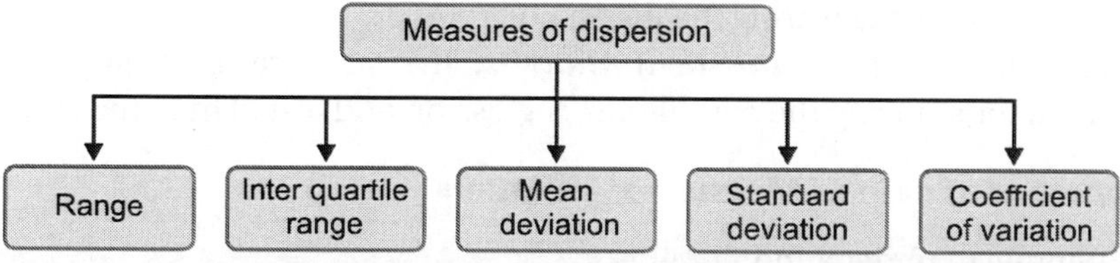

Fig. 14.1: Classification of measures of dispersion

The measures of dispersion are

1. Range
2. Inter quartile Range
3. Mean Deviation
4. Standard Deviation
5. Coefficient of Variation

Concept of Variation

The measures of central tendency such as mean, median, and mode are based on the real value of items of a series and are called Averages of the First Order. The measures of variation are called Averages of the Second Order. To study dispersion, deviations of the size of items from the central tendency are calculated and averaged so as to give an additional knowledge about the formation and composition of the given series. Since the deviations on the basis of central position, are to be averaged, it is known as averages of the second order. The average discovers the representative value of a series and the dispersion finds how individual values are scattered away from the central tendency.

An average by itself has little significance unless the degree of variation in the distribution is known. If the variation is small, an average becomes meaningful and useful; and if the variation is large, the average has only limited significance. In brief, dispersion is a lack of uniformity in the sizes of items of group, and is useful for ascertaining to what extent the average is typical or representative.

Purposes of Measurement of Variation

To test the Reliability of an Average: If the variation is small, an average becomes meaningful and useful; and if the variation is large, average is less reliable and it has only limited significance.

To Serve as a Basis for Control of Variability: When the causes of variation are known, it is easy to control the variation itself. The extreme values of the series influence the standard deviation. When we know to control and avoid those extreme values in an observation, the dispersion will be less and the observations are more or less homogenous.

To Compare Two or More Series with Regard to their Variability: The degree of uniformity or consistency of the data of two independent observations can be compared by measuring the dispersion.

To Facilitate Further Statistical Analysis: The measures of dispersion are essential for studying the correlation, regression and test of hypothesis, etc.

Properties of a Good Measure of Variation

- Simple to understand
- Easy to compute

- Rigidly defined
- Based on all observations
- Amenable for further treatment
- Not affected by extreme observations.

Range

Range is the simplest possible measure of dispersion and is defined as the difference between the values of the extreme items of a series. Thus the value of the range depends upon only the extreme values. It does not take account of any other values other than the extreme values. The occurrence of rare observation greatly influences the value of range. This can be calculated very easily and is easily understood. Thus,

Range = Highest value – Lowest value of the given observation

For grouped data, range is calculated by finding the difference between the lower limit of the first class interval and the upper limit of the last class interval.

Merits

- Like the mode, the range is easy to interpret and simple to compute.
- It is single valued.
- The utility of range is that it gives an idea of the variability very quickly.
- It is an absolute measure of dispersion.

Demerits

- Range is affected greatly by fluctuations of sampling.
- It is not based on all the observations.
- Its value is never stable, being based on only two values of the variable.
- It cannot be applied to open end classes.
- It is not suitable for mathematical treatment.
- Inclusion of any abnormal value in a series affect the range greatly.

For example, if we want to calculate the range of weight of children in a class which varies from 35 to 45 kg, the range is 10 kg. In the same class, if a child who is obese and whose weight is 60 kg (which is rare and abnormal), inclusion of the weight of this child leads to sudden rise of range to 25 kg. As such, range is mostly used as a rough measure of variability and is not considered as an appropriate measure in serious research studies. In spite of this limitation, the use of range is appropriate for certain types of data and certain purposes. The range of oxygen saturation, pulse, temperature and blood pressure which varies from time to time and in different circumstances. According to George W. Snedecor, 'A good guess of the population standard deviation can often be made from the range.' The following table can be referred to calculate the standard deviation when range is known.

If sample N is near this number	This σ is roughly estimated from dividing range by
5	2
10	3
25	4
100	5

(Statistical methods, Indian ed.1961, Allied Pacific, Mumbai, p44).

Example 1:

Find the range and coefficient of range of the weights of 10 children from the following data.

40 18 15 65 72 84 52 35 71 54

Arrange the data in ascending order.

15 18 35 40 52 54 65 71 72 84

Largest value = 84; Smallest value = 15

$$\text{Range} = L - S = 84 - 15 = 69$$

$$\text{Coefficient of Range} = \frac{L-S}{L+S} = \frac{84-15}{84+15} = \frac{69}{99} = 0.696$$

Example 2:

Find the range and coefficient of range of the marks obtained by 50 students given below:

Marks	No. of Students
20–40	10
40–60	20
60–80	15
80–100	05

Largest Value –100; Smallest value –20

Range = L – S = 100 – 20 = 80

$$\text{Coefficient of Range} = \frac{L - S}{L + S} = \frac{100 - 20}{100 + 20} = \frac{80}{120} = 0.667$$

Quartile Deviation or Interquartile Range

The interquartile range of the group of observation is the interval between the values of the upper quartile and the lower quartile for that group. By eliminating the lowest 25% and the highest 25% of items in a series, we are left with the central 50% which are ordinarily free from extreme values. Upper quartile of the group is the value above which 25% of the observation fall. Lower quartile is the value below which 25% of the observations fall. This measure gives us the range which covers the middle 50% of the observations. Unlike the range, the value given by this measure is unaffected by the extreme values. It is important to note that range cannot be computed from a frequency distribution with open end classes at both ends, so quartile deviation is a more suitable measure of dispersion than range. To obtain a measure of variation, we use the distance between the first and third quartiles, i.e. interquartile range, but generally take half of this distance, i.e. semi-interquartile range.

$$\text{Interquartile range} = Q_3 - Q_1$$

Semi-interquartile range or Quartile deviation = $\frac{Q_3 - Q_1}{2}$, where Q_1 = first or lower quartile; Q_3 = third or upper quartile.

Quartile deviation is an absolute measure of dispersion. The relative measure of dispersion, Coefficient of Quartile Deviation is calculated by using the formula = $\frac{Q_3 - Q_1}{Q_3 + Q_1}$

Example 3:

Calculate the semi-interquartile range and quartile coefficient from the following.

Age	20	30	40	50	60	70	80
No.	5	60	130	150	140	50	2

Age in Years	No. of members	Cumulative frequency
20	5	5
30	60	65
40	130	195
50	150	345
60	140	485
70	50	535
80	2	537

$$Q1 = \text{Value of } \frac{N+1}{4} \text{ th item}$$

$$\text{Value of } \frac{537+1}{4} \text{ th item} = \frac{538}{4} \text{ th item} = 134.5\text{th item} = 40 \text{ years}$$

Q3 = Value of $3\frac{N+1}{4}$ th item = $3 \times \frac{538}{4}$ th item = 3×134.5th item = 403.5th item = 60 years

$$\text{Quartile deviation} = \frac{Q_3 - Q_1}{2}$$

$$\text{Quartile deviation} = \frac{60 - 40}{2} = \frac{20}{2} = 10 \text{ years}$$

$$\text{Coefficient of Quartile deviation} = \frac{Q_3 - Q_1}{Q_3 + Q_1}$$

$$= \frac{60 - 40}{60 + 40} = \frac{20}{100} = 0.2$$

Merits

- It is easy to calculate.
- It can be easily understood.
- It is not affected by the extreme values.
- It has a special utility in measuring variation in case of frequency distribution with open end classes at both ends.

Demerits

- It is not based on all the observations.
- It is not the representative value of data.
- It is not capable of algebraic treatments.
- It is affected by sampling fluctuations.
- It gives only a rough measure.

Mean Deviation

Mean deviation is the average of difference of the values of items from some average of the series. It is arithmetic mean of deviations of the observation from the arithmetic mean. Such a difference is technically described as deviation. In calculating mean deviation we ignore the minus sign of deviations while taking their total for obtaining the mean deviation. The mean as the center of a distribution, it was shown that the sum of deviations for x values to the right of mean is equal to the negative of the sum of deviations for x values to the left of the mean and the sum of all deviations from the mean is therefore zero. However, if all deviations were treated as positive value, this property would disappear and mean deviation would become a meaningful index of a variability. Mean deviation can be computed from any one of the three averages such as mean, median and mode. Sometimes mode may be ill defined and as such mean deviation is computed from mean and median.

Mean deviation is, thus, obtained as under:

Mean deviation from mean $(\delta_{\bar{x}}) = \frac{\Sigma|Xi - \bar{x}|}{n}$, if deviations, $|Xi - \bar{X}|$, are obtained from arithmetic average.

Where δ = Symbol for mean deviation (pronounced as delta)

Xi = Xi th values of the variable X

N = Number of items

$\bar{X}$ = Arithmetic average

The formula to calculate Mean Deviation for grouped data is $(\delta_{\bar{x}}) = \frac{\Sigma f|Xi - \bar{x}|}{\Sigma f}$, Xi is the midpoint of the class interval and f is the frequency.

Coefficient of Mean Deviation

When mean deviation is divided by the average used in finding out the mean deviation itself, the resulting quantity is described as the coefficient of mean deviation. Coefficient of mean deviation is a relative measure of dispersion and is comparable to similar measure of other series. Mean deviation and its coefficient are used in statistical studies for judging the variability. It is a better measure of variability than range as it takes into consideration the values of all items of a series. Even then it is not a frequently used measure as it is not amenable to algebraic process.

$$\text{Coefficient of mean deviation} = \frac{\text{Mean deviation}}{\text{Mean or Median or Mode}} \times 100$$

Computation of Mean Deviation

The mean deviation is the mean of the items from an average (mean, median or mode) taking all deviations as positive, ignoring + or – sign.

Example 4:

Find the Mean deviation of 13 12 14 11 15

$$\text{Mean} = \frac{13+12+14+11+15}{5} = 65/5 = 13$$

x	13	12	14	11	15
$X-\bar{x}$	0	–1	1	–2	2

$$\text{Mean deviation from mean} = \frac{6}{5} = 1.2$$

$$\text{Coefficient of Mean deviation} = \frac{\text{Mean deviation}}{\text{Mean}} \times 100$$

$$= \frac{1.2}{13} \times 100 = 9.23$$

Example 5:

Mean Deviation-Discrete Series

Calculate the mean deviation from the following data.

x	2	4	6	8	10
f	1	4	6	4	1

Let us assume 17 as assumed mean.

x	f	fx	$\lvert x-\bar{x}\rvert$	$f\lvert x-\bar{x}\rvert$
2	1	2	4	4
4	4	16	2	8
6	6	36	0	0
8	4	32	2	8
10	1	10	4	4
Total	$N=\Sigma f=16$	$\Sigma fx=96$		$\Sigma f\lvert x-\bar{x}\rvert=24$

$$\text{Mean} = \frac{\Sigma fx}{\Sigma f} = \frac{96}{16} = 6$$

$$\text{Mean Deviation} = \frac{\Sigma f\lvert x-\bar{x}\rvert}{\Sigma f} = \frac{24}{16} = 1.5.$$

Example 6:

Calculate the mean deviation from the following data.

x	2–4	4–6	6–8	8–10
f	3	4	2	1

x	Mid value	f	fx	$\|X - \bar{x}\|$	$f\|X - \bar{x}\|$
2–4	3	3	9	2.2	6.6
4–6	5	4	20	0.2	0.8
6–8	7	2	14	1.8	3.6
8–10	9	1	9	3.8	3.8
Total		$N = \sum f = 10$	$\sum fX = 52$		$\sum f \|x - \bar{x}\| = 14.8$

$$\text{Mean} = \frac{\Sigma fx}{\Sigma f} = \frac{52}{10} = 5.2$$

$$\text{Mean Deviation} = \frac{\Sigma f|x-\bar{x}|}{\Sigma f} = \frac{14.8}{10} = 1.48.$$

Merits

- It is easy to understand and compute.
- Mean deviation is less affected by the extreme values as compared to standard deviation.
- It is based on all items of the series
- It is rigidly defined.
- It can be calculated from any measure of central tendency
- It is a better measure for comparison.

Demerits

- In mean deviation the signs of all deviations are taken as positive and therefore, it is not suitable for further algebraic treatments.
- It is rarely used in social sciences.
- It is often not useful for statistical inferences.

The Variance and Standard Deviation

It is already discussed that when the values are scattered the dispersion is more than they are less scattered. When this measure of dispersion is calculated from the mean it is known as variance. To compute variance, one must find the difference between each value with the mean i.e., to substract each value from the mean and square the resulting differences. Then add the squared difference of each observation and divide by the samples size minus one. This is denoted as S^2

$$S^2 = \frac{\Sigma(x-\bar{x})^2}{n-1}$$

The finite population variance (σ^2) can be calculated by the formula

$$\sigma^2 = \frac{\Sigma(x-\bar{x})^2}{N}$$

When we take the square root of the variance, we can obtain the standard deviation

$$S = \sqrt{s^2}$$

Standard Deviation

Standard deviation is most widely used and important measure of dispersion of a series and is commonly denoted by the symbol 'σ' (pronounced as sigma). Standard deviation is defined as the square-root of the average of squares of deviations, when such deviations for the values of individual items in a series are obtained from the arithmetic average. The deviation from mean is considered without its sign when calculating the mean deviation but in calculating the standard deviation it is squared (Table 14.1). The standard deviation together with arithmetic mean can describe a frequency distribution. A small standard deviation means a high degree of uniformity in the observations as well as homogeneity of the series. It is extremely useful in judging the representativeness of the mean.

Standard deviation is the positive square root of the average of squared deviations taken from arithmetic mean. It is worked out for an ungrouped data or series as under:

$$\text{Standard Deviation } (\sigma) = \sqrt{\frac{\Sigma(x-\bar{x})^2}{n}}$$

Alternatively, we can calculate using the formula, $(\sigma) = \sqrt{\frac{\Sigma x^2}{n} - \left[\frac{\Sigma x}{n}\right]^2}$

For grouped data, it is calculated as under:

$$\text{Standard deviation } (\sigma) = \sqrt{\frac{\Sigma f(x-\bar{x})^2}{\Sigma f}}$$

Variance is calculated by S^2

A large standard deviation means that the items are widely scattered. Under ordinarily circumstances the range, interquartile range, the mean deviation and the standard deviation differ in size. The interquartile range is usually the smallest followed by the mean deviation, the standard deviation and the range, in the order named.

In case of a normal distribution (which is discussed in detail in the later chapter) the sizes of the measures of dispersion bear a definite and known relationship, and in these distributions, the interquartile range is about 2/3 of standard deviation and the mean deviation is about 4/5 of standard deviation. The range has no fixed relation to standard deviation. But as a rough guide, it should not be less than the standard deviation. It should also not be more than 7 times the standard deviation.

Merits

- It is based on all the observatios.
- It is rigidly defined.
- The actual signs of deviations are used.
- It is the most important and widely used measures of dispersion.
- It is the basis for measuring sampling and statistical inferences.
- It has a greater mathematical significance and is capable of further mathematical treatment.

- It is least affected by fluctuation of sampling.
- It provides the unit measurement for the normal distribution.

Demerits

- It is comparatively difficult to compute.
- It is not simple to understand.
- It consumes much time and labor while computing it.
- It is affected by the value of every item in the series.

Uses of Standard Deviation

- In a normal distribution, it is used as a unit for measuring the distance between the mean and any given value of x.
- If we have the values of the mean and standard deviation, then we can calculate the standardized score(Z) by using this formula

$$Z = \frac{x - \overline{x}}{\sigma}$$

x = Values of the individual items

X = Mean

σ = Standard Deviation

Once the scores are standardized, we can compare the individual items, even though they are from different distributions.

- It enables us to determine with a great degree of accuracy, the percentage of values of a frequency distribution within specific ranges under a symmetrical bell shaped curve as shown below:
- About 68% of the values will fall within ± 1 standard deviation from mean.
- About 95% of the values will lie within ± 2 standard deviation from the mean.
- About 99% of the values will lie within ± 3 standard deviation from the mean.

Table 14.1: Comparison between mean deviation and standard deviation

Mean deviation	Standard deviation
Deviations are calculated from mean, median or mode	Deviations are calculated only from mean
Algebraic signs are ignored while calculating mean deviation	Algebraic signs are taken into account
It is simple to calculate	It is difficult to calculate
It lacks mathematical properties, because algebraic signs are ignored	It is mathematically sound, because algebraic signs are taken into account

Calculation of Standard Deviation – Individual Observations

Example 7:

Direct Method (when the deviations are taken from the actual arithmetic mean).

In case of simple series, the standard deviation can be obtained by the formula:

$$\text{Standard Deviation } (\sigma) = \sqrt{\frac{\Sigma(x-\bar{x})^2}{n}}$$

Find the standard deviation of 13 12 14 11 15

$$\text{Mean} = \frac{13+12+14+11+15}{5} = \frac{65}{5} = 13$$

x	13	12	14	11	15
$X-\bar{x}$	0	–1	1	-2	2
$(X-\bar{x})^2$	0	1	1	4	4

Summation of $(X-\bar{x})^2 = 10$

$$\text{Standard Deviation } (\sigma) = \sqrt{\frac{\Sigma(x-\bar{x})^2}{n}} - \sqrt{\frac{10}{5}} = \sqrt{2} = 1.414$$

Example 8:

When the deviations are taken from the assumed mean

Short cut method: The formula to calculate the standard deviation

$$= (\sigma) = \sqrt{\frac{\Sigma d^2}{n} - \left[\frac{\Sigma d}{n}\right]^2}$$

where d = x – A, A = assumed mean, n = total number of observations

The weight of 10 children are as follows:

20, 30, 35, 15, 25 12, 48, 45, 15, 55

In the above example, let us take the assumed mean as 25

x	20	30	35	15	25	12	48	45	15	55
d	-5	5	10	–10	0	–13	23	20	–10	30
d^2	25	25	100	100	0	169	529	400	100	900

$\Sigma d = 50; \Sigma d^2 = 2348$

$$(\sigma) = \sqrt{\frac{\Sigma d^2}{n} - \left[\frac{\Sigma d}{n}\right]^2} = \sqrt{\frac{2348}{10} - \left[\frac{50}{10}\right]^2}$$

$$= \sqrt{234.8 - [5]^2} = \sqrt{234.8 - 25} = \sqrt{209.8} = 14.48$$

Calculation of Standard Deviation–Discrete Series or Grouped Data

Example 9:

Assumed Mean Method or Short cut method

Weight (x)	15	16	17	18	19	20
No. of Children (f)	3	8	10	6	8	5

Let us assume 17 as assumed mean.

x	f	d = X – A	fd	d^2	fd^2
15	3	–2	–6	4	12
16	8	–1	–8	1	8
17	10	0	0	0	0
18	6	1	6	1	6
19	8	2	16	4	32
20	5	3	15	9	45
Total	N = Σf = 40		Σfd = 23		$\Sigma fd^2 = 103$

The formula to calculate the standard deviation = $(\sigma) = \sqrt{\frac{\Sigma fd^2}{n} - \left[\frac{\Sigma fd}{n}\right]^2}$

$$= \sqrt{\frac{103}{40} - \left[\frac{23}{40}\right]^2} = \sqrt{2.575 - [0.575]^2} = \sqrt{2.575 - 0.33} = \sqrt{2.245} = 1.498$$

Example 10:

Step Deviation Method

Systolic BP	102	106	110	114	118	122	126
No. of persons	3	9	25	35	17	10	1

Let us take the assumed mean A = 114

Then $d = \frac{x - A}{i}$, where i = class interval.

Systolic BP	f	$d = \frac{x - 114}{4}$	d^2	fd	fd^2
102	3	–3	9	–9	27
106	9	–2	4	–18	36
110	25	–1	1	–25	25
114	35	0	0	0	0
118	17	1	1	17	17
122	10	2	4	20	40
126	1	3	9	3	9
	N = 100			Σfd = –12	$\Sigma fd^2 = 154$

The formula to calculate the standard deviation = $(\sigma) = \sqrt{\frac{\Sigma fd^2}{n} - \left[\frac{\Sigma fd}{n}\right]^2} \times i$

$$= \sqrt{\frac{154}{100} - \left[\frac{-12}{100}\right]^2} \times 4 = \sqrt{1.54 - [-0.12]^2} \times 4 = \sqrt{1.54 - 0.0144} \times 4 = \sqrt{1.5256} \times 4$$

$$= 1.235 \times 4 = 4.94.$$

Calculation of Standard Deviation-Continuous Series: The standard deviation of a continuous series can be calculated by either Assumed Mean Method or Step Deviation Method.

Assumed Mean Method:

The formula to calculate the standard deviation = (σ) = $\sqrt{\frac{\Sigma fd^2}{n} - \left[\frac{\Sigma fd}{n}\right]^2}$ where $d = m - A$

A = Assumed Mean; m = Middle value, f = Frequency

Step Deviation Method:

The formula to calculate the standard deviation = (σ) = $\sqrt{\frac{\Sigma fd^2}{n} - \left[\frac{\Sigma fd}{n}\right]^2} \times i$ where $d = \frac{m - A}{i}$, where i = class interval.

Example 11:

The data on age and number of patients are given below. Calculate the standard deviation.

Age of patients	0–10	10–20	20–30	30–40	40–50
Frequency	6	8	10	12	10

Let us take the Assumed mean as 15.

Age of patients	m	Frequency (f)	d = m – A	fd	d^2	fd^2
0 –10	5	6	5 – 15 = –10	–60	100	600
10–20	15	8	15 – 15 = 0	0	0	0
20–30	25	10	25 – 15 = 10	100	100	1000
30–40	35	12	35 – 15 = 20	240	400	4800
40–50	45	10	45 – 15 = 30	300	900	9000
		N = 46	Σd = 50	Σfd = 580		Σfd^2 = 15400

The formula to calculate the standard deviation = (σ) = $\sqrt{\frac{\Sigma fd^2}{n} - \left[\frac{\Sigma fd}{n}\right]^2}$ where $d = m - A$

$$= \sqrt{\frac{15400}{46} - \left[\frac{580}{46}\right]^2} = \sqrt{334.78 - [12.61]^2} = \sqrt{334.78 - 159.01} = \sqrt{175.77} = 13.26$$

Example 12:

Step Deviation Method

Age of patients	0–10	10–20	20–30	30–40	40–50
Frequency	6	8	10	12	10

Let us take the Assumed mean as 25; i = 10

$$d = \frac{m-A}{i} = \frac{m-25}{10}$$

Age of patients	m	Frequency(f)	$d = \frac{m-25}{10}$	fd	d^2	fd^2
0–10	5	6	–2	–12	4	24
10–20	15	8	–1	–8	1	8
20–30	25	10	0	0	0	0
30–40	35	12	1	12	1	12
40–50	45	10	2	20	4	40
		N = 46		Σfd = 12		$\Sigma fd^2 = 84$

The formula to calculate the standard deviation = (σ) = $\sqrt{\frac{\Sigma fd^2}{n} - \left[\frac{\Sigma fd}{n}\right]^2} \times i$

where $d = \frac{m-A}{i}$ where i = class interval.

$$= \sqrt{\frac{84}{46} - \left[\frac{12}{46}\right]^2} \times 10 = \sqrt{1.83 - [0.26]^2} \times 10 = \sqrt{1.83 - 0.0676} \times 10 = \sqrt{1.76} \times 10$$

$$= 1.33 \times 10 = 13.3$$

Coefficient of Variation

The standard deviation is useful as a measure of variation within a given set of data. When we want to compare the dispersion in two sets of data which are measured in different units, the coefficient of variation is used. Also the coefficient of variation is used when we want to compare the data sets that have markedly different means. The Coefficient of Variation is the Standard Deviation expressed as a percentage of the arithmetic mean. When variability of the groups of observation is depend on the average size of the group and when the observations are in different units of measurement, this measure of dispersion is adopted to facilitate comparision of the relative variability in different groups. The formula for Coefficient of Variation (CV) for grouped and un grouped data is

$$CV = \frac{\text{Standard Deviation}}{\text{Mean}} \times 100$$

For example when we want to measure the dispersion of height and weight in samples the coefficient of variation is used. The height and weight are used in different units.

$$CV = \frac{\text{Standard Deviation}}{\text{Mean}} \times 100$$

Example 13:

Find the Coefficient of Variation

	Height	**Weight**
Mean	145 cm	48 kg
Standard deviation	5	5

$$\text{Coefficient of variation for height} = \frac{5}{145} \times 100 = \frac{500}{145} = 3.45$$

$$\text{Coefficient of variation for weight} = \frac{5}{48} \times 100 = \frac{500}{48} = 10.4$$

In both height and weight, the measure of dispersion, i.e. the standard deviation is same. But the coefficient of variation is different. The variation is more in weight than the height.

To Recapitulate

Example 14:

Suppose we are given weights of 10 infants as

8.5 kg, 9 kg, 9.4 kg, 10 kg, 8.8 kg, 9 kg, 8.9 kg, 9.8 kg, 9.5 kg, 9 kg

Calculate the Measures of Dispersion for the data given above:

Calculation of Range: Range = Highest value – Lowest value

Range = 10 – 8.5 = 1.5

Range = 1.5

Calculation of Mean Deviation:

$$\text{Mean} = \frac{8.5+9+9.4+10+8.8+9+8.9+9.8+9.5+9}{10} = \frac{91.9}{10} = 9.19$$

Mean value $(\overline{x})$ = 9.2

x value	$\lvert x - \overline{X} \rvert$
8.5	8.5 – 9.2 = 0.7
9.0	9.0 – 9.2 = 0.2
9.4	9.4 – 9.2 = 0.2
10	10 – 9.2 = 0.8
8.8	8.8 – 9.2 = 0.4
9.0	9 .0 – 9.2 = 0.2
8.9	8.9 – 9.2 = 0.3
9.8	9.8 – 9.2 = 0.6
9.5	9.5 – 9.2 = 0.3
9.0	9.0 – 9.2 = 0.2
Total	3.9

$\Sigma\lvert Xi - \overline{X}\rvert$ = 3.9

Mean deviation = 3.9/10 = 0.39

Mean deviation = 0.39

Calculation of Standard deviation:

x-value	$x - \overline{X}$	$(x - \overline{x})^2$
8.5	8.5 – 9.2 = –0.7	0.49
9.0	9.0 – 9.2 = –0.2	0.04
9.4	9.4 – 9.2 = 0.2	0.04
10	10 – 9.2 = 0.8	0.64
8.8	8.8 – 9.2 = –0.4	0.16
9.0	9 .0 – 9.2 = –0.2	0.04
8.9	8.9 – 9.2 = –0.3	0.09
9.8	9.8 – 9.2 = 0.6	0.36
9.5	9.5 – 9.2 = 0.3	0.09
9.0	9.0 – 9.2 = –0.2	0.04
Total		1.99

$$\text{Variance} = 1.99/9 = 0.22$$

$$\text{Standard deviation} = \sqrt{Variance}$$

$$\text{Standard deviation} = \sqrt{\frac{1.99}{9}}$$

$$\text{Standard deviation} = \sqrt{\frac{\Sigma(x-\overline{x})^2}{n-1}}$$

$$\text{Standard deviation} = \sqrt{0.22} = 0.47$$

$$\text{Coefficient of variation} = \frac{\text{Standard Deviation}}{\text{Mean}} \times 100$$

$$\text{Coefficient of variation} = \frac{0.47}{9.2} \times 100 = 0.0511 \times 100 = 5.11$$

Example 15:

Calculate the measures of dispersion for the below mentioned data

Class Interval	Frequency
21–30	11
31–40	14
41–50	12
51–60	**24**
61–70	14
71–80	17
81–90	8

CI	f	x	fx	$(x-\bar{x})$	$(x-\bar{x})^2$	$f(x-\bar{x})^2$	$f\|X-\bar{x}\|$
21–30	11	25.5	280.5	25.5 – 55.4 = –29.9	894.01	11 × 894.01 = 9834.11	328.9
31–40	14	35.5	497.0	35.5 – 55.4 = –19.9	396.01	14 × 396.01 = 5544.14	278.6
41–50	12	45.5	546.0	45.5 – 55.4 = –9.9	98.01	12 × 98.01 = 1176.12	118.8
51–60	24	55.5	1332.0	55.5 – 55.4 = 0.1	0.01	24 × 0.01 = 0.24	2.4
61–70	14	65.5	917.0	65.5 – 55.4 = 10.1	102.01	14 × 102.01 = 1428.14	141.4
71–80	17	75.5	1283.5	75.5 – 55.4 = 20.1	404.01	17 × 404.01 = 6868.17	341.7
81–90	8	85.5	684.0	85.5 – 55.4 = 30.1	906.01	8 × 906.01 = 7248.08	240.8
	100		**5540**			**32099**	**1452.6**

$$\textbf{Mean} = \frac{\Sigma fx}{\Sigma f} = \frac{5540}{100} = \mathbf{55.4}$$

$$\text{Mean deviation} = \frac{\Sigma f\,|Xi-\bar{x}|}{\Sigma f}$$

$$\text{Mean deviation} = \frac{1452.6}{100} = 14.53$$

$$\text{Standard deviation } (\sigma) = \sqrt{\frac{\Sigma f(x-\bar{x})^2}{\Sigma f}} = \sqrt{\frac{32099}{100}} = \sqrt{320.99}$$

$$= 17.92$$

Standard deviation = 17.92

Variance = 320.99

Calculation using Step Deviation Method:

Let us take the Assumed mean as 55.5; i = 9

$$d = \frac{m-A}{i} = \frac{m-55.5}{10}$$

CI	m	Frequency(f)	$d = \frac{m-55.5}{10}$	fd	d^2	fd^2
21–30	25.5	11	–3	–33	9	99
31–40	35.5	14	–2	–28	4	56
41–50	45.5	12	–1	–12	1	12
51–60	55.5	24	0	0	0	0
61–70	65.5	14	1	14	1	14
71–80	75.5	17	2	34	4	68
81–90	85.5	8	3	24	9	72
		100		$\Sigma fd = -1$		$\Sigma fd^2 = 321$

The formula to calculate the standard deviation = $(\sigma) = \sqrt{\frac{\Sigma fd^2}{n} - \left[\frac{\Sigma fd}{n}\right]^2} \times i$

where $d = \frac{m-A}{i}$ where i = class interval.

$$= \sqrt{\frac{321}{100} - \left[\frac{-1}{100}\right]^2} \times 10 = \sqrt{3.21-[-0.01]^2} \times 10 = \sqrt{3.21-0.0001} \times 10$$

$$= \sqrt{3.21} \times 10 = 1.79 \times 10$$

Standard Deviation = 17.91

Calculate the standard deviation.

Class Interval	Frequency
65–71	08
72–78	28
79–85	34
86–92	22
93–99	05
100–106	01
107–113	02

CI	f	X	fX	$(X - \bar{x})$	$(X - \bar{x})^2$	$f(X - \bar{x})^2$
65–71	08	68	544	68 – 82 = –14	196	1568
72–78	28	75	2100	75 – 82 = –7	49	1372
79–85	34	82	2788	82 – 82 = 0	0	0
86–92	22	89	1958	89 – 82 = 7	49	1078
93–99	05	96	480	96 – 82 = 14	196	980
100–106	01	103	103	103 – 82 = 21	441	441
107–113	02	110	220	110 – 82 = 28	784	1568
	100		**8193**			7007

$$\textbf{Mean} = \frac{\Sigma fx}{\Sigma f} = \frac{8193}{100} = \mathbf{81.9}$$

$$\text{Standard deviation } (\sigma) = \sqrt{\frac{\Sigma f(x-\bar{x})^2}{\Sigma f}} = \sqrt{\frac{7007}{100}} = \sqrt{70.07} = 8.4$$

Variance = 70.07

Standard deviation = 8.4

Example 17:

Weight:	53.9	69.0	43.8	61.8	55.3	69.6	60.3	59.0	56.4	66.2	58.8	49.7	54.6	58.8
Height:	158	164	148	158	150	168	160	160	158	168	160	158	160	164

For each variable, compute the standard deviation and coefficient of variation Which set of measurements is more variable weight or height? On what do you base your answer.

For the variable weight

Weight (x)	$(x - \bar{x})$	$(X - \bar{X})^2$
53.9	–4.47	19.98
69	10.63	113
43.8	–14.57	212.28
61.8	3.43	11.76

Weight (x)	$(x - \bar{x})$	$(X - \bar{X})^2$
55.3	–3.07	9.42
69.6	11.23	126.11
60.3	1.93	3.72
59	0.63	0.4
56.4	–1.97	3.88
66.2	7.83	61.31
58.8	0.43	0.18
49.7	–8.67	75.17
54.6	–3.77	14.21
58.8	0.43	0.18
$\Sigma x = 817.2$	Total	651.63

$$N = 14$$

$$\bar{x} = \frac{\Sigma X}{N} = \frac{817.2}{14} = 58.37$$

$$\text{Standard deviation} = \sqrt{\frac{\Sigma(x - \bar{x})^2}{n}} = \sqrt{\frac{651.63}{14}} = \sqrt{46.55}$$

$$= 6.822$$

$$\text{Variance} = 46.55$$

$$\text{Coefficient of variation} = \frac{6.822}{58.36} \times 100 = \frac{682.2}{58.36} = 11.70$$

For variable height

Calculate the standard deviation and coefficient of variation.

Height(x)	$(x - \bar{x})$	$(X - \bar{X})^2$
158	–1.57	2.4649
164	4.43	19.6249
148	–11.57	133.8649
158	–1.57	2.4649
150	–9.57	91.5849
168	8.43	71.0649
160	0.43	0.1849
160	0.43	0.1849
158	–1.57	2.4649
168	8.43	71.0649
160	0.43	0.1849
158	–1.57	2.4649
160	0.43	0.1849
164	4.43	19.6249
2234	Total	417.4286

$$\text{Mean} = \frac{\Sigma X}{n} = \frac{2234}{14} = 159.57$$

$$\text{Standard deviation} = \sqrt{\frac{\Sigma(x-\bar{x})^2}{n}} = \sqrt{\frac{417.43}{14}} = \sqrt{29.82} = 5.46$$

$$\text{Variance} = 29.82$$

$$\text{Coefficient of variation} = \frac{5.46}{159.57} \times 100 = \frac{546}{159.57} = 3.42$$

Weight is more variable than height.

Example 18:

The BMI scores of 20 adolescents are given below.

21.2 20.4 22.8 22.0 23.4 24.5 25.2 23.6 20.6 22.2 21.6 21.9
22.5 22.8 23.4 23.4 22.8 23.1 24.1 22.9

Compute variance, standard deviation and coefficient of variation

BMI(x)	$(x-\bar{x})$	$(X-\bar{X})^2$
21.2	–1.52	2.31
20.4	–2.32	5.38
22.8	0.08	0.01
22	–0.72	0.52
23.4	0.68	0.46
24.5	1.78	3.17
25.2	2.48	6.15
23.6	0.88	0.77
20.6	–2.12	4.49
22.2	–0.52	0.27
21.6	–1.12	1.25
21.9	–0.82	0.67
22.5	–0.22	0.05
22.8	0.08	0.01
23.4	0.68	0.46
23.4	0.68	0.46
22.8	0.08	0.01
23.1	0.38	0.14
24.1	1.38	1.90
22.9	0.18	0.03
454.4		28.53

$$\bar{x} = \frac{\Sigma X}{n} = \frac{454.4}{20} = 454.4/20 = 22.72$$

$$\text{Standard deviation} = \sqrt{\frac{\Sigma(x-\bar{x})^2}{n}}$$

$$\text{Standard deviation} = \sqrt{\frac{28.53}{20}} = \sqrt{1.43} = 1.20$$

$$\text{Variance} = 1.43$$

$$\text{Coefficient of variation} = \frac{\sigma}{\bar{x}} \times 100$$

$$\text{Coefficient of variation} = \frac{1.20}{22.72} \times 100 = \frac{120}{22.72} = 5.28$$

$$\text{Coefficient of variation} = 5.28$$

Example 19:

Compute the mean and standard deviation for the following distribution. The data represents the number of days stay in a hospital as follows:

Days	1	2	3	4	5	6
No.	20	40	50	40	30	20

X	f	fx	$(X - \bar{x})$	$(x - \bar{x})^2$	$f(x - \bar{x})^2$
1	20	20	–2.4	5.76	115.2
2	40	80	–1.4	1.96	78.4
3	50	150	–0.4	0.16	8.0
4	40	160	0.6	0.36	14.4
5	30	150	1.6	2.56	76.8
6	20	120	2.6	6.76	135.2
	200	680			428.0

$$\text{Mean } (\bar{x}) = \frac{\Sigma fx}{\Sigma f} = \frac{680}{200} = 3.4$$

$$\text{Standard deviation} = \sqrt{\frac{\Sigma f(x - \bar{x})^2}{\Sigma f}} = \sqrt{\frac{428}{200}} = \sqrt{2.14} = 1.462$$

Example 20:

Calculate coefficient of variation for the following data

Age of children attended a clinic 9, 12, 10, 11, 8

x	$(x - \bar{x})$	$(x - \bar{x})^2$
9	–1	1
12	2	4
10	0	0
11	1	1
8	–2	4
50		10

$$\bar{x} = \frac{\Sigma x}{n} = \frac{50}{5} = 50/5{=}10$$

$$\text{Standard deviation} = \sqrt{\frac{\Sigma(x - \bar{x})^2}{n}} = \sqrt{\frac{10}{5}} = \sqrt{2} = 1.414$$

$$\text{Coefficient of variation} = \frac{\sigma}{\bar{x}} \times 100$$

$$\text{Coefficient of variation} = \frac{1.414}{10} \times 100 = 14.14$$

$$\text{Coefficient of variation} = 14.14$$

Example 21:

Calculate standard deviation for the following data

17, 20, 15, 13, 25

x	$(x - \bar{x})$	$(x - \bar{x})^2$
17	−1	1
20	2	4
15	−3	9
13	−5	25
25	7	49
90		88

$$\bar{x} = \frac{\Sigma x}{n} = \frac{90}{5} = 18$$

$$\text{Standard deviation} = \sqrt{\frac{\Sigma(x-\bar{x})^2}{n}} = \sqrt{\frac{88}{5}} = \sqrt{17.6} = 4.19$$

Example 22:

Calculate standard deviation for the following data 3, 6, 7, 5, 4

x	$(x - \bar{x})$	$(x - \bar{x})^2$
3	−2	4
6	1	1
7	2	4
5	0	0
4	−1	1
25		10

$$\bar{x} = \frac{\Sigma x}{n} = \frac{25}{5}$$

$$\text{Standard deviation} = \sqrt{\frac{\Sigma(x-\bar{x})^2}{n}} = \sqrt{\frac{10}{5}} = \sqrt{2} = 1.414$$

Application in Research

Range gives quick idea about the minimum and the maximum value of the data. When we write our findings, we write with the standard deviation with the mean value. For example, we write that the samples had a mean knowledge score of 60 with the standard deviation of 6. We should understand that the average knowledge score is 60% and the sample knowledge score is deviated for the value of 6. A large standard deviation score indicates that the data are very much scattered from the mean whereas a small standard deviation score indicates that the data are almost similar and are less scattered. The mean and standard deviation value helps to understand and describe the nature of samples' data. Mean and standard deviation are the important sample statistics which are used in estimation of parameters and hypothesis testing.

SUMMARY

- A measure of dispersion conveys information regarding the amount of variability present in a set of data. If all the values are same, there is no dispersion.
- The measures of dispersion are range, interquartile range, mean deviation, standard deviation and coefficient of variation. Range is the simplest possible measure of dispersion and is defined as the difference between the values of the extreme items of a series. For grouped data, range is calculated by finding the difference between the lower limit of the first class interval and the upper limit of the last class interval.
- The interquartile range of the group of observation is the interval between the values of the upper quartile and the lower quartile for that group. Upper quartile of the group is the value above which 25% of the observation fall. Lower quartile is the value below which 25% of the observations fall.
- Mean deviation is the average of difference of the values of items from some average of the series. It is arithmetic mean of deviations of the observation from the arithmetic mean.
- Standard deviation is the positive square root of the average of squared deviations taken from arithmetic mean. It is worked out for an ungrouped data or series by using the formula: Standard Deviation (σ) = $\sqrt{\frac{\Sigma(x-\overline{x})^2}{n}}$. For grouped data, it is calculated using the formula: Standard deviation (σ) = $\sqrt{\frac{\Sigma f(x-\overline{x})^2}{\Sigma f}}$.
- Variance is calculated by S^2. A large standard deviation means that the items are widely scattered.
- The Coefficient of Variation is the Standard Deviation expressed as a percentage of the arithmetic mean.

EXERCISE

I. State whether the following statements are True or False:
   1. Coefficient of variation is expressed in same units as the original data.
   2. Variance is the square of standard deviation.
   3. Mean deviation can be a negative value.
   4. Median divides the total frequency into two equal parts.
   5. Range is the best measure of dispersion.
   6. Quartile deviation is more suitable in case of open end deviation.

II. Solve the problems
   1. Find the range of weight of 10 students from the following:
      40 10 15 65 50 60 40 35 55 40

2. Compute the quartile deviation and its coefficient from the following data.

Height in inches	58	59	60	61	62	63	64
No. of students	14	20	32	30	20	22	10

3. Calculate the mean deviation (deviation from mean)

X	2	4	6	8	10
f	2	8	10	8	2

4. Calculate the mean deviation (deviation from mean)

Size of the item	Frequency
3–4	3
4–5	7
5–6	20
6–7	50
7–8	40
8–9	30
9–10	10

5. Calculate the range and standard deviation for the following data
   12 20 15 22 16 14 21 17
6. Calculate the range and standard deviation for the following data

Classes	10–20	20–30	30–40	40–50	50–60
Frequency	6	7	10	8	4

7. Students in college A has scored an average of 68 marks with the standard deviation of 4 marks. Students in college B has scored an average of 70 with the standard deviation of 6. Find which college students' performance is more consistent.
8. Calculate the standard deviation for the following frequency distribution

Class Interval	0–4	4–8	8–12	12–16
Frequency	4	8	2	2

9. Find the standard deviation and coefficient of variation for the following data.

Size	10	11	12	13	14	15	16
Frequency	2	7	11	15	10	4	1

10. Calculate the Mean Deviation and Standard Deviation

Age	20–25	25–30	30–35	35–40	40–45
No. of staffs	50	40	35	20	20

11. Calculate the standard deviation from the following data.

Class interval	5–10	10–15	15–20	20–25	25–30
Frequency	20	10	30	40	20

12. Calculate the coefficient of variation for the following.

	Hospital A	Hospital B
No. of Staffs	200	160
Average monthly income	₹ 7500	₹ 8000
Standard deviation	₹ 50	₹ 30

Find in which hospital there is a greater variability in payment?

13. Calculate the coefficient of variation for the following.

	Village A	Village B
No. of People	2000	1500
Average income	₹ 3000	₹ 2800
Variance	₹ 100	₹ 81

15 Measures of Skewness and Kurtosis

OBJECTIVES

After reading this chapter, you will be able to:
- Explain the measures of skewness
- Explain the measures of kurtosis

INTRODUCTION

In the distribution of data, the measures of location and dispersion are quantitative concepts. We have learned the technique of calculating the measures of location and dispersion when the series of data are given. It is easy to calculate the above vlaues for any given series of data by forming frequency distribution and tabulation. The measures of dispersion fail to reveal whether the scatter of values on either side of the mean is symmetrical or not. At the same time, when these data are plotted on a graph, it may give rise to frequency polygon which assumes a shape. The graphic features of a distribution are most commonly described in terms of two properties called ***skewness*** and ***kurtosis***.

MEASURES OF SKEWNESS (ASYMMETRY)

The word 'skewness' means 'lack of symmetry' or 'absence of symmetry'. It helps us to study the shape of the distribution. Skewness is a measure that refers to the extent of symmetry or asymmetry in a distribution.

A distribution is said to be symmetrical when its mean, median and mode are identical. When the portion of a frequency polygon to the right of the mean is the mirror image of the portion to the left, the distribution is said to be ***symmetrical distribution***. The normal distribution assumes a bell-shaped curve and symmetrical in nature. The mean, median and mode are identical in a normal distribution (Fig. 15.1A). But, practically, a frequency distribution may not be normal and may be asymmetrical in nature. The curve may be deviated to either right or left side. If more observations lie on one side of the mean than on the other side, the distrbution is said to be skewed. If more observations lie to the left of the mean, the distribution is typically balanced (at the mean) by a long tail to the right and the distribution is said to be positively skewed or skewed to the right (Fig. 15.1C). If more observations lie on the right side of the mean, the longer tail extends to the left

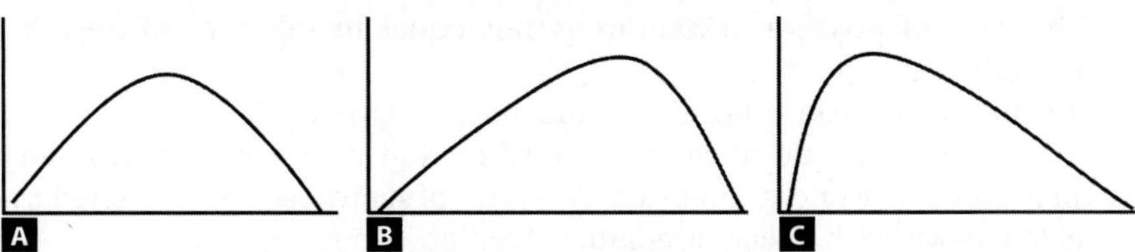

Figs 15.1A to C: A. Normal distribution, **B.** Negatively skewed, **C.** Positively skewed

and the distribution is said to be negatively skewed or skewed to the left (Fig. 15.1B). A distribution which is not symmetrical is said to be an ***asymmetrical distribution***. It is also known as ***skew distribution***.

In statistics, the scores that are far above or below the middle score of any distribution are called the ***extreme scores***. In normal distribution, the extreme scores have a relatively low frequency. In the language of statistics, the far left and right portions of a normal curve containing the relatively low frequency, extreme scores are called the ***tails of the distribution***.

A skewed distribution is similar in shape to a normal distribution except that it is not symmetrical. The left half of the polygon is not a mirror image of the right half. Instead, a skewed distribution has only one pronounced tail.

A negatively skewed distribution contains extreme low scores that have low frequency, but does not contain extreme high scores that have low frequency. On the other hand, a positively skewed distribution contains extreme high scores that have low frequency, but does not contain extreme low scores that have low frequency.

If the curve has a longer tail towards the right or when the curve of the distribution is deviated to the right side, the skewness will be positive since the mean will be greater than the mode or median. If the curve has a longer tail towards the left side or when the curve of the distribution is deviated to the life side, the skewness will be negative since the mean will be less than the median or mode.

An unimodal distribution can be divided into three parts—the ***left tail***, the ***middle part*** and the ***right tail***. In case of symmetrical distribution, the two tails are of equal length. But in asymmetrical distribution, one tail is longer than the other. A bimodal distribution is symmetrical distribution that contains two distinct humps reflecting relatively high-frequency scores. At the center of each hump is a score that occurs more frequently than the surrounding scores and technically the center scores in each hump have the same frequency. Such a distribution would occur with test scores, for example, most students scoring around 60 or 80, with fewer students failing or scoring 70s or 90s.

Tests of Skewness

The skewness is present if :

- Mean ≠ Median ≠ Mode
- The quartiles are not equidistant from Median

- The sum of positive deviations is not equal to the sum of negative deviations.
- The frequencies on either side of the mode are unequal.

The calculation of the measures of the direction and degree of asymmetry are measures of skweness. Thus, the measures of skewness are calculated by

a. Mean–Mode; b. Mean–Median; c. Median–Mode

In case of positive skewness, we have (Mode) Z < (Median) M < (Mean) $\overline{X}$ and in case of negative skewness, we have X < M < Z. Skewness is measured as follows:

Skewness = $\overline{X}$ - Z and its coefficient is worked out by dividing the skewness by standard deviation, which is known as Pearonian Coefficient of Skewness.

$$= \frac{\overline{X}-Z}{\sigma} = \frac{\text{Mean}-\text{Mode}}{\text{Standard deviation}}$$

$$\text{Mode} = 3\text{ Median} - 2\text{ Mean}$$

$$= \frac{\text{Mean}-(3\text{ Median}-2\text{ Mean})}{\text{Standard deviation}}$$

In case mode is not well-defined, then we can work out skewness by :

Skewness = 3(X - M) and its coefficient is worked out by dividing the skewness by the σ value.

$$= \frac{3(\overline{X}-M)}{\sigma} = \frac{3(\text{Mean}-\text{Median})}{\text{Standard deviation}}$$

Interpretation of Pearson's Coefficient of Skewness

- Its value is rarely very high and usually lies between -1 and +1.
- When its value is zero, there is no skewness.
- When its value is negative, the distribution is negatively skewed.
- When its value is positive, the distribution is positively skewed.

Type of distribution	Skewness
Symmetrical distribution	Zero
Distribution skewed to right	Positive
Distribution skewed to left	Negative

Karl Person's Coefficient of Skewness Based on Mean

Example 1:

The weights of 10 children are as follows:

20, 30, 35, 15, 25 12, 48, 45, 15, 55

The mean can be calculated by the following formula:

$$x = A + \frac{\Sigma d}{n}$$

A = Assumed mean

n = Number of items

Σd = (X – A), i.e. the sum of deviation of each item from the assumed mean.

In this example, let us take the assumed mean as 25

Weight (X)	d = (X – A)	d²
20	20 – 25= –5	25
30	30 – 25 = 5	25
35	35 – 25 = 10	100
15	15 – 25= –10	100
25	25 – 25 = 0	0
12	12 – 25 = –13	169
48	48 – 25 = 23	529
45	45 – 25 = 20	400
15	15 – 25 = –10	100
55	55 – 25 = 30	900
Total	50	2348

$$\bar{x} = A + \frac{\Sigma d}{n}$$

$$x = 25 + \frac{50}{10} = 25 + 5 = 30$$

$$\text{Standard Deviation} = \sqrt{\frac{\Sigma d^2}{n} - \left[\frac{\Sigma d}{n}\right]^2} = \sqrt{\frac{2348}{10} - \left[\frac{50}{10}\right]^2}$$

$$= \sqrt{234.8 - 25} = \sqrt{209.8} = 14.4844$$

$$\text{Skewness} = \frac{\bar{X} - \text{Mode}}{\sigma} = \frac{30 - 15}{14.5} = \frac{15}{14.5} = 1.03$$

Example 2:

Weight (X)	No. of children (f)	d = (X – a)	fd	fd²
15	3	–2	–6	12
16	8	–1	–8	08
17	10	0	0	0
18	6	1	6	06
19	8	2	16	32
20	5	3	15	45
Total	40		23	103

Let us assume 17 as assumed mean.

$$\bar{x} = A + \frac{\Sigma fd}{n}$$

$$\bar{x} = 17 + \frac{23}{40}$$

$$\bar{x} = 17 + 0.575 = 17.58$$

$$\text{Standard deviation} = \sqrt{\frac{\Sigma fd^2}{N} - \left[\frac{\Sigma fd}{N}\right]^2} = \sqrt{\frac{103}{40} - \left[\frac{23}{40}\right]^2}$$

$$= \sqrt{2.58 - [0.575]^2} = \sqrt{2.58 - 0.33} = \sqrt{2.25} = 1.5$$

$$= \frac{\overline{X} - \text{Mode}}{\sigma} = \frac{17.58 - 17}{1.5} = \frac{0.58}{1.5} = 0.387$$

Example 3:

The marks scored by 9 students in two subjects were as given below. Determine which subject mark is more skewed.

Subject	Mean	Standard Deviation	Mode
Nursing Management	55	16	58
Nursing Research	53	15.5	49

$$\text{Nursing Management} = \frac{\overline{X} - \text{Mode}}{\sigma} = \frac{55 - 58}{16} = \frac{-3}{16} = -0.188$$

$$\text{Nursing Research} = \frac{\overline{X} - \text{Mode}}{\sigma} = \frac{53 - 49}{15.5} = \frac{4}{15.5} = 0.258$$

The distribution of marks of Nursing Research is more skewed.

Karl Person's Coefficient of Skewness Based on Median

Example 4:

Age of patients	Frequency (f)	Cumulative frequency
0–10	6	6
10–20	8	14
20–30	**10**	**24**
30–40	12	36
40–50	10	46
Total	46	

In this let us assume 25 as the assumed mean

Age of patients	Frequency (f)	Mid-value (x)	d = x – A	fd	fd²
0–10	6	5	5 – 25 = -20	–120	2400
10–20	8	15	15 – 25 = –10	–80	800
20–30	10	25	25 – 25 = 0	0	0
30–40	12	35	35 – 25 = 10	120	1200
40–50	10	45	45 – 25 = 20	200	4000
Total	46			120	8400

$$\overline{x} = \overline{x} = A + \frac{\Sigma fd}{n}$$

$$= 25+\frac{120}{46} = 25 + 2.6 = 27.6$$

$$N/2 = 46/2 = 23$$

The median item lies in the range 20–30.

$$\text{Median} = L+\frac{\frac{N}{2}-F}{f}\times c$$

$$= 20+\frac{23-14}{10}\times 10$$

$$= 20 + \frac{9}{10}\times 10 = 20 + 0.9 \times 10$$

$$\text{Median} = 29.$$

$$\text{Standard Deviation} = \sqrt{\frac{\Sigma fd^2}{N}-\left[\frac{\Sigma fd}{N}\right]^2} = \sqrt{\frac{8400}{46}-\left[\frac{120}{46}\right]^2}$$

$$= \sqrt{2.58-[2.61]^2} = \sqrt{182.61-6.81} = \sqrt{175.8}$$

$$= 13.26$$

$$= \frac{3(\bar{X}-M)}{\sigma} = \frac{3(\text{Mean}-\text{Median})}{\text{Standard deviation}}$$

$$= \frac{3(27.6-29)}{13.26} = \frac{3\times -1.4}{13.26} = \frac{-4.2}{13.26} = -0.317$$

Example 5:

Calculate the coefficient of skewness for the data given below and test whether the two distributions have the same degree of skewness.

	Mean	Median	Standard Deviation
Distribution 1	100	90	10
Distribution 2	90	80	10

Coefficient of Skewness for Distribution 1 = $\frac{3(\bar{X}-M)}{\sigma} = \frac{3(100-90)}{10} = \frac{3\times 10}{10} = \frac{30}{10} = 3.$

Coefficient of Skewness for Distribution 2 = $\frac{3(\bar{X}-M)}{\sigma} = \frac{3(90-80)}{10} = \frac{3\times 10}{10} = \frac{30}{10} = 3.$

Hence, both the distributions have the same degree of skewness.

MEASURES OF KURTOSIS

It is the measure of 'flat-toppedness' or 'peakedness' of a curve. These measures show the extent to which the ditribution (when plotted on a graph) is more peaked or less peaked than the normal curve. In a frequency distribution, when the curve is unusually peaked, it is known as leptokurtic (Fig. 15.2A). In leptokurtic distribution, most of the observations are concentrated near the mode. If, on the other hand, the curve is more flat-topped than normal, it is known as platykurtic (Fig. 15.2C). The normal curve is known as mesokurtic

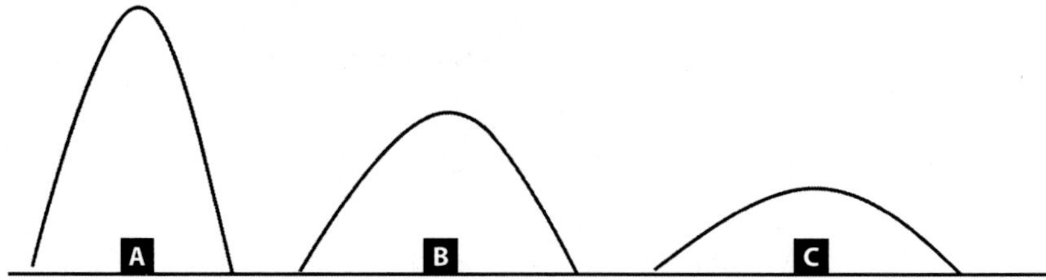

Figs 15.2A to C: **A.** Leptokurtic, **B.** Mesokurtic, **C.** Platykurtic

(Fig. 15.2B). The condition of peakedness or of flat-toppedness itself is known as kurtosis or excess.

> The words 'kurtosis', 'leptokurtic', 'mesokurtic' and 'platykurtic' are derived from Greek. 'Kurtosis' means 'curvature'; 'leptos' means 'slender'; 'mesos' means 'middle' and 'platys' means 'broad'.

Significance of Kurtosis

Kurtosis of the population influences the type of average to use for a sample. If the population is very leptokurtic, the median is appropriate; if the population is approximately mesokurtic, the arithmetic mean should always be used; if the population is very platykurtic, the mid range (i.e. the arithmetic mean of the smallest and the largest items) should be used. Kurtosis is generally greater when the observations cluster within one standard deviation of the mean and it is zero if the observations lie exactly at the mean.

SUMMARY

- The calculation of the measures of the direction and degree of asymmetry are measures of skewness. The normal distribution assumes a bell-shaped curve and is symmetrical in nature. The mean, median and mode are identical in a normal distribution.
- When the curve of the distribution is deviated to the right side, skewness will be positive since the mean will be greater than the mode or the median. When the curve of the distribution is deviated to the left side, skewness will be negative since the mean will be less than the median or mode.
- In case of positive skewness, we have (Mode) $Z <$ (Median) $M <$ (Mean) X and in case of negative skewness, we have $X < M < Z$.
- Kurtosis is the measure of 'flat-toppedness' or 'peakedness' of a curve. These measures show the extent to which the distribution (when plotted on a graph) is more peaked or less peaked than the normal curve. Based on the peakedness of the curve, a distribution may be classified as leptokurtic, mesokurtic and platykurtic.

EXERCISE

- Calculate Karl Pearson's Coefficient of Skewness for the following data of marks obtained by five students.

1	2	3	4	5
10	16	33	20	16

- Calculate Karl Pearson's Coefficient of Skewness for the following data:

X	10–15	15–20	20–25	25–30	30–35	35–40	40–45	45–50
f	8	14	16	20	30	32	15	6

- Calculate Karl Pearson's Coefficient of Skewness
  Mean = 72; Median = 75 and Standard deviation = 12
- From a moderately skewed distribution of retail price for Nurse's shoes, it is found that the mean price is ₹ 200 and the median price is ₹ 180. If the coefficient of variation is 20% find the pearsonian coefficient of skewness of the distribution.
- Calculate the standard deviation from the following information.
  Mean = 45; Median = 48 and Coefficient of skewness = –0.4.

16 Measures of Relationship—Correlation Coefficient

OBJECTIVES

After reading this chapter, you will be able to:

- List the measures of relationship
- Explain the meaning of correlation coefficient
- List the types of correlation
- Explain the methods of studying the correlation

INTRODUCTION

In research, a researcher may want to study about single variable or sometimes more than one variable. When a researcher wants to study more than one variable, she may be interested to study the relationship between the two variables. Practically, two variables may be related or unrelated. For example, we have studied that there exists some relationship between age and blood pressure, height and weight, food intake and weight gain, intelligence and test score, etc. When studying the relationship, one can study the nature and strength of relationships between variables. There are two statistical techniques, such as correlation and regression analysis available to study the relationship between two variables.

If we have the data on two variables, i.e. for every measurement of a variable, X, if we have corresponding value of a second variable Y, in such a situation, we are generally interested in knowing:

(i) whether there exists any correlation or association between the two variables, and

(ii) whether one of the two variables is the cause and the other the effect.

The first question is answered by the use of correlation and association techniques and the second question by the technique of regression (Fig. 16.1). Correlation analysis is the study of relationship between two or more variables. It is the co-variation of two variables. The measure of correlation is called ***correlation coefficient***.

MEASURES OF RELATIONSHIP

In our observation of data, we can find some relationship between the variables. In order to find the relationship, we have to have observation for each variable and the relationship is computed using the two observations which is the measure of two variables. For example, there is a relationship between height and weight. The relationship can be assessed in terms of nature and strength. Correlation coefficient is used to investigate the relationship between the two variables.

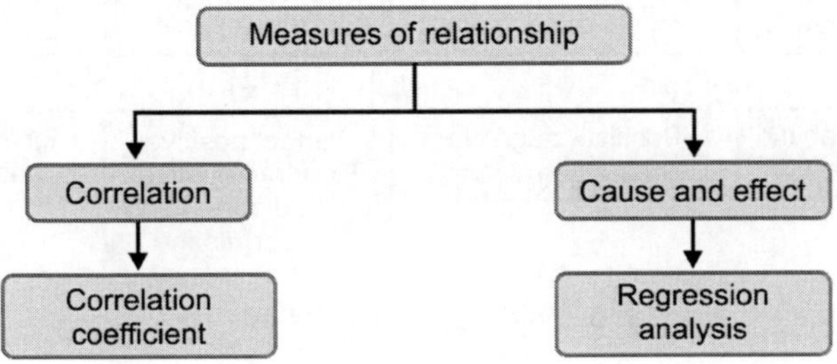

Fig. 16.1: Classification of measures of relationship

CORRELATION

Correlation is the relationship between two variables such that a change in one variable results in a direct or inverse change in the other variable. Also the variables are said to be correlated if greater the magnitude of change in one variable corresponds to greater the magnitude of change in the other variable. However, if the second variable does not change by a change in the first, then these variables are called statistically independent, e.g. the increase in rainfall does not affect the students' marks in nursing subject and, hence, these are statistically independent.

According to Ya Lun Chou, "Correlation analysis is to determine the degree of relationship between variables."

According to AM Tuttle, "Correlation is an analysis of the covariation between two or more variables."

Correlation attempts to determine the degree of relationship between the variables.

Significance of Study of Correlation

- In nursing, we study many variables and try to find the relationship between them in order to understand the nature of variables and also manipulate and see whether change in one variable causes change in another variable.
- We can test whether the relationship is statistically significant and can reduce the level of uncertainty in our prediction.
- Sampling error can also be calculated.
- Correlation is the basis for the concept of regression and ratio of variation.

Types of Correlation

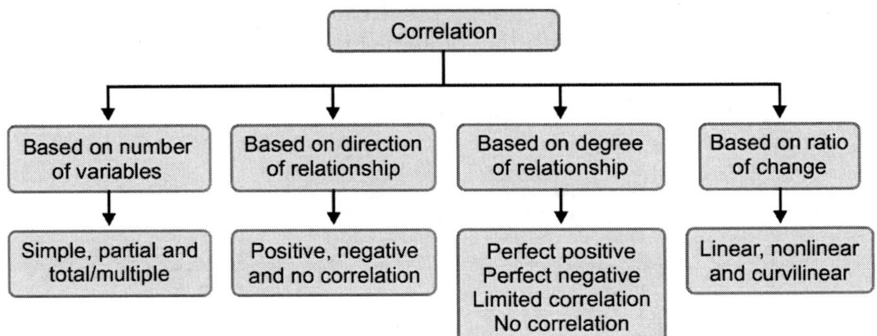

Fig. 16.2: Types of correlation

Based on the Number of Variables Studied

- ***Simple correlation:*** The study of the relationship between only two variables is known as ***simple correlation***. Examples height and weight.
- ***Partial correlation:*** The study of two variables excluding other variables is known as ***partial correlation***.
- ***Total correlation:*** In this, all variables are taken into consideration and usually more than two variables are included. Examples height, weight and food intake (Fig. 16.2).

Based on the Direction of Relationship

- ***Positive or negative correlation:*** When an increase (or decrease) in one variable corresponds to an increase (or decrease) in the other variable, then the correlation is said to be positive (or direct). If the two variables move together in the same direction, the correlation is called ***positive correlation***. It is negative (or inverse) when increase (or decrease) in one vatriable corresponds to decrease (or increase) in the other variable. In negative correlation, the two variables tend to move in opposite direction.
- ***Linear or nonlinear correlation:*** If the change in one variable is always a fixed ratio to the change in the other variable, the correlation is said to be linear. If the change in one variable is not normal to the ratio of the change in the other variable then the correlation is said to be ***nonlinear*** or ***curvilinear (Fig. 16.2)***.
- ***Degree of correlation:*** To find the degree of correlation, correlation coefficient is to be calculated. The different degrees of correlation are as follows:

(a) ***Perfect correlation:*** If the two variables change in the same direction ie with the increase in one, the other also increases and vice versa, and in the same ratio, then there is perfect positive correlation. The correlation cofficient is +1.

If the two variables change in the same ratio, but in opposite directions, i.e. with the increase in one, the other decreases and vice versa, there is a perfect negative correlation and the correlation coefficient is –1.

(b) ***Absence of correlation:*** If the change in one variable has no effect on the other variable, then the correlation is completely absent and we call it ***no correlation***. The correlation coefficient is zero.

(c) ***Limited correlation:*** If r is not equal to 0, –1, and 1 it is said to be limited correlation. In this, the correlation coefficient lies numerically between 0 and 1. $0 < r < 1$ or $-1 < r < 0$.

If r is positive, it is positive correlation and if r is negative, it is negative correlation.

The limited correlation is of the following three degrees.

- ***High degree:*** $\pm 0.75 < r < \pm 1$. If r lies between ± 0.75 and ± 1.0, it is high degree.
- ***Moderate degree:*** If r lies between ±0.25 and ±0.75, then it is of moderate degree.
- ***Low degree:*** 0 and ± 0.25, it is low degree.
- ***Spurious correlation:*** In a small sample, the correlation is due to pure chance. A high degree of mathematical correlation can be obtained even at the time when there is no relationship between the variables. For example, there might be a high degree of relationship between the number of pregnant mother and the car produced. It may be only a chance of coincidence and such type of correlation is called nonsensical or spurious correlation. There is no logical relationship.

Measurement of Correlation

Correlation can be studied through the following methods:

1. Scatter diagram
2. Simple graph
3. Cross tabulation
4. Charles Spearman's coefficient of correlation (rank correlation)
5. Karl Pearson's coefficient of correlation

Scatter Diagram

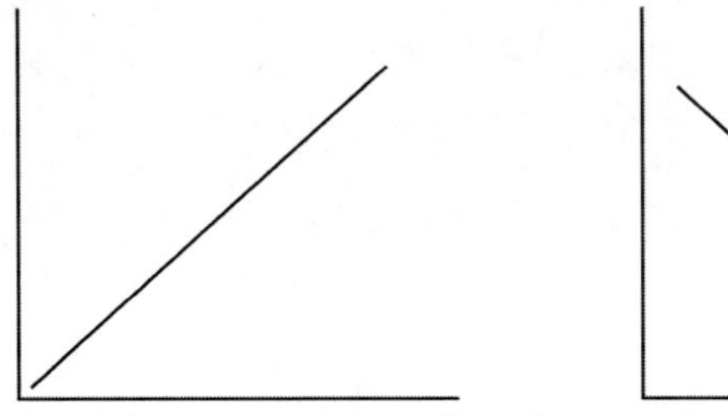

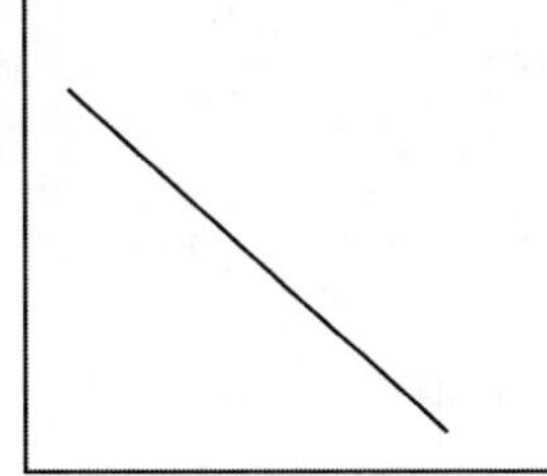

Perfect Positive Correlation (r = 1) Perfect Negative Correlation (r = –1)

This is the simplest method of finding out whether there is any relationship present between two variables by plotting the value on a chart, known as scatter diagram. It is studied by plotting the values on a graph paper. One variable is plotted on the horizontal axis (x) and the other is plotted on the vertical (y) axis. We can assess the correlation by connecting the dots. This graph is known as ***scatter diagram***. It is in the form of dots. So, it is also called ***dotograph***. When the values of the two variables are marked in a graph, we can analyze the relationship between the two variables by assessing the nature of the scattering or clustering of data. The configuration of the point on the graph will indicate the nature of the relationship. If the plotted points form a straight line running from the lower left-hand corner to the upper right-hand corner, then there is a perfect positive correlation. On the other hand, when this straight line shows a downward trend, i.e. from left upper to right lower, we can understand that it shows a negative relationship.

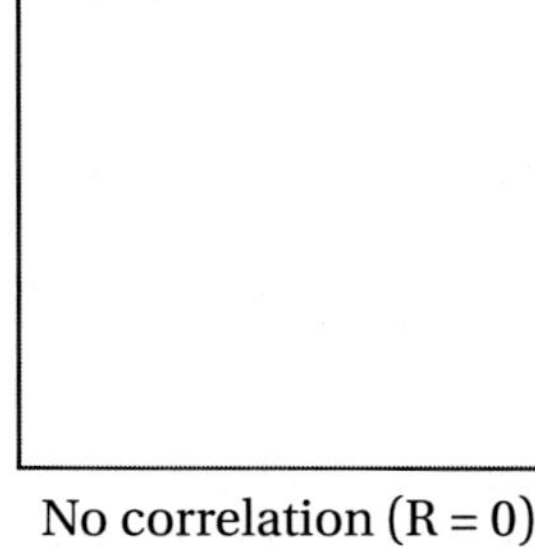

No correlation (R = 0)

If the points or dots lie scattered randomly, the absence of any relationship between these is suggested. If, on the other hand, the points lie clustered along a line or curve, existence of the relationship is suggested.

In case of a linear relationship between the variables, there is a tendency of the data to lie cluster along a straight line, known as the ***regression line***. Sometimes, there might be a curvilinear relationship too between the variables. It is often good idea to create a scatter diagram of the data before computing correlation, to see if the relationship between two variables is linear. If it is linear, the scatter plot will more or less resemble a straight line. While a scatter plot can aid in detecting linear or curvilinear relationships, it is often true that significant correlations may exist even though they cannot be detected by visual analysis alone. Scatter diagram is one of the easy and simple methods to study the relationship. Also it is not affected by the extreme values. The limitation of this is that it only gives a rough idea about the relationship.

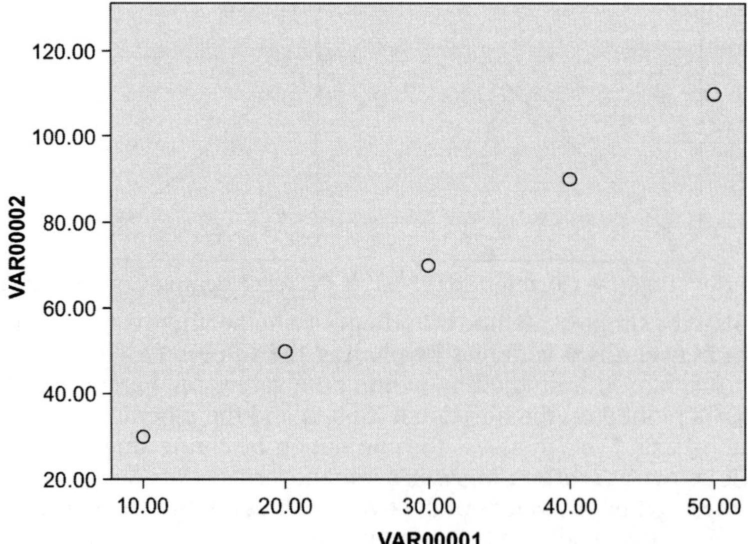

Scatter diagram showing the perfect positive relationship between two variables (r = 1).

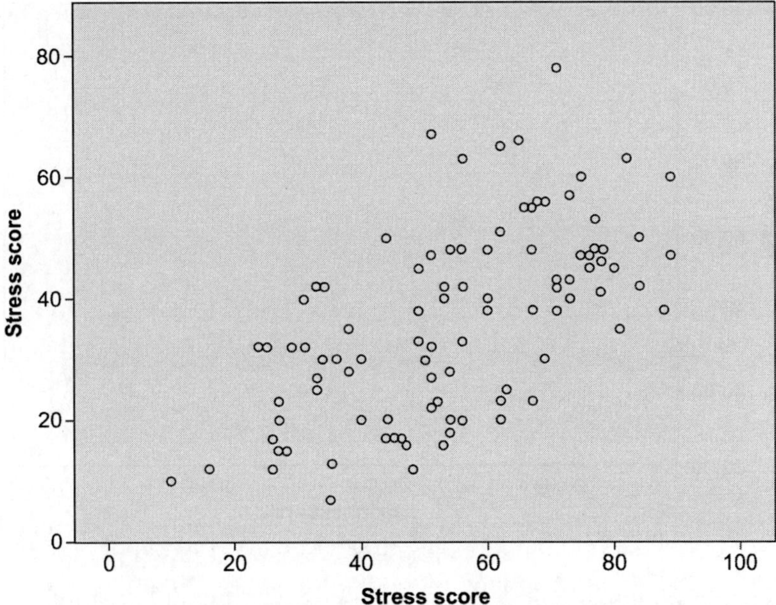

Scatter diagram showing the positive relationship between aggression and stress in children. The calculated r value is 0.626 (Correlation is significant at 0.01 level).

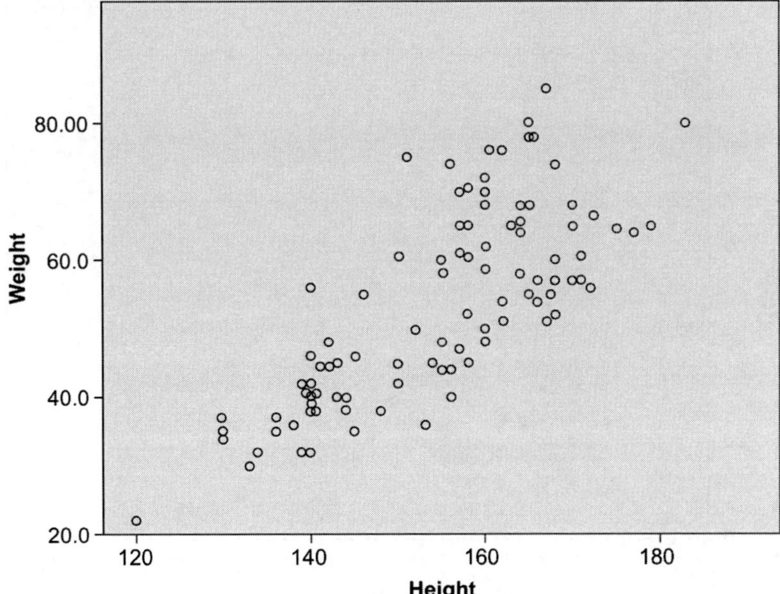

Scatter diagram showing the positive relationship between height and weight of the children. The calculated r value is 0.77 (Correlation is significant at 0.01 level).

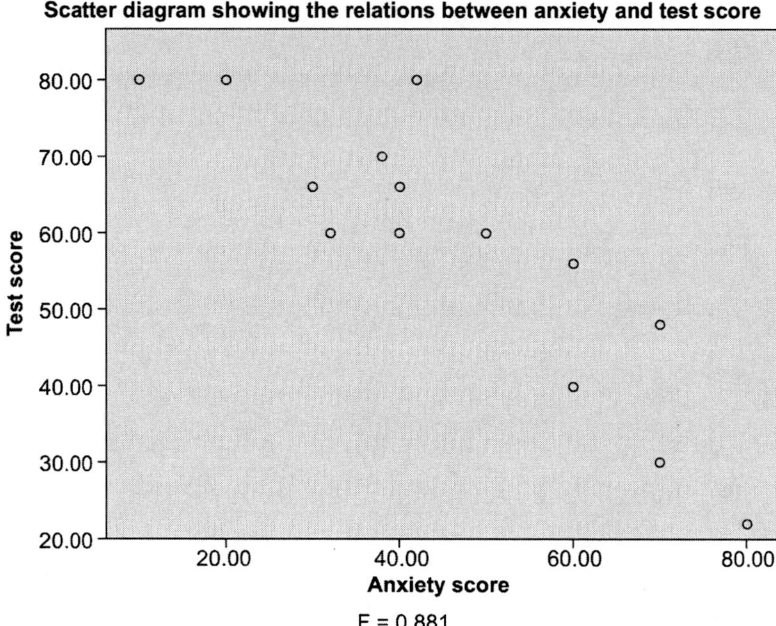

Scatter diagram showing the negative relationship between the anxiety and test score (r = – 0.881)

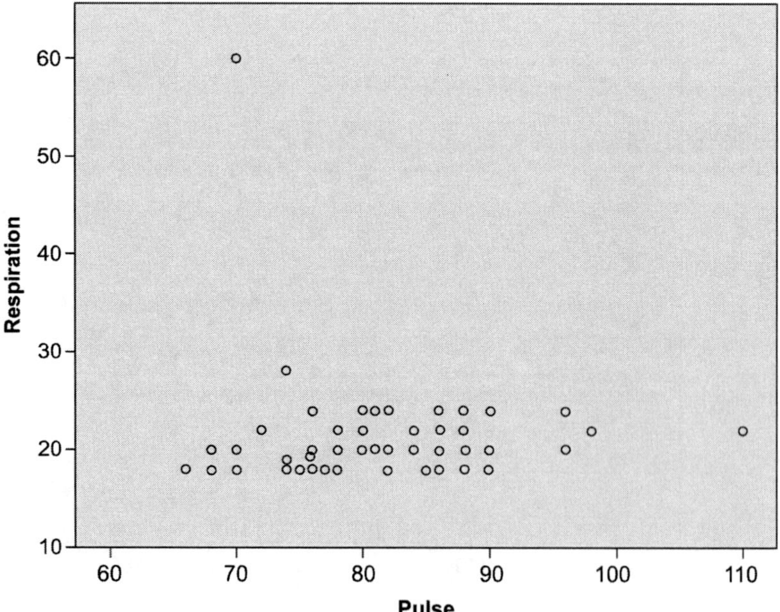

Scatter diagram showing the relationship between pulse and respiration of the children. The calculated r value is – 0.024.

Simple Graph

The values of the two variables are plotted on a graph paper. We get two curves, one for x variables and another for y variables. These two curves reveal the direction and closeness of the two curves and also reveal whether or not the variables are related. If both the curves move in the same direction, i.e. parallel to each other, either upward or downward, correlation is said to be positive. On the other hand, if they move in the opposite direction, then the correlation is said to be negative.

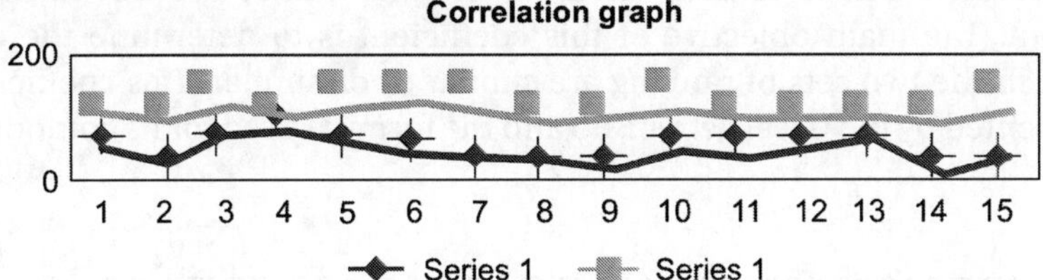

The above method is used in case of time series. This method also does not reveal the extent to which the variables are related.

Cross Tabulation

Cross-tabulation approach is specially useful when the data are in nominal form. Under it, we classify each variable into two or more categories and then cross-classify the variables in these sub-categories. Then we look for interactions between them, which may be symmetrical, reciprocal or asymmetrical. A symmetrical relationship is one in which the two variables vary together, but we assume that neither variable is due to the other. A reciprocal relationship exists when the two variables mutually influence or reinforce each other. Asymmetrical relationship is said to exist if one variable (the independent variable) is responsible for another variable (the dependent variable). The cross-classification procedure begins with a two-way table, which indicates whether there is or there is not an interrelationship between the variables.

Spearman's Coefficient of Correlation (or Rank Correlation)

In our day-to-day life, we may come across certain characteristics/variables which are not measurable in quantitative terms, e.g. honesty, character, beauty, etc.—also, its human tendency to rank objects, characteristics or items in order of its merits. We even rank individuals based on their performance, their talents, functional ability, etc. Similarly, various objects, such as advertisements, color combinations, jokes and pictures may be put in order of merit for aesthetic quality, beauty, humor or some other characteristics. Ranking can also be applied to numerical data (e.g. scores). We may give rank 1 to the individual with the highest score, 2 to the next lower, and so on. Spearman's coefficient of correlation (also called ***rank correlation***) is the technique of finding the degree of correlation in all such cases of ordinal data. Charles Spearman's coefficient of correlation (or rank correlation) is the technique of determining the degree of correlation between two variables in case of ordinal data, where ranks are given to the different values of the variables. Rank correlation is a nonparametric technique for measuring relationship between paired observations of two variables when data are in the ranked form. It can be used when the data are irregular or extreme items are erratic or inaccurate. The result of rank correlation is only an approximate one, because under ranking method, original values are not taken into account. The main objective of this coefficient is to determine the extent to which the two sets of ranking are similar or dissimilar. This coefficient is represented by the Greek letter Rho and the formula used for its computation is:

$$\text{Spearman's coefficient of corrrelation (or r)} = 1-\left[\frac{6\sum d_i^2}{n(n^2-1)}\right]$$

Where d_i = difference between ranks of ith pair of the two variables.

n = number of pairs of observations.

or

$$\rho = 1-\left[\frac{6\sum d^2}{N^3-N}\right]$$

where ρ represents Spearman's coefficient, Σd^2 the sum of the squared differences between pairs of ranks and N the number of pairs of observations.

The value of this coefficient always lies between +1 and –1. If the concordance between rankings is perfect, Σd^2 will equal 0 and ρ will be +1. If the discordance is perfect (Σd^2) will always be twice (N^3 – N) and ρ will be –1.

Two points are of interest when applying the rank correlation coefficient. First, it does not matter whether we rank the observation in ascending or descending order. However, we must use the same rule of ranking for both variables. Second, if two (or more) observations have the same value, we assign to them the mean rank.

Merits of Rank Correlation Coefficient

- It is simple to understand and easy to calculate.
- It is very useful if the data are qualitative in nature, such as intelligence, beauty, etc.
- If ranks are given, it is easy to calculate.

Demerits of Rank Correlation

- It cannot be used in case of bivariate distribution.
- If the number of items are more, assigning rank becomes difficult and also the calculation is difficult.

Karl Pearson's Coefficient of Correlation

Karl Pearson's coefficient of correlation (or simple correlation) is the most widely used method of measuring the degree of relationship between two variables. This coefficient assumes the following:

- There is linear relationship between the two variables;
- The two variables are casually related, which means that one of the variables is independent and the other one is dependent;
- A large number of independent causes are operating in both variables so as to produce a normal distribution;
- If the error of measurement is reduced to the minimum, the coefficient of correlation is more reliable.

Karl Pearson's coefficient of correlation, also known as simple linear correlation or the Product Moment, is used to discover the extent of correspondence of movement or concomitant variation in the paired values of any two series. Such variation (in the same or in opposite direction) may exist in a number of cases, such as age and blood pressure, height and weight, supply and price, and so on. It should, however, be remembered that, by itself, correlation establishes only covariation. It does not determine which variables may be the cause of the other or covariables of the two may be due to a third variable or it may be the result of chance.

Karl Pearson's coefficient of correlation can be worked out thus:

$$\text{Karl Pearson's coefficient of correlation (or r)} = \frac{\sum(x_i-\bar{x})(y_i-\bar{y})}{n\,\sigma_x\,\sigma_y}$$

Alternatively, the formula can be written as:

$$r = \frac{1/n\Sigma xy - \bar{x}\,\bar{y}}{Sx\ Sy}$$

Sx is standard deviation of x and is Sy standard deviation of y.

or $$r = \frac{\Sigma xy}{\sqrt{\Sigma x^2\ \Sigma y^2}}$$

$$x = (x-\bar{x})$$
$$y = (y-\bar{y})$$

The value of 'r' lies between ±1. Positive values of r indicates positive correlation between the two variables (i.e. changes in both variables take place in the same direction), whereas negative values of 'r' indicate negative correlation, i.e. changes in the two variables taking place in the opposite directions. A zero value of 'r' indicates that there is no correlation between the two variables. When r = (+)1, it indicates perfect positive correlation and when it is (–)1, it indicates perfect negative correlation, meaning thereby that variations in independent variable (X) explain 100% of the variations in the dependent variable (Y). We can also say that for a unit change in independent variable, if there happens to be a constant change in the dependent variable in the same direction, then correlation will be termed as ***perfect positive.*** But if such change occurs in the opposite direction, the correlation will be termed as perfect negative. The value of 'r' nearer to +1 or –1 indicates high degree of correlation between the two variables.

It should, however, be remembered at the time of interpreting this coefficient that it is not a measurement on a scale of equal units. Hence, one cannot say that a correlation of +0.9 is three times as close a relationship as +0.3 or an increase in correlation, say, from +0.3 to +0.5 in one case is the same as an increase from +0.6 to +0.8 in another case. One can say only that in both the cases, there is an increase in the closeness of the variables but not necessarily to the same degree. It is to be noted that r = 0 does not mean that there does not exist any relation between two variates. The variates may be related other than nonlinear relation.

Merits

- Karl Pearson's method is the most popular mathematical method used for measuring the degree of relationship.
- The coefficient of correlation summarizes in one figure the degree of correlation and its direction.
- Moreover, we can estimate the value of the dependent variable from the known value of the independent variable.

Demerits

- The assumption of linear relationship between variables is not affected, whether it is correct or not.
- Like standard deviation, the value of the coefficient is unduly affected by extreme items.

Coefficient of Correlation and Probable Error

To find out the reliability or the significance of the value of pearsonian coefficient of correlation, probable error is used.

Probable Error of r = $0.6745\frac{1-r^2}{N}$, where 0.6745 is a constant number.

r = Pearsonian coefficient of correlation

N = Number of pairs

The limits for population correlation coefficient are r ± P.E(r).

Functions of Probable Error

- If the value of r is less than the probable error, the value of r is not at all significant.
- If the value of r is more than six times the probable error (r = 6PE), the value of r is significant.
- If the probable error is less than 0.3, the correlation should not be considered at all.
- If the probable error is small, the correlation is definitely existing.

Conditions for the Use of Probable Error

- The number of items should be large enough. When the number of pairs of observation is small, the probable error may lead to fallacious conclusions.
- The distribution should have a normal bell-shaped curve.
- The items in the sample must have been selected by random sample method and in an unbiased manner.

Standard error is considered better than the probable error and the formula is:

$$\text{Standard Error of r} = \frac{1-r^2}{\sqrt{N}}$$

- ***Partial Correlation:*** A partial correlation coefficient measures the relationship between any two variables, when all other variables connected with those two are kept constant. It is the process of finding the correlation between two variables after the influence of other variables has been controlled for. Suppose, if we want to assess the correlation between the intelligence and the test performance, we can keep the year of study as a constant, since a 4th-year student can do better than the first-year student.

Purposes of Correlation Analysis

- It helps in studying the relationship between two variables.
- It measures the degree of relationship between the variables.
- The relationship can be tested for its significance.
- For ethical and practical considerations, some relationships can be studied only through a correlational design.
- It is useful for discovering a new relationship.
- It is conducted in natural setting unlike laboratory experiments which creates artificial situation.
- It provides greater external validity.
- It is the basis for the concept of regression (dealt in detail in Chapter 17).

Limitations of the Coefficient of Correlation 'r'

- The above formula for r applies only when the relationship between the variables (X and Y) is linear.
- The coefficient does not establish any causal relationship between the variables, that is to say, it does not prove which is the dependent and which is the explanatory variable.

  Knowledge of the value of r alone does not enable us to predict the value of Y from X. A high correlation between variables Y and X may describe any one of the following situations:
  - Variation in X is the cause of variation in Y;
  - Variation in Y is the cause of variation in X;
  - There is two-way causation;
  - There is another common factor (Z) that affects X and Y in such a way as to show a close relation between them;

- The correlation between X and Y is due to chance. This is called ***spurious correlation***, which does not show any causal relationship between the variables involved. Thus, a high correlation found between the number of births and the number of murders in a country does not mean that one is determined by the other. It simply shows that the two figures covary.

Correlation does not necessarily indicate causation. Sometimes causation is clear. If height and weight are correlated, it is clear that additional height causes additional weight. Gaining weight is not known to increase one's height. There are other settings where direction of causality is likely but open to question. Sometimes it is difficult to have any idea of what causes what. For example, hard work and productivity is correlated. Does hard work result in productivity or else productivity leads to hard work?

Example 1:

Find out the correlation coefficient for the weight (x) and height (y) of seven adolescent boys.

Weight (kg)	32	52	44	38	57	65	52
Height (cms)	139	158	155	148	170	158	168

(x)	**(y)**	**X^2**	**Y^2**	**xy**	**$(x-\bar{x})$**	**$(x-\bar{x})^2$**	**$(y-\bar{y})$**	**$(y-\bar{y})^2$**	**$(x-\bar{x})(y-\bar{y})$**
32	139	1024	19321	4448	−16.6	275.56	−17.6	309.76	292.16
52	158	2704	24964	8216	3.4	11.56	1.4	1.96	4.76
44	155	1936	24025	6820	−4.6	21.16	−1.6	2.56	7.36
38	148	1444	21904	5624	−10.6	112.36	−8.6	73.96	91.16
57	170	3249	28900	9690	8.4	70.56	13.4	179.56	112.56
65	158	4225	24964	10270	16.4	268.96	1.4	1.96	22.96
52	168	2704	28224	8736	3.4	11.56	11.4	129.96	38.76
Total 340	1096	17286	172302	53804		771.72		699.72	569.72
Mean 48.6	156.6	2469.43	24614.57	7686.29					

The formula to calculate the r value is:

$$r = \frac{\Sigma(x-\bar{x})(y-\bar{y})}{\sqrt{\Sigma(x-\bar{x})^2\ \Sigma(y-\bar{y})^2}}$$

$$r = \frac{569.72}{\sqrt{771.72 \times 699.72}} = \frac{569.72}{\sqrt{539987.92}}$$

$$\frac{569.72}{734.84} = 0.775 = 0.76$$

The correlation coefficient value is 0.76

$$r = \frac{1/n\Sigma xy - \bar{x}\,\bar{y}}{Sx\ Sy}$$

$$\bar{x} = \frac{340}{7} = 48.6$$

$$\bar{y} = \frac{1096}{7} = 156.6$$

$$Sx = \sqrt{\frac{\Sigma x^2}{n} - \left[\frac{\Sigma x}{n}\right]^2}$$

$$Sx = \sqrt{2469.43 - (48.6)^2}$$

$$= \sqrt{2469.43 - 2361.96} = \sqrt{107.47} = 10.37$$

$$Sy = \sqrt{\frac{\Sigma y^2}{n} - \left[\frac{\Sigma y}{n}\right]^2} = \sqrt{24614.57 - (156.6)^2}$$

$$= \sqrt{24614.57 - 24523.56} = \sqrt{91.01} = 9.54$$

$$r = \frac{7686.29 - 48.6 \times 156.6}{10.37 \times 9.54} = \frac{7686.29 - 7610.76}{10.37 \times 9.54}$$

$$= \frac{75.53}{98.93} = 0.76$$

The correlation coefficient value is 0.76

Example 2:

Find out the correlation coefficient for the mother's gestational age and their baby's crown heel length.

Gestational age	31	38	34	40	42	37	35	40	42	41
Crown heel length	46.4	47.2	47.4	47.8	48.4	46.4	47.8	48.2	48	48

(x)	(y)	X^2	Y^2	xy	$(x-\bar{x})$	$(x-\bar{x})^2$	$(y-\bar{y})$	$(y-\bar{y})^2$	$(x-\bar{x})(y-\bar{y})$
31	46.4	961	2152.96	1438.4	–7	49	–1.16	1.3456	8.12
38	47.2	1444	2227.84	1793.6	0	0	–0.36	0.1296	0
34	47.4	1156	2246.76	1611.6	–4	16	–0.16	0.0256	0.64
40	47.8	1600	2284.84	1912	2	4	0.24	0.0576	0.48
42	48.4	1764	2342.56	2032.8	4	16	0.84	0.7056	3.36
37	46.4	1369	2152.96	1716.8	–1	1	–1.16	1.3456	1.16
35	47.8	1225	2284.84	1673	–3	9	0.24	0.0576	–0.72
40	48.2	1600	2323.24	1928	2	4	0.64	0.4096	1.28
42	48	1764	2304	2016	4	16	0.44	0.1936	1.76
41	48	1681	2304	1968	3	9	0.44	0.1936	1.32
Total 380	475.6	14564	22624	18090.2	0	124		4.464	17.4
Mean 38.0	47.56	1456.4	2262.4	1809.02					

The formula to calculate the r value is:

$$r = \frac{\Sigma(x-\bar{x})(y-\bar{y})}{\sqrt{\Sigma(x-\bar{x})^2 \, \Sigma(y-\bar{y})^2}}$$

$$r = \frac{17.4}{\sqrt{124 \times 4.464}} = \frac{17.4}{\sqrt{553.54}}$$

$$\frac{17.4}{23.53} = 0.74$$

The correlation coefficient value is 0.74

$$r = \frac{1/n\Sigma xy - \bar{x}\,\bar{y}}{Sx\ Sy}$$

$$\bar{x} = \frac{380}{10} = 38$$

$$\bar{y} = \frac{475.6}{10} = 47.56$$

$$Sx = \sqrt{\frac{\Sigma x^2}{n} - \left[\frac{\Sigma x}{n}\right]^2}$$

$$Sx = \sqrt{1456.4 - (38)^2} = \sqrt{1456.4 - 1444}$$

$$= \sqrt{12.4} = 3.52$$

$$Sy = \sqrt{\frac{\Sigma y^2}{n} - \left[\frac{\Sigma y}{n}\right]^2} = \sqrt{2262.4 - (47.56)^2}$$

$$= \sqrt{2262.4 - 2261.95} = \sqrt{0.45} = 0.67$$

$$r = \frac{1809.02 - 38 \times 47.56}{3.52 \times 0.67} = \frac{1809.02 - 1807.28}{2.36} = \frac{1.74}{2.36} = 0.74$$

The correlation coefficient value is 0.74

Example 3:

Find out the correlation coefficient.

x	10	20	30	40	50
y	30	50	70	90	110

(x)	(y)	X^2	Y^2	xy	$(x - \bar{x})$	$(y - \bar{y})$	$(x - \bar{x})^2$	$(y - \bar{y})^2$	$(x - \bar{x})(y - \bar{y})$
10	30	100	900	300	−20	−40	400	1600	800
20	50	400	2500	1000	−10	−20	100	400	200
30	70	900	4900	2100	0	0	0	0	0
40	90	1600	8100	3600	10	20	100	400	200
50	110	2500	12100	5500	20	40	400	1600	800
Total 150	350	5500	28500	12500			1000	4000	2000
Mean 30	70	1100	5700	2500					

The formula to calculate the r value is:

$$r = \frac{\Sigma(x - \bar{x})(y - \bar{y})}{\sqrt{\Sigma(x - \bar{x})^2\ \Sigma(y - \bar{y})^2}}$$

$$r = \frac{2000}{\sqrt{1000 \times 4000}} = \frac{2000}{\sqrt{4000000}}$$

$$\frac{2000}{2000} = 1.0$$

The correlation coefficient value is 1

$$r = \frac{1/n\Sigma xy - \bar{x}\,\bar{y}}{Sx\,Sy}$$

$$\bar{x} = \frac{150}{5} = 30$$

$$\bar{y} = \frac{350}{5} = 70$$

$$Sx = \sqrt{\frac{\Sigma x^2}{n} - \left[\frac{\Sigma x}{n}\right]^2}$$

$$Sx = \sqrt{1100-(30)^2} = \sqrt{1100-900} = \sqrt{200} = 14.14$$

$$Sy = \sqrt{\frac{\Sigma y^2}{n} - \left[\frac{\Sigma y}{n}\right]^2} = \sqrt{5700-(70)^2}$$

$$= \sqrt{5700-4900} = \sqrt{800} = 28.28$$

$$r = \frac{2500 - 30 \times 70}{14.14 \times 28.28} = \frac{2500-2100}{399.88} = \frac{400}{399.88} = 1$$

The correlation coefficient value is 1.

Example 4:

Find out the correlation coefficient for duration of service (x) and the job satisfaction (y).

Duration	2	3	1	5	8	10	6	12	4
Job satisfaction	76	80	50	70	60	60	70	60	70

x	**y**	**X^2**	**Y^2**	**xy**	**$(x-\bar{x})$**	**$(x-\bar{x})^2$**	**$(y-\bar{y})$**	**$(y-\bar{y})^2$**	**$(x-\bar{x})(y-\bar{y})$**
2	76	4	5776	152	–3.67	13.4689	9.78	95.6484	–35.8926
3	80	9	6400	240	–2.67	7.1289	13.78	189.8884	–36.7926
1	50	1	2500	50	–4.67	21.8089	–16.22	263.0884	75.7474
5	70	25	4900	350	–0.67	0.4489	3.78	14.2884	–2.5326
8	60	64	3600	480	2.33	5.4289	–6.22	38.6884	–14.4926
10	60	100	3600	600	4.33	18.7489	–6.22	38.6884	–26.9326
6	70	36	4900	420	0.33	0.1089	3.78	14.2884	1.2474
12	60	144	3600	720	6.33	40.0689	–6.22	38.6884	–39.3726
4	70	16	4900	280	–1.67	2.7889	3.78	14.2884	–6.3126
Total 51	596	399	40176	3292		110.001		707.5556	–85.3334
Mean 5.67	66.22	44.3	4464	365.8					

The formula to calculate the r value is:

$$r = \frac{\Sigma(x-\bar{x})(y-\bar{y})}{\sqrt{\Sigma(x-\bar{x})^2\,\Sigma(y-\bar{y})^2}}$$

$$r = \frac{-85.3334}{\sqrt{110 \times 707.56}} = \frac{-85.3334}{\sqrt{77831.6}} = \frac{-85.33}{278.98} = -0.310$$

The correlation coefficient value is –0.31

$$r = \frac{1/n\Sigma xy - \bar{x}\,\bar{y}}{Sx\ Sy}$$

$$\bar{x} = \frac{51}{9} = 5.67$$

$$\bar{y} = \frac{596}{9} = 66.22$$

$$Sx = \sqrt{\frac{\Sigma x^2}{n} - \left[\frac{\Sigma x}{n}\right]^2}$$

$$Sx = \sqrt{44.3 - (5.67)^2} = \sqrt{44.3 - 32.15}$$

$$= \sqrt{12.15} = 3.49$$

$$Sy = \sqrt{\frac{\Sigma y^2}{n} - \left[\frac{\Sigma y}{n}\right]^2} = \sqrt{4464 - (66.22)^2}$$

$$= \sqrt{4464 - 4385.09} = \sqrt{78.9} = 8.88$$

$$r = \frac{365.8 - 5.67 \times 66.22}{3.49 \times 8.88} = \frac{365.8 - 375.47}{30.99} = \frac{-9.67}{30.99} = -0.31$$

The correlation coefficient value is –0.31.

Example 5:

Anxiety score	40	30	70	80	60	42	38	32
Test score	66	66	48	22	56	80	70	60

x	y	X^2	Y^2	xy	$(x-\bar{x})$	$(x-\bar{x})^2$	$(y-\bar{y})$	$(y-\bar{y})^2$	$(x-\bar{x})(y-\bar{y})$
40	66	1600	4356	2640	–9	81	7.5	56.25	–67.5
30	66	900	4356	1980	–19	361	7.5	56.25	–142.5
70	48	4900	2304	3360	21	441	–10.5	110.25	–220.5
80	22	6400	484	1760	31	961	–36.5	1332.25	–1131.5
60	56	3600	3136	3360	11	121	–2.5	6.25	–27.5
42	80	1764	6400	3360	–7	49	21.5	462.25	–150.5
38	70	1444	4900	2660	–11	121	11.5	132.25	–126.5
32	60	1024	3600	1920	–17	289	1.5	2.25	–25.5
Total 392	468	21632	29536	21040		2424		2158	–1892
Mean 49	58.5	2704	3692	2630					

The formula to calculate the r value is:

$$r = \frac{\Sigma(x-\bar{x})(y-\bar{y})}{\sqrt{\Sigma(x-\bar{x})^2\ \Sigma(y-\bar{y})^2}}$$

$$r = \frac{-1892}{\sqrt{2424 \times 2158}} = \frac{-1892}{\sqrt{5230992}} = \frac{-1892}{2287.14} = -0.83$$

The correlation coefficient value is –0.83

$$r = \frac{1/n\Sigma xy - \bar{x}\,\bar{y}}{Sx\ Sy}$$

$$\bar{x} = \frac{44}{8} = 49$$

$$\bar{y} = \frac{124}{8} = 58.5$$

$$Sx = \sqrt{\frac{\Sigma x^2}{n} - \left[\frac{\Sigma x}{n}\right]^2}$$

$$Sx = \sqrt{2704 - (49)^2} = \sqrt{2704 - 2401} = \sqrt{303} = 17.41$$

$$Sy = \sqrt{\frac{\Sigma y^2}{n} - \left[\frac{\Sigma y}{n}\right]^2} = \sqrt{3692 - (58.5)^2}$$

$$= \sqrt{3692 - 3422.25} = \sqrt{269.75} = 16.42$$

$$r = \frac{2630 - 49 \times 58.5}{17.41 \times 16.42} = \frac{2630 - 2866.5}{285.87} = \frac{-236.5}{285.87}$$

$$= -0.827 = -0.83$$

The correlation coefficient value is –0.83

Example 6:

In a study, physical risk score and the fetal outcome score were calculated for a pregnant woman. Calculate the degree of relationship between the two variables and interpret.

Physical risk	16	2	6	4	5	2	7	2
Fetal outcome	12	18	16	14	14	20	10	20

x	y	X^2	Y^2	xy	$(x-\bar{x})$	$(x-\bar{x})^2$	$(y-\bar{y})$	$(y-\bar{y})^2$	$(x-\bar{x})(y-\bar{y})$
16	12	256	144	192	10.5	110.25	-3.5	12.25	-36.75
2	18	4	324	36	-3.5	12.25	2.5	6.25	-8.75
6	16	36	256	96	0.5	0.25	0.5	0.25	0.25
4	14	16	196	56	-1.5	2.25	-1.5	2.25	2.25
5	14	25	196	70	-0.5	0.25	-1.5	2.25	0.75
2	20	4	400	40	-3.5	12.25	4.5	20.25	-15.75
7	10	49	100	70	1.5	2.25	-5.5	30.25	-8.25
2	20	4	400	40	-3.5	12.25	4.5	20.25	-15.75
Total 44	124	394	2016	600		152		94	-82
Mean 5.5	15.5	49.25	252	75					

The formula to calculate the r value is:

$$r = \frac{\Sigma(x-\bar{x})(y-\bar{y})}{\sqrt{\Sigma(x-\bar{x})^2\ \Sigma(y-\bar{y})^2}}$$

$$r = \frac{-82}{\sqrt{152 \times 94}} = \frac{-82}{\sqrt{14288}} = \frac{-82}{119.53} = -0.686 = -0.69$$

The correlation coefficient value is –0.69

$$r = \frac{1/n\Sigma xy - \bar{x}\,\bar{y}}{Sx\,Sy}$$

$$\bar{x} = \frac{44}{8} = 5.5$$

$$\bar{y} = \frac{124}{8} = 15.5$$

$$Sx = \sqrt{\frac{\Sigma x^2}{n} - \left[\frac{\Sigma x}{n}\right]^2}$$

$$Sx = \sqrt{49.25 - (5.5)^2} = \sqrt{49.25 - 30.25} = \sqrt{19} = 4.36$$

$$Sy = \sqrt{\frac{\Sigma y^2}{n} - \left[\frac{\Sigma y}{n}\right]^2} = \sqrt{252 - (15.5)^2}$$

$$= \sqrt{252 - 240.25} = \sqrt{11.75} = 3.43$$

$$r = \frac{75 - 5.5 \times 15.5}{4.36 \times 3.43} = \frac{75 - 85.25}{14.95} = \frac{-10.25}{14.95}$$

$$= -0.686 = -0.69$$

The correlation coefficient value is –0.69.

Example 7:

Find the correlation coefficient:

X	1	3	2	4	5	3	4	3	2	3
Y	1.5	2.5	2	3	3.5	2	3.5	2	2	3

x	y	X^2	Y^2	xy	$(x-\bar{x})$	$(x-\bar{x})^2$	$(y-\bar{y})$	$(y-\bar{y})^2$	$(x-\bar{x})(y-\bar{y})$
1	1.5	1	2.25	1.5	–2	4	–1	1	2
3	2.5	9	6.25	7.5	0	0	0	0	0
2	2	4	4	4	–1	1	–0.5	0.25	0.5
4	3	16	9	12	1	1	0.5	0.25	0.5
5	3.5	25	12.25	17.5	2	4	1	1	2
3	2	9	4	6	0	0	–0.5	0.25	0
4	3.5	16	12.25	14	1	1	1	1	1
3	2	9	4	6	0	0	–0.5	0.25	0
2	2	4	4	4	–1	1	–0.5	0.25	0.5
3	3	9	9	9	0	0	0.5	0.25	0
Total 30	25	102	67	81.5		12		4.5	6.5
Mean 3	2.5	10.2	6.7	8.15					

The formula to calculate the r value is:

$$r = \frac{\Sigma(x-\bar{x})(y-\bar{y})}{\sqrt{\Sigma(x-\bar{x})^2\,\Sigma(y-\bar{y})^2}}$$

$$r = \frac{6.5}{\sqrt{12 \times 4.5}} = \frac{6.5}{\sqrt{54}} = \frac{6.5}{7.35} = 0.884 = 0.88$$

The correlation coefficient value is 0.88

$$r = \frac{1/n\Sigma xy - \bar{x}\,\bar{y}}{Sx\,Sy}$$

$$\bar{x} = \frac{30}{10} = 3$$

$$\bar{y} = \frac{25}{10} = 2.5$$

$$Sx = \sqrt{\frac{\Sigma x^2}{n} - \left[\frac{\Sigma x}{n}\right]^2}$$

$$Sx = \sqrt{10.2 - (3)^2} = \sqrt{10.2 - 9} = \sqrt{1.2} = 1.1$$

$$Sy = \sqrt{\frac{\Sigma y^2}{n} - \left[\frac{\Sigma y}{n}\right]^2} = \sqrt{6.7 - (2.5)^2}$$

$$= \sqrt{6.7 - 6.25} = \sqrt{0.45} = 0.67$$

$$r = \frac{8.15 - 3 \times 2.5}{1.1 \times 0.67} = \frac{8.15 - 7.5}{0.74} = \frac{0.65}{0.74} = 0.878 = 0.88$$

The correlation coefficient value is 0.88.

Example 8:

Calculate coefficient of correlation between age and mean hemoglobin values of children.

Age	8–9	9–10	10–11	11–12	12–13	13–14	14–15	15–16	16–17	17–18
Hb	16.5	15.8	15.0	14.9	14.8	15	14.6	13.8	12.8	12.6

Age	**x**	**y**	**X^2**	**Y^2**	**xy**	**$(x-\bar{x})$**	**$(x-\bar{x})^2$**	**$(y-\bar{y})$**	**$(y-\bar{y})^2$**	**$(x-\bar{x})(y-\bar{y})$**
8-9	8.5	16.5	72.25	272.25	140.25	–4.5	20.25	1.9	3.61	–8.55
9-10	9.5	15.8	90.25	249.64	150.1	–3.5	12.25	1.2	1.44	–4.2
10-11	10.5	15	110.25	225	157.5	–2.5	6.25	0.4	0.16	–1
11-12	11.5	14.9	132.25	222.01	171.35	–1.5	2.25	0.3	0.09	–0.45
12-13	12.5	14.8	156.25	219.04	185	–0.5	0.25	0.2	0.04	–0.1
13-14	13.5	15	182.25	225	202.5	0.5	0.25	0.4	0.16	0.2
14-15	14.5	14.6	210.25	213.16	211.7	1.5	2.25	0	0	0
15-16	15.5	13.8	240.25	190.44	213.9	2.5	6.25	–0.8	0.64	–2
16-17	16.5	12.8	272.25	163.84	211.2	3.5	12.25	–1.8	3.24	–6.3
17-18	17.5	12.6	306.25	158.76	220.5	4.5	20.25	–2	4	–9
Total	I 30	145.8	1772.5	2139.14	1864		82.5		13.38	–31.4
Mean	13	14.58	177.25	213.9	186.4					

The formula to calculate the r value is:

$$r = \frac{\Sigma(x-\bar{x})(y-\bar{y})}{\sqrt{\Sigma(x-\bar{x})^2\,\Sigma(y-\bar{y})^2}}$$

$$r = \frac{-31.4}{\sqrt{82.5 \times 13.38}} = \frac{-31.4}{\sqrt{1103.85}} = \frac{-31.4}{33.22} = -0.95$$

The correlation coefficient value is –0.95

$$r = \frac{1/n\Sigma xy - \bar{x}\,\bar{y}}{Sx\,Sy}$$

$$\bar{x} = \frac{130}{10} = 13$$

$$\bar{y} = \frac{145.8}{10} = 14.58$$

$$Sx = \sqrt{\frac{\Sigma x^2}{n} - \left[\frac{\Sigma x}{n}\right]^2}$$

$$Sx = \sqrt{177.25 - (13)^2} = \sqrt{177.25 - 169} = \sqrt{8.25} = 2.9$$

$$Sy = \sqrt{\frac{\Sigma y^2}{n} - \left[\frac{\Sigma y}{n}\right]^2} = \sqrt{213.9 - (14.58)^2}$$

$$= \sqrt{213.9 - 212.58} = \sqrt{1.32} = 1.15$$

$$r = \frac{186.4 - 13 \times 14.58}{2.9 \times 1.15} = \frac{186.4 - 189.54}{3.335} = \frac{-3.14}{3.335}$$

$$= -0.94$$

The correlation coefficient value is –0.94

Example 9:

Calculate the correlation coefficient between the temperature (X) and pulse (Y) given below.

Temperatures	102	101	100	99	98
Pulse	100	90	80	70	60

x	**y**	**X^2**	**Y^2**	**xy**	**$(x-\bar{x})$**	**$(x-\bar{x})^2$**	**$(y-\bar{y})$**	**$(y-\bar{y})^2$**	**$(x-\bar{x})(y-\bar{y})$**
102	100	10404	10000	10200	2	4	20	400	40
101	90	10201	8100	9090	1	1	10	100	10
100	80	10000	6400	8000	0	0	0	0	0
99	70	9801	4900	6930	–1	1	-10	100	10
98	60	9604	3600	5880	–2	4	-20	400	40
Total 500	400	50010	33000	40100		10		1000	100
Mean 100	80	10002	6600	8020					

The formula to calculate the r value is:

$$r = \frac{\Sigma(x-\bar{x})(y-\bar{y})}{\sqrt{\Sigma(x-\bar{x})^2\,\Sigma(y-\bar{y})^2}}$$

$$r = \frac{100}{\sqrt{10 \times 1000}} = \frac{100}{\sqrt{10000}} = \frac{100}{100} = 1$$

The correlation coefficient value is 1

$$r = \frac{1/n\Sigma xy - \bar{x}\,\bar{y}}{Sx\,Sy}$$

$$\bar{x} = 100$$
$$\bar{y} = 80$$
$$Sx = \sqrt{\frac{\Sigma x^2}{n} - \left[\frac{\Sigma x}{n}\right]^2}$$
$$Sx = \sqrt{10002 - (100)^2} = \sqrt{10002 - 10000} = \sqrt{2} = 1.41$$
$$Sy = \sqrt{\frac{\Sigma y^2}{n} - \left[\frac{\Sigma y}{n}\right]^2} = \sqrt{6600 - (80)^2}$$
$$= \sqrt{6600 - 6400} = \sqrt{200} = 14.14$$
$$r = \frac{8020 - 100 \times 80}{1.41 \times 14.14} = \frac{8020 - 8000}{19.9} = \frac{20}{20} = 1$$

The correlation coefficient value is 1

There is a positive perfect correlation between the temperature and pulse.

Example 10:

Calculate the correlation coefficient between height (X) and weight (Y) given below.

Height (in inches)	57	59	62	63	64	65	55	58	57
Weight (in pounds)	113	117	126	126	130	129	111	116	112

x	**y**	**X²**	**Y²**	**xy**
57	113	3249	12769	6441
59	117	3481	13689	6903
62	126	3844	15876	7812
63	126	3969	15876	7938
64	130	4096	16900	8320
65	129	4225	16641	8385
55	111	3025	12321	6105
58	116	3364	13456	6728
57	112	3249	12544	6384
Total 540	1080	32502	130072	65016
Mean 60	120	3611.3	14452.4	7224

$$r = \frac{1/n\Sigma xy - \bar{x}\,\bar{y}}{Sx\ Sy}$$
$$\bar{x} = 60$$
$$\bar{y} = 120$$
$$Sx = \sqrt{\frac{\Sigma x^2}{n} - \left[\frac{\Sigma x}{n}\right]^2}$$
$$Sx = \sqrt{3611.3 - (60)^2} = \sqrt{3611.3 - 3600} = \sqrt{11.3} = 3.36$$
$$Sy = \sqrt{\frac{\Sigma y^2}{n} - \left[\frac{\Sigma y}{n}\right]^2} = \sqrt{14452.4 - (120)^2}$$
$$= \sqrt{14452.4 - 14400} = \sqrt{52.4} = 7.24$$

$$r = \frac{7224 - 60 \times 120}{3.36 \times 7.24} = \frac{7224 - 7200}{24.32} = \frac{24}{24.32} = 0.99$$

The correlation coefficient value is 1

There is a positive perfect correlation between height and weight.

Example 11:

Calculate the correlation coefficient between age (X) and systolic BP (Y) given below.

Age	30	40	50	60	70
Systolic BP	120	126	142	146	150

x	**y**	**X²**	**Y²**	**xy**
30	120	900	14400	3600
40	126	1600	15876	5040
50	142	2500	20164	7100
60	146	3600	21316	8760
70	150	4900	22500	10500
Total 250	684	13500	94256	35000
Mean 50	136.8	2700	18851.2	7000

$$r = \frac{1/n\Sigma xy - \bar{x}\,\bar{y}}{Sx\;Sy}$$

$$\bar{x} = 50$$

$$\bar{y} = 136.8$$

$$Sx = \sqrt{\frac{\Sigma x^2}{n} - \left[\frac{\Sigma x}{n}\right]^2}$$

$$Sx = \sqrt{2700 - (50)^2} = \sqrt{2700 - 2500} = \sqrt{200} = 14.14$$

$$Sy = \sqrt{\frac{\Sigma y^2}{n} - \left[\frac{\Sigma y}{n}\right]^2} = \sqrt{18851.2 - (136.8)^2}$$

$$= \sqrt{18851.2 - 18714.24} = \sqrt{136.96} = 11.7$$

$$r = \frac{7000 - 50 \times 136.8}{14.14 \times 11.7} = \frac{7000 - 6840}{165.44} = \frac{160}{165.4} = 0.97$$

The correlation coefficient value is 1

There is a positive perfect correlation between age and systolic blood pressure.

Calculation of Rank Correlation

Spearman's coefficient of corrrelation (or r) $= 1 - \left[\frac{6\sum d_i^2}{n(n^2 - 1)}\right]$

Example 12:

Two judges in a dance competition ranked 8 entries as follows. Calculate the correlation coefficient.

Judge 1	1	3	5	2	4	6	8	7
Judge 2	3	2	4	1	6	5	7	8

x	**y**	**d**	**d^2**
1	3	–2	4
3	2	1	1
5	4	1	1
2	1	1	1
4	6	–2	4
6	5	1	1
8	7	1	1
7	8	–1	1
		$\sum d^2$	14

$$r = 1 - \left[\frac{6\sum d_i^2}{n(n^2-1)}\right]$$

$$r = 1 - \frac{6 \times 14}{8(8^2-1)} = 1 - \frac{84}{8 \times 63} = 1 - \frac{84}{504}$$

$$= 1 - 0.167 = 0.833$$

Example 13:

Two judges in a fancy dress competition ranked 10 participants as follows. Calculate the correlation coefficient.

X	1	10	3	4	9	7	6	8	5	2
Y	4	7	6	5	8	9	3	10	2	1

x	**y**	**d**	**d^2**
1	4	–3	9
10	7	3	9
3	6	–3	9
4	5	–1	1
9	8	1	1
7	9	–2	4
6	3	3	9
8	10	–2	4
5	2	3	9
2	1	1	1
		$\sum d^2$	56

$$r = 1 - \left[\frac{6\sum d_i^2}{n(n^2-1)}\right]$$

$$r = 1 - \frac{6 \times 56}{10(10^2-1)} = 1 - \frac{336}{10 \times 99} = 1 - \frac{336}{990}$$

$$= 1 - 0.34 = 0.66$$

Example 14:

Calculate the rank correlation for the following:

x	40	30	70	80	60	42	38	32
y	66	68	48	22	56	80	70	60

x	**Rank x(r_1)**	**Y**	**Rank y(r_2)**	**$d = r_1 - r_2$**	**d^2**
40	5	66	4	1	1
30	8	68	3	5	25
70	2	48	7	–5	25
80	1	22	8	–7	49
60	3	56	6	–3	9
42	4	80	1	3	9
38	6	70	2	4	16
32	7	60	5	2	4
				$\sum d^2$	138

$$r = 1 - \left[\frac{6\sum d_i^2}{n(n^2-1)}\right]$$

$$r = 1 - \frac{6 \times 138}{8(8^2-1)} = 1 - \frac{828}{8 \times 63} = 1 - \frac{828}{504}$$

$$= 1 - 1.64 = -0.64$$

Example 15:

X	10	12	18	12	12	16	20	14
Y	14	16	20	14	12	10	22	18

x	**Rank x(r_1)**	**Y**	**Rank y(r_2)**	**$d = r_1 - r_2$**	**d^2**
10	1	14	3.5	–2.5	6.25
12	3	16	5	–2	4
18	7	20	7	0	0
12	3	14	3.5	–0.5	0.25
12	3	12	2	1	1
16	6	10	1	5	25
20	8	22	8	0	0
14	5	18	6	–1	1
				$\sum d^2$	37.5

- ***Equal or repeated ranks:*** When two or more items have equal values, it is difficult to give ranks to them. In that case, the items are given the average of the ranks they would have received, if they are not tied. For example, if three individuals are placed in the second place, they are each given the rank $\frac{2+3+4}{3}=\frac{9}{3}=3$, which is common rank to be assigned; and the next rank will be 5; if two individuals are placed in 8th place, they are each given the rank $\frac{8+9}{2}=\frac{17}{2}=8.5$ and the next rank will be 10. In this case, a slightly different formula is used when there is more than one item having the same value. The formula is:

$$= 1-6\left[\frac{\Sigma d^2+\frac{1}{12}(m^3-m)+\frac{1}{12}(m^3-m)...}{n^3-n}\right]$$

12 is repeated 3 times in x items and hence m = 3 and 14 are repeated 2 times in y items and, hence, m = 2. Therefore, the formula is:

$$= 1-6\left[\frac{37.5+\frac{1}{12}(3^3-3)+\frac{1}{12}(2^3-2)...}{8^3-8}\right]$$

$$= 1-6\left[\frac{37.5+\frac{1}{12}(27-3)+\frac{1}{12}(8-2)...}{512-8}\right]$$

$$= 1-6\left[\frac{37.5+\frac{1}{12}(24)+\frac{1}{12}(6)}{512-8}\right]$$

$$= 1-6\left[\frac{37.5+2+0.5}{512-8}\right]$$

$$1-6\left[\frac{40}{504}\right] = 1-\frac{240}{504} = 1 - 0.476 = 0.524$$

Example 16:

Compute rank correlation:

X	116	135	121	130	124	128
Y	128	132	130	130	127	125

x	Rank x(r_1)	Y	Rank y(r_2)	$d = r_1 - r_2$	d^2
116	1	128	3	−2	4
135	6	132	6	0	0

x	Rank x(r_1)	Y	Rank y(r_2)	$d = r_1 - r_2$	d^2
121	2	130	4.5	−2.5	6.25
130	5	130	4.5	0.5	0.25
124	3	127	2	1	1
128	4	125	1	3	9
				$\sum d^2$	20.5

130 is repeated 2 times in y items and, hence, m = 2. Therefore, the formula is:

$$= 1-6\left[\frac{20.5+\frac{1}{12}(2^3-2)}{6^3-6}\right]$$

$$= 1-6\left[\frac{20.5+\frac{1}{12}(8-2)}{216-6}\right]$$

$$= 1-6\left[\frac{20.5+\frac{6}{12}}{210}\right]$$

$$1-6\left[\frac{20.5+0.5}{210}\right] = 1-6\left[\frac{21}{210}\right]=1-\left[\frac{126}{210}\right] = 1 - 0.6 = 0.4$$

Example 17:

The following are the intelligence quotient and the achievement score of 10 nursing students. Calculate the rank correlation coefficient.

IQ score	100	100	110	140	150	130	100	120	140	110
Achievement score	35	40	25	55	85	90	65	55	45	50

x	Rank x(r_1)	Y	Rank y(r_2)	$d = r_1 - r_2$	d^2
100	2	35	2	0	0
100	2	40	3	−1	1
110	4.5	25	1	3.5	12.25
140	8.5	55	6.5	2	4
150	10	85	9	1	1
130	7	90	10	-3	9
100	2	65	8	-6	36
120	6	55	6.5	−0.5	0.25
140	8.5	45	4	4.5	20.25
110	4.5	50	5	−0.5	0.25
				$\sum d^2$	84

In x items, 100 is repeated 3 times (m = 3); 110 is repeated 2 times (m = 2); 140 is repeated 2 times (m = 2). In y items, 55 is repeated 2 times (m = 2). Therefore, the formula is:

$$= 1-6\left[\frac{\Sigma d^2 + \frac{1}{12}(m^3 - m) + \frac{1}{12}(m^3 - m)...}{n^3 - n}\right]$$

$$= 1-6\left[\frac{84 + \frac{1}{12}(3^3 - 3) + \frac{1}{12}(2^3 - 2) + \frac{1}{12}(2^3 - 2) + \frac{1}{12}(2^3 - 2)}{10^3 - 10}\right]$$

$$= 1-6\left[\frac{84 + \frac{1}{12}(27 - 3) + \frac{1}{12}(8 - 2) + \frac{1}{12}(8 - 2) + \frac{1}{12}(8 - 2)}{1000 - 10}\right]$$

$$1-6\left[\frac{84 + \frac{24}{12} + \frac{6}{12} + \frac{6}{12} + \frac{6}{12}}{990}\right] = 1-6\left[\frac{84 + 2.0 + 0.5 + 0.5 + 0.5}{990}\right]$$

$$= 1-\frac{6 \times 87.5}{990} = 1-\frac{525}{990} = 1 - 0.530 = 0.47$$

Application in Nursing Research

In research, any given r value indicates the value of correlation coefficient. The value will range from –1 to +1. One should not come into conclusion by seeing the r value itself. The r value might show either positive or negative or no relationship. In case of either positive or negative relationship, one should check whether it is statistically significant or not. If it is not statistically significant, it may be due to pure chance. The researcher should decide which method to adopt to calculate the correlation coefficient. A scatter diagram can give an idea of what might be the relationship. Based on the scale of measurement, one can choose pearson's r or spearman's rank correlation. If two variables are measured in ratio scale, pearson's r can be used. If the variables are ranked or are in other scale of measurement, rank correlation method is used. Also while deciding to calculate correlation coefficient, one must check for the fulfillment of the assumptions of correlation coefficient. Also if data on variables are extreme, it is better to use rank correlation method. The r value simply denotes the degree and strength of relationship and if we want to find out the cause and effect relationship, we should use regression analysis.

SUMMARY

- The relationship between two variables such that a change in one variable results in a direct or inverse change in the other and also greater the magnitude of change in one variable corresponds to greater the magnitude of change in the other, then the variables are said to be correlated or the relationship between the variables is called ***correlation***.
- Correlation attempts to determine the degree of relationship between the variables. Correlation is an analysis of the covariation between two or more variables.

- When an increase (or decrease) in one variable corresponds to an increase (or decrease) in the other variable, then the correlation is said to be positive (or direct). It is negative (or inverse) when increase (or decrease) in one vatriable corresponds to decrease (or increase) in the other variable.
- If the two variables change in the same direction, i.e. with the increase in one, the other also increases and vice versa, and in the same ratio, then there is perfect positive correlation. The correlation coefficient is +1.
- If the two variables change in the same ratio, but in opposite directions, i.e. with the increase in one, the other decreases and vice versa, there is a perfect negative correlation and the correlation coefficient is –1.
- If the change in one variable has no effect on the other variable, then the correlation is completely absent and we call it no correlation. The correlation coefficient is zero.
- If the change in one variable is always a fixed ratio to the change in the other variable, the correlation is said to be linear. If the change in one variable is not to the ratio of the change in the other variable, then the correlation is said to be nonlinear or curvilinear.
- Correlation can be studied through (a) Scatter diagram, (b) Simple graph, (c) Cross tabulation, (d) Charles Spearman's coefficient of correlation (rank correlation) and (e) Karl Pearson's coefficient of correlation; whereas cause and effect relationship can be studied through simple regression equations.
- The value of 'r' lies between ±1. Positive values of r indicate positive correlation between the two variables (i.e. changes in both variables take place in the same direction), whereas negative values of 'r' indicate negative correlation, i.e. changes in the two variables taking place in the opposite directions. A zero value of 'r' indicates that there is no correlation between the two variables.

EXERCISE

- In a study, the weight of young adults and their stress score was measured. Calculate the r value and interpret the findings.

Stress score	60	40	70	30	58	62	70	68
Weight in kg	50	48	52	55	46	47	42	55

- In a study, data on students' intelligence and their test performance was calculated. Find if there is any correlation and interpret the findings.

Intelligence	89	92	95	94	96	90	98	92
Test score	68	76	78	80	78	78	82	72

- In a study, sample's age and pulse was calculated. Calculate the r value and interpret the findings.

Age in years	22	36	40	44	48	50	55	60	28	30
Pulse rate	96	80	78	78	76	78	72	72	82	86

- Calculate the correlation coefficient for the data given below and interpret the findings.

Stress score	60	80	36	48	50	42	71	22	28	30
Performance score	70	40	78	46	60	70	42	66	70	68

- The ranking of 9 students in Research and Statistics are as follows. Calculate the rank correlation.

Research	2	4	1	3	6	5	9	8	7
Statistics	4	9	5	6	3	1	2	7	8

- The ranking of 10 participants by two judges in a drawing competition is given below. Calculate the correlation coefficient.

Judge A	2	3	4	6	5	8	7	9	10	1
Judge B	3	6	4	5	1	9	10	8	7	2

- Calculate the rank correlation for the data given below.

X	10	12	12	16	18	14	14	14	20	22
Y	16	18	18	24	28	20	22	22	26	20

- Calculate the rank correlation for the data given below.

X	100	110	120	120	130	140	150	160	180	190
Y	120	130	140	150	150	160	180	100	110	170

- Calculate the correlation coefficient by Pearsonian method. The values of age and their mean weight is given.

Age	11–14	14–16	16–18	18–20	20–22	22–24
Mean weight	42	50	56	58	58	60

- Calculate the correlation coefficient for age of the children and their mean height (cms).

Age	5–6	6–7	7–8	8–9	9–10	10–11	11–12	12–13
Mean height	112	118	124	126	130	134	139	145

- Calculate the correlation coefficient for the data given below.

X	2.5	3.8	4.6	5.8	6.9	7.2	8.1
Y	8.1	6.8	5.2	9.1	4.2	6.3	5.3

- Calculate the correlation coefficient between pain and pulse rate for the data given below.

Pain	4	8	2	6	6	8	2	4
Pulse	86	98	72	90	96	100	74	76

- Find the correlation between the age of candidates and their enrolment into MSc (N) degree program.

Age	22–24	25–27	28–30	31–33	34–36	37–39
No. of candidates	24	22	12	8	6	2

- Find the correlation between the spiritual well-being score and youth risk behavior score.

Spiritual well-being	18	10	5	8	12	10	16	10
Youth risk behavior score	4	10	8	10	6	12	10	8

17 Measures of Relationship—Regression Analysis

OBJECTIVES

After reading this chapter, you will be able to:
- Explain simple regression
- Explain the relationship between the correlation and regression
- List the types of regression analysis
- Explain the application of regression analysis in Nursing
- Construct two regression equations

INTRODUCTION

Correlation and the regression analysis are the measures of relationship. Correlation deals with the covariation of two variables which does not explain the cause and effect relationship. There are many times when we know about one characteristic of a particular phenomenon, we can have some ideas as to the nature of another characteristic. There is a relationship between the height and weight of the human being. If a person's height is given, we can predict the weight of the person. If IQ (intelligence quotient) is given, we can get the clue about the academic performance of a person. Sometimes our inferences are correct, other times not. Simple regression helps us to make inferences. Regression analysis is helpful in ascertaining the probable form of the relationship between variables, and it is used to predict or estimate the value of one variable corresponding to a given value of another variable. The ideas of regression were first elucidated by the English scientist Sir Francis Galton in reports of his research on heredity. He described a tendency of adult offspring, having short or tall parents, to revert back toward the average height of the general population. He first used the word reversion and later to regression, to refer to this phenomenon.

REGRESSION ANALYSIS

The statistical method which helps us to estimate the unknown value of one variable from the known value of the related variable is called ***regression***. Regression is the measures of the average relationship between two or more variables in terms of the original units of the data. Literally regression means going back or stepping back. The estimation of regression is called

regression analysis. In calculation of regression, two values are involved, one independent variable and the other dependent variable. In regression analysis value of dependent variable can be calculated from the independent variable. For example, if we calculate the regression between the aggression (dependent variable) and the duration of playing violent video games (independent variable), we can estimate the value of aggression based on the values of duration of playing violent video games.

Relationship between the Correlation and Regression Lines

In case of perfect positive correlation (r = 1) or perfect negative correlation (r = -1), the two line will coincide with each other and there will be only one regression line. In either cases, if we connect the dots or draw a line of correlation which will coincide with the regression line.

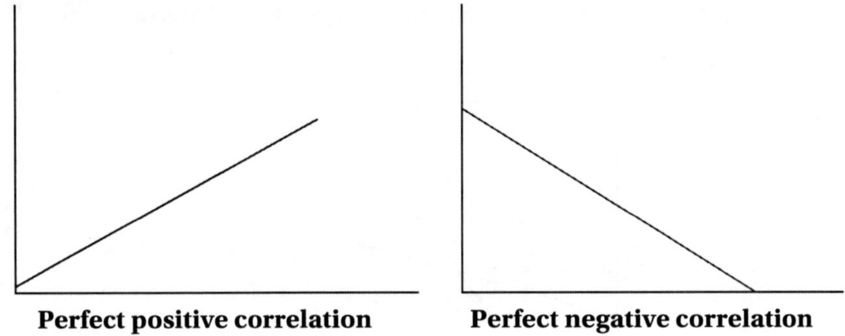

Perfect positive correlation **Perfect negative correlation**

If there is no correlation between the variables in case if both variables are independent of each other, in such cases both the regression lines cut each other at right angles.

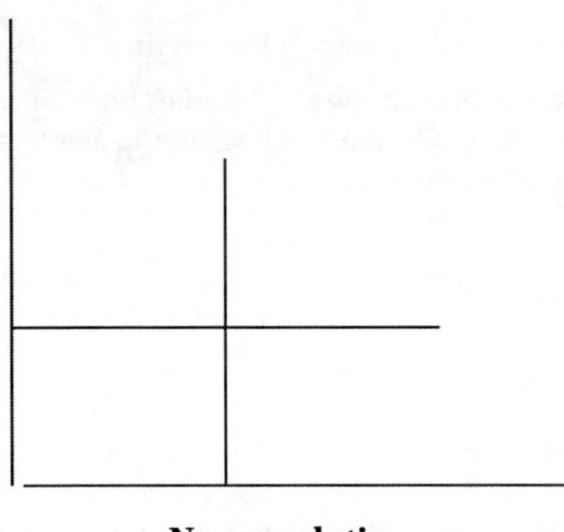

No correlation

If the regression lines are nearer to each other, then there is a high degree of correlation. If the regression lines are farther away from each other, then there is lesser degree of correlation (Table 17.1).

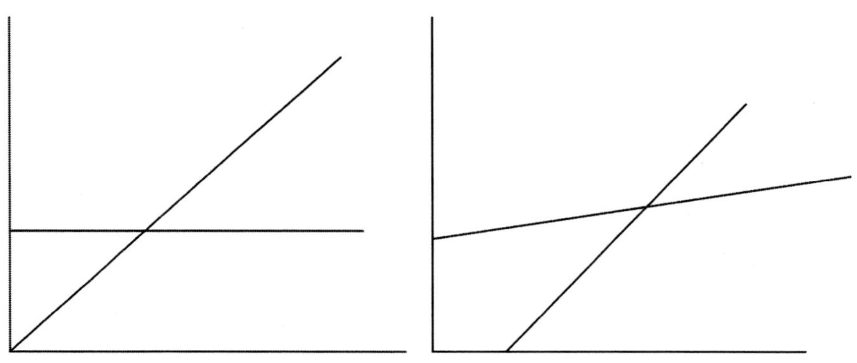

High degree of correlation **Low degree of correlation**

The regression lines cut each other at the point of average of X and Y. If a perpendicular line is drawn from the point of intersection to the X axis the average value of X is obtained. Similarly if a perpendicular line is drawn from the point of intersection to the Y axis, the average value of Y is obtained.

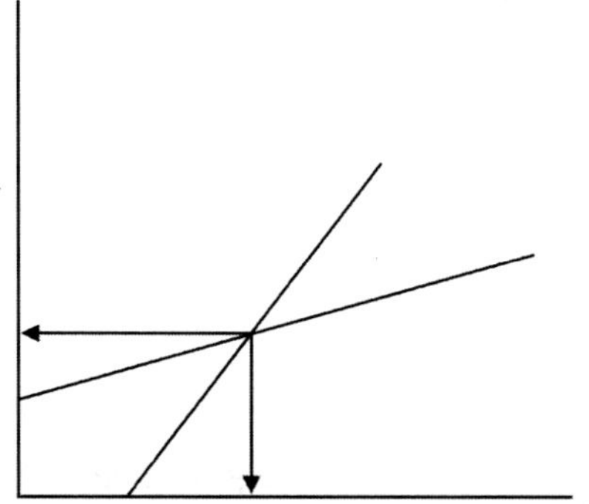

Regression lines showing averages

Table 17.1: Difference between correlation and regression

S. No.	Correlation	Regression
1	It studies the covariation of two variables. They tell us whether these two variables move in same or reverse direction	It studies how the variables regress or go back to the average
2	It measures the degree of covariation as correlation coefficient	It measures or predicts the value of one variable (dependent variable) when the value of the other variable (independent variable) is known
3	Correlation between two variables is not necessarily the cause and effect relationship	It presumes one variable as a cause and the other as its effect. The independent variable might influence the dependent variable and as such we can estimate the values of dependent variable by projecting the relationship between them

contd...

contd...

S. No.	Correlation	Regression
4	Correlation coefficient varies from −1 to + 1	The regression coefficient is positive when correlation coefficient is positive and the regression coefficient is negative when the correlation coefficient is negative
5	Both the variables x and y are random variables	Here x is a random variable and y is a fixed variable. Sometimes both variables may be random variables
6	It has limited application, because it is confined only to linear relationship between the variables	It has wider application, as it studies linear and nonlinear relationship between the variables

Types of Regression Analysis

Regression thus implies going back or returning towards the mean. There are three types of regression analysis. They are as follows:

1. ***Simple and multiple:*** Simple regression analysis involves the study of only two variables at a time whereas multiple regression analysis involves study of more than two variables.
2. ***Linear and nonlinear:*** In linear regression, the regression line is a straight line whereas in nonlinear regression, the regression line is not a straight line.
3. ***Total and Partial:*** In total regression analysis, all the variables are included in the analysis where as in partial only few are included excluding the unrelevant variables.

Importance of Regression Analysis

- The cause and effect relations are indicated from the study of regression analysis.
- It establishes the rate of change in one variable in terms of the changes in another variable.
- It helps in prediction and thus it can estimate the values of unknown quantities.
- It helps in determining the coefficient of correlation.
- It enables us to study the nature of relationship between the variables.

Regression Equations

Regression shows a relationship between the average values of two variables. Thus regression is very helpful in estimating and predicting the average value of one variable for a given value of the other variable. The estimate or prediction may be made with the help of a regression line which shows the average value of one variable x for a given value of the other variable y. The best average value of one variable associated with the given value of the other variable may also be estimated or predicted by means of an equation and the equation is known as ***Regression equation***.

The relationships between variables can be expressed in terms of mathematical/algebraic equations. As there are two regression lines, there are two regression equations. The two regression lines are as follows:

- Regression line of X on Y which shows the regression of X on Y.
- Regression line of Y on X which shows the regression of Y on X.

Regression line of X on Y which shows the regression of X on Y

It is the line which gives the best estimate for the values of x for a specified value of y. It is given by

$$\mathbf{x} - \bar{x} = r\frac{\sigma x}{\sigma y}(y - \bar{y})$$

$\bar{x}$ Mean of x series

$\bar{y}$ Mean of y series

r is correlation coefficient

σx standard deviation of x series

σy standard deviation of y series

It also can be written in the form of

- **X = a + bY**

Here 'a' and 'b' are two unknown constants. The constant 'a' shows the level of the fitted line. It is the distance between the point of origin and point where the regression line touches the Y axis. The constant 'b' shows the slop of the line.

The values of 'a' and 'b' in the above equation are found with the help of normal equations:

$$\sum X = na + b\sum Y$$
$$\sum XY = a\sum Y + b\sum Y^2$$

'n' is the number of observed pairs of value. $\sum X$, $\sum Y$, $\sum XY$, $\sum Y^2$ are the totals and they are computed from the value of two variables X and Y. Thus we can fit a least square line.

Regression line of Y on X which shows the regression of Y on X

$$\mathbf{y} - \bar{y} = r\frac{\sigma y}{\sigma x}(x - \bar{x})$$

It also can be written in the form of

$$\mathbf{Y = a + bX.}$$

where 'a' is the intercept of the line and 'b' is the slope of the line Y on X.

This line Y = a + bX is used to describe the dependence of one characteristic (y) upon the other characteristics(X). Here 'a' and 'b' are numerical unknown constants and parameters of the line X and Y represents the value of the two characteristics and once they are known we can calculate a predicted value of Y for any given value of X by direct substitution. It is evident that two regression lines can be constructed for every set of data, one each to describe the dependence of one characteristic on the other. This method is called the ***method of least squares***. 'b' is known as ***regression coefficient*** which shows a change expected in 'y' for unit of change in 'x'. The above line describes the dependence of 'y' on 'x' and b is the regression coefficient of 'y' on 'x'.

The value of 'a' and 'b' are found with the help of normal equations.

$$\Sigma Y = na + b\Sigma X$$
$$\Sigma XY = a\Sigma X + b\Sigma X^2$$

Regression Coefficients

There are two regression coefficients b_{xy} and $b_{yx.}$ Te regression coefficient of Y on X is: b_{yx} $r\frac{\sigma y}{\sigma x}$ and that of X on Y is b_{xy} $r\frac{\sigma x}{\sigma y}$. The properties of regression coefficients are as follows:

- The correlation coefficient is the geometric mean of the regression coefficients, i.e. $r\sqrt{byx \times bxy}$.
- If one of the regression coefficients is greater than unity, then the other is less than unity.
- Arithmetic mean of the regression coefficients is greater than the correlation coefficient. Both regression coefficients will have the same sign, i.e. either both are positive or both are negative.
- The sign of correlation coefficient is same as that of regression coefficients, i.e. $r > 0$ if $b_{xy} > 0$ and $b_{yx} > 0$; and $r < 0$ if regression coefficients are negative.

Properties of Linear Regressions

- The two regression lines X on Y and Y on X always intersect at their means $(\bar{x}\,\bar{y})$.
- Since $r^2 = b_{xy} \times b_{yx} => r = \sqrt{byx \times bxy}$, then r, b_{xy}, b_{yx} all have the same sign.
- If $r = 0$, then the regression coefficients are zero.
- The regression line become identical if $r = \pm 1$. If $r = 0$, then these lines are perpendicular to each other.

In any linear regression equation, the value of 'b' (known as the regression coefficient) shows the number of units increase (or decrease) in the dependent variable which accompany an increase of one unit in the independent variable. This value thus determines the slope of the line. If this value is positive, it means that the line is rising as we move toward higher values of X. If this value is negative, it means that the line is falling as we move toward higher values of X.

It must be noted, however, that the equation $Y = a + bX$ can be used only when Y is to be predicted from a given X. But when we want to predict X for a given Y, we need another equation $X = a + bY$ unless the correlation is perfect and there is a single regression line. Moreover, the two predicting equations should be used for estimating for those values of X and Y only which fall within the given series or are not very much outside of it. The reason is simple. We should not expect the same straight line trend to hold good in respect of the unknown data on either side of the series. The regression applies within the range of the observed data.

After the determination of the least square regression line, we need to know how 'good' is the fit of this line to the sample observations of Y on X, that is to say, we need to measure the dispersion of observations around the regression line. This knowledge is essential, because the closer the observations to the line, the better the goodness of fit, that is, the better is the explanation of the variations of Y by the changes in the explanatory variable X. A measure of the goodness of fit is the square of the correlation coefficient, r^2, which shows the percentage of the total variation of the dependent variable that can be explained by the independent variable X. It is called the ***coefficient of determination***. Thus, if $r^2 = 0.9$, this means that the regression line gives a good fit to the observed data, since this line explains 90% of the total variation of the Y values around their mean. The remaining 10% of the total variation in Y is unaccounted for by the regression line and is attributed to other factors. Once the regression equation has been obtained, it must be evaluated to determine whether it adequately describes the relationship between the two variables and whether it can be used effectively for prediction and estimation purposes.

Calculation of Regression Coefficients

There are two regression coefficients b_{xy} and b_{yx}. The regression coefficient of Y on X is: $b_{yx} = r\frac{\sigma y}{\sigma x}$ and that of X on Y is $b_{xy} = r\frac{\sigma x}{\sigma y}$.

Method 1

$$b_{yx} = r\frac{\sigma y}{\sigma x} = \frac{1/n\Sigma xy - \bar{x}\,\bar{y}}{Sx\ SY} X \frac{\sigma y}{\sigma x}$$

$$b_{yx} = \frac{1/n\Sigma xy - \bar{x}\,\bar{y}}{Sx\ SY} X \frac{\sigma y}{\sigma x}$$ (delete standard deviation of y from numerator and denominator)

$$b_{yx} = \frac{1/n\Sigma xy - \bar{x}\,\bar{y}}{Sx\ Sx} = \frac{\frac{\Sigma xy}{n} - \bar{x}\,\bar{y}}{\frac{\Sigma x^2}{n} - \frac{(\Sigma x)^2}{n^2}} = \frac{\Sigma xy - n\bar{x}\,\bar{y}}{\Sigma x^2 - n(\bar{x})^2}$$

$$b_{yx} = \frac{\Sigma xy - n\bar{x}\,\bar{y}}{\Sigma x^2 - n(\bar{x})^2}$$

or

Method 2

$$b_{yx} = r\frac{\sigma y}{\sigma x} = \frac{\Sigma xy}{\sqrt{\Sigma x^2}\sqrt{\Sigma y^2}} X \frac{\sigma y}{\sigma x}$$ (delete standard deviation of y from numerator and denominator)

In this method, $X = (x - \bar{x}); Y = (y - \bar{y});$

$$b_{yx} = \frac{\Sigma xy}{\Sigma x^2}; \qquad b_{xy} = \frac{\Sigma xy}{\Sigma y^2}.$$

Example 1:

Construct the two regression equations from the data given below.

X	2	4	6	8	10	12	14	16
Y	1	3	5	7	9	11	13	15

Method 1: Regression equation of Y on X

$$\text{Y on X} = Y = a + bX$$

The two normal equations to evaluate a and b are:

$$\Sigma Y = na + b\Sigma X$$
$$\Sigma XY = a\Sigma X + b\Sigma X^2$$

X	Y	X^2	Y^2	XY
2	1	4	1	2
4	3	16	9	12
6	5	36	25	30
8	7	64	49	56
10	9	100	81	90
12	11	144	121	132
14	13	196	169	182
16	15	256	225	240
$\Sigma X = 72$	$\Sigma Y = 64$	$\Sigma X^2 = 816$	$\Sigma Y^2 = 680$	$\Sigma XY = 744$

Substitute the values

$$\Sigma Y = na + b\Sigma X$$
$$64 = 8a + 72b \text{-----------} 1$$
$$\Sigma XY = a\Sigma X + b\Sigma X^2$$
$$744 = 72a + 816b \text{--------} 2$$

Divide equations 1 & 2 by 8

$$8 = a + 9b \text{-------------} 3$$
$$93 = 9a + 102b \text{---------} 4$$

Multiplying equation (3) by 9

$$72 = 9a + 81b \text{----------} 5$$
$$93 = 9a + 102b \text{---------} 4$$

Subtracting the equation 4 from 5

$$-21 = -21b$$
$$b = -21/-21 = 1$$
$$b = 1$$

Substitute the value of b in equation 1

$$64 = 8a + 72b \text{---------} 1$$
$$64 = 8a + 72$$
$$64 - 72 = 8a$$
$$8a = -8$$
$$a = -8/8 = -1.$$
$$Y = a + bX$$
$$Y = -1 + X$$
$$Y = X - 1$$

The regression equation of X on Y = **X = a + bY.**

The two normal equations to evaluate a and b are:

$$\Sigma X = na + b\Sigma Y$$
$$\Sigma XY = a\Sigma Y + b\Sigma Y^2$$

Substitute the values

$$\Sigma X = na + b\Sigma Y$$
$$72 = 8a + 64b\text{-------}6$$
$$\Sigma XY = a\Sigma Y + b\Sigma Y^2$$
$$744 = 64a + 680b\text{---}7$$

Divide equation 7 by 8

$$93 = 8a + 85b\text{-------}8$$

Subtract equation 8 from 6.

$$-21 = -21b$$
$$b = -21/-21 = 1$$

Substitute the value of b

$$72 = 8a + 64b\text{-------}6$$
$$72 = 8a + 64$$
$$8a = 72 - 64$$
$$8a = 8$$
$$a = 8/8 = 1$$
$$X = a + bY.$$
$$X = 1 + Y$$
$$X = Y + 1$$

$$b_{yx} = \frac{\Sigma xy - n\bar{x}\,\bar{y}}{\Sigma x^2 - n(\bar{x})^2} = \frac{744 - 8 \times 9 \times 8}{816 - 8 \times 9 \times 9}$$

$$= \frac{744 - 576}{816 - 648} = \frac{168}{168} = 1$$

Method 2

$$\Sigma X = 72; \Sigma Y = 64; n = 8$$
$$\text{Mean of X} = 72/8 = 9$$
$$\text{Mean of Y} = 64/8 = 8$$

Calculation of regression coefficient

$$r\frac{\sigma y}{\sigma x} = \frac{\Sigma XY}{\Sigma y^2} = 168/168 = 1$$

X	X–9	Y	Y–8	X^2	Y^2	XY
2	–7	1	-7	49	49	49
4	–5	3	-5	25	25	25
6	–3	5	-3	9	9	9
8	–1	7	-1	1	1	1
10	1	9	1	1	1	1
12	3	11	3	9	9	9
14	5	13	5	25	25	25
16	7	15	7	49	49	49
$\Sigma X = 72$		$\Sigma Y = 64$		$\Sigma X^2 = 168$	$\Sigma Y^2 = 168$	$\Sigma XY = 168$

Regression line of Y on X which shows the regression of Y on X.

$$y - \bar{y} = r\frac{\sigma y}{\sigma x}(x - \bar{y})$$

$$y - 8 = \frac{\Sigma XY}{\Sigma y^2}(x - 9)$$

$$\frac{\Sigma XY}{\Sigma y^2} = 168/168 = 1$$

$$Y-8 = X-9$$
$$Y = X-9+8$$
$$Y = X-1$$

Regression line of X on Y which shows the regression of X on Y

$$x - \bar{x} = r\frac{\sigma x}{\sigma y}(y - \bar{y})$$

$$X - 9 = \frac{\Sigma XY}{\Sigma x^2}(Y - 8)$$

$$\frac{\Sigma XY}{\Sigma x^2} = 168/168 = 1$$

$$X - 9 = Y - 8$$
$$X = Y - 8 + 9$$
$$X = Y + 1$$

Example 2:

Construct the two regression equations from the data given below.

X	1	2	3	4	5	6
Y	2	1	3	2	4	3

Regression equation of Y on X

$$Y = a + bX$$

The two normal equations to evaluate a and b are:

$$\Sigma Y = na + b\Sigma X$$
$$\Sigma XY = a\Sigma X + b\Sigma X^2$$

X	**Y**	**X^2**	**Y^2**	**XY**
1	2	1	4	2
2	1	4	1	2
3	3	9	9	9
4	2	16	4	8
5	4	25	16	20
6	3	36	9	18
$\Sigma X = 21$	$\Sigma Y = 15$	$X^2 = 91$	$\Sigma Y^2 = 43$	$\Sigma XY = 59$

Substitute the values

$$\Sigma Y = na + b\Sigma X$$

$$15 = 6a + 21b\text{----------}1$$
$$\Sigma XY = a\Sigma X + b\Sigma X^2$$
$$59 = 21a + 91b\text{--------}2$$

Multiplying equation (1) by 21

$$315 = 126a + 441b\text{------}3$$

Multiplying equation (2) by 6

$$354 = 126a + 546b\text{------}4$$

Subtracting the equation 4 from 3

$$39 = 0 + 105b$$
$$105b = 39$$
$$b = 39/105 = 0.37$$
$$Y = a + 0.37X$$
$$15 = 6a + 21(0.37)\text{-----}1$$
$$15 = 6a + 7.77$$
$$6a = 15–7.77$$
$$6a = 7.23$$
$$a = 7.23/6$$
$$a = 1.21$$
$$Y = 1.21 + 0.37X$$

Regression of X on Y

$$X = a + bY.$$

Normal equation

$$\Sigma X = na + b\Sigma Y$$
$$\Sigma XY = a\Sigma Y + b\Sigma y^2$$

Substitute the values

$$\Sigma X = na + \Sigma Y$$
$$21 = 6a + 15b\text{----------}5$$
$$\Sigma XY = a\Sigma Y + b\Sigma y^2$$
$$59 = 15a + 43b\text{---------}6$$

Multiplying equation (5) by 43, we get

$$903 = 258a + 645b\text{------}7$$

Multiplying equation (6) by 15, we get

$$885 = 225a + 645b\text{------}8$$

Subtracting the equation 8 from 7

$$18 = 33a$$
$$a = 18/33 = 0.55$$
$$21 = 6a + 15b\text{----------}5$$

Substituting the a value in equation 5

$$21 = 6(0.55) + 15b$$
$$21 = 3.3 + 15b$$
$$15b = 21 - 3.3$$
$$15b = 17.7$$
$$b = 17.7/15 = 1.18$$
$$X = 0.55 + 1.18Y$$

$$b_{yx} = \frac{\Sigma xy - n\bar{x}\,\bar{y}}{\Sigma x^2 - n(\bar{x})^2} = \frac{59 - 6 \times 3.5 \times 2.5}{91 - 6 \times 3.5 \times 3.5}$$

$$= \frac{59 - 52.5}{91 - 73.5} = \frac{6.5}{17.5} = 0.37$$

X	X – 3.5	Y	Y – 2.5	X²	Y²	XY
1	–2.5	2	–0.5	6.25	0.25	1.25
2	–1.5	1	–1.5	2.25	2.25	2.25
3	–0.5	3	0.5	0.25	0.25	–0.25
4	0.5	2	–0.5	0.25	0.25	–0.25
5	1.5	4	1.5	2.25	2.25	2.25
6	2.5	3	0.5	6.25	0.25	1.25
$\Sigma X = 21$		$\Sigma Y = 15$		$X^2 = 17.5$	$\Sigma Y^2 = 5.5$	$\Sigma XY = 6.5$

Mean of X = 21/6 = 3.5

Mean of Y = 15/6 = 2.5

The equation of regression line of Y on X is:

$$\mathbf{y} - \bar{y} = r\frac{\sigma y}{\sigma x}(x - \bar{x})$$

$$r\frac{\sigma y}{\sigma x} = \frac{\Sigma xy}{\Sigma x^2} = \frac{6.5}{17.5} = 0.37$$

$$\mathbf{y} - 2.5 = 0.37\ (x - 3.5)$$

$$y - 2.5 = 0.37\ x - 1.29$$

$$y = 0.37x - 1.29 + 2.5$$

$$y = 0.37x + 1.21$$

Regression equation of X on Y

$$\mathbf{x} - \bar{x} = r\frac{\sigma x}{\sigma y}(y - \bar{y})$$

Regression Coefficient

$$r\frac{\sigma x}{\sigma y} = \frac{\Sigma XY}{\Sigma y^2}\ 6.5/5.5 = 1.18$$

$$\mathbf{x} - \bar{x} = r\frac{\sigma x}{\sigma y}(y - \bar{y})$$

$$\mathbf{x - 3.5} = 1.18\ (y - 2.5)$$

$$x - 3.5 = 1.18y - 2.95$$

$$x = 1.18y - 2.95 + 3.5$$

$$x = 1.18y + 0.55$$

Example 3:

Find the regression equation of systolic BP(Y) on age (X) using the following data.

Age(X)	30	40	50	60	70
Systolic BP(Y)	120	126	142	146	150

Estimate the BP for the age of 57 years.

Method 1: Regression equation of Y on X

$$Y = a + bX$$

The two normal equations to evaluate a and b are:

$$\Sigma Y = na + b\Sigma X$$

$$\Sigma XY = a\Sigma X + b\Sigma X^2$$

X	Y	X^2	Y^2	XY
30	120	900	14400	3600
40	126	1600	15876	5040
50	142	2500	20164	7100
60	146	3600	21316	8760
70	150	4900	22500	10500
$\Sigma X = 250$	$\Sigma Y = 684$	$\Sigma X^2 = 13500$	$\Sigma Y^2 = 94256$	$\Sigma XY = 35000$

684 = 5a + 250b---------1

35000 = 250a + 13500b-----2

Multiply equation 1 by 50

34200 = 250a + 12500b-----3

Subtract equation 2 from 3

800 = 1000b

b = 800/1000 = 0.8

Substitute b value in equation 1

$$684 = 5a + 250b$$
$$684 = 5a + 250 \times 0.8$$
$$684 = 5a + 200$$
$$5a = 684 - 200$$
$$5a = 484$$
$$a = 484/5 = 96.8$$

Regression equation = y = 96.8 + 0.8x.

Method 2

X	**Y**	**X – 50**	**X^2**	**Y – 136.8**	**Y^2**	**XY**
30	120	–20	400	–16.8	282.24	336
40	126	–10	100	–10.8	116.64	108
50	142	0	0	5.2	27.04	0
60	146	10	100	9.2	84.64	92
70	150	20	400	13.2	174.24	264
$\Sigma X = 250$	$\Sigma Y = 684$		$\Sigma X^2 = 1000$		$\Sigma Y^2 = 684.8$	$\Sigma XY = 800$

$$\bar{x} = 250/5 = 50$$
$$\bar{y} = 684/5 = 136.8$$

Regression coefficient

$$r\frac{\sigma y}{\sigma x} = \frac{\Sigma xy}{\Sigma x^2} = \frac{800}{1000} = 0.8$$

Regression line Y(BP) on X(Age)

$$\mathbf{y} - \bar{y} = r\frac{\sigma y}{\sigma x}(x - \bar{x})$$

$$Y - 136.8 = 0.8\,(x - 50)$$
$$Y - 136.8 = 0.8\,(X - 50)$$
$$Y - 136.8 = 0.8X - 40$$
$$Y = 0.8X - 40 + 136.8$$

$$Y = 0.8X + 96.8$$

When $X = 57$

$$Y = 0.8(57) + 96.8$$

$$Y = 45.6 + 96.8 = 142.4$$

When age is 57 years the BP is 142.4

Example 4:

From the following data, construct the two regression equations. What is the probable value of aggression when the children play for 20 hours per week?

Sample No.	Score on aggression inventory (%)	Hours spent in a week
1	60	6
2	48	4
3	70	8
4	30	6
5	64	10
6	72	12

Method 1: Regression equation of Y on X

$$Y = a + bX$$

normal equation

$$\Sigma Y = na + b\Sigma X$$

$$\Sigma XY = a\Sigma X + b\Sigma X^2$$

Y	X	Y^2	X^2	XY
60	6	3600	36	360
48	4	2304	16	192
70	8	4900	64	560
30	6	900	36	180
64	10	4096	100	640
72	12	5184	144	864
Total 344	46	20984	396	2796

Substitute the values

$$\Sigma Y = na + b\Sigma X$$

$$344 = 6a + 46b \text{-----------} 1$$

$$\Sigma XY = a\Sigma X + b\Sigma X^2$$

$$2796 = 46a + 396b \text{--------} 2$$

Multiplying equation (1) by 46

$$15824 = 276a + 2116b \text{---} 3$$

Multiplying equation (2) by 6

$$16776 = 276a + 2376b \text{-----} 4$$

Subtracting the equation 4 from 3

$$16776 = 276a + 2376b \text{---} 5$$

$$15824 = 276a + 2116b \text{----} 3$$

$$952 = 260b$$
$$b = 952/260 = 3.66$$
$$b = 3.7$$

Substituting the value of 'b' in equation 1

$$344 = 6a + 46b$$
$$344 = 6a + 46x(3.7)$$
$$344 = 6a + 170.2$$
$$6a = 344 - 170.2$$
$$6a = 173.8$$
$$a = 173.8/6$$
$$a = 28.96$$
$$Y = a + bX$$
$$Y = 28.96 + 3.7X$$

Regression of X on Y

$$X = a + bY.$$

Normal equation

$$\Sigma X = na + b\Sigma Y$$
$$\Sigma XY = a\Sigma Y + b\Sigma y^2$$

Substitute the values

$$\Sigma X = na + \Sigma Y$$
$$46 = 6a + 344b\text{---------}5$$
$$\Sigma XY = a\Sigma Y + b\Sigma y^2$$
$$2796 = 344a + 20984b\text{----}6$$

Multiplying equation (5) by 344, we get

$$15824 = 2064a + 118336b\text{---------}7$$

Multiplying equation (6) by 6, we get

$$16776 = 2064a + 125904b\text{---------}8$$

Subtracting 8 from 7

$$-952 = -7568b$$
$$b = 952/7568 = 0.126 = 0.13$$

Substituting the value of b in equation 5

$$46 = 6a + 344b$$
$$46 = 6a + 344 \times 0.13$$
$$6a = 46 - 44.72$$
$$6a = 1.28$$
$$a = 1.28/6 = 0.21$$
$$X = a + bY$$
$$X = 0.21 + 0.13Y$$

Regression equation of Y on X = Y= 28.96 + 3.7X

Regression equation of X on Y = X = 0.21 + 0.13Y

Method 2

Mean value of $x = 46/6 = 7.66$

Mean value of $y = 344/6 = 57.3$

X	**x – 7.7**	**Y**	**Y – 57.3**	**Y²**	**X²**	**XY**
6	–1.6	60	2.7	7.29	2.56	–4.32
4	–3.6	48	–9.3	86.49	12.96	33.48
8	0.4	70	12.7	161.29	0.16	5.08
6	–1.6	30	–27.3	745.29	2.56	43.68
10	2.4	64	6.7	44.89	5.76	16.08
12	4.4	72	14.7	216.09	19.36	64.68
Total 46		344		1261.34	43.36	158.68

$$\mathbf{y} - \bar{y} = r\frac{\sigma y}{\sigma x}(x - \bar{x})$$

$$r\frac{\sigma y}{\sigma x} = \frac{\Sigma xy}{\Sigma x^2} = \frac{158.68}{43.36} = 3.7$$

$$\mathbf{y} - 57.3 = 3.7\,(x - 7.66)$$

$$\mathbf{y} - 57.3 = 3.7x - 28.34$$

$$y = 3.7x - 28.34 + 57.3$$

$$y = 3.7x + 28.96$$

Regression equation of X on Y

$$\mathbf{x} - \bar{x} = r\frac{\sigma x}{\sigma y}(y - \bar{y})$$

Regression Coefficient

$$r\frac{\sigma x}{\sigma y} = \frac{\Sigma XY}{\Sigma y^2} = 158.68/1261.34 = 0.1258 = 0.13$$

$$\mathbf{x} - \bar{x} = r\frac{\sigma x}{\sigma y}(y - \bar{y})$$

$$x - 7.66 = 0.13\,(y - 57.3)$$

$$x - 7.66 = 0.13y - 7.45$$

$$x = 0.13y - 7.45 + 7.66$$

$$x = 0.13y + 0.21$$

What is the probable value of aggression (Y) when the children play for 20 hours (X) per week.

We know the X value, i.e. hours of playing violent video game = 20 hours

$$Y = 28.96 + 3.7X$$

$$Y = 28.96 + 3.7 \times 20$$

$$Y = 28.96 + 74 = 102.96$$

Example 5:

Construct the regression equation for the following data

X	2	4	6	8	5
Y	5	8	9	10	8

Method 1

X	Y	X^2	Y^2	XY
2	5	4	25	10
4	8	16	64	32
6	9	36	81	54
8	10	64	100	80
5	8	25	64	40
Total 25	40	145	334	216

Regression equation of Y on X

$$Y = a + bX$$

Normal equation

$$\Sigma Y = na + b\Sigma X$$
$$\Sigma XY = a\Sigma X + b\Sigma X^2$$

Substitute the values

$$\Sigma Y = na + b\Sigma X$$
$$40 = 5a + 25b\text{-----------}1$$
$$\Sigma XY = a\Sigma X + b\Sigma X^2$$
$$216 = 25a + 145b\text{--------}2$$

Multiplying equation (1) by 5

$$200 = 25a + 125b\text{--------}3$$

Subtracting the equation 1 from 2

$$216 = 25a + 145b$$
$$200 = 25a + 125b$$
$$16 = 20b$$
$$b = 16/20 = 0.8$$

Substituting the value of 'b' in equation 1

$$40 = 5a + 25b$$
$$40 = 5a + 25x(0.8)$$
$$40 = 5a + 20$$
$$5a = 40 - 20$$
$$5a = 20$$
$$a = 20/5$$
$$a = 4$$
$$Y = a + bX$$
$$Y = 4 + 0.8X$$

Regression of X on Y

$$X = a + bY.$$

Normal equation

$$\Sigma X = na + b\Sigma Y$$
$$\Sigma XY = a\Sigma Y + b\Sigma y^2$$

Substitute the values

$$\Sigma X = na + \Sigma Y$$
$$25 = 5a + 40b\text{---------}4$$
$$\Sigma XY = a\Sigma Y + b\Sigma y^2$$
$$216 = 40a + 334b\text{------}5$$

Multiplying equation (4) by 8, we get

$$200 = 40a + 320b\text{------}6$$

Subtracting equation 6 from 5

$$216 = 40a + 334b$$
$$200 = 40a + 320b$$
$$16 = 14b$$
$$b = 16/14 = 1.14$$

Substitution of the value of 'b' in equation (4)

$$25 = 5a + 40b$$
$$25 = 5a + 40 \times (1.14)$$
$$25 = 5a + 45.6$$
$$5a = 25 - 45.6$$
$$5a = -20.6$$
$$a = -20.6/5 = -4.12$$
$$X = -4.12 + 1.14Y$$

Regression equation of Y on X = $Y = 4 + 0.8X$

Regression equation of X on Y = $X = -4.12 + 1.14Y$

Method 2

Mean value of X = 5

Mean value of Y = 8

X	Y	X – 5	X²	Y – 8	Y²	XY
2	5	–3	9	–3	9	9
4	8	–1	1	0	0	0
6	9	1	1	1	1	1
8	10	3	9	2	4	6
5	8	0	0	0	0	0
Total 25	40		20		14	16

$$\mathbf{y} - \bar{y} = r\frac{\sigma y}{\sigma x}(x - \bar{x})$$

$$r\frac{\sigma y}{\sigma x} = \frac{\Sigma xy}{\Sigma x^2} = \frac{16}{20} = 0.8$$

$$\mathbf{y} - 8 = 0.8\,(x - 5)$$

$$\mathbf{y} - 8 = 0.8x - 4$$

$$y = 0.8x - 4 + 8$$

$$y = 0.8x + 4$$

Regression equation of X on Y

$$\mathbf{x} - \bar{x} = r\frac{\sigma x}{\sigma y}(y - \bar{y})$$

Regression Coefficient

$$r\frac{\sigma x}{\sigma y} = \frac{\Sigma XY}{\Sigma y^2}\ 16/14 = 1.14$$

$$\mathbf{x} - \bar{x} = r\frac{\sigma x}{\sigma y}(y - \bar{y})$$

$$x - 5 = 1.14\,(y - 8)$$

$$x - 5 = 1.14y - 9.12$$

$$x = 1.14y - 9.12 + 5$$

$$x = 1.14y - 4.12$$

If X = 7 what is the probable value of Y?

$$Y = 4 + 0.8X$$

$$Y = 4 + 0.8(7)$$

$$Y = 4 + 5.6 = 9.6$$

If X = 10 what is the probable value of Y?

$$Y = 4 + 0.8X$$

$$Y = 4 + 0.8(10)$$

$$Y = 4 + 8 = 12$$

Example 6:

Construct the regression equation for the following data

X	20	10	40	80	60
Y	50	50	80	120	90

X	Y	X^2	Y^2	XY
20	50	400	2500	1000
10	50	100	2500	500
40	80	1600	6400	3200
80	120	6400	14400	9600
60	90	3600	8100	5400
Total 210	390	12100	33900	19700

Regression equation of Y on X

$$Y = a + bX$$

Normal equation

$$\Sigma Y = na + b\Sigma X$$
$$\Sigma XY = a\Sigma X + b\Sigma X^2$$

Substitute the values

$$\Sigma Y = na + b\Sigma X$$
$$390 = 5a + 210b\text{-----------}1$$
$$\Sigma XY = a\Sigma X + b\Sigma X^2$$
$$19700 = 210a + 12100b\text{-----}2$$

Multiplying equation (1) by 42

$$16380 = 210a + 8820b\text{------}3$$

Subtracting the equation 3 from 2

$$3320 = 3280b$$
$$b = 3320/3280 = 1.01$$
$$b = 1.01$$

Substituting the value of 'b' in equation 1

$$390 = 5a + 210b$$
$$390 = 5a + 210 \times 1.01$$
$$390 = 5a + 212.1$$
$$5a = 390 - 212 = 178$$
$$a = 178/5 = 35.6$$
$$Y = 35.6 + 1.01X$$

Regression of X on Y

$$X = a + bY.$$

Normal equation

$$\Sigma X = na + b\Sigma Y$$
$$\Sigma XY = a\Sigma Y + b\Sigma y^2$$

Substitute the values

$$\Sigma X = na + \Sigma Y$$
$$210 = 5a + 390b\text{---------}4$$
$$\Sigma XY = a\Sigma Y + b\Sigma y^2$$
$$19700 = 390a + 33900b\text{---}5$$

Multiplying equation (4) by 78, we get

$$16380 = 390a + 30420b\text{---}6$$

Subtracting equation 6 from 5

$$3320 = 3480b$$
$$b = 3320/3480$$
$$b = 0.95$$

Substitution of the value of 'b' in equation (4)

$$210 = 5a + 390b$$
$$210 = 5a + 390 \times 0.95$$
$$210 = 5a + 370.5$$

$$5a = -160.5$$
$$a = -160.5/5 = -32.1$$
$$X = -32.1 + 0.95Y$$

Regression equation of Y on X = Y = 35.6 + 1.01X

Regression equation of X on Y = X = −32.1 + 0.95Y

If X = 7 what is the probable value of Y?

$$Y = 35.6 + 1.01X$$
$$Y = 35.6 + 1.01 \times 7$$
$$Y = 35.6 + 7.07$$
$$Y = 42.67$$

If X = 10 what is the probable value of Y?

$$Y = 35.6 + 1.01 \times 10$$
$$Y = 35.6 + 10.1$$
$$Y = 45.7$$

Example 7:

Find out the regression equation for duration of service (x) and the job satisfaction (y).

Duration (X)	2	3	1	5	8	10	6	12	4
Job satisfaction (Y)	76	80	50	70	60	60	70	60	70

If X = 15 years find out the job satisfaction score.

x	y	X^2	Y^2	xy	$(x-\bar{x})$	$(x-\bar{x})^2$	$(y-\bar{y})$	$(y-\bar{y})^2$	$(x-\bar{x})(y-\bar{y})$
2	76	4	5776	152	−3.67	13.4689	9.78	95.6484	−35.8926
3	80	9	6400	240	−2.67	7.1289	13.78	189.8884	−36.7926
1	50	1	2500	50	−4.67	21.8089	−16.22	263.0884	75.7474
5	70	25	4900	350	−0.67	0.4489	3.78	14.2884	−2.5326
8	60	64	3600	480	2.33	5.4289	−6.22	38.6884	−14.4926
10	60	100	3600	600	4.33	18.7489	−6.22	38.6884	−26.9326
6	70	36	4900	420	0.33	0.1089	3.78	14.2884	1.2474
12	60	144	3600	720	6.33	40.0689	−6.22	38.6884	−39.3726
4	70	16	4900	280	−1.67	2.7889	3.78	14.2884	−6.3126
Total 51	596	399	40176	3292		110.001		707.5556	−85.3334
Mean 5.67	66.22	44.3	4464	365.8					

Method 1: Regression equation of Y on X = Y = a + bX

Normal equation

$$\Sigma Y = na + b\Sigma X$$
$$\Sigma XY = a\Sigma X + b\Sigma X^2$$

Substitute the values

$$\Sigma Y = na + b\Sigma X$$
$$596 = 9a + 51b\text{-----------}1$$
$$\Sigma XY = a\Sigma X + b\Sigma X^2$$
$$3292 = 51a + 399b\text{--------}2$$

Multiplying equation (1) by 51

$$30396 = 459a + 2601b\text{-----}3$$

Multiplying equation (2) by 9

$$29628 = 459a + 3591b\text{----}4$$

Subtracting 4 from 3

$$768 = 0 + (-990)b$$
$$b = 768/-990$$
$$b = -0.78$$

Substituting the value of 'b' in equation 1

$$596 = 9a + 51b\text{-----------}1$$
$$596 = 9a + 51\ (-0.78)$$
$$596 = 9a - 39.78$$
$$9a = 596 + 39.78$$
$$a = 635.78/9$$
$$a = 70.64$$
$$Y = a + bX$$
$$Y = 70.64 - 0.78X$$

Method 2

$$\mathbf{y} - \bar{y} = r\frac{\sigma y}{\sigma x}\ (x - \bar{x})$$

$$r\frac{\sigma y}{\sigma x} = \frac{\Sigma xy}{\Sigma x^2} = \frac{-85.33}{110} = -0.78$$

$$Y - 66.22 = -0.78(x - 5.67)$$
$$Y - 66.22 = -0.78x + 4.42$$
$$Y = -0.78x + 4.42 + 66.22$$
$$Y = -0.78x + 70.64$$
$$Y = 70.64 - 0.78x$$

When $x = 15$

$$Y = 70.64 - 0.78\ (15)$$
$$Y = 70.64 - 11.7$$
$$Y = 58.94$$

Example 8:

Construct the regression line Y on X and find the value of Y if X is 75

Anxiety score	40	30	70	80	60	42	38	32
Test score	66	66	48	22	56	80	70	60

x	y	X^2	Y^2	xy	$(x-\bar{x})$	$(x-\bar{x})^2$	$(y-\bar{y})$	$(y-\bar{y})^2$	$(x-\bar{x})(y-\bar{y})$
40	66	1600	4356	2640	–9	81	7.5	56.25	–67.5
30	66	900	4356	1980	–19	361	7.5	56.25	–142.5
70	48	4900	2304	3360	21	441	–10.5	110.25	–220.5
80	22	6400	484	1760	31	961	–36.5	1332.25	–1131.5
60	56	3600	3136	3360	11	121	–2.5	6.25	–27.5
42	80	1764	6400	3360	–7	49	21.5	462.25	–150.5
38	70	1444	4900	2660	–11	121	11.5	132.25	–126.5
32	60	1024	3600	1920	–17	289	1.5	2.25	–25.5
Total 392	468	21632	29536	21040		2424		2158	–1892
Mean 49	58.5	2704	3692	2630					

Method 1: Regression equation of Y on X = Y = a + bX

Normal equation

$$\Sigma Y = na + b\Sigma X$$
$$\Sigma XY = a\Sigma X + b\Sigma X^2$$

Substitute the values

$$\Sigma Y = na + b\Sigma X$$
$$468 = 8a + 392b\text{------------}1$$
$$\Sigma XY = a\Sigma X + b\Sigma X^2$$
$$21040 = 392a + 21632b\text{-------}2$$

Multiplying equation (1) by 49

$$22932 = 392a + 19208b\text{-------}3$$

Subtracting 3 from 2

$$-1892 = 0 + 2424b$$
$$b = -1892/2424$$
$$b = -0.78$$

Substituting the value of 'b' in equation 1

$$468 = 8a + 392b\text{------------}1$$
$$468 = 8a + 392\,(-0.78)$$
$$468 = 8a - 305.76$$
$$8a = 468 + 305.76$$
$$a = 773.76/8$$
$$a = 96.72$$
$$Y = a + bX$$
$$Y = 96.72 - 0.78X$$

Method 2

$$y - \bar{y} = r\frac{\sigma y}{\sigma x}(x - \bar{x})$$

$$r\frac{\sigma y}{\sigma x} = \frac{\Sigma xy}{\Sigma x^2} = \frac{-1892}{2424} = -0.78$$

$$Y - 58.5 = -0.78\,(x - 49)$$
$$Y - 58.5 = -0.78x + 38.22)$$
$$Y = -0.78x + 38.22 + 58.5$$
$$Y = -0.78x + 96.72$$
$$Y = 96.72 - 0.78x$$

When $X = 75$

$$Y = 96.72 - 0.78\,(75)$$
$$Y = 96.72 - 58.5$$
$$Y = 38.22$$

Example 9:

Construct regression equation Y on X for the below mentioned data.

Gestational age	31	38	34	40	42	37	35	40	42	41
Crown heel length	46.4	47.2	47.4	47.8	48.4	46.4	47.8	48.2	48	48

(x)	(y)	X^2	Y^2	xy	$(x-\bar{x})$	$(x-\bar{x})^2$	$(y-\bar{y})$	$(y-\bar{y})^2$	$(x-\bar{x})(y-\bar{y})$
31	46.4	961	2152.96	1438.4	−7	49	−1.16	1.3456	8.12
38	47.2	1444	2227.84	1793.6	0	0	−0.36	0.1296	0

(x)	(y)	X^2	Y^2	xy	$(x-\bar{x})$	$(x-\bar{x})^2$	$(y-\bar{y})$	$(y-\bar{y})^2$	$(x-\bar{x})(y-\bar{y})$
34	47.4	1156	2246.76	1611.6	–4	16	–0.16	0.0256	0.64
40	47.8	1600	2284.84	1912	2	4	0.24	0.0576	0.48
42	48.4	1764	2342.56	2032.8	4	16	0.84	0.7056	3.36
37	46.4	1369	2152.96	1716.8	–1	1	–1.16	1.3456	1.16
35	47.8	1225	2284.84	1673	–3	9	0.24	0.0576	–0.72
40	48.2	1600	2323.24	1928	2	4	0.64	0.4096	1.28
42	48	1764	2304	2016	4	16	0.44	0.1936	1.76
41	48	1681	2304	1968	3	9	0.44	0.1936	1.32
Total 380	475.6	14564	22624	18090.2	0	124		4.464	17.4
Mean 38.0	47.56	1456.4	2262.4	1809.02					

Method 1: Regression equation of Y on X = Y = a + bX

Normal equation

$$\Sigma Y = na + b\Sigma X$$
$$\Sigma XY = a\Sigma X + b\Sigma X^2$$

Substitute the values

$$\Sigma Y = na + b\Sigma X$$
$$475.6 = 10a + 380b \text{-----------} 1$$
$$\Sigma XY = a\Sigma X + b\Sigma X^2$$
$$18090.2 = 380a + 14564b \text{-------} 2$$

Multiplying equation (1) by 38

$$18072.8 = 380a + 14440b \text{------} 3$$

Subtracting 2 from 3

$$17.4 = 0 + 124b$$
$$b = 17.4/124$$
$$b = 0.14$$

Substituting the value of 'b' in equation 1

$$475.6 = 10a + 380b \text{-----------} 1$$
$$475.6 = 10a + 380\ (0.14)$$
$$475.6 = 10a + 53.2$$
$$10a = 475.6 - 53.2$$
$$a = 422.4/10$$
$$a = 42.24$$
$$Y = a + bX$$
$$Y = 42.24 + 0.14X$$

Method 2

$$\mathbf{y} - \bar{y} = r\frac{\sigma y}{\sigma x}(X - \bar{x})$$

$$r\frac{\sigma y}{\sigma x} = \frac{\Sigma xy}{\Sigma x^2} = \frac{17.4}{124} = 0.14$$

$$Y - 47.56 = 0.14\ (x - 38)$$
$$Y - 47.56 = 0.14x - 5.32)$$
$$Y = 0.14x - 5.32 + 47.56$$
$$Y = 0.14x + 42.24$$

Application of Regression Analysis in Nursing

It is used to estimate the value of unknown variable when we know the value of the other variable when both are correlated. If we know that aggression and playing violent video games are correlated we can estimate the value of aggression from the playing of violent video games. If we know that weight and dietary intake is correlated then we can estimate the amount of diet should be taken to achieve certain weight. Thus, regression analysis predicts the values of dependent variable from the values of independent variables.

In simple regression and correlation, the two variables of interest should be measured in the same individual. Suppose we want to study the relationship between the height and weight of 10 individuals, then we should measure the height and weight from each of these 10 samples. It is not sensible to measure the height of 10 individuals and weight of another 10 individuals and correlate. The sample regression equation should not be used to predict or estimate outside the range of values of the independent variable represented in the sample. Calculating outside the range of equation is called ***extrapolation***.

MULTIPLE REGRESSION ANALYSIS

Studies made on relationship between several variables simultaneously are termed as multiple correlation. In multiple correlation, we study three or more variables at a time to see the effect of all the independent factors on dependent factor. Multiple regression analysis represents an extension of two variables to three or more variables. In multiple regression, instead of one independent variable, two or more independent variables are used to estimate the values of dependent variable. Multiple regression is the appropriate method of analysis when the research problem involves a single metric dependent variable presumed to be related to two or more metric independent variables. The objective of multiple regression analysis is to predict the changes in the dependent variable in response to changes in the independent variables. It is the extension of simple linear regression. While simple regression shows the influence of one variable on another, multiple regression analysis shows the influence of two or more variables on a designated dependent variable. In multiple regression, it is assumed that a linear relationship exists between some variable Y which is known as the ***dependent variable***, and k independent variables, X_1, X_2, X_3,............X_k. The independent variables are sometimes referred to as explanatory variable, because of their use in explaining the variation in Y. They are also called ***predictor variables***, because of their use in predicting Y. In multiple regression analysis, any number of variables may be used as predictors. It is important to find variables that significantly influence the dependent variable.

In simple regression analysis, the equation Y = a + bX describes the relationship between the two variable X and Y. In multiple regression, we must extend that equation, adding one term for each new variable. Thus, when we have two independent variables, the formula would be:

$$Y = a + b_1X_1 + b_2X_2$$

We continue to use X for the independent variable but we add a subscript to distinguish between them. The values of the constants (a, b_1, b_2......) in the above equation are determined by the usual method of least squares.

The normal equations are as follows:

$$\Sigma y = Na + b_1\Sigma X_1 + b_2\Sigma X_2$$
$$\Sigma x_1y = a\Sigma X_1 + b_1\Sigma X_1^2 + b_2\Sigma X_1X_2$$
$$\Sigma x2y = a\Sigma X_2 + b_1X_1X_2 + b_2\Sigma X_2^2$$

It may be noted that the number of normal equations would depend upon the number of independent variables. If there are two independent variables, then 3 equations, if there are 3 independent variables then 4 equations and so on, are used.

The coefficient of Multiple Linear Correlation is represented by **R.**

Multiple correlation coefficient is a non negative coefficient. Its value ranges between 0 and 1. It cannot assume a minus value.

Example 10:

Calculate the multiple regression equation and estimate the rent for a two bedroom apartment 2 kms from downtown.

Rent Y	No. of rooms X_1	Distance X_2	X_1Y	X_2Y	X_1X_2	X_1^2	X_2^2	Y^2
360	2	1	720	360	2	4	1	129600
1000	6	1	6000	1000	6	36	1	1000000
450	3	2	1350	900	6	9	4	202500
525	4	3	2100	1575	12	16	9	275625
350	2	10	700	3500	20	4	100	122500
300	1	4	300	1200	4	1	16	90000
2985	18	21	11170	8535	50	70	131	1820225

The equations to solve are

$$y = a + b_1x_1 + b_2x_2$$
$$\Sigma y = Na + b_1\Sigma X_1 + b_2\Sigma x_2$$
$$\Sigma x_1y = a\Sigma x_1 + b_1\Sigma x_1^2 + b_2\Sigma x_1x_2$$
$$\Sigma x_2y = a\Sigma x_2 + b_1x_1x_2 + b_2\Sigma x_2^2$$
$$2985 = 6a + 18b_1 + 21b_2 \text{-----------------} 1$$
$$11170 = 18a + 70b_1 + 50b_2 \text{--------------} 2$$
$$8535 = 21a + 50b_1 + 131b_2 \text{-------------} 3$$

Multiply equation 1 by 18

$$53730 = 108a + 324\ b_1 + 378b_2 \text{----------} 4$$

Multiply equation 2 by 6

$$67020 = 108a + 420b_1 + 300b_2 \text{---------} 5$$

Subtract 5 from 4

$$-13290 = -96b_1 + 78b_2 \text{-------------------} 6$$

Multiply equation 1 by 21

$$62685 = 126a + 378b_1 + 441b_2 \text{---------} 7$$

Multiply equation 3 by 6

$$51210 = 126a + 300b_1 + 786b_2 \text{----------} 8$$

Subtract 8 from 7

$$11475 = 78b_1\text{-}345b_2 \text{---------------------} 9$$

Divide equations 6 and 9 by 3

$$-4430 = -32b_1 + 26b_2$$
$$3825 = 26b_1 - 115b_2$$

Again divide by 2

$$-2215 = -16b_1 + 13b_2 \text{-------------}10$$
$$1912.5 = 13b_1 - 57.5b_2 \text{------------}11$$

Multiply 10 by –13

$$28795 = 208b_1 - 169b_2 \text{------------}12$$

Multiply 11 by 16

$$30600 = 208b_1 - 920b_2 \text{------------}13$$

Subtract 12 from 13

$$1805 = -751b_2$$
$$\mathbf{b_2 = 1805/-751 = -2.40}$$

Substitute b_2 in equation 10

$$-2215 = -16b_1 + 13b_2$$
$$-2215 = -16b_1 + 13 \times -2.40$$
$$-2215 = -16b_1 - 31.2$$
$$-16b_1 = +31.2 - 2215$$
$$-16b_1 = -2183.8$$
$$\mathbf{b_1 = 2183.8/16 = 136.5}$$

Substitute b_1 and b_2 in equation 1

$$2985 = 6a + 18b_1 + 21b_2 \text{-----------}1$$
$$2985 = 6a + 18 \times 136.5 + 21 \times (-2.40)$$
$$2985 = 6a + 2457 - 50.4$$
$$2985 = 6a + 2406.6$$
$$6a = 2985 - 2406.6 = 578.4$$
$$\mathbf{a = 578.4/6 = 96.4}$$

Regression equation

$$y = a + b_1x_1 + b_2x_2$$
$$y = 96.4 + 136.5x_1 + (-2.40)x_2$$

If $X_1 = 2; X_2 = 2$

$$y = 96.4 + 136.5x_1 + (-2.40)x_2$$
$$y = 96.4 + 136.5 \times 2 + (-2.40) \times 2$$
$$y = 96.4 + 273 - 4.80$$
$$y = 364.6$$

Example 11:

Calculate the multiple regression equation for the below mentioned data. Estimate the number of patients who would visit when there are 10 specialty services in a clinic with a distance of 5 kms.

No. of patients Y	Specialty OPD services X_1	Distance X_2	X_1Y	X_2Y	X_1X_2	X_1^2	X_2^2	Y^2
50	3	1	150	50	3	9	1	2500
60	4	2	240	120	8	16	4	3600
100	6	2	600	200	12	36	4	10000
100	8	4	800	400	32	64	16	10000
200	8	3	1600	600	24	64	9	40000
Total 510	29	12	3390	1370	79	189	34	66100

The equations to solve are

$$y = a + b_1x_1 + b_2x_2$$
$$\Sigma y = Na + b_1\Sigma X_1 + b_2\Sigma x_2$$
$$\Sigma x_1y = a\Sigma x_1 + b_1\Sigma x_1{}^2 + b_2\Sigma x_1x_2$$
$$\Sigma x_2y = a\Sigma x_2 + b_1x_1x_2 + b_2\Sigma x_2^2$$
$$510 = 5a + 29b_1 + 12b_2\text{----------------}1$$
$$3390 = 29a + 189b_1 + 79b_2\text{-------------}2$$
$$1370 = 12a + 79b_1 + 34b_2\text{-------------}3$$

Multiply equation 1 by 29

$$14790 = 145a + 841\ b_1 + 348b_2\text{--------}4$$

Multiply equation 2 by 5

$$16950 = 145a + 945b_1 + 395b_2\text{---------}5$$

Subtract 5 from 4

$$-2160 = -104b_1 - 47b_2\text{-------------------}6$$

Multiply equation1 by 12

$$6120 = 60a + 348b_1 + 144b_2\text{-----------}7$$

Multiply equation 3 by 5

$$6850 = 60a + 395b_1 + 170b_2\text{-----------}8$$

Subtract 8 from 7

$$-730 = -47b_1 - 26b_2\text{---------------------}9$$

Multiply 6 by 26

$$-56160 = -2704b_1 - 1222b_2\text{-------------}10$$

Multiply 9 by 47

$$-34310 = -2209b_1 - 1222b_2\text{-------------}11$$

Subtract 11 from 10

$$21850 = 495\ b_1$$
$$\mathbf{b_1 = 21850/495 = 44.14}$$

Substitute b1 in equation 6

$$-2160 = -104\,(44.14) - 47b_2$$
$$-2160 = -4590.56 - 47b_2$$
$$-47b_2 = -2160 + 4590.56$$
$$-47b_2 = 2430.56$$
$$b_2 = 2430.56/47$$
$$b_2 = -51.71$$

Substitute b_1 and b_2 in equation 1

$$510 = 5a + 29b_1 + 12b_2\text{----------------}1$$
$$510 = 5a + 29\,(44.14) + 12(-51.71)$$
$$510 = 5a + 1280.06 - 620.52$$
$$5a = 510 - 1280.06 + 620.50$$
$$5a = 1130.5 - 1280.06$$
$$5a = -149.56$$
$$a = -149.56/5 = -29.9$$

Regression equation

$$y = a + b_1x_1 + b_2x_2$$
$$y = -29.9 + 44.14x_1 + (-51.71x_2)$$

If, $x_1 = 10;\ x_2 = 5$

$$y = -29.9 + 44.14x_1 + (-51.71x_2)$$
$$y = -29.9 + 44.14 \times 10 + (-51.71) \times 5$$
$$y = -29.9 + 441.4 - 258.6$$
$$y = 441.4 - 288.5$$
$$y = 152.9 = 153$$

Example 12:

The following data has been gathered from a random sample of adolescent boys who were playing violent video games. What would be the aggression score if a boy spends 2 hours per week for 1 year.

Sample No.	Score on Aggression Inventory	Hours Spent in a week X_1	Duration of playing in years X_2
1	60	6	3
2	48	4	2
3	70	8	5
4	30	6	2
5	64	10	4
6	72	12	5
7	44	6	2
8	68	8	4
9	38	6	2
10	56	4	6

Y	X_1	X_2	X_1y	X_2y	X_1x_2	X_1^2	X_2^2	y^2
60	6	3	360	180	18	36	9	3600
48	4	2	192	96	8	16	4	2304
70	8	5	560	350	40	64	25	4900
30	6	2	180	60	12	36	4	900
64	10	4	640	256	40	100	16	4096
72	12	5	864	360	60	144	25	5184
44	6	2	264	88	12	36	4	1936
68	8	4	544	272	32	64	16	4624
38	6	2	228	76	12	36	4	1444
56	4	6	224	336	24	16	36	3136
550	70	35	4056	2074	258	548	143	32124

The normal equations to solve are

$$y = a + b_1x_1 + b_2x_2$$
$$\Sigma y = Na + b_1\Sigma X_1 + b_2\Sigma x_2$$
$$\Sigma x_1y = a\Sigma x_1 + b_1\Sigma x_1^2 + b_2\Sigma x_1x_2$$
$$\Sigma x_2y = a\Sigma x_2 + b_1x_1x_2 + b_2\Sigma x_2^2$$
$$550 = 10a + 70b_1 + 35b_2 \text{---------------}1$$
$$4056 = 70a + 548b_1 + 258b_2 \text{------------}2$$
$$2074 = 35a + 258b_1 + 143b_2 \text{------------}3$$

Multiply equation 1 by 7

$$3850 = 70a + 490b_1 + 245b_2 \text{------------}4$$

Subtract equation 2 from 4

$$3850 = 70a + 490b_1 + 245b_2 \text{------------}4$$
$$4056 = 70a + 548b_1 + 258b_2 \text{------------}2$$
$$-206 = -58b_1 - 13b_2 \text{--------------------}5$$

Multiply equation 3 by 2

$$4148 = 70a + 516b_1 + 286b_2 \text{------------}6$$

Subtract equation 6 from 2

$$4056 = 70a + 548b_1 + 258b_2 \text{------------}2$$
$$4148 = 70a + 516b_1 + 286b_2 \text{------------}6$$
$$-92 = 32b_1 - 28b_2 \text{--------------------}7$$

Divide equation 7 by 2

$$-46 = 16b_1 - 14b_2 \text{---------------------}8$$

Multiply equation 5 by 14

$$-2884 = -812b_1 - 182b_2 \text{-----------------}9$$

Multiply equation 8 by 13

$$-598 = 208b_1 - 182b_2 \text{---------------}10$$

Subtract equation 10 from 9

$$-2884 = -812b_1 - 182b_2$$
$$-598 = 208b_1 - 182b_2$$
$$-2286 = 1020\,b_1$$
$$b_1 = -2286/1020 = -2.24$$

Substitute b_1 in equation 8

$$-46 = 16 \times -2.24 - 14b_2$$
$$-46 = -35.84 - 14b_2$$
$$-14b_2 = 35.84 - 46$$
$$-14b_2 = -10.16$$
$$b_2 = -10.16/-14 = 0.73$$

Substitute b_1 and b_2 in equation 1

$$550 = 10a + 70b_1 + 35b_2 \text{---------------}1$$
$$550 = 10a + 70 \times -2.24 + 35 \times 0.73$$
$$550 = 10a - 156.8 + 25.55$$
$$550 = 10a - 131.25$$
$$10a = 550 + 131.25$$
$$10a = 681.25$$
$$a = 681.25/10 = 68.13$$

Regression equation

$$y = a + b_1x_1 + b_2x_2$$
$$y = 68.13 - 2.24x_1 + 0.73x_2$$

If $x_1 = 2; x_2 = 1$

$$y = 68.13 - 2.24x_1 + 0.73x_2$$
$$y = 68.13 - 2.24 \times 2 + 0.73 \times 1$$
$$y = 68.13 - 4.48 + 0.73$$
$$y = 68.86 - 4.48$$
$$y = 64.38$$

SUMMARY

- The statistical method which helps us to estimate the unknown value of one variable from the known value of the related variable is called regression. Regression is the measures of the average relationship between two or more variables in terms of the original units of the data.
- The types of regression analysis are simple vs multiple, linear vs non linear and total vs partial.
- The relationships between variables can be expressed in terms of mathematical/ algebraic equations. As there are two regression line, there are two regression

equations. The two regression lines are regression line of X on Y which shows the regression of X on Y and regression line of Y on X which shows the regression of Y on X.

- Studies made on relationship between several variables simultaneously are termed as multiple correlation. Multiple regression analysis represents an extension of two variables to three or more variables.

EXERCISE

- Construct the regression line for the following

x	10	20	30	40	50
y	30	50	70	90	110

- Construct the regression line for the following

Duration	2	3	1	5	8	10	6	12	4
Job satisfaction	76	80	50	70	60	60	70	60	70

- In a study, physical risk score and the fetal outcome score was calculated for a pregnant women. Calculate the degree of relationship between the two variables and interpret.

Physical risk	16	2	6	4	5	2	7
Fetal Outcome	12	18	16	14	14	20	10

- Construct the regression line for the following

X	1	3	2	4	5	3	4	3	2	3
Y	1.5	2.5	2	3	3.5	2	3.5	2	2	3

- Construct the regression line for the data given below

Birthweight	Gestational age	Hb level of the mother
1.5	34	10
2.2	36	11
3.0	38	11.5
2.6	38	10
2.5	40	9.5
3.0	39	11

- Construct the regression line for the data given below

Achievement	Intelligence	Attendance
80	95	100
60	88	80
90	98	100
40	86	70
84	96	80
70	84	88

18 Probability Distribution

OBJECTIVES

After reading this chapter, you will be able to:

- Explain the concept of probability and probability distributions
- Understand binomial distribution
- Explain Poisson distribution
- Explain the concept of normal distribution
- Understand sampling distribution and central limit theorem
- Understand the application of probability distributions

INTRODUCTION

Probability theory was originated from gambling theory. The theory of probability provides the foundation for statistical inference. The concept of probability is not new to us. In our day-to-day life we apply and often use the term probability. We measure the probability of the occurrence of some event by a number between zero and one. The probability is one when an event is certain to occur and the probability is zero when the event is unlikely to occur. The more likely the event, the probability value is closer to one and the more unlikely the event the probability is closer to zero.

The subject of probability theory is the foundation upon which all of statistics is built providing a means for modeling populations, experiments, or almost anything else that could be considered a random phenomenon. Through these models statisticians are able to draw inferences about populations, inferences based on examination if only a part of the whole. Analyze these three statements.

When you jump from height, you will fall down.

When a coin is tossed, you may get either tail or head.

When you participate in a game, you may probably win.

It is impossible to run since he had fractured leg.

In the first statement there is a certainty. In the second statement, the chance is 50%. In the third statement, there is an uncertainty. In the fourth statement, there is an impossibility. In statistics, the numerical measurement of the certainty is one; impossibility is zero and uncertainty ranges from 0-1.

Today the probability theory has been used in all fields to a great extent. It is extensively used in commerce and economics. The theory of probability provides a numerical measure of the element of uncertainty.

Applications of Probability

- It is the base on which the law of statistical regularity and the law of inertia of large numbers are formed.
- Tests of significance are derived.
- It forms the base for the decision theory.
- It helps in foreseeing the uncertainties and chances of success.

PROBABILITY AND PROBABILITY DISTRIBUTIONS

The term probability is a commonly used one, to mean 'chance' or 'likelihood' of the occurrence of an event. In statistics, the term probability is used in a more precise sense. It is expressed numerically. The symbol to denote probability is P. The probability is measured in a probability scale.

Probability Scale

Absolute certainty	1.0	e.g. A stone thrown up will come down to earth
	0.9	
	0.8	
	0.7	
	0.6	
Equally likely	0.5	e.g. When a coin is tossed, the 'Head' will turn up
	0.4	
	0.3	
	0.2	
	0.1	
Absolute impossibility	0.0	e.g. I will travel to the sun tomorrow.

The probability scale runs from 0 to 1. There is no probability lesser than 0, that is, there is no negative probability and there is no probability greater than unity, i.e. 1. The word probable is used very commonly in everyday language to mean something which is very likely to happen. Probability is a measure or estimation of how likely it is that something will happen or that a statement is true. It is a measure of chance. Sometimes we may need to measure or quantify a chance. The concept of probability helps in fulfilling this need adequately. Probabilities are given a value between 0 (0% chance or will not happen) and 1 (100% chance or will happen). The higher the degree of probability, the more likely the event is to happen, or, in a longer series of samples, the greater the number of times such event is expected to happen. In day-to-day life, we may face with uncertainties or we may not sure about the outcome of any particular trial. But in a long run, one can predict the outcome. In physical and biological sciences, one may come across the phenomena of uncertainty and a long term regularity. For example, in the science of genetics, in the long run one can predict the percentage of offspring will be male and female. In genetic disorders, we are able to predict the probability of developing the genetic disorders in the family.

Definition of Probability

The chance of occurrence of any particular event is known as probability.
The probability scale: Chance is measured on a probability scale having zero at one end and one at the other end. It ranges from absolute certainty to absolute impossibility. The other point on the probability scale falling between zero and one indicates the relative chance of occurrence of the event. Each possible outcome of an experiment is called an event. A group of events said to be exhaustive if it includes all the possible events. A group of events is said to be equiprobable events if there is equal chance for each event in the group to occur.

Measurement of Probability

Classical probability: When a coin is tossed what is the probability of getting head or tail? One can expect either head or tail since there is only one possibility out of two when each time a coin is tossed. Same way what is the probability that a baby will be a male or female? Here the probability will be 1/2. This is otherwise known as the probability of outcome.
Frequency probability: In a long observation or study, one can measure the probability even in more complex situations. The estimate of probability of a specified outcome based on a series of independent trials is given by

$$\text{Probability} = \frac{\text{The number of times the outcome occurred}}{\text{Total number of trials}}$$

Sometimes this probability is referred to as statistical probability, frequency or empirical probability.

Look at the data given below in the table.

Prevalence of no. of children in the family in a selected community:

No. of children	No. of family
No children	28
1	257
2	823
3	542
4	60
5	20
Total	1730

Find out the probability distribution for the given information:

No. of children	No. of family
No children	0.02
1	0.15
2	0.48
3	0.31
4	0.03
5	0.01
Total	1.00

What is the probability that a randomly selected family to have 3 children?
The probability of a randomly selected family to have 3 children is 0.31.
What is the probability that a randomly selected family to have 1 child or 3 children?
To answer this addition rule is to be followed.

$$P\,(1 \text{ or } 3) = P\,(1) + P\,(3)$$
$$= 0.15 + 0.31 = 0.46$$

What is the probability that a randomly selected family is the one without a child?
The answer is 0.02
The probability distribution is the study of distribution of all values of a variable relative to its total values.

Laws of Probability

There are two important laws of probability which are used to find out the probability in complex situations where the events concerned are independent.
Additional law: If an event can occur in any one of several mutually exclusive ways, the probability of that event is sum of the individual probabilities of the different ways in which it can occur.

$$P(A \text{ or } B) = P(A + B)$$
$$= P\,(A) + P(B)$$

Example 1:

When we toss a dice, what is the probability of getting 4 or 6?

The probability of getting 4 = 1/6 or P (4) = 1/6
The probability of getting 6 = 1/6 or P (6) = 1/6

$$P\,(4 \text{ or } 6) = P\,(4) + P\,(6)$$
$$= \frac{1}{6} + \frac{1}{6} = \frac{2}{6} = \frac{1}{3}$$

Example 2:

What is the probability of getting an even number when a dice is thrown?
When a dice is thrown, the possibilities are 1, 2, 3, 4, 5 and 6.
The even numbers are 2, 4, and 6. So the probability of getting an even number is $= \frac{3}{6} = \frac{1}{2}$

Example 3:

A box contains 5 white ball and 10 blue ball. What is the probability of drawing a blue ball? What is the probability of getting a white or blue ball?
The total number of equally likely and exhaustive cases = n = 5 + 10 = 15

Number of favorable cases = 10

$$\text{Probability of drawing a blue ball} = \frac{10}{15} = \frac{2}{3}$$

$$\text{The probability of getting white ball} = \frac{5}{15} = \frac{1}{3}$$

$$\text{The probability of getting blue ball} = \frac{2}{3}$$

$$\text{The probability of getting white or blue ball} = \frac{2}{3} + \frac{1}{3} = \frac{3}{3} = 1$$

Multiplication Law: The probability of the simultaneous occurrence of 2 or more independent events is the product of the individual probabilities.

$$P\ (A \text{ and } B) = P\ (AB)$$
$$= P\ (A) \times P(B)$$

Example 4:

In tossing 2 coin what is the probability of getting tail in both coin?

$$\text{Probability of tail in one coin} = \frac{1}{2}$$

$$\text{Probability of tail in another coin} = \frac{1}{2}$$

$$\text{The probability of tail in both coins} = \frac{1}{2} \times \frac{1}{2} = \frac{1}{4}$$

Example 5:

In rolling a dice what is the probability of getting a 2 and 4?

$$\text{The probability of getting 2} = \frac{1}{6}$$

$$\text{The probability of getting 4} = \frac{1}{6}$$

$$\text{The probability of getting 2 and 4} = \frac{1}{6} \times \frac{1}{6} = \frac{1}{36}$$

Example 6:

A university has to select an examiner from a list of 30 persons. Eight of them from Chennai, 10 of them with more than 10 years of experience and 5 of them working in a post graduate teaching institution. What is the probability of the university selecting an examiner with more than 10 years of experience and working in post graduate teaching institution from Chennai.

Probability of selecting an examiner from Chennai = $\frac{8}{30}$

Probability of selecting an examiner with more than 10 years of experience

$$= \frac{10}{30}$$

Probability of selecting an examiner who is working in PG institution

$$= \frac{5}{30}$$

The probability of the university selecting an examiner with more than 10 years of experience and working in post graduate teaching institution from Chennai =

$$\frac{8}{30} \times \frac{10}{30} \times \frac{5}{30} = \frac{4}{270} = \frac{2}{135} = 0.015$$

Probability Distribution

When we draw inference from the sample, we consider the sampling distribution and the probability values. The statisticians have established theoretical distribution and the probability values. Mathematical models have been developed, the required probabilities are calculated and made available in tables for certain types of distributions such as binomial distribution, poisson distribution and normal distribution.

Theoretical or probability distributions refer to mathematical models of expected frequencies of a finite number of observations of a variable with associated probabilities. They are based on mathematical functions (Fig. 18.1).

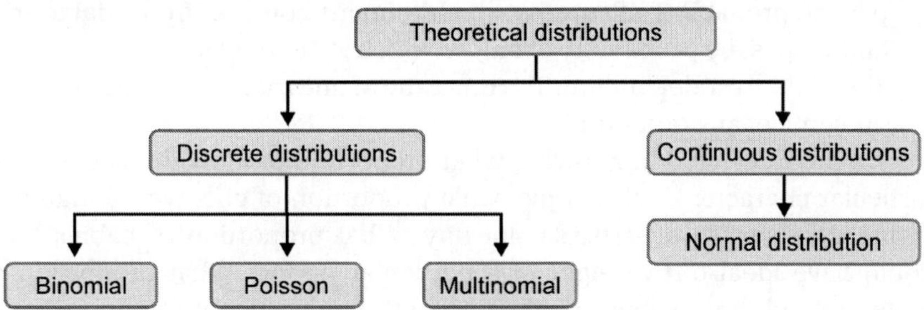

Fig. 18.1: Classification of theoretical distributions

A random variable is said to be discrete if it takes only a finite or an infinite but countable number of values. Tossing a coin or throwing a dice are the examples of discrete random variables. A continuous random variable is a random variable that can take on any value in an interval of two numbers. Weight and hemoglobin values are the examples of continuous random variable. When we collect data on some variable and make a frequency distribution, which is known as observed frequency distribution. In the introduction chapters, we have learned how to make frequency distribution of observed data. On the other hand, the statisticians/mathematicians had developed expected frequency distribution or theoretical frequency distributions based on the previous experience or theoretical considerations. One can compare the actual or observed frequency distribution with the theoretical or expected frequency distributions and check the discrepancy between these two is due to sampling fluctuation or some bias. This concept helps in hypothesis testing.

Binomial Distribution

Binomial distribution is a discrete probability distribution which is obtained when the probability of the happening of an event is same in all the trials, and there are only two events in each trial. For example, the probability of getting a head, when a coin is tossed a number of times, must remains same in each toss, i.e. $p = 1/2$.

This distribution was discovered by a Swiss mathematician, James Bernoulli and is also known as Bernoulli distribution. When a random process or experiment, called a trial, can result in only one of two mutually exclusive outcomes, such as dead or alive, sick or well, male or female, the trial is called a Bernoulli trial.

The Bernoulli Process

- A sequence of Bernoulli trials forms a Bernoulli process under the following conditions.
- Each trial results in one of two possible, mutually exclusive outcomes.
- One of the possible outcomes is denoted (arbitrarily) as a success, and the other is denoted a failure.
- p is the probability of success which remains constant from trial to trial and $1 - p$ is the probability of failure which is denoted as q.
- The trials are independent. The outcome of one trial is not affected by the outcome of any other trial.

We are interested in knowing what proportion of individuals possess a particular character. For example, what proportion of girls would maintain normal Hb level in a particular locality. What proportion of babies born would have ideal birth weight in a particular period. What proportion of students would score above distinction in the university exam. An estimate of this proportion is calculated on the basis of a suitably drawn sample from this population and the corresponding sampling distribution. In this type of problem the sampling distribution is given by a theoretical frequency distribution known as Binomial distribution.

The formula for binomial distribution is

$$C_r^n\, p^r\, q^{n-r} \text{ where } C_r^n = \frac{n!}{r!(n-r)!}$$

r is the number of occurrence of the event

P is the probability of occurrence of the event

q is the probability of non occurrence of the event

n is the size of the sample

n and p in the distribution are called the parameters of the distribution.

The mean and variance of binomial distribution for r successes in n trials is given as follows:

$$\text{Mean} = np$$
$$\text{Variance} = npq$$
$$\text{Standard deviation} = \sqrt{npq}$$

Binomial distribution is symmetrical if $p = q = 0.5$

It is positively skewed if $p < 0.5$ and it is negatively skewed if $p > 0.5$

The binomial distribution depends on the parameters of p or q, the probability of occurrence or non occurrence. The distribution will be symmetrical if $p = q$. It is skewed or asymmetric if $p \neq q$. The mode of the binomial distribution is equal to that value of X which has the largest frequency. The shape and location of a binomial distribution changes as p changes for given n or n changes for a given p.

Example 7:

In a population of postnatal mother, 20% of deliveries are by cesarean section. We can say that the probability of a delivery by cesarean section is 0.2. If we randomly select any five postnatal mother, what is the probability that exactly two of them would have undergone cesarean section?

The number of combinations of n objects that can be formed by taking r of them at a time is given by; $p = 0.2$, $n = 5$, $r = 2$

$$C_r^n = \frac{n!}{r!(n-r)!}$$

$$C_2^5 = \frac{5!}{2!(5-2)!} = \frac{5 \times 4 \times 3 \times 2 \times 1}{2! \times 3!} = \frac{5 \times 4 \times 3 \times 2 \times 1}{2 \times 1 \times 3 \times 2 \times 1} = 10$$

In this example, $r = 2$, the number of successes; the number of failures, $n - r = 5 - 2 = 3$. The probability of obtaining exactly r successes in n trials is $C_r^n p^r q^{n-r}$

$$= 10 \times (0.2)^2 \times (0.8)^3$$
$$= 10 \times 0.04 \times 0.512 = 0.2048$$

Example 8:

In a metro city, 30% of population developed skin diseases. If a random sample of size 12 is selected from this population, what is the probability that it will exactly contain 5 individuals with skin disease?

The probability of individuals with skin disease is 0.3.

Using the binomial distribution formula, we can find the probability as follows; $q = 0.7$, $n = 12$, $r = 5$

$$C_r^n = \frac{n!}{r!(n-r)!}$$

$$C_5^{12} = \frac{12!}{5!(12-5)!} = \frac{12 \times 11 \times 10 \times 9 \times 8 \times 7 \times 6 \times 5 \times 4 \times 3 \times 2 \times 1}{5 \times 4 \times 3 \times 2 \times 1 \times 7 \times 6 \times 5 \times 4 \times 3 \times 2 \times 1}$$

$$= \frac{12 \times 11 \times 10 \times 9 \times 8}{5 \times 4 \times 3 \times 2 \times 1} = 792$$

The probability of selecting 5 individuals with skin disease is calculated by using the formula, $C_r^n p^r q^{n-r}$

$$= 792 \times (0.3)^5 \times (0.7)^7$$
$$= 792 \times .00243 \times 0.0823 = 0.158$$

Using binomial table: When the sample size, n is large, the calculation of probability value is tedious. Probabilities for different values of n, p, and r have been tabulated, and one can use this table to find the probability value. When r = 5; n = 12 and p = 0.3, the table value can be calculated by the following.

In table, locate p = 0.3 for n = 12, we find that $p(r < 5) = 0.8822$ and $p(r < 4) = 0.7237$. By subtracting the later value from the first value (0.8822 – 0.7237), we get 0.1585. We can see that the answer is the same.

Example 9:

The average percentage of failure in Anatomy and Physiology examination is 40. What is the probability that out of 5 candidates, at least 4 passed in the examination?

The number of pass in the examination may be minimum 4 or all of them may pass.

$$P = 1 - q$$

$$q = \frac{40}{100} = 0.4$$

$$P = 1 - 0.4 = 0.6$$

The formula for binomial distribution is

$$C_r^n P^r q^{n-r} \text{ where } C_r^n = \frac{n!}{r!(n-r)!}$$

The probability of 4 or all passing in the examination

$$P(x \geq 4) = P(x = 4) + P(x = 5)$$

$$= P(4) + P(5)$$

$$= C_4^5 (0.6)^4 (0.4)^1 + C_5^5 (0.6)^5$$

(the value for C_4^5 is calculated using the formula

$$\frac{n!}{r!(n-r)!}, \text{ i.e. } \frac{5!}{4!\,(5-4)!} = \frac{5!}{4! \times 1!} = \frac{5 \times 4 \times 3 \times 2 \times 1}{4 \times 3 \times 2 \times 1 \times 1} = 5$$

$$= (5 \times 0.13)\,(0.4) + (1 \times 0.078)$$

$$= 0.26 + 0.078 = 0.338$$

Example 10:

The incidence of occupational disease in an industry is such that the workers have a 10% chance of suffering from it. What is the probability that out of 5 workers, 3 or more will develop the disease?

$$P = 10/100 = 0.1$$

$$q = 1 - P$$

$$q = 1 - 0.1 = 0.9$$

The formula for binomial distribution is where n = 5

$$C_r^n P^r q^{n-r} \text{ where } C_r^n = \frac{n!}{r!(n-r)!}$$

The probability of passing 3 or more will develop the disease

$$P(x \geq 3) = P(x = 3) + P(x = 4) + P(x = 5)$$
$$= P(3) + P(4) + P(5)$$
$$= C_3^{\,5}(0.1)^3(0.9)^2 + C_4^{\,5}(0.1)^4(0.9) + C_5^{\,5}(0.1)^5$$

(the value for $C_3^{\,5}$ is calculated using the formula

$$\frac{n!}{r!(n-r)!}. \text{ i.e. } \frac{5!}{3!(5-3)!} = \frac{5!}{3! \times 2!} = \frac{5 \times 4 \times 3 \times 2 \times 1}{3 \times 2 \times 1 \times 1 \times 2} = 10$$

$$= 10(0.001)(0.81) + 5(0.0001)(0.9) + 1(0.00001)$$
$$= 0.0081 + 0.00045 + 0.00001 = 0.0086$$

Example 11:

In a certain adolescent girls population, 15% of them are anemic. If a random sample of 10 adolescent girls were selected, find the probability that five or less will be anemic.

$$p(x \leq 5) = 0.9986$$

Six or more will be anemic

$$p(x \geq 6) = 1 - p(x \leq 5) = 1 - 0.9986 = 0.0014$$

Between 5 and 8 inclusive will be anemic.

$$p(5 \leq x \leq 8) = p(x \leq 9) - p(x \leq 4) = 1 - 0.9901 = 0.0099$$

Application of Binomial Distribution

In order to use binomial distribution, there are certain conditions to be met. They are as follows:

- The data collected on a variable must be discrete. It should be a complete number such as 1, 2, 3, 4, etc. and it should not be 1.8, 2.6, etc.
- There are only two alternatives or possible outcomes or occurrence. For example, either pass or fail, head or tail, success or failure, etc.
- The number of trials should be small and finite.
- Each trial should be repeated under the same conditions.
- The trials or events must be independent. The occurrence of one happening must not affect the others.
- p is the probability of success from trial to trial, is fixed and q is the probability of failure, is equal to 1-p. This is the same in all the trials.

Poisson Distribution

Poisson distribution was discovered by a French Mathematician Siméon Denis Poisson. It is also a discrete distribution and is widely used. It is different from binomial distribution that the n is large and p is very small. In binomial distribution, the sample size is definite and one can count the number of times a certain event is observed whereas in Poisson distribution, one cannot count the number of times an event occur or does not occur. For example, accident in an industry, person killed in road accidents, no. of flight hijack, no. of air crash, etc.

There are situations in which the number of times an event occur can be counted but the number of times the event did not occur cannot be counted. Yet counting the number of times the event did not occur is meaningless. For example, counting the number of times the rainfall occurred in a particular period is useful whereas the number of times the rainfall did not occur may not be useful. Counting the number of times the children in a particular locality suffered from fever is useful whereas the number of times children did not develop fever is meaningless.

Thus n, the total of trials in regard to a given event, is not known, the binomial distribution is inapplicable. Poisson distribution is made use of in such cases where p is very small. We mean that the chance of occurrence of that event is very small. The probability of observing one spell, two spells, etc in a given sample, can theoretically be found out by the use of Poisson distribution. The formula for Poisson distribution is

$$= \frac{e^{-\lambda}\lambda^{x}}{x!}$$

The Greek letter (lamda) is called the parameter of the distribution and is the average number of occurrences of the random event in the interval. The symbol 'e' is the constant (to four decimals) 2.7183.

x is the number of times the event occurs

λ is the mean of the distribution

$$x! = 1 \times 2 \times 3 \times 4 \times \ldots\ldots \times x$$

If the mean is known, all the frequencies can be found out theoretically.

The Poisson distribution arises when the events being counted occur

- Independently
- Such that the probability that two or more events simultaneously occur is zero
- Randomly in time or space
- Uniformly (that is the mean number of event in an interval is directly proportional to the length of the interval).

In Poisson distribution, as 'n' moves towards infinity and 'p' moves towards zero and np or mean remains constant. The mean and variance is the same in Poisson distribution.

$$\text{Mean} = np = m = \lambda$$
$$\text{Variance} = np = m = \lambda$$
$$\text{Standard Deviation} = \sqrt{np} = \sqrt{m}$$

Application of Poisson Distribution

- The random variable X must be discrete
- A dichotomy exists
- n is large and p is small (close to zero). If p is zero, then the distribution is j-shaped and unimodal
- Statistical independence is assumed. The occurrence of one event should not affect the occurrence of the other.

This distribution is positively skewed to the left. With the increase in the value of the mean, 'm' the distribution shifts to the right and the skewness diminishes. If n is large and p is small, this distribution gives a close approximation to binomial distribution. Since the arithmetic mean of Poisson is same as that of binomial, so the Poisson distribution can be used instead of binomial if n or p is not known. Poisson distribution has only one parameter, m, the arithmetic mean. Thus, the entire distribution can be determined once the arithmetic mean is known.

Example 12:

If the random variable X follows a Poisson distribution with the mean of 3.4, find p (x = 5).

$$\lambda = 3.4$$

The formula for Poisson distribution is = $\frac{e^{-\lambda}\lambda^{x}}{x!}$

$$p\,(x = 5) = \frac{e^{-3.4}3.4^{5}}{5!}$$

$$= \frac{(0.04979 \times 0.6703)(3.4 \times 3.4 \times 3.4 \times 3.4 \times 3.4)}{5 \times 4 \times 3 \times 2 \times 1}$$

$$= \frac{(0.0334)(454.35)}{120} = \frac{15.18}{120}$$

$$= 0.126$$

Example 13:

Find the probability that at most 5 defective thermometers will be found in a box of 200, if it is known that 2% of such thermometers are expected to be defective. (e – 4 = 0.0183)

$$\lambda = n^{*}p = 200^{*}0.02 = 4$$

The formula for Poisson distribution is = $\frac{e^{-\lambda}\lambda^{x}}{x!}$

P(x < 5)= P(0) + P(1) + P(2) + P(3) + P(4) + P(5)

$$= e^{-4}\left(\frac{4^0}{0!}+\frac{4^1}{1!}+\frac{4^2}{2!}+\frac{4^3}{3!}+\frac{4^4}{4!}+\frac{4^5}{5!}\right)$$

$$= 0.0183\left(1+4+\frac{16}{2}+\frac{64}{6}+\frac{256}{24}+\frac{1024}{120}\right)$$

$$= 0.0183(1 + 4 + 8 + 10.67 + 10.67 + 8.53)$$
$$= 0.0183 \times 42.87 = 0.7845$$

The value can be calculated using cumulative Poisson distribution table(look at $\lambda = 4$ and x = 5). The table value is 0.785.

Example 14:

It is known from past experience that in a certain hospital there are on the average 4 falls/accidents per month. Find the probability that in a given year there will be less than 4 accidents. Assume Poisson distribution.

$$\lambda = 4$$

The formula for Poisson distribution is $= \dfrac{e^{-\lambda}\lambda^{x}}{x!}$

The required probability that there will be less than 4 accidents is given as:

$$\begin{aligned} p(x < 4) &= P(0) + P(1) + P(2) + P(3) \\ &= e^{-4}\left(\frac{4^0}{0!}+\frac{4^1}{1!}+\frac{4^2}{2!}+\frac{4^3}{3!}\right) \\ &= 0.0183\left(1+4+\frac{16}{2}+\frac{64}{6}\right) \\ &= 0.0183(1 + 4 + 8 + 10.67) \\ &= 0.0183 \times 23.67 = 0.4336 \end{aligned}$$

Example 15:

The average number of patients who appeared at a medical OPD of a certain hospital per minute is 2. Find the probability that during a given minute (a) No patient appears; (b) Three or more patient appears.

$$\lambda = 2$$

The formula for Poisson distribution is $= \dfrac{e^{-\lambda}\lambda^{x}}{x!}$

(a) No patient appears

$$p(0) = 0.1353$$

(b) Three or more patient appears

$$\begin{aligned} p(x \geq 3) &= 1 - [P(0) + P(1) + P(2)] \\ &= 1 - e^{-2}\left[1+\frac{2^1}{1!}+\frac{2^2}{2!}\right] \\ &= 1 - [0.1353 \times (1 + 2 + 2)] = 1 - 0.1353 \times 5 \\ &= 1 - 0.6765 = 0.3235 \end{aligned}$$

Example 16:

A small life insurance company has determined that on the average it receives 6 death claims per day. Find the probability that the company receives at least seven death claims on a randomly selected day.

$$\lambda = 6$$

The formula for Poisson distribution is $= \dfrac{e^{-\lambda}\lambda^{x}}{x!}$

$$P(x \geq 7) = 1 - P(x \leq 6)$$

Referring to the cumulative Poisson distribution table, for $\lambda = 6$; $x = 6$ the value is 0.606

$$P(x \geq 7) = 1 - 0.606 = 0.394$$

Example 17:

The number of traffic accidents that occurs on a particular stretch of road during a month follows a Poisson distribution with a mean of 4. Find the probability that less than two accidents will occur on this stretch of road during a randomly selected month.

$$\lambda = 4$$

The formula for Poisson distribution is = $\frac{e^{-\lambda}\lambda^x}{x!}$

$$P(x < 2) = P(x = 0) + P(x = 1)$$

$$= e^4\left(\frac{4^0}{0!}+\frac{4^1}{1!}\right)$$

$$= 0.0183(1 + 4)$$

$$= 0.0183(5)$$

$$= 0.0183 \times 5 = 0.0915$$

Example 18:

In a town 10 accidents took place in a span of 50 days. Assuming that the number of accidents per day follows the Poisson distribution, find the probability that there will be three or more accidents in a day.

$$n = 10;\ p = 10/50 = 0.2$$

$$m = n \times p = 10 \times 0.2 = 2$$

$$x = \text{Three or more}$$

The formula for Poisson distribution is = $\frac{e^{-\lambda}\lambda^x}{x!}$

$$p(x \geq 3) = 1 - [P(0) + P(1) + P(2)]$$

$$= 1 - e^{-2}\left[1+\frac{2^1}{1!}+\frac{2^2}{2!}\right]$$

$$= 1 - [0.1353 \times (1 + 2 + 2)]$$

$$= 1 - 0.1353 \times 5$$

$$= 1 - 0.6765 = 0.3235$$

Normal Distribution

The binomial and poisson distribution are discrete probability distributions. The Binomial and Poisson distribution deal with the occurrence of distinct events such as the number of male babies, number of heads in the coins, number babies with diarrhea, etc. There are many situations in which the quantity that is studied is continuous in magnitude. The variables such as height, weight, temperature, test performance are examples of quantities that vary continuously. These characteristics adopts a frequency distribution known as normal (Gaussian) distribution. The formula for normal distribution is

$$= \frac{1}{\sqrt{2\pi\sigma^2}}\exp\left\{-\frac{(x-\mu)^2}{2\sigma^2}\right\}$$

The normal distribution is an important continuous probability distribution. The normal probability model was developed by one of the greatest mathematicians of all time Johann Friedrich Carl Gauss (1777-1855). Most mathematician of Gauss period were interested in applying mathematics to real world problems, such as in Astronomy and navigation. Knowing that data obtained through observation and measurement contained errors due to the imprecision of the measuring instruments, Gauss studied many different sets of such data and noticed that they all possessed certain common characteristics. In general each set of observations was symmetric about some central value and the farther from this central value, the fewer and fewer such observations there were. Based on such studies Gauss was able to develop a mathematical model that could be used to describe these sets of data. Gauss called the mathematical model, the normal probability model and the distribution of errors the normal probability distribution.

Three characteristics of the distributions described by the normal probability model.

1. A normal distribution is symmetric.
2. A normal distribution extends indefinitely to the right and to the left of the mean always getting closer and closer to the horizontal axis but never quite reaching it.
   (That is observations that are farther from the mean have smaller relative frequencies than observations that are closer to the mean).
3. The total area under the normal distribution is 1. By symmetry, this means that one half of the area is to right of the mean and one half is to the left.

It is symmetrical due to the fact that p = q. Even when p is not equal to q, it can be a normal distribution when n is large. All normal distributions have the same bell shaped appearance and differ from each other only in their particular mean and standard deviation values. The mean indicates where the distribution is located on the horizontal axis, whereas the standard deviation indicates the extent to which the scores tend to cluster about the mean.

We can calculate measures of location, variability and relationship (mean, standard deviation and correlation) just as we can on a sample taken from that population. When computed for populations the values of such descriptive measures are called parameters when computed for samples, they are called statistics.

We denote statistics by Roman letters and parameters by Greek letters. Symbols for common statistics and parameters

X = M= Sample mean	μ = Population mean
s^2 = Sample Variance	σ^2= Population Variance
s = Sample Standard deviation	σ = Population Standard deviation
r = Sample correlation	ρ = Population Correlation

Importance of Normal Curve: Normal distribution is of fundamental importance in statistical theory. The binomial and poisson distribution are also can be approximated by a normal curve.

The central limit theorem of the normal distribution states that as the sample size increases, the mean of the sample approaches the normal distribution. It helps us to draw inferences about the universe by making sample studies.

Standard normal distribution: The standard normal distribution is a normal distribution with a mean of 0 and a standard deviation of 1. Normal distributions can be transformed to standard normal distributions by the formula: $z = \frac{X - \mu}{\sigma}$ where X is an individual value; μ is the mean and σ is the standard deviation. The standard normal distribution is sometimes called the z distribution. A z score always reflects the number of standard deviations above or below the mean a particular score is. For instance, if a person scored 70 on a test with a mean of 50 and a standard deviation of 10, then he scored 2 standard deviations above the mean. Converting the test scores to z scores, an X of 70 would be z = 70–50/10 = 2.

So, a z score of 2 means the original score was 2 standard deviations above the mean. Note that the z distribution will only be a normal distribution if the original distribution (X) is normal. Applying the formula $z = \frac{X - \mu}{\sigma}$ will always produce a transformed distribution with a mean of zero and a standard deviation of one. However, the shape of the distribution will not be affected by the transformation. If X is not normal then the transformed distribution will not be normal either. One important use of the standard normal distribution is for converting between scores from a normal distribution and percentile ranks.

Areas under portions of the standard normal distribution are shown below. About 0.68 (0.34 + 0.34) of the distribution is between –1 and 1 while about 0.96 of the distribution is between –2 and 2.

Characteristics of Normal Curve

- It is symmetrical.
- The curve on either side of the mean is a mirror image of the other side.
- It is a bell shaped curve.
- The number of values above and below mean are equal.
- The height is maximum at the mean value
- The mean, median and mode will be equal.
- It is unimodal.
- μ and σ are the parameters of the normal distribution.
- It is mesokurtic.
- The range is unlimited, infinite in both directions,
- The both end or tail of the curve never touches its horizontal axis but the curve approaches more and more closely.
- No portion of the curve lies below the x axis.
- The normal distribution is also called the Gaussian distribution.

- A normal curve with 0 mean and unit standard deviation is known as Standard Normal curve.
- It has the most important property of relationship. The maximum ordinate is at the mean; and at various standard deviations the distances are in a fixed proportion to the ordinate at the mean. The following table gives the area under the normal probability curve for some important value of Z.

Distance from the mean ordinate in terms of $\pm \sigma$	Area under the curve
$Z = \pm 0.6745$	$50\% = 0.50$
$Z = \pm 1.0$	$68.26\% = 0.6826$
$Z = \pm 1.96$	$95\% = 0.95$
$Z = \pm 2.00$	$95.44\% = 0.9544$
$Z = \pm 2.58$	$99\% = 0.99$
$Z = \pm 3.0$	$99.73\% = 0.997$

By rewriting

- About 68% of the values will fall within ± 1 standard deviation from mean.
- About 95% of the values will lie within ± 2 standard deviation from the mean.
- About 99% of the values will lie within ± 3 standard deviation from the mean.

Computation of areas under normal probability curve.

Example 19:

Given the standard normal distribution find the area under the curve, above the Z axis between $Z = -\infty$ and $Z = 2$. Find the table value for $Z = 2$

$$Z = 2 = 0.9772.$$

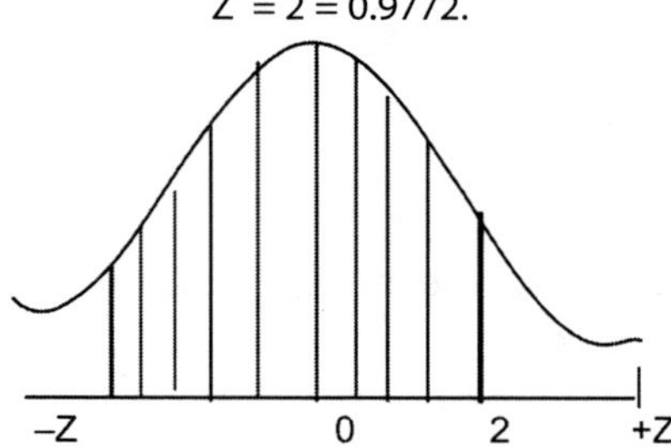

Example 20:

Find the area under the curve above the Z axis.

Between $Z = -\infty$ and $Z = 2.91 = 0.9982$

Between $Z = -\infty$ and $Z = 3.55 = 0.9998$

Example 21:

What is the probability that a Z picked at random from the population of Z's will have a value between –2.00 and +2.00?

Standard normal curvature showing $p(-2 < Z < 2)$

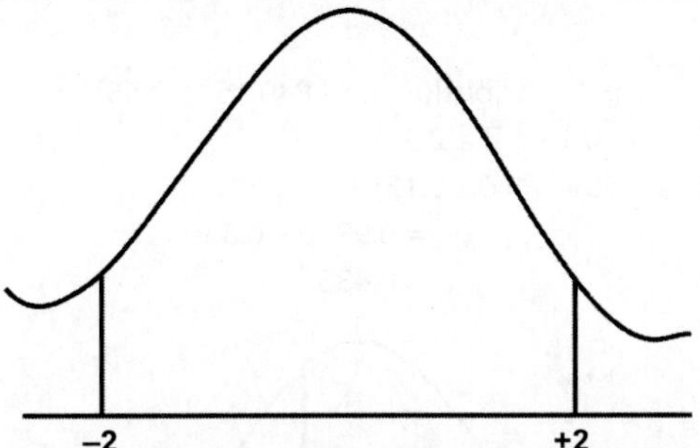

The value of $-\infty$ and 2.00, which is found by locating 2 in the left most column of the table. We find this area to be 0.9772.

The value between $-\infty$ and 2 = 0.9772

We need to subtract the area to the left of −2 which can be found referring to the table. The value is 0.0228. 0.9772 − 0.0228 = 0.9544.

Example 22:

What proportion of Z values are between −3 and 1.53.

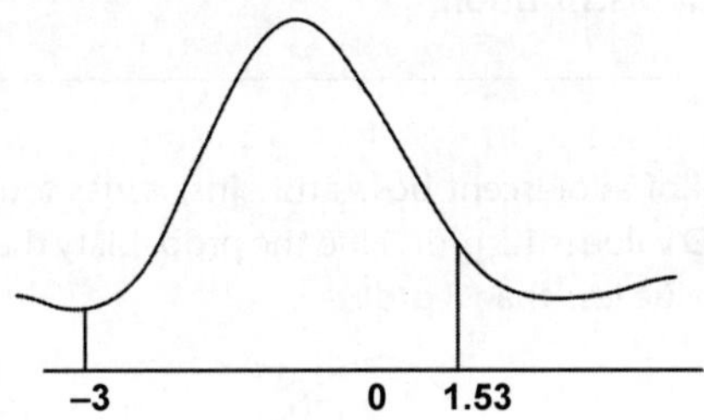

Z value between $-\infty$ and 1.53 = 0.9370

Z value between $-\infty$ and −3 = 0.0013

= 0.9370 − 0.0013

= 0.9357

Example 23:

Given the standard normal distribution, find $P(Z \geq 2.82)$

Z value between ∞ and 2.82 = 0.9976

$P(Z \geq 2.82) = 1 - 0.9976$

$P(Z \geq 2.82) = 0.0024$

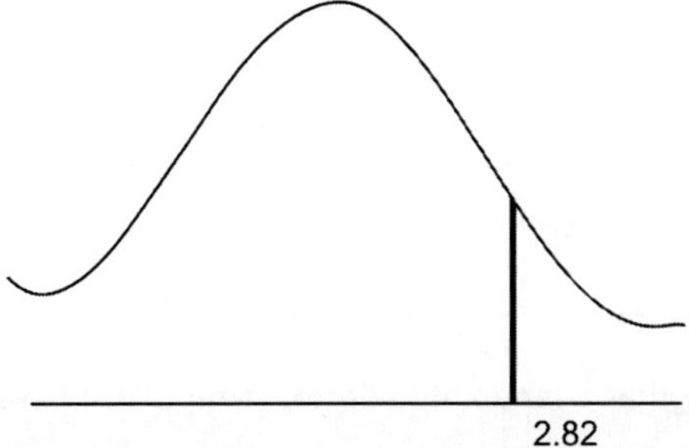

Example 24:

Given the standard normal distribution, find P (0.15 to 2.55).

$$P\ (0.15 \leq Z \geq 2.55)$$

$$P\ (Z \leq 2.55) - P\ (Z \geq 0.15)$$

$$= 0.9946 - 0.5596$$

$$= 0.435$$

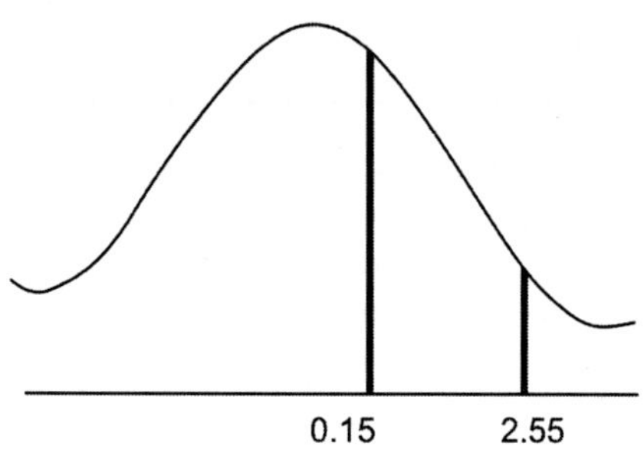

Application of Normal Distribution

Example 25:

In a study on Hb level of adolescent boys and girls, it was found that the mean Hb value is 10.2 and the SD value is 1.5 g/dL. Find the probability that a randomly selected sample will have Hb value less than 8 g/dL.

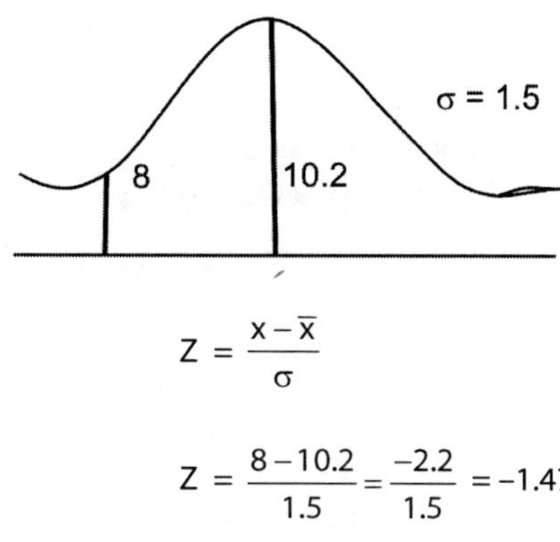

$$Z = \frac{x - \overline{x}}{\sigma}$$

$$Z = \frac{8 - 10.2}{1.5} = \frac{-2.2}{1.5} = -1.47$$

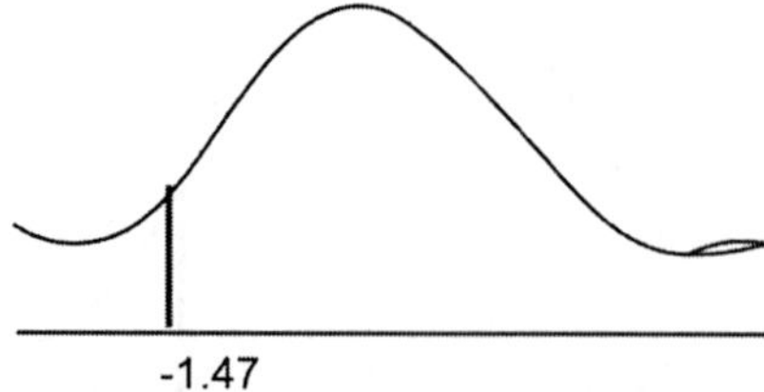

The probability that a randomly selected sample will have Hb value less than 8 g/dL = 0.0708

Example 26:

It is assumed that the height of a certain population of adolescents is normally distributed. The height is 155 cm and the SD is 6 cm. What is the probability that a person picked at random from this group will be between 148–158 cm tall?

$$\sigma = 6 \text{ cm}$$

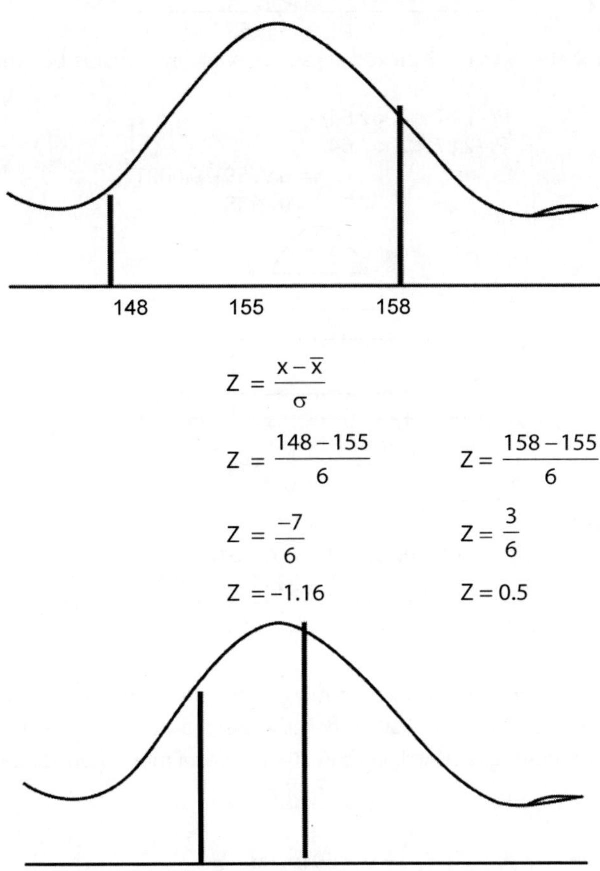

$$Z = \frac{x - \overline{x}}{\sigma}$$

$$Z = \frac{148-155}{6} \qquad Z = \frac{158-155}{6}$$

$$Z = \frac{-7}{6} \qquad Z = \frac{3}{6}$$

$$Z = -1.16 \qquad Z = 0.5$$

The area between –1.16 and 0.5 = P(–1.16 ≤ Z ≤ 0.5)

$= (Z \leq 0.5) - P(Z \leq -1.16)$

$= 0.6915 - 0.1230$

$= 0.5685$

Example 27:

Find the area under the curve between Z = 0 and Z = 1.53

$Z = 0$

$Z = 1.53$

Z value between 0 and 1.53 $= 0.9370 - 0.5000$

$= 0.4370$

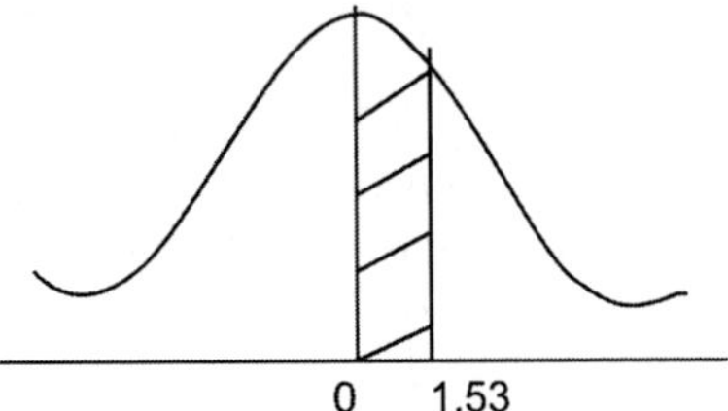

2. The Probability that a Z picked at random will have a value between Z = −2.87 and Z = 2.64

$$P(-2.87 < Z < 2.64)$$

$$P(-2.87 < Z < 2.64)$$

$$= 0.9959 - 0.0021$$

$$= 0.9938$$

-2.87 2.64

0.9938

3. P(Z ≥ 0.65)

$$P(Z \geq 0.65) = 1 - P(Z \leq 0.65)$$

$$= 1 - 0.7422 = 0.2578$$

Example 28:

The marks obtained in a certain examination follow normal distribution with mean 45 and standard deviation 10. If 1000 students appeared at the examination, calculate the number of students scoring less than 50 marks and more than 75 marks.

$$Z = \frac{x - \overline{X}}{\sigma}$$

If $x = 50$ marks

$$Z = \frac{50 - 45}{10} = \frac{5}{10} = 0.5$$

$$P(z < 0.5) = 0.5 + 0.1915 = 0.6915$$

$$\text{Number of students} = 0.6915 \times 1000 = 691.5$$

$$Z = \frac{75 - 45}{10} = \frac{30}{10} = 3$$

$$P(z < 0.5) = 1 - (0.5 + 0.4987) = 1 - 0.9987 = 0.0013$$

$$\text{Number of students} = 0.0013 \times 1000 = 1.3$$

SAMPLING DISTRIBUTION

Imagine that you have got the birth weight of 10,000 newborns. Using lottery method, pick up 30 newborn's birth weight and calculate the mean value. Like this, if you pick up 50 times, each 30 samples and calculate the mean value, you will get 50 mean value. When you formulate frequency distribution for this 50 mean values, the resulting distribution is known as sampling distribution of mean. Likewise you can formulate the sampling distribution of standard deviation. The distribution of all possible values of a statistic is called the sampling distribution or the probability distribution of that statistic. The distribution of all possible values that can be assumed by some statistic, computed from samples of the same size randomly drawn from the same population, is called the sampling distribution of that statistic. We are often concerned with sampling distribution in sampling analysis. If we take certain number of samples and for each sample compute various statistical measures such as mean, standard deviation, etc. then we can find that each sample may give its own value for the statistic under consideration. All such values of a particular statistic, say mean, together with their relative frequencies will constitute the sampling distribution of the particular statistic, say mean. Accordingly, we can have sampling distribution of mean, or the sampling distribution of standard deviation or the sampling distribution of any other statistical measure. It may be noted that each item in a sampling distribution is a particular statistic of a sample. The sampling distribution tends quite closer to the normal distribution if the number of samples is large. The significance of sampling distribution follows from the fact that the mean of a sampling distribution is the same as the mean of the universe. Thus, the mean of the sampling distribution can be taken as the mean of the universe.

The sampling distribution can be constructed by the following.

- From a finite population of size N, randomly draw all possible samples of size n.
- Compute the statistic of interest for each sample.
- List in one column the different distinct observed values of the statistic and in another column list the corresponding frequency of occurrence of each distinct observed values of the statistic.

The sampling distribution of statistic has several well-defined properties. This distribution has the following important properties:

(a) The distribution of mean will be normal. The arithmetic mean of the sampling distribution is the same as the mean of the universe from which samples were taken.

(b) The variance of the distribution of mean will be equal to the variance of the population divided by the sample size.

(c) The sampling distribution of mean has a standard deviation which is called the standard error. Like all standard deviations, it measures how spread out or dispersed the sample means are. It indicates the accuracy we are likely to get if we use a sample mean to estimate the population mean. A distribution of sample means that is less spread out or has a small standard error is a better estimator of the population mean than a distribution of sample means that is widely dispersed and has a large standard error.

(d) The standard error is equal to the population standard deviation divided by the square root of the sample size. This equations easily shows how one can reduce standard error by increasing the size of the sample, i.e. N.

(e) The sampling distribution of means is normally distributed regardless of the shape of the population from which samples have been drawn. This relationship between the shape of the population distribution and the shape of the sampling distribution is called the central limit theorem. It allows us to develop a method in which we can use the mean of our sample to estimate the population mean. For example, if we compute an interval of 2 standard errors, the interval will include 95.5% of all the sample means. A statistician would describe this by saying, 'We are 95.5% confident that the interval contains the population mean.' This theoretical concept is basic to our study of interval construction and statistical inference.

CENTRAL LIMIT THEOREM

Given a population with a mean μ and finite variance σ^2, the sampling distribution of mean, computed from samples of size n from this population, will have mean μ and variance σ^2/n and will be approximately normally distributed when the sample size is large. In order to apply central limit theorem, how large should be the sample? The size of the sample needed depends on the extent of non normality present in the population. One rule of thumb states that, in most practical situations a sample size of 30 is satisfactory. In general, the approximation to normality of the sampling distribution of mean becomes better and better as the sample size increases.

Summary of Sampling Distribution of Mean

- Sampling is from a normally distributed population with a known population variance:
  - ❒ $\mu_{\bar{x}} = \mu$
  - ❒ $\sigma_{\bar{x}} = \frac{\sigma}{\sqrt{N}}$
  - ❒ The sampling distribution of x is normal.
- Sampling is from a non normally distributed population with a known population variance:
  - ❒ $\mu_{\bar{x}} = \mu$
  - ❒ $\sigma_{\bar{x}} = \frac{\sigma}{\sqrt{N}}\sqrt{\frac{N-n}{N-1}}$
  - ❒ The sampling distribution of $\bar{x}$ is approximately normal.

SUMMARY

- Probability theory was originated from gambling theory. The theory of probability provides the foundation for statistical inference.
- We measure the probability of the occurrence of some event by a number between zero and one. The probability is one when an event is certain to occur and the probability is zero when the event is unlikely to occur. The more likely the event, the probability value is closer to one and the more unlikely the event the probability is closer to zero.
- The chance of occurrence of any particular event is known as probability. Chance is measured on a probability scale having zero at one end and one at the other end. It ranges from absolute certainty to absolute impossibility.
- If an event can occur in any one of several mutually exclusive ways, the probability of that event is sum of the individual probabilities of the different ways in which it can occur. P(A or B) = P(A + B) = P(A) + P(B).
- The probability of the simultaneous occurrence of 2 or more independent events is the product of the individual probabilities. P (A and B) = P(AB) = P(A) × P(B).
- Theoretical or probability distributions refer to mathematical models of expected frequencies of a finite number of observations of a variable with associated probabilities. They are based on mathematical functions.
- Binomial distribution is a discrete probability distribution which is obtained when the probability of the happening of an event is same in all the trials and there are only two events in each trial. The formula for binomial distribution is $C_r^n p^r q^{n-r}$ where $C_r^n = \frac{n!}{r!(n-r)!}$
- Poisson distribution was discovered by a French mathematician Simen Denis Poisson. It is also a discrete distribution and is widely used. It is different from binomial distribution that the n is large and p is very small. The formula for Poisson distribution is $= \frac{e^{-\lambda}\lambda^x}{x!}$
- The normal distribution is an important continuous probability distribution. The normal probability model was developed by Johann Friedrich Carl Gauss. The formula for normal distribution is

$$\frac{1}{\sqrt{2\pi\sigma^2}}\exp\left\{-\frac{(x-\mu)^2}{2\sigma^2}\right\}$$

- The standard normal distribution is a normal distribution with a mean of 0 and a standard deviation of 1. Normal distributions can be transformed to standard normal distributions by the formula, $z = \frac{X-\mu}{\sigma}$.

EXERCISE

- A class consists of 25 students. Five of them are male and the remaining are female. Ten of them are staying in a hostel and rest of them are day scholars. Five of them were above average performers. What is the probability of selecting a female staying in a hostel and who is above average performer?
- In a college vehicle, 20 PBBSc (N), 10 MSc (N) students were sitting. What is the probability of 3 PBBSc (N) and 2 MSc (N) students were called by the teacher?

- In a mess hall 5 staff nurses and 10 student nurses are eating. If one of them is selected, find the chance that the person selected is a staff nurse.
- In an auditorium, 100 students are sitting. 30 of them are Diploma students and 70 of them are of UG students. Forty of them are staying in a hostel. Sixty of them are in uniform. What is the probability of calling one UG student, staying in hostel and who is in uniform?
- In a faculty meeting, 20 PG teachers and 10 UG teachers are attending. What is the probability of selecting 4 PG teachers and 2 UG teachers team for some special task?
- In an ICU, there are 6 graduate nurses and 4 Diploma nurses working. What is the probability that two staff nurses selected are graduate?

Binomial distribution

- In a survey of nursing students pursuing a master degree, 80% stated that they need to be given job in the college within one month after receiving the degree. If a sample of 15 is selected, find the probability that the number expecting promotion within a month after receiving their degree is
  Five; at least 7 ; No more than 4 and Between six and 8 inclusive.
- In a children population, 60% of them suffer from hook work infestation. If a random sample of 8 is selected, find the probability that exactly 4 children will be with hook worm infestation.
- In a college, 30% of them are day scholars. If 10 students are selected randomly, what is the probability that 5 or more will be the day-scholars?
- In a hostel, 40% of the children are first born. If 5 children are selected randomly, what is the probability that 3 or more children are first born?

Poisson distribution

- In a certain population an average of 10 new cases of skin cancer are diagnosed each year. If the annual incidence of skin cancer follows a Poisson distribution, find the probability that in a given year the number of newly diagnosed cases of skin cancer will be (a) Exactly 8; (b) At least 6 and (c) between 4 and 6.
- In a certain population, an average of 12 new cases of Osteosarcoma are diagnosed each year. If this incidence follows a Poisson distribution, find the probability that in a given year the number of newly diagnosed cases of Osteosarcoma will be (a) Exactly 6 ; (b) At least 5 and (c) No more than 8.
- Suppose the number of babies born during an 8-hour shift at a hospital's maternity wing follows a Poisson distribution with a mean of 6 hour. Find the probability that five babies are born during a particular 1-hour period in this maternity wing.

Normal distribution

- Given the standard normal deviation , find?
  - The area under the curve between $Z = 0$ and $Z = 1.53$
  - The probability that a Z picked at random will have a value between $Z = -2.87$ and $Z = 2.64$
  - $P(Z \geq 0.65)$
  - $P(Z \geq -0.65)$
  - $P(Z < -2.33)$
  - $P(Z < 2.33)$
  - $P(-1.96 \leq Z \leq 1.96)$
  - $P(-2.58 \leq Z \leq 2.58)$
  - $P(Z = 0.74)$
- Given the following probabilities find Z_1
  - $P(Z \leq Z_1) = 0.0055$
  - $P(Z > Z_1) = 0.384$

- $P(-2.67 \le Z \le Z_1) = 0.9718$
- $P(Z_1 \le Z \le 2.98) = 0.1117$

- The age at onset of juvenile diabetes is approximately normally distributed with a mean of 10.2 years and a standard deviation of 2 years. A child has come down with the disease. Find the probability that the child is:
  (a) between the ages of 8.2 and 12.2; (b) Over 11 years of age and (c) under 12 years of age.
- If the hemoglobin values for certain adolescent girls population is normally distributed with a mean of 11.8 g/dL and a standard deviation of 0.8 g/dL, find the probability that an adolescent girl picked at random from this population will have a hemoglobin value of
  (a) Between 10 and 12 g/dL (b) Greater than 12 g/dL (c) Less than 9 g/dL
- If the weight of infants is approximately normally distributed with a mean of 8.5 kg and standard deviation of 1 kg, find the probability that the weight of the infants is (a) Between 7 and 9.5 kg; (b) Greater than 11 kg and (c) Less than 7.5 kg.
- If IQs of children admitted to a mentally retarded school are approximately normally distributed with a mean of 50 and a standard deviation of 10. If a child is picked at random, find the probability that the IQ of the child is
  (a) Between 55 and 65; (b) Less than 40 and (c) Greater than 60.
- Assume the mean height of children to be 65 cm with a variance of 10.5 cm. How many children in a school of 1000 would you expect to be over 70 cm tall?
- The scores made by a candidate in a certain test are normally distributed with mean 500 and standard deviation 100. What percentage of candidate receives the scores between 400 and 600?

19 Estimation of Parameters

OBJECTIVES

After reading this chapter, you will be able to:

- Understand the difference between the parameter and statistics
- Expalin the concept of sampling distribution
- Explain the concept of standard error
- Explain point estimation and interval estimation
- Compute point and interval estimates

INTRODUCTION

As discussed earlier, it is not possible to conduct study on the population. But it is possible to draw conclusion for the population based on the information provided by the study on samples. This is called statistical inference. Statistical inference may be of two kinds. They are parameter estimation and hypothesis testing. Parameter estimation is concerned with obtaining numerical values of the parameter from a sample. In parameter estimation we use some formula in which we substitute the observations of the sample in order to obtain a numerical estimate of the population parameters. This chapter deals with the estimation of parameters.

Estimation of Parameters

In most statistical research studies, population parameters are usually unknown and have to be estimated from a sample. Parameter refers to the measures or values of the population. Parameter estimation is concerned with obtaining numerical values of the parameter from a sample. One must understand the difference between the parameter and the statistics (Table 19.1).

Table 19.1: Difference between the parameter and statistic

S. No	Parameter	Statistic
1.	A parameter is a characteristic of a population. When such measures from the samples describe the characteristics of a population, they are known as parameter(s).	A statistic is a characteristic of a sample. The mean, median, mode or the like ones from samples are called statistic(s) since they describe the characteristics of a sample.
2.	Population mean is denoted as μ	Sample mean is denoted as $\overline{X}$

contd...

contd...

S. No	Parameter	Statistic
3.	Population standard deviation is denoted as σ_p	Sample standard deviation is denoted as σ_s
4.	μ and σ_p are conventionally called as estimates since these values are estimated using sample statistics	$\overline{X}$ and σ_s are referred to as estimators which helps to estimate population parameters
5.	Values derived from the statistics of the samples	Values derived from the data collected from the samples

Also, one must have the knowledge on sampling distribution, standard error and central limit theorem which are of fundamental importance in parameter estimation.

Sampling Distribution

The distribution of all possible values of a statistic is called the ***sampling distribution*** or the ***probability distribution*** of that statistic. The distribution of all possible values that can be assumed by some statistic, computed from samples of the same size randomly drawn from the same population, is called the sampling distribution of that statistic. We can have sampling distribution of mean, or the sampling distribution of standard deviation or the sampling distribution of any other statistical measure. The mean of a sampling distribution is the same as the mean of the universe. Thus, the mean of the sampling distribution can be taken as the mean of the universe. The sampling distribution of statistic has several well-defined properties. The distribution of mean will be normal. The arithmetic mean of the sampling distribution is the same as the mean of the universe from which samples were taken. The variance of the distribution of mean will be equal to the variance of the population divided by the sample size. The sampling distribution of mean has a standard deviation which is called the ***standard error***. Like all standard deviations, it measures how spread out or dispersed the sample means are. It indicates the accuracy we are likely to get if we use a sample mean to estimate the population mean. A distribution of sample means that is less spread out or has a small standard error is a better estimator of the population mean than a distribution of sample means, that is widely dispersed and has a large standard error. The relationship between the shape of the population distribution and the shape of the sampling distribution is called the ***central limit theorem***. It allows us to develop a method in which we can use the mean of our sample to estimate the population mean.

When sampling is from a normal population, the means of samples drawn from such a population are themselves normally distributed. But when sampling is not from a normal population, the size of the sample plays a critical role. When the sample size n is small, the shape of the distribution will depend largely on the shape of the parent population, but as n gets large (more than 30), the shape of the sampling distribution will become more and more like a normal distribution, irrespective of the shape of the parent population.

The central limit theorem assures that the sampling distribution of the mean approaches normal distribution as the sample size increases. The significance of the central limit theorem lies in the fact that it permits us to use sample statistics to make inferences about population parameters without knowing anything about the shape of the frequency distribution of that population.

Standard Error

The standard deviation of sampling distribution of a statistic is known as its standard error (SE) and is considered the key to sampling theory. The utility of the concept of standard error in statistical induction arises on account of the following reasons:

The standard error helps in testing whether the difference between observed and expected frequencies could arise due to chance. The criterion usually adopted is that if a difference is less than 3 times the S.E., the difference is supposed to exist as a matter of chance and if the difference is equal to or more than 3 times the S.E., chance fails to account for it, and we conclude the difference as significant difference. This criterion is based on the fact that at $\overline{X} \pm 3$ (SE) the normal curve covers an area of 99.73%. Sometimes the criterion of 2 SE, is also used in place of 3 SE. Thus the standard error is an important measure in significance tests or in examining hypotheses. If the estimated parameter differs from the calculated statistic by more than 1.96 times the SE, the difference is taken as significant at 5% level of significance. This, in other words, means that the difference is outside the limits, i.e. it lies in the 5% area (2.5% on both sides) outside the 95% area of the sampling distribution. The product of the critical value at a certain level of significance and the SE is often described as ***Sampling Error*** at that particular level of significance.

The standard error gives an idea about the reliability and precision of a sample. The smaller the SE, the greater the uniformity of sampling distribution and hence, greater is the reliability of sample. Conversely, the greater the SE, the greater the difference between observed and expected frequencies. In such a situation the unreliability of the sample is greater. The size of SE, depends upon the sample size to a great extent and it varies inversely with the size of the sample. If double reliability is required, i.e. reducing SE, to half of its existing magnitude, the sample size should be increased four-fold.

The standard error enables us to specify the limits within which the parameters of the population are expected to lie with a specified degree of confidence. Such an interval is usually known as confidence interval. The following table gives the percentage of samples having their mean values within a range of population mean (μ) ± SE

Range	Percentage Values
μ ± 1 SE	68.27%
μ ± 2 SE	95.45%
μ ± 3 SE	99.73%
μ ± 1.96 SE	95.00%
μ ± 2.5758 SE	99.00%

Confidence level and significance level : The confidence level or reliability is the expected percentage of times that the actual value will fall within the stated precision limits. Thus, if we take a confidence level of 95%, then we mean that there are 95 chances in 100 (or .95 in 1) that the sample results represent the true condition of the population within a specified precision range against 5 chances in 100 (or .05 in 1) that it does not. Precision is the range within which the answer may vary and still be acceptable; confidence level indicates the likelihood that the answer will fall outside that range. We can always remember that if the confidence level is 95%, then the significance level will be (100–95), i.e. 5%; if the confidence level is 99%, the significance level is (100–99), i.e. 1%, and so on. We should also remember that the area of normal curve within precision limits for the specified confidence level constitute the acceptance region and the area of the curve outside these limits in either direction constitutes the rejection regions.

Point and Interval Estimation

The estimate of a population parameter may be one single value or it could be a range of values. From the sample we attempt to estimate the true but unknown values of the population parameters. Such estimates may be either point estimates or interval estimates. A statistic used as an estimate of a parameter, and presented as a single number, is known as a ***point estimate.*** Thus, to say that 50 kg which is the average weight of a sample of 5 students randomly drawn from a class of 100 students is also the average weight of the entire class. It is described that we state not only our best single estimate, or point estimate, but also a pair of estimates, one above our point estimate and the other below it and assert with a certain degree of confidence that the parameter would lie within this stated interval. This method is called an ***interval estimate.***

If we want to be very confident of our stated limits we must make them rather wide, but if we are willing to take a big chance we can put them close together. It is customary in research to choose the 95% confidence level. This means that in repeated sampling, the confidence limits computed from the sample would include the true population parameter in 95% of the cases. In the other 5% of the cases, the population parameter will fall outside the confidence limits.

The researcher usually makes these two types of estimates through sampling analysis such as point or interval estimates. The researcher must know the various properties of a good estimator so that he can select appropriate estimators for his study.

Essential Properties of the Estimators

Property of Unbiasedness: An estimator should on an average be equal to the value of the parameter being estimated. An estimator is said to be unbiased if the expected value of the estimator is equal to the parameter being estimated. The sample mean ($\overline{X}$) is the most widely used estimator of the population mean (μ).

Property of efficiency: An estimator should have a relatively small variance. The most efficient estimator is the one which has the smallest variance.

Property of sufficiency: An estimator should use as much as possible the information available from the sample.

Property of consistency: An estimator should approach the value of population parameter as the sample size becomes larger and larger.

Keeping in view the above stated properties, the researcher must select appropriate estimator(s) for the study.

Point Estimation

A statistic used as an estimate of a parameter, and presented as a single number, is known as point estimate. The average weight, 52 kg calculated from a sample of 10 selected from a class of 100 is the point estimate which is also the average weight of the entire class. Point estimate is concerned with the sample mean ($\overline{X}$) which is the best estimator of the population mean (μ). For example, in a population of 500 students, select 10 students randomly and calculate their mean weight which is $\overline{X} = 45$ kg. Replace these students weight and select another 10 students randomly and find the mean weight which may be 50 kg. Likewise, you repeat it many times and find the value of the mean. We go on drawing such samples till we accumulate a large number of means (weight) of samples of 10. Each such sample mean is a separate point estimate of the population mean and the mean of the distribution of the sample means is equal to the population mean. This is true in case of large samples as per the dictates of the central limit theorem. In the first example, there might be a chance of error and one cannot say that how confidently we could say that 52 kg is the mean of the entire class, i.e. the population mean weight. To avoid this problem, one must construct a confidence interval or limits so that one can say that the value may lie in between the confidence limits. This method is known as interval estimation.

Interval Estimation in the case of Large Samples

In the case of large samples the concepts of the normal curve and the standard deviation help a researcher in making an interval estimate of the population parameter. It has been found that the frequency distribution of a sample statistic such as mean, median, standard deviation, etc. (called the sampling distribution) is so close to the normal distribution that we can use the sample statistics and the standard deviation of the sampling distribution (called the standard error) to make probability statements based on areas under the normal curve. Any sample statistic ± 1 standard error of that sample statistic tells us a range within which 68.27% of such statistics will be. A range of ± 1.96 standard errors will include 95% of all the sample statistics and a range of ± 3 standard errors will include 99.73% of all the sample statistics. Percentages of area covered by different values of standard errors are known from Z Table (Table in Appendix).

The following is a list of the formulae for obtaining standard errors of some important statistics:

- Standard error of Mean $= \dfrac{\sigma_p}{\sqrt{N}}$, where N stands for the number of observations and σ_p stands for the standard deviation of the population.

If population σ is not known, then the sample standard deviation can be used whenever N is large.

- Standard error of Median = $\frac{1.2533\sigma}{\sqrt{N}}$
- Standard error of Standard Deviation = $\frac{\sigma_p}{\sqrt{2N}}$ or $\frac{\sigma_s}{\sqrt{2N}}$ where population σ is not known.
- Standard error of Coefficient of Correlation = $\frac{1-r^2}{\sqrt{N}}$ [Provided that the value of N is large – say not less than 100 and provided also that the value of r is close to ± 0.5 and not very high (.80 or more) or not very low (.20 or less)].

  It can be shown mathematically that the standard deviation of a random sample underestimates (is smaller than) the corresponding population standard deviation, but this negative bias is quite small, whenever N is large. So, it is ignored. But when N is small, correction is made in the formula for computing the σ of a sample to get a better approximation to the σ_p, the corrected formula becomes $\sigma = \sqrt{\frac{\Sigma d^2}{N-1}}$ instead of the usual formula $\sigma = \sqrt{\frac{\Sigma d^2}{N}}$.
- Standard error of Regression Coefficient of Y on X (i.e. byx) = $\frac{\sigma_y\sqrt{1-r^2}}{\sigma_x\sqrt{N}}$.
- Standard error of Regression Coefficient of X on Y (i.e. bxy) = $\frac{\sigma_x\sqrt{1-r^2}}{\sigma_y\sqrt{N}}$.
- Standard error of Regression Estimate of Y on X = $\sigma_y\sqrt{1-r^2}$.
- Standard error of Regression Estimate of X on Y = $\sigma_x\sqrt{1-r^2}$.
- Standard error of Rank Correlation coefficient = $\frac{1}{\sqrt{N-1}}$.
- Standard error of the difference between the Means of two samples or SE $(\overline{X}_1 - \overline{X}_2) = \sqrt{\frac{\sigma_1^2}{N_1}+\frac{\sigma_2^2}{N_2}}$ (where population standard deviation is not known).
- Standard error of the difference between two Standard Deviations or SE $(\sigma_1 - \sigma_2) = \sqrt{\frac{\sigma_1^2}{2N_1}+\frac{\sigma_2^2}{2N_2}}$.
- Standard error of Variance = $\sigma_2\sqrt{\frac{2}{N}}$

Interval Estimation (Large Sample)

Example 1:

$n = 50 \ \bar{x} = 11 \ \sigma = 1.5$

$\bar{x} \pm z \text{ SE}$

$$\text{Standard error of Mean} = \frac{\sigma_p}{\sqrt{N}}$$

$11 \pm 1.96 \times 1.5/\sqrt{50}$

$11 \pm 1.96 \times 1.5/7.1$

$11 - 1.96 \times 0.21$

11 ± 0.4

$11.4 - 10.6$

Inference: Using the sample value, estimated population value should lie between 10.6 and 11.4 at 95% confidence or at 5% level of significance.

Substitute z score 2.58 for 99% confidence level and 3.29 for 99.9% confidence level.

$11 \pm 2.58 \times 1.5/\sqrt{50}$

$11 \pm 2.58 \times 1.5/7.1$

$11 \pm 2.58 \times 0.21$

11 ± 0.54

$11.54 - 10.46$

Using the sample value, estimated population value should lie between 10.46 and 11.54 at 99% confidence or at 1% level of significance.

$11 + 3.29 \times 1.5/\sqrt{50}$

$11 + 3.29 \times 1.5/7.1$

$11 - 3.29 \times 0.21$

11 ± 0.69

$11.69 - 10.31$

Using the sample value, estimated population value should lie between 10.31 and 11.69 at 99% confidence or at 1% level of significance.

Example 2:

$n = 80 \ \bar{x} = 16 \ \sigma = 2.5$

$\bar{x} \pm z \text{ SE}$

$$\text{Standard error of Mean} = \frac{\sigma_p}{\sqrt{N}},$$

$11 \pm 1.96 \times 2.5/\sqrt{80}$

$11 \pm 1.96 \times 2.5/8.9$

$11 - 1.96 \times 0.28$

11 ± 0.55

$11.55 - 10.45$

Inference: Using the sample value, estimated population value should lie between 10.45 and 11.55 at 95% confidence or at 5% level of significance.

Substitute z score 2.58 for 99% confidence level and 3.29 for 99.9% confidence level.

Example 3:

For a normal population with a known variance of 185, a sample of 64 individuals leads to 217 as an estimate of the mean:

(a) Find the standard error of the mean.

(b) Establish an interval estimate that should include the population mean 68.3% of the time.

$\sigma_p^2 = 185 \therefore \sigma_p = \sqrt{185} = 13.60$ N = 64 Mean = 217

(c) Standard error of Mean = $\frac{\sigma_p}{\sqrt{N}} = \frac{13.60}{\sqrt{64}} = 1.70$

(d) We have to establish an interval estimate that should include the population mean 68.3% of the time. A 68.3% confidence level will include 34.15% of the area on either side of the mean of the sampling distribution. We consider that 0.3415 of the area under the normal curve is contained between the mean and a point 1 stand error to the right of the mean. Therefore, we know that (2) (0.3415) = 68.3 of the area is located between plus and minus 1 standard error from the mean and that our confidence limits are:

$\bar{X} \pm 1$ standard error

or 217 ± 1.7 = 218.7 and 215.3

Example 4:

Miss. Sudha is interested in purchasing a mixie. She randomly selects 50 advertisements and finds that the average price of a mixie in the sample is ₹ 2,500. She knows that the standard deviation of mixie prices in this city is ₹ 200.

(a) Establish an interval estimate for the average price of a mixie so that Miss Sudha can be 68.3% certain that the population mean lies within this interval.

(b) Establish an interval estimate for the average price of a mixie so that Miss Sudha can be 95.5% certain that the population mean lies within this interval.

$\sigma = 200 \quad N = 50 \quad \bar{X} = 2500$

SE of Mean = $\frac{\sigma_p}{\sqrt{N}} = \frac{200}{\sqrt{50}} = 200/7.07 = 28.3$

(a) Mean ± SE = 2500 ± 28.3 = ₹ 2528.3, ₹ 2471.7

(b) Mean ± 2 SE = 2500 ± 2 (28.3) = 2500 ± 56.6 = ₹ 2556.6, ₹ 2443.4.

Example 5:

The standard deviation of the life of 80 BP apparatus was 18 years. Find the confidence interval for the whole lot at 95% and 99% confidence levels.

Here, the standard deviation of the population is not known. So we can use the

Standard Error of standard deviation = $\frac{\sigma_s}{\sqrt{2N}}$

$= \frac{18}{\sqrt{2 \times 80}} = 18/\sqrt{160} = 18/12.7$

$= 1.42$

Confidence limits at 95% level are

$= 18 \pm 1.96 \times 1.42$

$= 18 \pm 2.8$

Confidence limits at 99% level are

$$= 18 \pm 2.58 \times 1.42$$
$$= 18 \pm 3.7$$

Example 6:

Correlation between the intelligence and test score was studied among 500 students and it was found to be + 0.72. Within what limits does it hold true for universe?

The standard error of correlation coefficient is $\frac{1-r^2}{\sqrt{N}}$

$$= \frac{1-(0.72)^2}{\sqrt{500}} = \frac{1-0.52}{22.4} = \frac{0.48}{22.4} = 0.02$$

The correlation in the universe cannot deviate from the correlation in the sample by more than thrice the standard error, i.e. 0.06. Hence, the correlation in the universe most probably lies within 0.72 + 0.06, that is 0.78 – 0.66.

Example 7:

A coefficient of correlation found between the height of sons and fathers in a sample of 1600 is 0.8. Within what limits does it hold true for the universe?

The standard error of correlation coefficient is $\frac{1-r^2}{\sqrt{N}}$

$$= \frac{1-(0.8)^2}{\sqrt{1600}} = \frac{1-0.64}{40} = \frac{0.36}{40} = 0.009$$

The correlation in the universe cannot deviate from the correlation in the sample by more than thrice the standard error, i.e. 0.027. Hence, the correlation in the universe most probably lies within 0.8 ± 0.027, that is 0.827 – 0.773.

Interval Estimation in the Case of Small Samples

Z statistic and the Standard Normal Curve are applied only when the size of the sample is large. They are not used in situations where the size of the sample is small, i.e. less than 30 items. The reason is that when the sample is small the sampling distribution of a statistic (e.g. $\overline{X}$), though symmetrical is not normal. In this case the researcher can apply another distribution based on the Student's t-statistics provided that the parent population is normal.

Student's t-distribution differs from normal distribution in being a little flatter and more widely dispersed. This means it takes somewhat more than ± 2 standard errors to include 95% of all sample means in such a distribution.

t-tables have been worked out which contain values of the number of standard errors needed for a particular confidence interval for all possible sample sizes upto 30. These values are given with reference to the degrees of freedom. The number of degrees of freedom is the sample size less one, i.e. (N - 1). Where N > 30 the t-distribution approaches the standard normal distribution and so one may use Z instead of t.

It should, however, be remembered that in the case of small samples the use of relatively wide confidence intervals makes parameter estimation less precise. Therefore, small samples are more used for hypothesis testing than for estimating parameter values.

Example 8:

For the following sample sizes and confidence levels, find the appropriate t values for constructing confidence intervals:

(a) N = 29; 95%
(b) N = 8; 98%
(c) N = 13; 90%
(d) N = 12; 95%
(e) N = 24; 99%
(f) N = 10; 99%
(g) N = 20; 95%

[(a) 2.048 (b) 2.998 (c) 1.782 (d) 2.201 (e) 2.807 (f) 3.250 (g) 2.093]

Example 9:

Given the following sample sizes and t values used to construct confidence intervals, find the corresponding confidence levels:

(a) N = 27 ; t = ± 2.056
(b) N = 5 ; t = ± 2.132
(c) N = 18 ; t = ± 2.898
(d) N = 15 ; t = ± 1.761
(e) N = 20; t = ± 2.093

[(a) 95% (b) 90% (c) 98% (d) 90% (e) 95%]

Example 10:

$n = 8 \ \bar{x} = 8 \ \sigma = 1.5$

$\bar{x} \pm t\,SE$

Standard error of Mean $= \dfrac{\sigma_p}{\sqrt{N}}$

$$= \frac{1.5}{\sqrt{8}} = 1.5/2.83 = 0.53$$

degrees of freedom = n – 1 = 8 – 1 = 7

The critical value of t for 95% confidence interval or at 5% level of significance is 2.365 for 7 df.

Thus 95% confidence interval for population mean is

$$\bar{x} \pm t\,SE = 8 \pm (2.365)(0.53)$$

$$8 \pm 1.253 = 6.747 - 9.253$$

Using the sample value, estimated population value should lie between 6.747 and 9.253 at 95% confidence or at 5% level of significance.

Example 11:

A random sample of 10 individuals chosen from a group gives their average height equal to 67″ and the standard deviation 3.13″. What are the limits within which the average height of the whole group can be expected to lie at 95% confidence?

$$SE\,\bar{x} = \frac{\sigma}{\sqrt{N}} = \frac{3.13}{\sqrt{10}} = 0.99$$

$$= \bar{x} \pm t\,SE$$

For 9 degrees of freedom the table value of t at 95% confidence level is 2.26. Thus, our 95% confidence limits are 67 ± (2.26) (0.99) or 64.76 and 69.24.

Example 12:

Seven staff nurses were randomly sampled and it was determined that the distances they traveled from their houses to hospital had an average of 39.2 miles per week and a sample standard deviation of 3.2 miles per week. Construct a 95% confidence interval for the population mean.

$$SE\,\bar{x} = \frac{\sigma}{\sqrt{N}} = \frac{3.2}{\sqrt{7}} = 1.2095$$

95% confidence interval $= \bar{x} \pm t\,SE$

Table value of t for 6 degrees of freedom at 95% confidence level is 2.44

$$= 39.2 \pm (2.44)\,(1.2095)$$
$$= 39.2 \pm 2.9512$$
$$= (36.25, 42.15) \text{ miles.}$$

Example 13:

A random sample of 27 pairs from a normal universe gives a correlation coefficient of 0.6 . What are the limits within which the r of the entire universe can be expected to be at 95% confidence?

The standard error of r in small samples is given by the formula $\sqrt{\frac{1-r^2}{N-2}}$

$$SE\,r = \frac{\sqrt{1-(0.6)^2}}{\sqrt{27-2}} = \frac{\sqrt{.64}}{\sqrt{25}} = \frac{0.8}{5} = .16$$

For 25 degrees of freedom the table value of t at 95% confidence level is 2.06. Thus, our 95% confidence limits are 0.6 ± (2.06) (0.16) or 0.2704 and 0.9296. But sometimes this formula gives the limits of r which are out of question in actual practice.

Interval Estimation in the Case of Attributes–Proportions

Unlike variables where a phenomenon is quantitatively measured, in the case of attributes (e.g. male-female, literate-illiterate, married-single and so on) one only counts the presence or absence of a particular attribute. The presence of an attribute is generally called a ***success*** and its absence is called a ***failure***.

Theoretically, the binomial distribution is the correct distribution to use in constructing confidence intervals in the case of attributes (or proportions of occurrences in a population). However, fortunately, as the sample size increases, the binomial can be approximated by an appropriate normal distribution.

(a) SE of the number of successes = $\sqrt{Npq}$ where N stands for the size of the sample, p for the probability of success, i.e. the sample proportion having the desired attribute, and q for the probability of failure, i.e. the sample proportion not having the desired attribute 'q' is always equal to (1 – p).

Example 14:

In a survey of 150 student nurses, it was found that 42% of them reported that they were unable to start IV line at single prick.

(a) Estimate the standard error of the proportion.
(b) Construct a 99% confidence interval for the true proportion student nurses who cannot establish IV line at single prick.

$$N = 150,\ p = 0.42,\ q = 1 - 0.42 = 0.58$$

$$SE_p = \sqrt{\frac{pq}{N}} = \sqrt{\frac{(0.42)(0.58)}{150}} = 0.0403$$

$$\text{99\% confidence interval} = p \pm 2.58\ SE_p$$

$$\text{or } 0.42 \pm 2.58\ (0.0403)$$

$$\text{or } 0.42 \pm 0.104\ (0.316, 0.524)$$

Example 15:

500 apples are taken at random from a large basket and 50 are found to be bad. Estimate the proportion of bad apples in the basket and assign limits within which the percentage most probably lies.

The proportion of bad apples in the given sample = $\frac{50}{500} = 0.1$

Hence, p = 0.1 and q = 1 – 0.1 = 0.9

$$SE\ p = \sqrt{\frac{pq}{N}} = \sqrt{\frac{0.1 \times 0.9}{500}} = \sqrt{\frac{0.09}{500}} = 0.013$$

The limit within which percentage of bad apples lies

$$= [p \pm 3\ (0.013)] \times 100]$$

A sample statistics and a range of plus or minus 3 standard deviation (Standard error) will include 99.73% of all the sample statistics.

$$= [0.1 \pm 0.039] \times 100]$$

$$= (0.139) \times 100 \text{ and } (0.061 \times 100)$$

$$= 13.9 \text{ and } 6.1$$

Thus, assuming the conditions of simple random sampling the percentage of bad apples in consignment almost certainly lies between 6.1 and 13.9.

Example 16:

In a survey, out of 100 children, 30% of children found to be playing violent video games. Estimate to the population using 95%, 99% and 99.9%.

n = 100 p = 0.3 q = 1 – 0.3 = 0.7

$$p + z\sqrt{pq/n}$$

$$0.3 \pm 1.96 \times \sqrt{0.3 \times 0.7/100}$$

$$0.3 \pm 1.96 \times 0.05$$
$$0.3 \pm 0.098$$
$$0.4 - 0.2\ (40\% - 20\%)$$

Inference: Using this sample value, estimated population value should lie between 38.98 and 21.02 at 95% confidence or 5% level of significance.

$$p \pm z\sqrt{pq/n}$$
$$0.3 \pm 2.58 \times 0.05$$
$$0.3 \pm 0.13$$
$$0.43 - 0.17\ (43\% - 17\%)$$

Inference: Using this sample value, estimate population value should lie between 41.82 and 18.18 at 99% confidence or 1% level of significance.

$$p \pm z\sqrt{pq/n}$$
$$0.3 \pm 3.29 \times 0.05$$
$$0.3 \pm 0.16$$
$$0.46 - 0.14\ (46\% - 14\%)$$

Inference: Using this sample value, estimate population value should lie between 45.07 and 14.93 at 99.9% confidence or 0.1% level of significance.

Example 17:

A study was conducted among 68, +2 students and 32% of them stated that their choice of course for undergraduate program is BSc (N). Find the confidence limits for the population proportion of +2 students choice of their course for undergraduate program.

$n = 68$ $p = 32\%$ or 0.32 $q = 1 - p = 1 - 0.32 = 0.68$

and the standard variate (z) for 95% confidence is 1.96 (as per the normal curve area table).

Thus, 95% confidence interval for the proportion of +2 students choice of their UG course in the population is

$$p \pm z\sqrt{pq/n}$$
$$0.64 \pm 1.96\sqrt{\frac{0.32 \times 0.68}{68}}$$
$$0.64 \pm 1.96\sqrt{0.0032}$$
$$0.64 \pm 1.96 \times 0.057$$
$$0.64 + 0.11$$
$$0.75 - 0.53$$

The lower confidence limit is 53%

Upper confidence limit is 75%

SUMMARY

- Parameter refers to the measures or values of the population. Parameter estimation is concerned with obtaining numerical values of the parameter from a sample.
- Population mean is denoted as μ whereas sample mean is denoted as $\overline{X}$. Population standard deviation is denoted as σ_p, whereas sample standard deviation is denoted as σ_s.
- μ and σ_p are conventionally called as 'estimators'. $\overline{X}$ and σ_s are referred to as 'estimates'.

- The distribution of all possible values of a statistic is called the sampling distribution or the probability distribution of that statistic. The distribution of all possible values that can be assumed by some statistic, computed from samples of the same size randomly drawn from the same population, is called the sampling distribution of that statistic.
- The relationship between the shape of the population distribution and the shape of the sampling distribution is called the central limit theorem. The significance of the central limit theorem lies in the fact that it permits us to use sample statistics to make inferences about population parameters without knowing anything about the shape of the frequency distribution of that population.
- The standard deviation of sampling distribution of a statistic is known as its standard error (SE) and is considered the key to sampling theory. The standard error helps in testing whether the difference between observed and expected frequencies could arise due to chance. The confidence level or reliability is the expected percentage of times that the actual value will fall within the stated precision limits.
- A statistic used as an estimate of a parameter, and presented as a single number, is known as a point estimate. A pair of estimates, one above the point estimate and the other below it and assert with a certain degree of confidence that the parameter would lie within this stated interval is known as an interval estimate.

EXERCISES

- In a survey among 100 adolescent children, 30% of children found to be suffering from hookworm infestation. Estimate to the population using 95%, 99% and 99.9%.
- In a survey among 200 school children, 40% of them suffered from dental caries. Estimate to the population using 95%, 99% and 99.9%.
- In a study of vitamin A deficiency among school children, 144 or 41.4% of the 348 children were found to have vitamin A deficiency. Estimate their number in the population of 3480 children.
- In a sample of 548 children 150 were found to be vegetarian. Estimate their number in the population.
- A random sample of 10 individuals chosen from a group gives their average weight equal to 60 kg with the standard deviation of 5.8 kg. What are the limits within which the average weight of the whole group can be expected to lie at 95% confidence?
- A study was conducted among +2 children regarding their attitude towards the nursing as a profession. In a sample of 400 students taken from the population of 4000 students, 80 of them had favorable attitude and the remaining had unfavorable attitude towards nursing. Estimate the number with favorable attitude in the population.
- The mean number of accidental falls of patient to occur in 8 randomly selected months in a big hospital was 24 and the standard deviation in the sample was 6 accidental falls. Construct a 95% confidence interval for the mean number.
- In a patient satisfaction survey, 80 patients were contacted and 58% of them were extremely satisfied by the care provided by the hospital. Find the confidence limits for the proportion of patients satisfied in the population, given a confidence level equal to 95%.
- 8 women were randomly selected and it was determined that the time they spent for exercise per week on an average is 4 hours and a standard deviation of 2 hour. Construct a 95% confidence interval for the population mean.

- A random sample of 12 pairs from a normal universe gives a correlation coefficient of 0.6. What are the limits within which the r of the entire universe can be expected to lie at 95% confidence?
- For the following sample sizes, and confidence levels, find the appropriate t values for constructing confidence intervals:
  - N = 12; 95%
  - N = 22; 90%
  - N = 8; 99%
  - N = 10; 95%
  - N = 18; 90%
  - N = 25; 95%

20 Hypothesis Testing

OBJECTIVES

After reading this chapter, you will be able to:

- Explain the concepts of hypothesis testing
- Explain the procedure of hypothesis testing
- Understand Type I and Type II error
- Understand one tailed and two tailed tests
- List various parametric and non-parametric tests used to test hypothesis.

INTRODUCTION

Hypothesis means less than the thesis. It is an important instrument in research. In a general meaning, hypothesis is an assumption or supposition to be proved or disproved. But in research, it is a tentative or predictive statement which predicts the relationship between two or more variables which are amenable to testing by scientific methods. A sample investigation produces results; and with these results, decisions are made on the population. Hypothesis is an assumption which may or may not be true about a population parameter. Therefore, we may conduct a test to judge significance whether the difference is due to sampling. The purpose of hypothesis testing is to facilitate the researcher to arrive at a conclusion concerning a population by examining a sample from that population. Testing of hypothesis requires the researcher's ability to think critically, formulate null and alternative hypothesis and test it based on the sample data. Hypothesis enables the researcher to make probability statements about population parameter(s).

The word 'parameter' is used to denote the values of population whereas the term 'statistic' refers to the values of the sample.

Concept of Hypothesis Testing

A hypothesis is the formal statement of the expected relationship (s) between two or more variables (Burns & Groove).

According to polit 'A hypothesis is a tentative prediction or explanation of the relationship between two or more variables.'

A hypothesis is a conjectural statement of the relationship between two or more variables (Kerlin, 1986).

A hypothesis may be defined simply as a statement about one or more populations. The hypothesis is frequently concerned with the parameters of the populations about which the statement is made. Hypothesis testing is a systematic way of checking or testing an idea or concept formed about a group or population. This is done by collecting data from the samples and subjecting them to the statistical analysis. A hospital administrator may hypothesize that the average length of stay of patients admitted to the hospital is six days. A faculty in a college may hypothesize that a specific teaching methodology will result in improved scores and pass percentage. A pharmacologist may hypothesize that a particular drug may be effective in 95% of the cases. By means of hypothesis testing one determines whether or not such statements are compatible with available data. In statistics one must be familiar with the null hypothesis and alternative hypothesis.

Null hypothesis (H_o): It is referred to as a statistical hypothesis. A null hypothesis is used for the purpose of statistical testing and interpreting statistical outcomes. It is usually formulated for the purpose of being rejected. The null hypothesis states that there is no difference between two variables. The level of significance for rejection or acceptance of the null hypothesis is arbitrarily determined before hand by the researcher.

Null hypothesis is akin to the legal principle that a man is innocent until he is proved guilty. It constitutes a challenge and the function of research is to give the facts a chance to refute (or fail to refute) this challenge. This type of hypothesis is especially useful in tests of statistical significance.

Alternative hypothesis (H_a): It is a rival hypothesis for null hypothesis and this is the one the researcher wishes to prove. Alternative hypothesis is just the negation of the null hypothesis. A null hypothesis is the one a researcher wishes to reject and alternative hypothesis includes all other possibilities. For example if the null hypothesis is that the individual and group health education are equally good, then the alternative hypothesis is that either the individual health education is better than the group health education or group health education is better than the individual health education. Or else both are not good.

In research, if we reject null hypothesis, we are accepting alternative hypothesis. Also, if we accept null hypothesis, we are rejecting the alternative hypothesis. Both null hypothesis and alternative hypothesis are chosen before the sample is drawn.

Procedure of Hypothesis Testing

The procedure for testing a hypothesis concerning the value of population parameters includes the following steps:

- Identify the problem
- Formulate the null and alternative hypotheses
- Choose the level of significance of the test
- Choose the location of the critical region
- Choose the appropriate test statistic (for example, Z, t, $\mathcal{X}^2$, F) and find from the relevant table the critical value of the chosen statistic, that is the value that defines the boundary of the critical region.

- Compute from the sample observations the observed value (or sample value, or empirical value) of the chosen statistic, using the relevant formula
- Compare the sample value of the chosen statistic with the theoretical (table) value that defines the critical region. If the observed value of the statistic falls in the critical region or rejection region, we reject the null hypothesis. Otherwise we accept the null hypothesis.

Identify the Problem or Deciding What we Want to Test

The first step in testing hypothesis is deciding what we want to test or check.

Think of a person Mr. A who is being accused of stealing. Here we want to check that Mr. A is a thief.

In another situation, we may want to test or prove that the mean hemoglobin value of adolescent girls in a community is 12.0 g/dL.

Formulate the Null Hypothesis (H_o) and the Alternative Hypothesis (H_a)

The second step is stating the hypothesis in a way so that it is amenable for testing. In general we formulate null hypothesis. In the example mentioned above, when we want to prove that Mr. A is a thief, we can do this by assuming that Mr. A is innocent or not a thief, since there is a possibility that he may be innocent.

Thinking that Mr. A is innocent, it is the responsibility to provide all the evidences to prove that he is guilty.

We should remember here that the only reason we are testing the null hypothesis is to prove what we think is wrong. Here thinking that Mr. A is innocent is wrong. The null hypothesis here is Mr. A is innocent. The assumption which a researcher is trying to reject is called the null hypothesis and is symbolized H_0.

The alternate hypothesis is stated to say what we think about null hypothesis is wrong. Here the alternate hypothesis is Mr. A is guilty or Mr. A is a thief.

In the example of Hb value of adolescent girls, the null hypothesis is stated as follows:

The mean Hb value of the adolescent girls in a community is equal to 12.0 g/dL. By stating like this we are directed to test whether what we have stated or assumption about population is true or not. The null hypothesis (H_0), stated as the null, is a statement about a population parameter, such as the population mean, that is assumed to be true.

The alternate hypothesis is stated as the mean hemoglobin value is not equal to or greater than or lesser than 12.0 g/dL. We place the burden on the researcher to conduct a study to show evidence that the null hypothesis is unlikely to be true. Regardless, we always make a decision about the null hypothesis (that it is likely or unlikely to be true). A decision made in hypothesis testing centers on the null hypothesis. This means two things in terms of making a decision:

1. Decisions are made about the null hypothesis. A researcher conducts a study showing evidence that this assumption is unlikely (we reject the null hypothesis) or fails to do so (we retain the null hypothesis).
2. The bias is to do nothing. In the above example, the guilty may be let go free than punishing him, researchers would rather do nothing than make statements that are not correct. For this reason, we assume the null hypothesis is correct, thereby placing the burden on the researcher to demonstrate that the null hypothesis is not likely to be correct.

The assumption which a researcher is trying to reject is called the null hypothesis and is symbolized H_0, or 'H sub-zero'. When a null hypothesis is rejected, the conclusion the researcher accepts is called the alternative hypothesis and is symbolized as H_a ('H sub-a'). The null hypothesis is sometimes referred to as a hypothesis of no difference, since it is a statement of agreement with (or no difference from) conditions presumed to be true in the population of interest. Usually the alternative hypothesis and the research hypothesis are the same, and in fact the two terms are used interchangeably.

When null hypothesis is a type which indicates some quantitative value, the sign such as =, <, > must be present in the hypothesis. These signs help in decision making regarding one tail or two tail test. Suppose if we want to test that certain population hemoglobin mean value is not equal to 15 g/dL, then our null hypothesis would be.

$H_0 : \mu = 15$ and our alternative hypothesis would be either $H_a : \mu \neq 15$, $H_a : \mu > 15$ and $Ha : \mu < 15$.

As a rule of thumb, what we want to conclude as a result of the test usually should be placed in alternative hypothesis. The null and alternative hypothesis are complementary.

Choose the Level of Significance of the Test

In this case, the claim or idea is that the mean hemoglobin value of adolescent girls in a community is 12.0 g/dL. In order to test whether this is true or not we need to collect data, i.e. Hb value from adolescents girls. Most samples should have a Hb value of 12.0 or closer if the claim we are testing is true. So at what point do we decide that the discrepancy between the sample mean and 12.0 g/dL is so big that the claim we are testing is likely not true? We answer this question in this step of hypothesis testing. To set the criteria for a decision, we state the level of significance for a test. In hypothesis testing, we collect data to show that the null hypothesis is not true, based on the likelihood of selecting a sample mean from a population (the likelihood is the criterion). The likelihood or level of significance is typically set at 5% in behavioral research studies. When the probability of obtaining a sample mean is less than 5% if the null hypothesis were true, then we conclude that the sample we selected is too unlikely and so we reject the null hypothesis.

Level of significance, or significance level, refers to a criterion of judgment upon which a decision is made regarding the value stated in a null hypothesis. The criterion is based on the probability of obtaining a statistic measured in a sample if the value stated in the null hypothesis were true.

The alternative hypothesis helps us to decide the placement of the level of significance in tail. Remember that we know that the sample mean will equal the population mean on average if the null hypothesis is true. All other possible values of the sample mean are normally distributed (central limit theorem). The empirical rule tells us that at least 95% of all sample means fall within about 2 standard deviations (SD) of the population mean, meaning that there is less than a 5% probability of obtaining a sample mean that is beyond 2 SD from the population mean. For the adolescent girls of Hb levels, we can look for the probability of obtaining a sample mean beyond 2 SD in the upper tail (greater than 12 g/dL), the lower tail (less than 12 g/dL), or both tails (not equal to 12 g/dL).

It is to be noted that acceptance or rejection of hypothesis is based upon the information supplied by the sample and what is indicated by a particular sample may not always be true in respect of the population. Hence, in making a decision the researcher can never be 100% sure that he will make the right decision. In fact, there are four possible situations which may arise. The researcher may make a correct decision by (a) accepting the null hypothesis when it is true or by (b) rejecting the null hypothesis when it is false. The researcher may also make a wrong decision by a (a) rejecting the null hypothesis when it is true, or by (b) accepting the null hypothesis when it is false. The former of these two wrong decisions is known as the Type I error or the 'rejection error' and the latter is known as the Type II error or the 'acceptance error'. All these four situations are shown in a tabular form thus:

Null hypothesis is actually	**Null hypothesis is**	
	Accepted	Rejected
True	Correct decision (No error)	Wrong decision (Type I error)
False	Wrong decision (Type II error)	Correct decision (No error)

By rewriting

Reject the null hypothesis when it is true – Type I error = α

Accept the null hypothesis when it is false – Type II error = β

Accept the null hypothesis when it is true – Correct decision

Reject the null hypothesis when it is false – Correct decision

A level of significance represents the probability of committing Type I error. This probability is denoted by the Greek letter α (alpha). It is obvious that every researcher wants this probability to be small. Conventionally, this probability is fixed at 5% before a test is made, and more rarely at 1%. 5% level of significance gives a value which has a rare chance of coming up only once in 20 trails. Similarly, 1% level of significance gives a value which has the chance of coming up only once in 100 trials. Hence, none of these values can be considered by the researcher as substantially supporting his null hypothesis. So, when these values appear he rejects the hypothesis. This is why a level of significance is also called the region of rejection or the critical region. Needless to say that a researcher feels more confident in rejecting

H_0 at 1% level of significance than at 5% level of significance because in the former case the probability of his making a wrong decision (of rejecting the null hypothesis when it is actually true) is only one in a hundred (or 0.01). One can express this error thus:

Type I error or α = Probability (Rejecting H_0/H_0 is true)

The researcher can also fix the probability of committing the Type II error, i.e. accepting the null hypothesis when it is false. This probability which is denoted by the Greek letter β can be expressed thus:

Type II error or β = Probability (Accepting H_0/H_0 is false)

Every researcher likes β to be as small as possible. Alternatively, he likes 1 - β, i.e. the probability of rejecting the null hypothesis when it is false, to be as large as possible or to be as close to unity as possible. Thus, $(1-\beta)$ becomes the measure of how well the test is functioning or what is technically described as the power of the test.

Choose the Location of the Critical Region

The critical region which, as we have told, corresponds to the level of significance may be chosen either at the right end (right tail) of the distribution of the variable, or at the left tail, or half at each end of the distribution depending on the form in which the alternative hypothesis is expressed. In the first and second cases, we say that we conduct a one-tail test, in the third case, we say that we conduct a two-tail test.

The following rule of thumb may summaries the above description regarding the choice of the location of the critical region. Choose the location of the critical region on the basis of the direction at which the inequality sign points:

- If > (more than), choose the right tail as the critical region
- If < (less than), choose the left tail as the critical region
- If ≠ (not equal to), choose as two-tail as the critical region.

Choose the Appropriate Test Statistic

There are two types of tests: parametric and non parametric. For the application of parametric tests normality of distribution is crucial. If our assumptions of normality do not hold good or if our data are on the ordinal or nominal scale, these tests cannot be used. In these situations, several non parametric tests (which being without any model are also known as distribution-free tests) can be used.

Important parametric tests are the z-test, t-test, $\mathcal{X}^2$-test and F-test. The choice among them depends on the nature of the problem. Z-test is, however, the most frequently used test in research studies. It is generally used for comparing the mean of a sample with some hypothesized population mean or for judging the significance of difference between two sample means or for testing the significance of difference between two proportions of successes, and so on. Being based on the normal probability distribution, this test is generally used in the case of large samples.

T-test is based on t-distribution and is considered an appropriate test for judging the significance of a sample mean or of difference between the means of two samples in case of small samples when population variance is not known (and so we use variance of the sample as an estimate of the population variance).

$\mathcal{X}^2$-test is based on chi-square distribution and as a parametric test is used for comparing a sample variance with some hypothesized population variance.

F-test is based on F-distribution and is used for comparing the variance of two independent samples. This test is also used for judging the significance of the difference in the variance of more than two samples at one and the same time.

There are many nonparametric tests such as Median test, Mann-Whitney U-test, Sign-test, McNemar test and chi-square test etc. are also used in calculating test statistic.

Compute the Sample Value of the Chosen Test Statistic

After choosing any one of the test statistic, using an appropriate formula, one can calculate the test statistic from the data obtained from the sample. The test statistic, that is the value calculated from the data obtained from the sample helps in deciding whether to accept or reject the null hypothesis.

For example, we could select 100 adolescent girls and measure the Hb value and calculate the test statistic. The test statistic is a mathematical formula that allows researchers to determine the likelihood of obtaining sample outcomes if the null hypothesis were true. The value of the test statistic is used to make a decision regarding the null hypothesis which tells us how far, or how many standard deviations, a sample mean is from the population mean. The larger the value of the test statistic, the further the distance, or number of standard deviations, a sample mean is from the population mean stated in the null hypothesis.

Compare the Computed Value with its Table Value

The final step of our hypothesis testing is to compare the calculated value of the chosen statistic with its table value at the pre determined level of significance (5% or 1%). If the calculated value is less than the table value, we may accept our null hypothesis of 'no difference' and conclude that whatever difference we are observing between the sample and the hypothesized value is only due to sampling fluctuations. In other words, the difference is not statistically significant.

On the other hand, if the calculated value is more than the table value and falls in the critical region, it is obviously too large to have arisen by chance and so we may reject our null hypothesis of 'no difference' and conclude that the difference is real and statistically significant. Rejection of null hypothesis, however, does not imply that our alternative hypothesis is correct. It only suggests that the test does not support our hypothesis of 'no difference'.

We expect the sample mean to be equal to 12.0 g/dL. If the discrepancy between the sample mean and population mean is small, then we will likely decide that the claim we are testing is indeed true. If the discrepancy is too large, then we will likely decide to reject the claim as being not true. The probability of obtaining a sample mean, given that the value stated in the null hypothesis is true, is stated by the ***p value***. The p value is a probability: It varies between 0 and 1 and can never be negative. A *p* value is the probability of obtaining a sample outcome, given that the value stated in the null hypothesis is true. The p value for obtaining a sample outcome is compared to the level of significance. Significance, or statistical significance, describes a decision made concerning a value stated in the null hypothesis. When the null hypothesis is rejected, we reach significance. When the null hypothesis is retained, we fail to reach significance. When the p value is less than 5% ($p < .05$), we reject the null hypothesis. We will refer to $p < .05$ as the criterion for deciding to reject the null hypothesis, although note that when $p = .05$, the decision is also to reject the null hypothesis. When the p value is greater than 5% ($p > .05$), we retain the null hypothesis.

TWO-TAILED TESTS

Two-tailed tests are used when the directions of hypothesis is not known. When a null hypothesis is that the population mean is equal to 50 and the alternative hypothesis is that the population mean is not equal to 50, then the two-tailed tests are used. In two-tailed test, there are two rejection regions (critical regions) one on each tail of the curve which can be seen in the above diagram.

If the level of significance is 5% and the two-tailed test is to be used, the probability of the rejection area will be 0.05 (equally splitted on both tails of the curve as 0.025) and that of the acceptance region will be 0.95 as shown in the above curve.

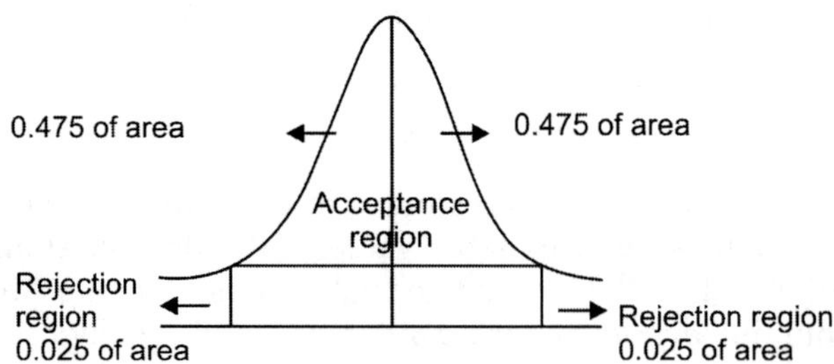

ONE-TAILED TEST

When a null hypothesis is that the population mean is equal to 50 and the alternative hypothesis is that the population mean is less than 50 or more than 50, then one tailed test is used. In case of any value less than some hypothesized value left tail test is used (only one rejection region 0.05 area on the left side which is illustrated below) and for more than the hypothesized value right tail test is used (only one rejection region, 0.05 area on the right tail only).

The region of rejection is the portion of a sampling distribution containing values that are considered too unlikely to occur to be representing the underlying raw score population. A critical value marks the edge of the region of rejection and thus defines the value required for a sample to fall in the region of rejection.

Nonsignificant indicates that results are not too unlikely to accept as being due to sampling error. In other words, the differences reflected by the results were likely to have occurred even if there is no real relationship in the population.

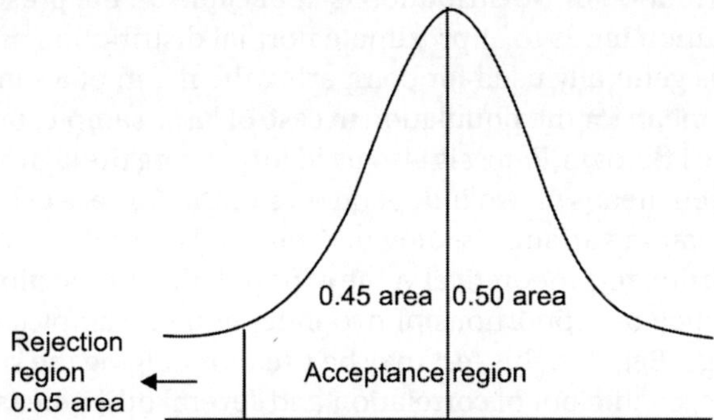

VARIOUS TESTS FOR HYPOTHESIS TESTING

All these tests are explained in detail in the further chapters.

Parametric Tests

The important parametric tests are: (1) Z-test; (2) t-test; (3) $\mathcal{X}^2$ - test, and (4) F-test. All these tests are based on the assumption of normality, i.e. the source of data is considered to be normally distributed. In some cases the population may not be normally distributed, yet the tests will be applicable on account of the fact that we mostly deal with samples and the sampling distributions closely approach normal distributions (Fig. 20.1).

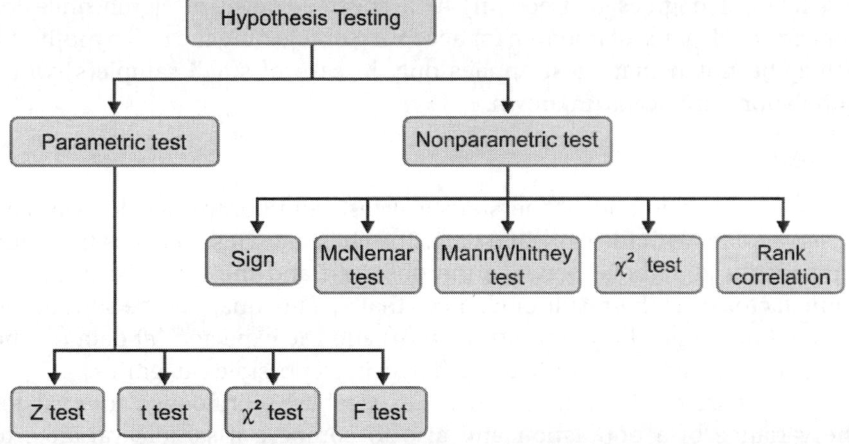

Fig. 20.1 Classification of various test for hypothesis testing

Z-test

Z-test is based on the normal probability distribution and is used for judging the significance of several statistical measures, particularly the mean. The relevant test statistic, Z, is worked out and compared with its probable value (to be read from table showing area under normal cruve) at a specified level of significance for judging the significance of the measure concerned. This is a most frequently used test in research studies. This test is used even when binomial distribution or t-distribution is applicable on the presumption that such a distribution tends to approximate normal distribution as 'n' becomes larger. Z-test is generally used for comparing the mean of a sample to some hypothesized mean for the population in case of large sample, or when population variance is known. Z-test is also used for judging the significance of difference between means of two independent samples in case of large samples, or when population variance is known. Z-test is also used for comparing the sample proportion to a theoretical value of population proportion or for judging the difference in proportions of two independent samples when n happens to be large. Besides, this test may be used for judging the significance of median, mode, coefficient of correlation and several other measures.

t-Test

t-Test is based on t-distributiion and is considered an appropriate test for judgjing the significance of a sample mean or for judging the significance of difference between the means of two sample in case of small sample(s) when population variance is not known. In case two samples are related, we use paired t-test (or what is known as difference test) for judging the significance of the mean of difference between the two related samples. It can also be used for judging the significance of the coefficients of simple and partial correlations. The relevant test statistisc, t, is calculated from the sample data and then compared with its probable value based on t-distribution (to be read from the table that gives probable values of t for different levels of significance for different degrees of freedom) at a specified level of significance for concerning degrees of freedom for accepting or rejecting the null hypothesis. It may be noted that t-test applies only in case of small sample(s) when population variance is unknown.

X^2-test

Chi square test is one of the statistical test commonly used to compare observed data with the expected data. The chi square test helps us to decide whether the difference between the observed and the expected is due to some factor or is the result of chance. That is, chi-square is the sum of the squared difference between observed (o) and the expected (e) data (or the deviation, d), divided by the expected data in all possible categories.

As a parametric test, it is used to establish confidence interval for the variance of a population and also to compare a sample variance to a theoretical population variance. It is used to test the hypothesis that the population variance is the same as the sample variance. The deviations of the observed numbers from those specified by the hypothesis form the basis of the chi-square. Each deviation is squared, each square is divided by the hypothetical or expected number and the results are added.

F-test

F distribution is a continuous probability distribution. It is also known as Snedecor's F distribution or the Fisher-Snedecor distribution. Suppose we take samples, of sizes N1 and N2 respetively from either a single population or two populations with the same variance. We calculate the variances for both samples (S_1^2 and S_2^2) and then find the ratio between these variances (S_1^2/S_2^2). If we do this for a very large number of pairs of samples, the ratios would form a distribution known as the F distribution, whose properties are known for various numbers of degrees of freedom, these being (N1–1) and (N2-1) for the two samples. In other words, tables of F, the ratio of S_1^2 to S_2^2 allows us to find the probability of obtaining F ratios above any given value, for two samples from the same population, or from two populations with the same variance. F-test is based on F-distribution and is used to compare the variance of the two-independent samples.

Nonparametric Test

Nonparametric tests procedure deals primarily with populations that are not normally distributed. Nonparametric tests do not make any assumptions about the shape of the population from which the sample scores were drawn and are, therefore, known as 'distribution free' tests.

These tests are much easier to learn and to apply than parametric tests. They are particularly useful in case of small samples—a feature which should be helpful to the researcher collecting pilot study data and to the researcher whose samples must be small because of their very nature (e.g. samples of persons with a rare form of mental illness). There are various nonparametric tests. They are as follows:

A. One-sample and Two-sample Tests

Appropriate for Nominal Data

Chi-square test: $\mathcal{X}^2$: As a nonparametric measure, it is used (i) as a test of goodness of fit, and (ii) as a test of independence. It can be used to determine if categorical data shows dependency or the two classifications are independent.

McNemar test: It is one of the important tests often used when data is nominal and two related samples. This test is useful with before-after measurement of the same subjects. The experiment is designed for the use of this test in such a way that the subjects initially are divided into equal groups as to their favorable and unfavorable views about something, practice or concept. After some treatment, the same number of subjects are asked to express their views about the given system whether they favor it or do not favor it. By using this test, we can assess any significant change in views of the same subjects before and after the treatment by developing a table in respect of the first and second measurement.

B. Appropriate for Ordinal Data

Sign test: It is quite simple to do and applies to both one-tailed and two-tailed tests. It is usually based on the binomial distribution. This test is used both in the study of single and paired samples. The sign test utilizes pair-wise comparisons of two different distributions to identify which is larger than which and then from this information it determines if the two distributions differ significantly from each other. The sign test sums all the positive signs, negative signs, and ties and then computes z score and a 'p' value associated with the frequency of the positives and negatives.

Wilcoxon signed rank test: Unlike the sign test which is based on only the number of plus or minus signs, this test utilizes both the signs and magnitudes of the differences. This makes it more sensitive and powerful than the ordinary sign test. Wilcoxon Signed Rank Test also applies both to single and paired samples.

Median test: Sign test and the wilcoxon test require the samples to be paired. If the samples are unpaired, as is very often the case, the use of these tests should be avoided. Median Test should be preferred in such situations. This test can be used even when more than 2 samples are being studied.

One-sample runs test: It is used to know whether the observations in a given series can be regarded as random. This is done by ascertaining the number of runs which are present in a series. A run is a sequence of like symbols which are followed and preceded by other kinds of symbols or no symbol on either side. A sequence of symbols exhibiting a pattern of symbols is usually indicative of lack of randomness.

Mann-Whitney U test: This is a very popular test amongst the rank sum tests. This test is used to determine whether two independent samples have been drawn from the same population. It uses more information than the sign test or the Fisher-Irwin test. This test applies under very general conditions and requires only that the populations sampled are continuous.

Spearman's rank correlation coefficient: Rank correlation is a nonparametric technique for measuring relationship between paired observations of two variables when data are in the ranked form. It can be used when the data are irregular or extreme items are erratic or inaccurate. The result of rank correlation is only an approximate one, because under ranking method original value are not taken into account. The main objective of this coefficient is to determine the extent to which the two sets of ranking are similar or dissimilar.

C. K-Sample Tests ($K \geq 3$)

Kruskal-Wallis test: The Kruskal Wallis H test is analogous to a one-way between subjects ANOVA for ranked data. It assumes that the study involves one independent variable and that there are three or more independent samples with at least five participants in each sample. The null hypothesis is that all conditions represent the same distribution of ranks in the population.

SUMMARY

- A hypothesis is the formal statement of the expected relationship (s) between two or more variables.
- A null hypothesis is used for the purpose of statistical testing and interpreting statistical outcomes. It is usually formulated for the purpose of being rejected. The null hypothesis states that there is no difference between two variables. The level of significance for rejection or acceptance of the null hypothesis is arbitrarily determined before hand by the researcher.
- Alternative hypothesis is just the negation of the null hypothesis. A null hypothesis is the one a researcher wishes to reject and alternative hypothesis includes all other possibilities.
- Type I error or is the probability of rejecting the null hypothesis when it is true. Type II error or β is the probability of accepting the null hypothesis when it is false.
- In choosing the location of critical region one can use two-tailed or one-tailed test. When the direction of hypothesis is not known one can use two-tailed test and if the direction is known one can use one-tailed test (left or right tail).
- There are various parametric and non-parametric tests used in calculating the test statistic. The important parametric tests are Z-test, t-test, F-test and Chi square-test. Some of the nonparametric tests are sign test, median test, Mc-Nemar test, Mann Whitney test and Chi square test.
- The final step of our hypothesis testing is to compare the calculated value of the chosen statistic with its table value at the pre-determined level of significance (5% or 1%). If the calculated value is less than the table value, we may accept our null hypothesis. On the other hand, if the calculated value is more than the table value and falls in the critical region, it is obviously too large to have arisen by chance and so we may reject our null hypothesis.

EXERCISE

Reason out:

- Why null hypothesis is formulated?
- Why do we fix alpha 0.05 in a research?
- When do you go for two-tailed test?
- What is the relation between the concept of normal distribution and hypothesis testing?
- What is type I and type II error?

21 Research Designs and its Statistical Application

OBJECTIVES

After reading this chapter, you will be able to:
- State the meaning of research design
- List the various research design
- Explain the research design and its statistical analysis.

INTRODUCTION

There are various research designs we use to conduct a research. Research design is a blue print of the study and it shows the researcher's overall plan in conducting a research. The selection of a particular research design depends upon the research problem, objectives and hypothesis. A researcher must think of pros and cons of all research designs and based on the research problem, he must choose the appropriate research design.

EXPERIMENTAL DESIGNS

In all disciplines, experimental designs are used in conducting research. Nursing is not an exception. A good experimental design must possess the two attributes such as internal validity and external validity. Internal validity in a research can be ensured by designing and conducting a research in such a way that the treatment alone brings some effect or changes in the outcome variable. The researcher must identify all those variables (extraneous variables) which can influence the outcome variable and try to eliminate the effect it can bring on the outcome variable. The condition which rules out the effects of other variables on the experiment is known as internal validity of the experiment. The effects of extraneous variable can be controlled by holding its effect constant for all subjects, balancing and statistical elimination. Another important attribute of a good experimental design is its external validity, that is its generalizability or representativeness. A given experiment has external validity to the extent that its results are generalizable beyond the conditions associated with the experiment. Kerlinger has proposed a principle for experimental study. This principle known as the Max Min Con principle directs researcher to:

1. Maximize the variance of a study's independent variable (in order to make the study externally valid)

2. Minimize the variance caused by unreliability of measures, and
3. Control the variance caused by nuisance or confounding variables (in order to make the study internally valid).

Single Sample Experiment

It is a design used when we have one group of samples and the experiment or treatment is given for the single group. We randomly select a group of samples and the subjects should be exposed to an intervention and its effectiveness is assessed by conducting the post test. Measurement is done at only one time which is after the intervention. For example, we would like to assess the effect of specific management regimen on blood sugar level among adults with diabetes mellitus. In this we can randomly select a group of samples with Diabetes mellitus and give them the treatment and their blood glucose level can be monitored. Then their results are compared with the standard values. We know the normal range of blood glucose level. Or their results can be compared with the adults with Diabetes mellitus who are on regular or routine treatment (which can be obtained from the past records or previous studies).

Suppose, if we knew that the blood glucose level of people with Diabetes mellitus who are on routine treatment is 130 g/dL. The obtained value is compared with this value and the inference is drawn.

In this study, the null hypothesis can be formulated as mentioned below:

Null hypothesis:

$H_o : \mu = 130$ mg/dL

$H_a : \mu \neq 130$ mg/dL

Suppose, in sample statistic the mean is 128 mg/dL.

Although we cannot determine whether the null hypothesis is true, we can determine how likely it is that a sample mean of 128 g/dL will occur through sampling error when the sample actually represents the population where μ is 130 g/dL.

The difference between the population mean (130 g/dL) and the sample mean (128 g/dL) can be attributed to the specific management regimen or the sampling error. We are not sure that the specific management regimen really worked or not. Here the problem can be tackled by increasing our confidence level that the specific management regimen has worked out well.

The Z test can be used at 95% confidence level or 5% level of significance.

Why Z test?

We have one group of randomly selected samples.

The dependent variable (blood glucose) is approximately normally distributed

We know the mean of the population

We know the true standard deviation of the population.

The formula to find out the significant difference of the mean $Z = \frac{\bar{x} - \mu}{\sigma / \sqrt{N}}$

$\bar{x}$ = Mean of the sample

μ = Mean of the population

$\sigma / \sqrt{N}$ = Standard Error of the mean.

In case of small samples, we can use t test. The formula is as follows:

$$\mathbf{t} = \frac{\overline{x} - \mu H_0}{SE}$$

Two Sample Experiment

In two sample experiment, two groups are involved, either two different groups or the same groups performance can be measured twice and compared for any difference. There are two types, such as, between subjects experiment and within subjects experiment.

Between Subjects Experiment

Between subjects design includes the selection of participants for two conditions and each participant serves in only one condition. We do not match the participants between the different conditions. In this design, we have one random sample of participants in one group or condition and another group of independent samples in another condition.

The conditions are

- A group of participants is selected for each condition, without regard for those selected in the other condition
- Each sample is limited to the particular group alone.
- No matching of samples is done, and
- We do not test the same participants in different conditions.

Controlling Subject Variables

We randomly assign participants to each condition. Randomization facilitates the balancing of subject variation by mixing them and assigning to two different groups.

Balancing Subject Variables

It needs random assignment of participants to each condition. This controls subject variables by randomly mixing them. Subject variables can be controlled by balancing and counter balancing. Balancing can be achieved by scrutinizing our inclusion criteria and including participant who met the inclusion criteria.

Though random assignment can balance the subject variation to some extent, we cannot entirely leave this task to randomization. We need to systematically balance or counter balance the confounding variable in each condition. For example, to balance the gender effect we can select the equal number of male and female participants for each condition or else we can test amongst equal number of male and female samples even in single condition.

Sometimes pre-measurement helps in balancing subject variables. For example, we can assess the IQ level of children then randomly assign them to different groups based on their IQ scores.

Limiting the Population

One of the approach is to limit the population based on the variable. For example, we can limit the population to only male or only female. We can limit the population through the selection criteria. We can pretest or scrutinize the participants before being included in the study. We can select a group of students with similar IQ score and test them for the effectiveness of various teaching methods on their performance.

For example, we may want to test the effect of cognitive training on IQ of the children. Here the subject variables may be the gender and IQ level itself.

This can be balanced by including equal number of male and female children and equal number of children with good and poor IQ.

The independent samples test is used for between subjects design.

Why independent samples t test?

- The dependent variable is measured on interval or ratio level of measurement.
- The sample drawn from the population assumes a normal distribution.
- The variance is estimated from the sample data.
- The population represented by the samples has homogeneous variance. i.e. homogeneity of variance.

Here we have μ_1 and μ_2 and $X_1$and X_2. Since there are two independent populations, it's quite natural that the sample and population mean of two conditions are not equal.

So, the alternative hypothesis is that Ha : $\mu_1 - \mu_2 \neq 0$.

The null hypothesis is that Ho : $\mu_1 - \mu_2 = 0$.

If we check the intervention in two conditions for the entire population, we will get only one μ. Here μ_1 and μ_2 are equal and the sample mean also should be equal. There should not be any difference or the difference between this is zero.

The formula to find the significant difference between two means is

$$= \frac{\overline{X}_1 - \overline{X}_2}{SE}$$

Standard Error of difference between two means = $\sigma_{(comb)} \times \sqrt{\frac{1}{N_1} + \frac{1}{N_2}}$

Within Subject Design

In between subjects design, the approach is to control the subject variables by random assignment and balancing and counter balancing. To gain greater control of subject variables, and reduce error, we can use within subject design. The individuals in one condition are comparable to those in the other conditions. We employ this approach when there is one or more crucial extraneous subject variable that must be controlled. Here, we can use two designs or methods to compare the same individuals on two conditions.

1. Matched group designs
2. Repeated measures designs.

Matched groups design: In a matched group design, each participant in one condition matches a participant in the other condition(s) on one or more extraneous subject variables. For example, if want to know the effect of two weight reduction diets among samples, we have to choose the samples and match them and assign them to two different weight reduction diets. The variables such as weight of the sample, BMI of the sample, gender of the sample can be matched. It is very difficult to find the participants who have the same score on the matching variable, we can rank order the participants based on a specific variable, create pairs using adjacent ranked scores.

For example, if we want to assess the effectiveness of two teaching strategies, we have to have two groups matched for each other. Here the extraneous variables such as the age, gender and IQ level of students can be matched. Here our task is to identify the important variables on which to match participants. Second we may not have valid and reliable method for measuring the matching variable.

The advantage to matching is that it ensures that in every condition there is a participant with virtually the same score on the subject variable(s) we wish to control. This keeps these variables constant across the conditions, eliminating this potential confounding. The disadvantage of this design is the need to pretest the samples in order to match the samples and one may have to settle for small sample size. Pretesting may communicate the study purpose and it may influence the study outcome. We may not know the important variables on which to match participants. Second, we may not have a valid and reliable method for measuring the matching variable.

Repeated measures designs: A repeated measures design is one in which measurements of the same variable are made on each subject on two or more different occasions. The different occasions during which measurements are taken may be either points in time or different conditions such as different treatments. Repeated measures design is used to control for variability among subjects. In such a design each subject serves as its own control. This design is used to see the samples' responses over time.

In matched groups design, we match the samples in each group in order to control the confounding variables. The confounding variables can be eliminated by matching as many as variables in participants. The other way is exposing the participants to all conditions. This technique is called as repeated measures. Repeated measures design is different from the multiple trials. In multiple trials, the same participant is repeatedly observed in one condition. With repeated measures, the same participant is observed in various conditions. For example, if we want to test the effectiveness of conventional method vs newer method in managing a chronic disease say example blood glucose level in diabetes mellitus, we have to expose the samples to the conventional method of treatment and we have to measure the blood glucose level. Then the same group has to be exposed to the newer treatment method and the blood glucose level should be measured. While doing so, the group can be divided into two based on certain variable, such as gender. A group of male can be exposed to conventional treatment and a group of females can be exposed to newer treatment and the two groups are exchanged and exposed to all conditions.

Treatment	Conventional treatment	Newer treatment
Conventional treatment	Male	Female
Newer treatment	Female	Male

A researcher may want to see the effect of yoga versus moderate walking on weight reduction in participants. In case of repeated measures design, the samples have to be exposed first to the yoga for a specific duration say example, two weeks and their weight before and after should be measured. The same sample can be asked to go for moderate walking for two weeks and their weight before and after can be measured.

The strength of repeated measures design is they eliminate potential confounding variable. The differences between the conditions is not due to differences in subject variables, because this design ensures each participant with the same characteristics, is in every condition. Repeated measures should keep subject variables constant, but individuals change from moment to moment. The participants are aware of all conditions. Because of repeated exposures, participants may be aware of the research itself which leads to unnatural behavior. Subject history and maturation will influence the responses. Subject history refers to the fact that participants continue to have a life and experience things that can change them and influence their responses. Subject maturation occurs when someone grows over a period of time and they change their responses also over a period of time. This two factors severely reduce the internal validity.

Repeated measures produce greater subject mortality. Since repeated measures involves the subject being exposed to various conditions, it naturally takes time. We may lose the subject before the study is completed. Repeated measures design may produce a order effects. It means the changes in response of the sample in relation to their participation in series of trials. This includes Practice effects—showing better performance over trials; Fatigue effects-showing poor performance on repeated trials; Carry over effects—the experience of any one trial that influences scores on subsequent trials; and Response sets—from previous trials, developing a habitual response for subsequent trials. The order effects can be counter balanced by half the participants performing condition 1 followed by condition 2 and the remaining participants perform condition 2 followed by condition 1. The order effects can be controlled by complete counter balancing and randomizing the order of conditions.

Complete Counter Balancing

Complete counter balancing is the process of balancing order effects by testing different participants with different orders, so that all possible orders are present. In case if we want to test at three different conditions such as A, B, and C; it will produce six possible orders.

ABC ACB BAC BCA CAB CBA

In case if we want to test at four different conditions such as A, B, C and D; it will produce 24 possible orders.

ABCD	ABDC	ACBD	ACDB	ADCB	ADBC	BACD
BADC	BCDA	BCAD	BDAC	BDCA	CDAB	CDBA
CBAD	CBDA	CABD	CADB	DABC	DACB	DBCA
DBAC	DCAB	DCBA				

Partial counter balancing is the process of balancing order effects by testing different participants using only some of the possible orders.

Randomization is the process of balancing order effects by randomly creating different orders under which different participants are tested.

A simple repeated measure may be a before and after experiment. For example, we want to know the effect of nutrition supplementation on hemoglobin level of adolescent girls.

We must check the hemoglobin level of adolescent girls before and after nutrition supplementation. The difference between this can be calculated and it is tested for significance. The formula to test is as follows:

$$t = \frac{\bar{d}}{\frac{\sigma_{diff}}{\sqrt{N}}}$$

Advantages

This design has the ability to control for extraneous variation among subjects. Fewer samples are needed and their responses over time can be measured. This design is used when subjects are scarce and expensive to recruit.

Disadvantage

There is a risk of carry over effect. This problem can be solved by allowing adequate time pass between treatments.

Another risk is position effect. On repeated measures, at the first measurement the samples may be more enthusiastic and participate well in the study whereas when they approach towards the end may be third or fourth measurement, they may not show much interest or involvement. The treatment given before the first measurement and the last measurement will be influenced by the subjects interest and participation. The position of the treatment has the effect.

Types of Repeated Measures Design

Single factor repeated measures design

The simplest repeated measures design is the one in which in addition to the treatment variable, one additional variable is considered. The reason for introducing this additional variables is to measure and isolate its contribution to the total variability among the observation. We refer to this additional variable as a factor. The factor here is the subjects. In the single factor repeated measures design, each subjects receives each of the treatments. The order in which the subjects are exposed to the treatments, when possible, is random, and the randomization is carried out independently for each subject.

Factorial design

The experiment in which two or more factors are investigated simultaneously is called a factorial experiment. The different designated categories of the factor are called levels. In this, we can see not only the effects of individual factors but also the interaction between the factors. Factorial designs can be of two types: (1) simple factorial designs and (2) complex factorial designs.

Simple factorial designs: In case of simple factorial designs, we consider the effects of two factors on the dependent variable. It is also termed as a 'two factor- factorial design.' Simple factorial design may either be a 2 × 2 simple factorial design, or it may be 3 × 4 or 5 × 3 design etc.

2 × 2 Simple Factorial Design

	Independent variable	
Dependent variable	**Treatment A**	**Treatment B**
Level 1	Cell 1	Cell 3
Level 2	Cell 2	Cell 4

As such there are four cells into which the sample is divided. Each of the four combinations would provide one experimental condition. Subjects are assigned at random to each treatment. The means for different cells may be obtained along with the means for different rows and columns.

Example of 2 × 2 Simple Factorial Design

	Independent variable	
Dependent variable	**Lecture**	**Demonstration**
Male	Cell 1	Cell 3
Female	Cell 2	Cell 4

If a teacher wants to study the effect of two teaching methods on gender influence, a simple 2 × 2 factorial design can be used.

4 × 3 Simple Factorial Design

This design includes four treatments of the experimental variable and three levels of control variable.

Control variable	Experimental variable			
	Intervention A	**Intervention B**	**Intervention C**	**Intervention D**
Level I	Cell 1	Cell 4	Cell 7	Cell 10
Level II	Cell 2	Cell 5	Cell 8	Cell 11
Level III	Cell 3	Cell 6	Cell 9	Cell 12

Example 1:

Control Variable	Experimental variable			
	Drug	**Hot application**	**Cold application**	**Placebo**
Mild Pain	Cell 1	Cell 4	Cell 7	Cell 10
Moderate Pain	Cell 2	Cell 5	Cell 8	Cell 11
Severe Pain	Cell 3	Cell 6	Cell 9	Cell 12

If a researcher wants to see the effect of four treatments on various levels of pain, she can use 4 × 3 factorial design.

Complex Factorial or Multifactor Design

Experiments with more than two factors at a time involve the use of complex factorial designs. A design which considers three or more independent variables simultaneously is called a complex factorial design. Multifactor design has advantage over single factor design. Multifactor design helps in assessing the interaction effect. An interaction is the influence of combining the levels from the two factors: It shows how the effect of one independent variable on the dependent variable depends on the level of the other independent variable that is present. The interaction of two factors is called a two way interaction. The two way interaction is the influence on scores when combining each level of factor A with each level of factor B. They are cost effective since it requires only an additional effort to study one more independent variable.

In case of three factors with one experimental variable having two treatments and two control variables, each one of which having two levels, the design will be termed as 2 × 2 × 2 complex factorial design.

2 × 2 × 2 Complex Factorial Design

		Experimental variable			
		Treatment A		**Treatment B**	
		Control Variable II		Control Variable II	
		Level I	Level II	Level I	Level II
Control Variable I	Level I	Cell 1	Cell 3	Cell 5	Cell 7
	Level II	Cell 2	Cell 4	Cell 6	Cell 8

Example 2:

		Experimental variable			
		Pharmacological therapy		**Non-pharmacological therapy**	
		Duration of Illness		Duration of Illness	
		Less than 2 years	More than 2 years	Less than 2 years	More than 2 years
Control Variable I	Male	Cell 1	Cell 3	Cell 5	Cell 7
	Female	Cell 2	Cell 4	Cell 6	Cell 8

A researcher may like to see the interaction between the pharmacological vs non-pharmacological therapy with the gender and the duration of illness.

Advantage

- Simultaneously, we can study the effect of more than one factor and it is time saving and effort.
- The interaction of the factors may be studied.
- Since the various factors are combined in one experiment, the results have a wider range of application.

Analysis of Variance and Between Subjects Design

Analysis of variance is the parametric procedure for determining whether significant differences exist in an experiment that contains two or more sample means. One-way ANOVA is performed when data are classified according to only one criterion, (only one independent variable is involved) and Two-way ANOVA is performed when data are classified according to two criteria.

In ANOVA, an independent variable is called as factor. The independent variable or factor may have different levels. For example, pain as an independent variable or factor may have different levels such as mild, moderate and severe. Perceived difficulty as easy, moderate and high or low, moderate and high. The symbol for number of levels in a factor is k.

In ANOVA, a factor that is studied using independent samples in all conditions is called a between subject factor. For example, an independent variable or factor is knowledge.

The knowledge on infection control measures can be studied among DGNM, B.Sc(N), PBBSc(N) groups. The mean knowledge score of all these three groups can be compared. A factor studied using dependent samples in all conditions is a within subject factor.

Assumptions of the One Way, Between Subjects ANOVA

- Each condition contains a random sample of interval or ratio scores.
- The population represented by the scores in each condition forms a normal distribution
- The variances of all populations represented in the study are homogeneous.

Assumptions of the Two Way Between Subjects Design

- All cells contain independent samples of participants.
- The dependent variable measures interval or ratio scores
- The populations represented by the data are approximately normally distributed.
- The represented populations all have homogeneous variance.

Analysis of Variance and Within Subjects Experiments

In this, there is only one independent variable in which we either match different subjects across the conditions or we repeatedly measure the same participants under all the levels of a factor. In two way within subjects design, we repeatedly measure the same group of participants in all conditions of two independent variables and we match participants in all cells. A two way mixed design has one within subjects factor and one between subjects factor. A three way design has 3 factors.

RANDOMIZED BLOCK DESIGN

This design was developed about 1925 by R A Fisher, who was seeking methods of improving agricultural field experiments. The randomized block design is a design in which the units (called experimental units) to which the treatments are applied are subdivided into homogenous groups called blocks, so that the number of experimental units in a block is equal to the number of treatments being studied. The treatments are then assigned at random to the experimental units within each block. It should be ensured that each treatment appears in every block and each block receives every treatment.

The main objective is to remove the error or variation attributable to each block, while assuring that treatment means will be free of block effects. The effectiveness of the design depends on the ability to achieve homogeneous blocks of experimental units. The ability to form homogeneous blocks depends on the researcher's knowledge of the experimental material. The randomized block design may be used when an experiment is carried out in more than one homogenous setting, for example schools of homogeneous type; hospitals of homogeneous type (each one referred as a block here) or when it is done at different point of time (point of time is referred to as block) or at different age groups.

For example,

School A*Meal Plan A	School B*Meal Plan B	School C*Meal Plan C
School B*Meal Plan A	School C*Meal Plan B	School A*Meal Plan C
School C*Meal Plan A	School A*Meal Plan B	School B*Meal Plan C

The technique for analyzing the data from a randomized complete block design is called two way analysis of variance.

Calculation of test statistic in ANOVA

It can be shown that the total sum of squares for the randomized complete block design can be partitioned into three components, one each attributable to treatments (SST_r), blocks (SSBl) and error (SSE). That is

SST = SSBl + SSTr + SSE

SSE = SST – SSBl – SSTr

LATIN SQUARE DESIGN

It is an experimental design used in agricultural research. Latin square design allows the researcher to control statistically the effects of two non interacting extraneous variables on the variable. The design requires that each extraneous variables be divided into as many levels as the independent variable. If independent variables are in three levels, the extraneous variables should also be divided into three levels so as to form a square.

A Latin square design is shown in the form of table with the rows and columns representing the various levels or divisions of the two extraneous variables. The levels of the independent variable are then so assigned to the cells in the table that each level appears once and only once, in each row and each column. Latin square designs are described on the basis of the number of levels in which the extraneous variables are divided. A design with each variable having been divided into three levels is called a 3 × 3 Latin square, into 4 levels is a 4 × 4 Latin square and so forth.

Suppose if we want to see the durability of a specific medical equipment say example, ventilator manufactured by three different manufacturers on three different users and three different maintenance. The first step in constructing a Latin square would be to construct a table. Since we have three levels of the independent variable (ventilator) and three levels of each of the two extraneous variables (user and maintenance) we can construct a 3 × 3 tables shown below. By randomly assigning the levels of the independent variable to the nine cells of the table, such that each of the three ventilator is assigned once and only once to each row and each column.

		Handled by		
		Doctors	**Nurses**	**Technicians**
Maintenance by	Supplier	A	B	C
	Hospital	B	C	A
	Third party	C	A	B

This design gives useful data about the average durability of various ventilator under various maintenance and various users. By averaging the values of a given column one obtains an unbiased estimate of mean durability under various users and by averaging the values of a given row, one obtains an unbiased estimate of mean durability under various maintenance. By averaging the values of a given letter (A, B, C) one obtains an unbiased estimate of mean durability of that ventilator under different users and different maintenance.

One major advantage of this design is that it controls the effects of the extraneous variables (user and maintenance) on the dependent variable (durability of ventilator). Another advantage of this design is that it economizes the use of test units. In the above example, if the researcher selects a factorial design, he will need more than 9 test units (ventilator).

This design suffers from two serious limitations. First, the requirement of dividing each extraneous variable into as many levels as the independent variable can sometimes pose problems for specific research tasks. Second, it does not detect the interaction effect between various levels of the two extraneous variables. In case where interaction is suspected, some form of a factorial design is required.

QUASI EXPERIMENTAL DESIGNS

A time series design is a repeated measures design in which participants, behavior is measured prior to the occurrence of an even and again after it has occurred. Although this sounds like a pre-test and post-test design, it is quasi experimental since the samples cannot be randomly assigned. We cannot randomly select people who will develop some rare form of cancer or who will experience earthquake. It is very difficult to have a control group. The various quasi experimental designs such as one group pre-test/ post-test design and non-equivalent control group design and designs based on duration of study such as interrupted time series design and multiple time series designs, longitudinal design, cross sectional design and cohort design are discussed under research design in part I.

CORRELATIONAL DESIGN

It examines the relationship/correlation between variables. In correlational design, we do not manipulate any variables. We simply measure two variables. Causality is not inferred from a correlational design because the order of occurrence of the variables is unknown. Variable X and Variable Y is measured and the relationship between these variables is found by calculating correlation coefficient (Table 21.1).

Correlational design has two flaws that severely reduce internal validity for concluding that differences in the X variable cause differences in Y scores. We cannot surely say that X occurred before Y. For example, in a study to establish the relationship between the violent video game playing and aggression, we cannot surely say that violent video game playing lead to aggression or aggression lead to the playing of violent video game in children. We are not sure about which variable occurred first.

Table 21.1: The difference between the experimental and correlational design

Experimental design	Correlational design
It examines whether a particular intervention is effective and does intervention bring any changes in the variable.	It examines the relationship/correlation between variables.
Variables are manipulated.	Variables are not manipulated.
Variables are measured before and after manipulation.	The two variables are measured simply.
Extraneous variables are controlled	Extraneous variables are not controlled.
It establishes the effectiveness of the intervention.	Cause and effect is not established.
It is done in controlled setting.	It is done in natural setting.

Second flaw is that we do not usually control extraneous variable. We do not randomly assign participants to a score on X variable. The participants differences on the X variable are likely to be confounded by differences in the participants. For example, in the above mentioned example, younger children's exposure may be less than older children. Teen age children may be more aggressive when compared to the young children.

In general, we mean that correlational study explains that changes in X causes changes in Y. But changes in Y may cause changes in X or some third variable may produce differences in both the X and Y scores. Therefore a single correlational study should not be interpreted as showing that changes in X causes changes in Y.

A correlational design may be preferred for several reasons.

Ethical and practical considerations: Some relationships can be studied only through a correlation design. For example, ethically we cannot randomly assign people to experience variables such as child abuse, infanticide, feticide, accidents, falls etc.

It is impossible to manipulate the variables: Correlational study can be conducted prior to the experimental studies. The relationship can be established initially before experimenting the variables.

Theoretically, a correlation coefficient may be as large as plus or minus 1, in real research such values do not occur. In correlational research, a coefficient around 0.50 is considered to be quite ok and coefficients above this value is impressive. If one gets the value of plus or minus one, one must check for possible errors in measurement and computation.

SUMMARY

- A good experimental design must possess the two attributes such as internal validity and external validity. Internal validity in a research can be ensured by designing and conducting a research in such a way that the treatment alone brings some effect or changes in the outcome variable. A given experiment has external validity to the extent that its results are generalizable beyond the conditions associated with the experiment.
- A single sample experiment is a design used when we have one group of samples and the experiment or treatment is given for the single group. We randomly select a group of samples and the subjects should be exposed to an intervention and its effectiveness are assessed by conducting the post-test.
- In two sample experiment, two groups are involved either two different groups or the same groups performance can be measured twice and compared for any difference. There are two types such as between subjects experiment and within subjects experiment.
- Between subjects design includes the selection of participants for two conditions and each participant serves in only one condition. Within subject design is used to gain greater control of subject variables, and reduce error. The individuals in one condition are comparable to those in the other conditions. We employ this approach when there is one or more crucial extraneous subject variable that must be controlled. There are two types of within subjects design such as matched group design and repeated measures designs.

- In a matched group design, each participant in one condition matches a participant in the other condition(s) on one or more extraneous subject variables.
- A repeated measures design is one in which measurements of the same variable are made on each subject on two or more different occasions. The different occasions during which measurements are taken may be either points in time or different conditions such as different treatments.
- The experiment in which two or more factors are investigated simultaneously is called a factorial experiment. Experiments with more than two factors at a time involve the use of complex factorial designs.
- The randomized block design is a design in which the units (called experimental units) to which the treatments are applied are subdivided into homogenous groups called blocks, so that the number of experimental units in a block is equal to the number of treatments being studied. The treatments are then assigned at random to the experimental units within each block. It should be ensured that each treatment appears in every block and each block receives every treatment.
- Latin square design allows the researcher to control statistically the effects of two non interacting extraneous variables on the variable. The design requires that each extraneous variables be divided into as many levels as the independent variable.
- Correlational design examines the relationship/correlation between variables. Causality is not inferred from a correlational design because the order of occurrence of the variables is unknown. Variable X and Variable Y is measured and the relationship between these variables is found by calculating correlation coefficient.

22 Z Distribution

OBJECTIVES

After reading this chapter, you will be able to:

- Understand Z Distribution
- Compute Z Statistic
- Test Hypothesis using Z Statistic

INTRODUCTION

Z distribution is just a special case of the normal distribution, with an idealized mean of 0 and standard deviation of 1. It is otherwise known as ***standard normal distribution***. The normal random variable of a standard normal distribution is called a ***standard score*** or a ***Z score***.

Z DISTRIBUTION

A Z distribution is the distribution produced by transforming an entire raw score distribution into Z scores. By transforming all raw scores into Z scores one can construct Z distribution. One may wonder how to transform raw score into z score. This is done by using the following formula:

$Z = \frac{X - \overline{X}}{\sigma}$. A Z score describes a raw score's location in terms of the number of standard deviations the score is from the mean.

Z distribution is a probability density function and especially a normal distribution that has a mean equal to zero and a standard deviation equal to one and that is used especially in testing hypotheses about means or proportions of samples drawn from population whose population standard deviations are known.

Every normal random variable **X** can be transformed or converted into a ***Z*** score via the following equation:

$$Z = \frac{X - \overline{X}}{\sigma}$$

Where, **X** is a normal random variable, μ is the mean and σ is the standard deviation.

The probability of getting a score between Z = –1 and Z = 1 is about **0.68**. That is, there's a 68% chance that if any variable X is taken from the population, its value will be between -1 and 1 standard distribution from the mean. The probability of getting a score between Z = -2 and Z = 2 is about **0.954,** or there's a 95.4% chance of getting a score between -2 and 2 standard deviations from the mean. The range associated with a 95% probability (which will be important later on) is Z = -1.96 to Z = 1.96 (Fig. 22.1).

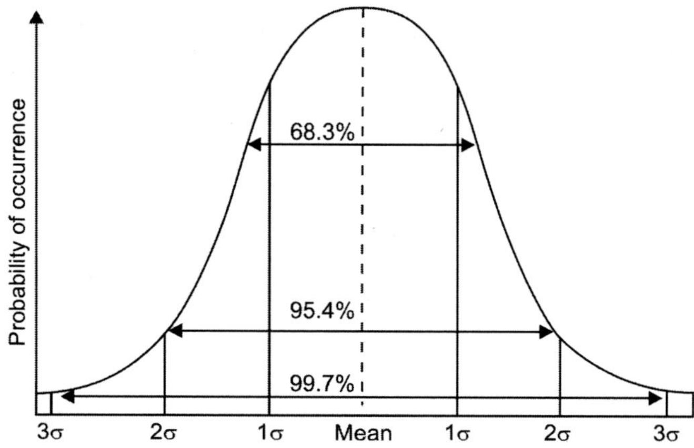

Fig. 22.1: Normal distribution

Z Test

Z test is based on the normal probability distribution and is used for judging the significance of several statistical measures, particularly the mean. The relevant test statistic, Z, is worked out and compared with its probable value (to be read from table showing area under normal curve) at a specified level of significance for judging the significance of the measure concerned. This is a most frequently used test in research studies. This test is used even when binomial distribution or t distribution is applicable on the presumption that such a distribution tends to approximate normal distribution as 'n' becomes larger. Z test is generally used in the following conditions, such as

- For comparing the mean of a sample to some hypothesized mean for the population in case of large sample, or when population variance is known.
- For judging the significance of difference between means of two independent samples in case of large samples, or when population variance is known.
- For comparing the sample proportion to a theoretical value of population proportion or for judging the difference in proportions of two independent samples when n happens to be large.
- For judging the significance of median, mode, coefficient of correlation and several other measures.

Hypothesis Testing of Mean Using Z Test

1. The population is infinite, sample size may be large or small and the standard deviation of the population is known, the significance of difference between the sample mean ($\bar{x}$) and the hypothesized mean (μ) can be expressed by

$$Z = \frac{\overline{x}-\mu}{\sigma_p/\sqrt{N}}.$$

When the standard deviation of the population is not known, the sample standard deviation is used in the formula.

2. Population is finite, sample size may be large or small and the standard deviation of the population is known.

$$Z = \frac{\overline{x}-\mu}{\frac{\sigma}{\sqrt{n}} \times \left(\frac{\sqrt{N-n}}{N-1}\right)}$$

One Sample Z Test

It is used when the distribution is normal distribution or n > 30 and standard deviation (σ) is known. Z is the distance from the mean in standard deviations. It is possible to calculate a minimum proportion of a population that falls within n standard deviations.

If the sample size is large (>30) or the population standard deviation is known, we use the Z distribution. If the sample size is small and the population standard deviation is unknown, we use the t distribution.

Where the population is infinite and the standard deviation of the population is known, the significance of difference between the sample mean ($\overline{x}$) and the hypothesized mean (μ) can be expressed by

$$Z = \frac{\overline{x}-\mu}{\sigma/\sqrt{N}}.$$

Two Sample Z Test

Two sample Z test is used when we want to compare the mean of two groups. It is used when normally distributed and two independent observations are made and σ1 and σ2 known.

$$\mathbf{Z} = \frac{\overline{x}_1 - \overline{x}_2}{SE}$$

$$S.E. (\overline{x}_1 - \overline{x}_2) = \sqrt{\frac{\sigma_1^2}{N_1} + \frac{\sigma_2^2}{N_2}} \text{ where}$$

σ_1^2 and σ_2^2 are the variances of the populations 1 and 2 and N_1 and N_2 are their sizes, where variances of the population are not known we can use sample variances.

One sample Z Test

Example 1:

A sample of 400 male students has the mean height of 67.47 inches. Can this sample be regarded as coming from a population with mean height 67.39 inches and standard deviation 1.3? Test at 5% level of significance.

Let our null hypothesis be that there is no difference between the two means or the sample can be regarded as coming from the population with mean height 67.39".

$N = 400 \quad \overline{x} = 67.47 \quad \mu = 67.39 \quad \sigma_p = 1.3$

Conditions

Population infinite, Sample size and mean is known; population mean and the standard deviation is also known.

The formula is

$$Z = \frac{\overline{x} - \mu}{\sigma/\sqrt{N}}.$$

What are the hypotheses?

Null hypothesis: Sample mean is equal to population mean, i.e. 67.39 inches.

Alternative hypothesis: Sample mean is not equal to population mean, i.e. 67.39 inches.

Symbolically, we can write it thus:

$H_0 : \mu H_0 = 67.39''$; $H_1 : \mu H_0^1 \neq 67.39''$;

What type of test is this?

No direction. So two tailed test.

What is the significance level?

Alpha = 0.05 level (two tailed test, each tail the area is 0.025)

What is the sample size?

n = 400

What is the standard error?

$SE = \sigma/\sqrt{N}$

$= 1.3/\sqrt{400} = 1.3/20 = 0.065$

What is the test statistic?

$$Z = \frac{\overline{x} - \mu}{\sigma/\sqrt{N}}.$$

$$Z = \frac{67.47 - 67.39}{1.3/\sqrt{400}} = \frac{0.08}{0.06} = 1.231.$$

What is the conclusion?

Is there evidence that the height is different from 67.39 inches?

This is a two–tailed test because in it the null hypothesis will be rejected if the sample value is found significantly higher or lower than the hypothesized value of the population parameter. This test is involving two rejection areas of 0.025 on either side of the mean. At 0.025 level of significance, the table value of Z = ± 1.96. The computed value of Z = 1.23 which being less than 1.96 falls in the acceptance region. Thus we accept our null hypothesis. The sample mean height is equal to population mean height 67.39 inches.

Example 2:

The mean life of a bulb in the over head projector is known to be 8000 hours and the standard deviation 500 hours. Engineers developed a new design of this to improve the mean life. A sample of 50 bulbs gives 8400 hours. Test at alpha 0.05 level whether the improvement shown by the sample is real or due to chance?

Conditions:

Population is infinite. Population mean and standard deviation, sample mean is known.

$N = 50 \quad \overline{x} = 8400 \quad \mu = 8000 \quad s_p = 500$

What are the hypotheses?

Null hypothesis: Sample mean (Mean life of new bulb) is equal to population mean, i.e. 8000 hours.

Alternative hypothesis: Sample mean is more than population mean, i.e. 8000 hours.

$H_0 : \mu H_0 = 8000; H_1 : \mu H_0 > 8000;$

What type of test is this?

There is a direction. So one tailed test.

What is the significance level?

Alpha = 0.05 level (one tailed test, right tail the area is 0.05)

What is the sample size?

n = 50

What is the standard error?

$SE = \sigma/\sqrt{N}$

$= 500/\sqrt{50} = 500/7.07 = 70.7$

What is the test statistic?

$$Z = \frac{\overline{X} - \mu}{\sigma/\sqrt{N}}.$$

$$= \frac{8400 - 8000}{500/\sqrt{50}} = \frac{400}{70.7} = 5.66$$

Z = 5.66

What is the conclusion?

Is there evidence that the improvement is real?

This is an upper tail or right tail test. Thus the rejection area which is equal to 0.05 area lies in the right tail. The Z value for the 0.45 area (acceptance region) is 1.645. The calculated Z value is more than the table value which falls in the rejection region. So we reject the null hypothesis. So we conclude that the higher mean of sample is probably a significant increase and not a result of chance.

Example 3:

You are working in a dietary department of the hospital. Your hospital prepares the nutrition supplement for children and the expected weight of one packet of nutrition supplement is 100 g. You want to check whether all packets are prepared in 100 g. You are taking a sample of 25 packets and its mean value is 104 g with the standard deviation of 10 g. Is there any evidence that weight is different from 100 g? You have selected alpha level of 0.05 as your significance level.

Conditions:

Population is infinite. We have population mean, sample mean and sample standard deviation.

What are the hypotheses?

Null hypothesis Sample mean is equal to population mean, i.e. 100 g.

Alternative hypothesis: Sample mean is not equal to population mean, i.e. 100 g.

What type of test is this?

No direction. So two-tailed test.

What is the significance level?

Alpha = 0.05 level (two-tailed test, each tail the area is 0.025)

What is the sample size?

n = 25

What is the standard error?

$SE = \sigma/\sqrt{N}$

$= 10/\sqrt{25} = 10/5 = 2$

What is the test statistic?

$$Z = \frac{\bar{x} - \mu}{\sigma/\sqrt{N}}.$$

$$= \frac{104 - 100}{10/\sqrt{25}} = \frac{4}{2} = 2.$$

$Z = 2$

What is the conclusion?

Is there evidence that the weight is different from 100 g?

The probability of getting a score between Z = –2 and Z = 2 is about **0.954,** or there's a 95.4% chance of getting a score between –2 and 2 standard deviations from the mean. The range associated with a 95% probability is Z = –1.96 to +1.96 or ± 1.96.

The calculated value is more than the table value. The calculated value lies in the rejection region. So, reject the null hypothesis. The sample mean is not equal to poplation mean, i.e. 100 g.

Example 4:

We are interested in analyzing the staff turnover in 20 hospitals. The past records show that the mean of annual turnover is 300 staff nurses with a standard deviation of 50 staff nurses. A sample of 10 of these hospitals is taken at random which gives a mean annual turnover as 280 staffs. Is the sample mean consistent with the population mean? Test at 5% level of significance.

Conditions:

Population is finite. Population mean and standard deviation, sample mean is known.

$N = 20; n = 10 \quad \bar{x} = 280 \quad \mu = 300 \quad s_p = 50$

What are the hypotheses?

Null hypothesis: Annual turnover of the sample is equal to annual turnover of the population, i.e. 300 staff nurses.

Alternative hypothesis: Annual turnover of the sample is not equal to annual turnover of the population.

$H_0 : \mu H_0 = 300$ staff nurses; $H_1 : \mu H_0 \neq 300$ staff nurses;

What type of test is this?

There is no direction. So two-tailed test.

What is the significance level?

Alpha = 0.05 level (two-tailed test, each tail the area is 0.025)

What is the sample size?

N = 20; n = 10

What is the standard error?

$SE = \sigma/\sqrt{N}$

$= 50/\sqrt{10} = 50/3.16 = 15.8$

What is the test statistic?

$$Z = \frac{\bar{x} - \mu}{\frac{\sigma}{\sqrt{n}} \times \left(\frac{\sqrt{N-n}}{N-1}\right)}$$

$$\frac{280 - 300}{\frac{50}{\sqrt{10}} \times \left(\frac{\sqrt{20-10}}{20-1}\right)} = \frac{-20}{15.8 \times \left(\frac{\sqrt{10}}{19}\right)} = \frac{-20}{15.8 \times \left(\frac{3.16}{19}\right)}$$

$$= \frac{-20}{15.8 \times 0.166} = \frac{-20}{2.62} = -7.63$$

$$Z = -7.63$$

What is the conclusion?

Is the sample mean consistent with the population mean? This is a two-tailed test. This test is involving two rejection areas of 0.025 on either side of the mean. At 0.025 level of significance, the table value of Z = ± 1.96. The computed value of Z = –7.63 which being less than –1.96 which falls in the rejection region. Thus, we reject our null hypothesis. The sample mean is not consistent with the population mean.

Example 5:

A random sample of 36 adolescent girls were taken and their mean hemoglobin was 12.2 g/dL. Test whether the samples have come from the population whose mean hemoglobin level was 13 g/dL with the standard deviation of 1 g/dL.

Conditions:

Population infinite, Sample size and mean is known; population mean and standard deviation is known.

The formula is $Z = \frac{\bar{x} - \mu}{\sigma/\sqrt{N}}$.

What are the hypotheses?

Null hypothesis: There is no difference between the sample mean and the population mean or the sample mean hemoglobin value is equal to 13 g/dL.

Alternative hypothesis: There is a difference between the sample mean and the population mean or the mean hemoglobin value is not equal to 13 g/dL.

Symbolically, we can write it thus:

Null Hypothesis: H_0: $\mu = 13$

Alternative hypothesis: H_a: $\mu \neq 13$

What type of test is this?

There is no direction. So it is a two-tailed test.

What is the significance level?

Alpha = 0.05 level (two-tailed test, each tail the area is 0.025)

What is the sample size?

n = 36

What is the standard error?

$$SE = \sigma/\sqrt{N}$$

$$= 1/\sqrt{36} = 1/6 = 0.17$$

What is the test statistic?

$$Z = \frac{\bar{x} - \mu}{\sigma/\sqrt{N}}.$$

$$Z = \frac{12.2 - 13}{1/\sqrt{36}} = \frac{-0.8}{0.17} = -4.71$$

What is the conclusion?

Is there evidence that the sample mean is equal to the population mean?

This is a two-tailed test. This test is involving two rejection areas of 0.025 on both side of the mean. At 0.05 level of significance, the table value of Z = ±1.96. The computed value of Z = –4.71 which being less than –1.96 falls in the rejection region. Thus, we reject our null hypothesis. There is a difference between the sample mean and the population mean or the mean hemoglobin value is not equal to 13 g/dL.

Two sample Z Test

When the mean of one sample is being compared with the mean of another sample, the standard error of the difference between two means is calculated as follows:

$$SE\ (\bar{x}_1 - \bar{x}_2) = \sqrt{\frac{\sigma_1^2}{N_1} + \frac{\sigma_2^2}{N_2}} \text{ where}$$

σ_1^2 and σ_2^2 are the variances of the populations 1 and 2 and N_1 and N_2 are their sizes, where variances of the population are not known we can use sample variances.

Example 6:

A researcher randomly selects two groups of mothers of 100 each. One group was taught on child abuse using mother to mother approach. The other group was taught on the same topic using structured teaching program by the researcher herself. The knowledge was assessed after the program. The mean knowledge score of group A is 80 with the standard deviation of 8. The mean knowledge score group B is 70 with the standard deviation of 10. Test the null hypothesis that there is no significant difference between group A and group B with regard to the gain in knowledge. Alpha = 0.05

Null hypothesis: There is no significant difference between group A and group B with regard to the gain in knowledge.

Alternative hypothesis: There is a significant difference between group A and group B with regard to the gain in knowledge.

Level of significance(α) = 0.05

Choosing the distribution and finding the critical value: A two-tailed test is appropriate since we are interested to know whether the two groups are equal or are not equal. The significance level of 0.05 corresponds to 0.025 of the rejection area will be at both tails. This test is involving two rejection areas of 0.025 on either side of the mean. At 0.025 level of significance, the table value of Z = ± 1.96.

$$SE\ (\bar{x}_1 - \bar{x}_2) = \sqrt{\frac{\sigma_1^2}{N_1} + \frac{\sigma_2^2}{N_2}} = \sqrt{\frac{(8)^2}{100} + \frac{(10)^2}{100}}$$

$$= \sqrt{\frac{64}{100} + \frac{100}{100}} = \sqrt{0.64 + 1} = \sqrt{1.64} = 1.28$$

$$\textbf{\textit{Calculation of Z}} = \frac{\bar{x}_1 - \bar{x}_2}{SE} = \frac{80-70}{1.28} = \frac{10}{1.28} = 7.81$$

Interpretation of the result: The table value of Z for acceptance area of 0.475 is 1.96. This is our acceptance region. The calculated value of mean (7.81) is outside this region. We should reject the null hypothesis. There is a significant difference between group A and group B with regard to the gain in knowledge.

Example 7:

A researcher randomly selects 50, II year nursing students each in two colleges. The researcher showed a movie on interpersonal relationship to Group A and none to group B. He assessed the samples' attitude towards interpersonal relationship for both groups. The mean score of group A is 110 with the standard deviation of 6 whereas the mean score of group B is 100 with the standard deviation of 8. Test is there any changes in the attitude between group A and B.

Alpha = 0.05

Null hypothesis: There is no significant difference between group A and group B with regard to the attitude.

Alternative hypothesis: There is a significant difference between group A and group B with regard to attitude.

Level of significance(α) =0.05

Choosing the distribution and finding the critical value: A two-tailed test is appropriate since we are interested to know whether the two groups are equal or are not equal. The significance level of 0.05 corresponds to 0.025 of the rejection area will be at both tails. Because the sample size is 50, Z distribution is used. On looking in the table of Z distribution, the table value of Z for acceptance area of 0.475 is 1.96.

$$SE(\bar{x}_1 - \bar{x}_2) = \sqrt{\frac{\sigma_1^2}{N_1} + \frac{\sigma_2^2}{N_2}} = \sqrt{\frac{(6)^2}{50} + \frac{(8)^2}{50}}$$

$$= \sqrt{\frac{36}{50} + \frac{64}{50}} = \sqrt{0.72 + 1.28} = \sqrt{2} = 1.414$$

Calculation of Z $= \frac{\bar{x}_1 - \bar{x}_2}{SE} = \frac{110 - 100}{1.414} = \frac{10}{1.414} = 7.07$

Interpretation of the result: The table value of Z for acceptance area of 0.475 is 1.96. This is our acceptance region. The calculated value of mean (7.07) is outside this region. We should reject the null hypothesis. There is a significant difference between group A and group B with regard to the change in attitude.

Example 8:

A sample of 300 nurses of one hospital showed a mean income of ₹ 9500 per month with standard deviation of ₹ 100. Another sample of 500 nurses from another hospital showed a mean income of ₹ 10,000 with standard deviation of ₹ 50. Is the difference between the two means statistically significant at 5% level?

Null hypothesis: There is no significant difference between the mean income of nurses from two hospitals.

Alternative hypothesis: There is a significant difference between the mean income of nurses from two hospitals.

Level of significance(α) = 0.05

Choosing the distribution and finding the critical value: A two-tailed test is appropriate since we are interested to know whether the two groups are equal or are not equal. The significance level of 0.05 corresponds to 0.025 of the rejection area will be at both tails. Because the sample size is 50, Z distribution is used. On looking in the table of Z distribution, the table value of Z for acceptance area of 0.475 is 1.96 on both sides.

$$S.E.(\bar{x}_1 - \bar{x}_2) = \sqrt{\frac{\sigma_1^2}{N_1} + \frac{\sigma_2^2}{N_2}} = \sqrt{\frac{(100)^2}{300} + \frac{(50)^2}{500}}$$

$$= \sqrt{\frac{10000}{300} + \frac{2500}{500}} = \sqrt{33.33 + 5} = \sqrt{38.33} = 6.19$$

Calculation of Z $= \frac{\bar{x}_1 - \bar{x}_2}{SE} = \frac{9500 - 10000}{6.19} = \frac{-500}{6.19} = -80.77$

Interpretation of the result: The significance level of 0.05 corresponds to 0.025 of the rejection area will be at both tails. This test is involving two rejection areas of 0.025 on either side of the mean. At 0.025 level of significance, the table value of $Z = \pm 1.96$. The calculated Z value falls outside the table value. Thus, we reject the null hypothesis. We conclude that there is a significant difference between the mean income of nurses from two hospitals.

Hypothesis Testing of Attributes

These tests comprise tests for number of successes and tests for proportion of successes. The sampling distributions in both the cases follow a binomial probability distribution but as the tests are mostly based on large samples, Z test is used.

Test for Number of Successes. Here, we should first calculate the standard error of the number of successes. As already mentioned, the formula is:

S.E. of number of successes = $\sqrt{Npq}$, where

N = Size of sample,

p = Probability of successes in each trial

q = (1–p), i.e. probability of failure.

Next, we should standardize the sample number of successes by dividing the difference between the observed number and the hypothesized number by the standard error. This will help us in knowing whether our sample number falls inside or outside the region of acceptance for the given level of confidence.

Example 9:

A coin is tossed 400 times and the head turns up 216 times. Test the hypothesis that the coin is unbiased at 5% level of significance.

Our null hypothesis is that the coin is unbiased. Thus, H_0: Heads = 200 and H_1: Heads ≠ 200.

$$\text{SE of the number of heads} = \sqrt{Npq} = \sqrt{(400)(0.5)(0.5)} = 10.$$

$$Z = \frac{\text{Observed No. of Heads} - \text{Hypothesized No.}}{\text{SE}}$$

$$= \frac{216 - 200}{10} = 1.6$$

This is a two-tailed test. Hence, 0.025 area of the normal curve of both tails is rejection area. Z value of 0.475 acceptance area on both sides is 1.96. Our Z value is less than this. Hence, our H_0 is true.

Example 10:

In a sample of 500 people from a village in Punjab, 280 are found to be rice eaters and 220 wheat eaters. Can we conclude that both the food grains are equally popular? Test at 1% level of significance.

H_0: Both food grain eaters are equal, i.e. 250; H_1: Both food grain eaters are not equal.

$$\text{SE} = \sqrt{Npq} = \sqrt{(500)(0.5)(0.5)} = 11.18$$

$$Z = \frac{220-250}{11.18} = -2.68$$

This is a two-tailed test with 0.005 rejection area on both sides. The acceptable area on both sides is 0.495. Z value for this area is ± 2.58. Our Z value falls outside the table value. Hence, we reject our null hypothesis. Both food grain eaters are not equal. Hence both food grains are not equally popular.

Example 11:

A wholesaler claims that only 4% of the thermometers sold by him are defective. A random sample of 400 thermometers contained 6% defective thermometers. Does this support the wholesaler's claim at 0.05 level of significance.

Let the H_0 be that there is no significant difference between the sample proportion and the claimed proportion of defective thermometers.

N = Size of sample – 400

p = 0.04 and q = 1–0.04 = 0.96.

Standard error of the proportion of defective thermometers

$$= \sqrt{\frac{pq}{N}} = \sqrt{\frac{0.04 \times 0.96}{400}} = \sqrt{\frac{0.0384}{400}} = \sqrt{0.000096} = 0.0098$$

Difference between the observed and expected proportions of defective thermometers

$$= \frac{6}{100} - \frac{4}{100} = \frac{2}{100} = 0.02$$

$$Z = \frac{\text{Difference between proportions}}{\text{Standard error of proportions}} = \frac{0.02}{0.0098} = 2.040$$

At 0.05 level of significance for a two-tailed test the table value of Z is ±1.96. The computer value of Z (2.040) falls in the rejection region. Thus, we reject the null hypothesis and conclude that the difference in proportions could not have arisen due to fluctuations of sampling. The sample does not support the wholesaler's claim.

SUMMARY

- Z distribution is just a special case of the normal distribution, with an idealized mean of 0 and standard deviation of 1. It is otherwise known as ***standard normal distribution***. The normal random variable of a standard normal distribution is called a standard score or a *z* score.
- A Z distribution is the distribution produced by transforming an entire raw score distribution into Z scores. By transforming all raw scores into Z scores one can construct Z distribution. A Z score describes a raw score's location in terms of the number of standard deviations the score is from the mean. Every normal random variable *X* can be transformed or converted into a *z* score via the following equation, $Z = \frac{x - \bar{x}}{\sigma}$ where x is a normal random variable, μ is the mean and σ is the standard deviation.
- Z test is based on the normal probability distribution and is used for judging the significance of several statistical measures, particularly the mean. The relevant test statistic, Z, is worked out and compared with its probable value (to be read from table

showing area under normal cruve) at a specified level of significance for judging the significance of the measure concerned.

- The population is infinite, sample size may be large or small and the standard deviation of the population is known, the significance of difference between the sample mean ($\overline{x}$) and the hypothesized mean (μ) can be expressed by

$Z = \dfrac{\overline{x} - \mu}{\sigma_p / \sqrt{N}}$, when the standard deviation of the population is not known, the sample standard deviation is used in the formula.

- The population is finite, sample size may be large or small and the standard deviation of the population is known, the formula to calculate the Z statistic is

$$Z = \frac{\overline{x} - \mu}{\dfrac{\sigma}{\sqrt{n}} \times \left\{\dfrac{\sqrt{N-n}}{N-1}\right\}}$$

- Two sample Z test is used when we want to compare the mean of two groups. It is used when normally distributed and two independent observations are made and σ_1 and σ_2 known. The formula to calculate the z statistic is $Z = \dfrac{\overline{x}_1 - \overline{x}_2}{SE}$, where SE $(\overline{x}_1 - \overline{x}_2) = \sqrt{\dfrac{\sigma_1^2}{N_1} + \dfrac{\sigma_2^2}{N_2}}$ where σ_1^2 and σ_2^2 are the variances of populations 1 and 2 and N_1 and N_2 are their sizes, where variances of the population are not known we can use sample variances.

EXERCISE

- A company manufactures sphygmomanometers. Their lives are normally distributed with the mean life of 25 years and standard deviation of 2.5 years. A change in the production process is believed to result in a better product. A test sample of 50 new BP apparatus had a mean life of 26 years. Can you conclude that the new product is significantly better than the old?
- A survey of 100 similar sized hospitals revealed a mean daily census in the pediatric service of 30 with a standard deviation of 6. Do these data provide sufficient evidence to indicate that the population mean is greater than 25? Let alpha = 0.05.
- Suppose it is known that the IQ scores of a certain population of adults are approximately normally distributed with a standard deviation of 15. A simple random sample of 25 adults drawn from this population had a mean IQ score of 105. On the basis of these data, can we conclude that the mean IQ score for the population is not 100? Test at alpha = 0.05.
- It was assumed that systolic blood pressures of a certain population of males are normally distributed with a standard deviation of 12. A simple random sample of 64 males from the population has a mean systolic blood pressure reading of 132. At the 0.05 level of significance, whether these data provide sufficient evidence for us to conclude that the population mean is greater than 130?
- A simple random sample of 16 adults drawn from a certain population of adults yielded a mean weight of 63 kg. Assume that weights in the population are approximately normally distributed with a variance of 49. Do the sample data provide sufficient evidence for us to conclude that the mean weight for the population is less than 70 kg? Let the probability of committing the type I error be 0.05.
- A personnel manager of a hospital believed that 16% of the staff nurses of the hospital work overtime every week. If the observed proportion of one week is 13%

in a random sample of 100 does this support the personnel manager's belief about the staff's overtime. Let alpha = 0.05.

- 100 students of a two college each were put to test in research and statistics. The results were as under.
  Statistics: Mean marks = 40; Standard deviation = 6.
  Research: Mean marks = 45; Standard deviation = 8.
  Test at 5% level of significance whether two average marks are in fact unequal.
- Two pharmacy companies released a drugs that provides analgesic effect for people. The first drug tested on 100 samples and produced an average of 10 hours relief and a standard deviation of 1.5 hours. The second drug was tested on 120 samples and produced an average pain relief of 9.5 hours and a standard deviation of 1.8 hours. At the 0.05 level of significance, does the second drug provide a significantly shorter period of relief?
- A survey of vegetable buying habits of housewives in a city in urban and a village in rural area gave the following results:

Area	Sample Size	Average weekly purchase on vegetables	Standard deviation
Urban city	200	₹ 400	₹ 40
Rural village	300	₹ 250	₹ 30

Test at 5% level of significance whether two average weekly expenditures are in fact equal.

- Two independent samples of observations were collected. For the first sample of 60 elements, the mean was 86 and the standard deviation 6. The second sample of 75 elements has a mean of 82 and a standard deviation of 9. Compute the estimated standard error of the difference between the two mean. Using alpha = 0.05, test the two samples can reasonably be considered to have come from populations with the same mean.

23 t Distribution

OBJECTIVES

After reading this chapter, you will be able to:

- Explain the concept of t distribution and t-test
- Understand the application of t-test
- Test hypothesis using t-test.

INTRODUCTION

The t distribution, also known as student's t distribution, is a sampling distribution derived from the parent normal distribution, introduced by WS Gossett, a statistician employed at the Guiness brewery. However, because the brewery did not allow employees to publish their research, Gossett's work on the t-test appears under the name ***student*** (and the t-test is sometimes referred to as 'Student's t-test'). Gossett was a chemist and was responsible for developing procedures for ensuring the similarity of batches of Guiness. The t-test was developed as a way of measuring how closely the yeast content of a particular batch of beer corresponded to the brewery's standard. It was specifically designed to evaluate statistical differences for samples of 30 or less. This t distribution is also a symmetric distribution about its mean. The shape of the t distribution varies according to the size of the sample or according to the degrees of freedom. When the size of the sample is large, the t distribution closely approximates the normal distribution.

t-test is based on t distribution and is considered an appropriate test for judging the significance of a sample mean or for judging the significance of difference between the means of two samples in case of small sample(s) when population variance is not known (in which case, we use variance of the sample as an estimate of the population variance). In case two samples are related, we use paired t-test (or what is known as ***difference test***) for judging the significance of the mean of difference between the two related samples. It can also be used for judging the significance of the coefficients of simple and partial correlations. The relevant test statistic, t is calculated from the sample data and then compared with its probable value which based on t distribution (to be read from the table that gives probable values of t for different levels of significance for different degrees of freedom) at a specified level of significance for concerning degrees of freedom for accepting or rejecting the null hypothesis. It may be noted that t-test applies only in case of small sample(s) when population variance is unknown.

APPLICATION OF t-TEST

One sample t-test: t-test is used in normal population or n < 30 and standard deviation (σ) is unknown. The one sample t-test, in which the level of outcome for a group is compared to a known standard, compares the mean score of a sample to a known value, usually the population mean (the average for the outcome of some population of interest). The basic idea of the test is a comparison of the average of the sample (observed average) and the population (expected average), with an adjustment for the number of cases in the sample and the standard deviation of the average.

Two sample t-test: The two sample t-test, where the outcome levels of two groups are compared to each other.

Paired t-test: It is used in normal population of differences or n < 30 and σ unknown.

Example for One Sample t-test

A study to assess the effectiveness of prenatal care program on birthweight of newborn babies among antenatal mothers of low-income group attending selected hospital in Chennai.

Research approach : Experimental
Research design : One group pre test and post test design

Variables

Independent variable : Prenatal care program
Dependent variable : Birth weight of newborn babies
Sample : Antenatal mothers of low-income group

Hypothesis

Null hypothesis : The difference between the birthweight of babies born to mothers who participated in the program and those born to other mothers of low-income group is zero.
The difference between the observed mean birthweight for program babies and the expected mean birthweight for low-income group mothers is zero.

Alternative hypothesis : The difference between the observed mean birthweight for program babies and the expected mean birthweight for poor women is not zero.

Here, t-test is used to compare the sample mean with the known population mean. One sample t-test is used.

Two Sample t-test

We often want to know whether the means of two populations on some outcome differ. For example, there are many questions in which we want to compare two categories of some categorical variable (e.g. compare males and females) or two populations receiving different treatments in context of an experiment. The two sample t-test is a hypothesis test for answering questions about the mean where the data are collected from two random samples of independent observations, each from an underlying normal distribution:

t-test is used to compare two groups of samples selected randomly. For example, to evaluate the effects of some intervention, program or treatment, a group of subjects is divided into two groups, t-test can be used. The group receiving the treatment to be evaluated is referred to as the treatment group, while those who do not are referred to as the control or comparison group. In this example, mothers who are part of the prenatal care program to reduce the likelihood of low birthweight is the treatment group, a control group comprised of women who do not take part in the program.

Returning to the two sample t-test, the steps to conduct the test are similar to those of the one sample test.

Example 1:

A study to assess the effectiveness of prenatal care program on birthweight of newborn babies among antenatal mothers of treatment group and control group attending selected hospital in Chennai.

Research approach : Experimental

Research design : Experimental and control group pre test and post test design

Variables

Independent variable : Prenatal care program

Dependent variable : Birth weight of newborn babies

Sample : Antenatal mothers

Hypothesis

Null hypothesis : The difference between the two groups is zero. Another way of stating the null hypothesis is that the difference between the mean birthweight of the babies born for the treatment group and the mean birthweight of the babies born for the control group of women is zero.

Alternative hypothesis : The difference between the observed mean birthweight for program babies and the expected mean birthweight for control group women is not zero.

ONE SAMPLE t-TEST

Example 2:

A nurse manager wants to recruit a large number of nurses for the hospital. She expects the average score on the aptitude test to be around 90. But on a review of 10 test results, the mean score is found to be 80 and the standard deviation is 10. The nurse manager wants to test her hypothesis at the 0.10 level of significance:

- ***Null hypothesis:*** The average score on aptitude test is equal to 90.
- ***Alternative hypothesis:*** The average score on aptitude test is not equal to 90.
- ***Level of significance (α)*** = 0.10

- ***Choosing the distribution and finding the critical value:*** Because the manager is interested in knowing whether the true mean score is larger or smaller than the hypothesized score, a two-tailed test is the appropriate one to use. The significance level of 0.10 will consist of two tails each containing 0.05 of the area under the t distribution. Because the sample size is 10, the degree of freedom is 9, i.e. 10–1. On looking at the table of t distribution, the critical value of t = 1.833.

Standard error of mean $= \frac{\sigma_s}{\sqrt{N}} = \frac{10}{\sqrt{10}} = \frac{10}{3.16} = 3.16$

Calculation of **t** $= \frac{\bar{x} - \mu H_0}{SE} = \frac{80-90}{3.16} = \frac{-10}{3.16} = -3.164$

Interpretation of the result: The critical value of t lies between ±1.833. This is our acceptance region. The calculated value of mean (–3.164) is outside this region. The nurse manager should reject the null hypothesis. The average score on aptitude test is not equal to 90.

Example 3:

Given a mean of 70, a sample size of 20 and a standard deviation of 8, test the hypothesis that the value of population mean is 60 against the alternative hypothesis that it is more than 60. Use the 0.025 significance level.

Null hypothesis: The mean score of population is 60.

Alternative hypothesis: The mean score of population is more than 60.

Level of significance (α) = 0.025

Choosing the distribution and finding the critical value: A one-tail test is appropriate. The significance level of 0.025 will be at the right side since the alternative hypothesis is more than type. Because the sample size is 20, the degree of freedom is 19, i.e. 20–1. On looking at the table of t distribution, the critical value of t = 2.093.

Standard error of mean (SE) $= \frac{\sigma_s}{\sqrt{N}} = \frac{8}{\sqrt{20}} = \frac{8}{4.47} = 1.79$

Calculation of t $= \frac{\bar{x} - \mu H_0}{SE} = \frac{70-60}{1.79} = \frac{10}{1.79} = 5.58$

Interpretation of the result: The critical value of t lies at 2.093. This is our acceptance region. The calculated value of mean (5.58) is outside this region. We should reject the null hypothesis. The sample study indicates that the population mean is more than 60.

Example 4:

A survey reported that the school children are on an average 5 kg overweight. To test this report, a random sample of 15 children were selected and their average excess weight was calculated, which was 6 kg and the standard deviation was 2 kg. Test the validity of the report at 0.01 level of significance.

Null hypothesis: The average excess weight (overweight) of school children is 5 kg.

Alternative hypothesis: The average excess weight (overweight) of school children is not equal to 5 kg.

Level of significance (α) = 0.01

Choosing the distribution and finding the critical value: A two-tailed test is appropriate. The significance level of 0.005 will be at both tails. Because the sample size is 15, the degree of freedom is 14, i.e. 15–1. On looking at the table of t distribution, the critical value of t = 2.977.

Standard error of mean (SE) $= \frac{\sigma_s}{\sqrt{N}} = \frac{2}{\sqrt{15}} = \frac{2}{3.87} = 0.52$

***Calculation of* t** $= \frac{\bar{x} - \mu H_0}{S.E} = \frac{6-5}{0.52} = \frac{1}{0.52} = 1.92$

Interpretation of the result: The critical value of t lies between ±2.977. This is our acceptance region. The calculated value of mean (1.92) is inside this region. We should accept the null hypothesis. The average excess weight (overweight) of school children is 5 kg.

Example 5:

An investigator is interested to study the amount of violence in movies. He has selected 10 movies and the number of violent scenes in each of the movies is as given below:

1	2	3	4	5	6	7	8	9	10
30	12	22	12	4	18	26	25	14	17

Is there any evidence that the number of violence scenes is less than 20 scenes?

Conditions:

Population is infinite. You have sample mean. Standard deviation is unknown.

What are the hypotheses?

Null hypothesis: The number of violent scenes is 20 or more.

Alternative hypothesis: The number of violent scenes is less than 20.

What type of test is this?

There is a direction. Here, the word less than is present. So, it is one-tailed test.

What is the significance level?

Alpha (α) = 0.05 level (one-tailed test, the left tail area is 0.05)

What is the sample size?

n = 10

What is the standard error?

$$SE = \frac{\sigma_s}{\sqrt{N}}$$

We have to find out the standard deviation.

$$\text{Mean} = \frac{30+12+22+12+4+18+26+25+14+17}{10}$$

$$= \frac{180}{10} = 18$$

X	$X - \bar{X}$	$(X - \bar{X})^2$
30	30 – 18 = 12	144
12	12 – 18 = –6	36
22	22 – 18 = 4	16
12	12 – 18 = –6	36
4	4 – 18 = –14	196

18	18 – 18 = 0	0
26	26 –18 = 8	64
25	25 –18 = 7	49
14	14 – 18 = –4	16
17	17 –18 = –1	1
		558/10 = 55.8

$$\text{Standard deviation} = \sqrt{\frac{\Sigma(X-\bar{X})^2}{n-1}} = \sqrt{\frac{558}{10-1}} = \sqrt{\frac{558}{9}} = \sqrt{62} = 7.9$$

$$SE = \frac{\sigma_s}{\sqrt{N}} = \frac{7.9}{\sqrt{10}} = \frac{7.9}{3.16} = 2.5$$

Level of significance (α) =0.05

Choosing the distribution and finding the critical value: A one-tailed test is appropriate. The significance level of 0.05 will be at left tail. Because the sample size is 10, the degree of freedom is 9, i.e. 10–1. On looking at the table of t distribution, the critical value of t = 1.833.

$$\textbf{\textit{Calculation of t}} = \frac{\bar{x} - \mu H_0}{SE} = \frac{18-20}{2.5} = \frac{-2}{2.5} = -0.8$$

Interpretation of the result: The critical value of t is 1.833. The calculated value of t (–0.8) is less than the table value. We should accept the null hypothesis. The number of violence scene is 20 or more.

TWO SAMPLE t-TEST

When the sample sizes are small, when we want to test the differences between two means, we first compute the standard error of the difference between the 2 sample means and then we must base our test on the t distribution. The standard error of the difference between two independent sample means are calculated as follow:

$$= \sigma_{(Comb)8}\sqrt{\frac{1}{N_1}+\frac{1}{N_2}} \quad \text{where, } \sigma_{(Comb)} = \sqrt{\frac{(N_1-1)\sigma_1^2(N_2-1)\sigma_2^2}{N_1+N_2-2}}$$

$$SE = \sqrt{\frac{(N_1-1)\sigma_1^2+(N_2-1)\sigma_2^2}{N_1+N_2-2}} \times \sqrt{\frac{1}{N_1}+\frac{1}{N_2}}$$

$$t = \frac{(\bar{x}_1-\bar{x}_2)-(\mu_1-\mu_2)}{\sqrt{\frac{(N_1-1)\sigma_1^2+(N_2-1)\sigma_2^2}{N_1+N_2-2}} \times \sqrt{\frac{1}{N_1}+\frac{1}{N_2}}} = \frac{(\bar{x}_1-\bar{x}_2)-(\mu_1-\mu_2)}{SE}$$

Example 6:

An attitude test is administered to 6 girls in school A and their mean attitude score is 60 with the standard deviation of 8. The same test is administered to 8 girls in school B and their mean attitude score is 70 with the standard deviation of 10. Test if there is any significant difference between the attitude score of two groups. Let α = 0.05.

Null hypothesis: There is no significant difference in mean attitude score between group A and group B.

Alternative hypothesis: There is a significant difference in mean attitude score between group A and group B.

Level of significance (α) = 0.05

Choosing the distribution and finding the critical value: A two-tailed test is appropriate since we are interested to know whether the two groups are equal or are not equal. The significance level of 0.05 corresponds to 0.025 and the rejection area will be at both tails. Because the sample size is small, t distribution is used. On looking at the table of t distribution, the table value of t for 12 [(6 + 8 – 2 = 12) ($N_1 + N_2 - 2$)] degree of freedom is 2.179.

Standard error of difference between two means

$$= \sqrt{\frac{(N_1-1)\sigma_1^2+(N_2-1)\sigma_2^2}{N_1+N_2-2}} \times \sqrt{\frac{1}{N_1}+\frac{1}{N_2}}$$

$$= \sqrt{\frac{(6-1)(8)^2+(8-1)(10)^2}{6+8-2}} \times \sqrt{\frac{1}{6}+\frac{1}{8}} = \sqrt{\frac{5\times 64+7\times 100}{12}} \times \sqrt{\frac{8+6}{48}}$$

$$= \sqrt{\frac{320+700}{12}} \times \sqrt{\frac{14}{48}} = \sqrt{\frac{1020}{12}} \times \sqrt{0.292} = \sqrt{85} \times 0.543 = 9.22 \times 0.543 = 5.00$$

Calculation of t $= \frac{\bar{x}_1-\bar{x}_2}{SE} = \frac{60-70}{5} = \frac{-10}{5} = -2$

Interpretation of the result: The table value of t for acceptance area is ± 2.179. This is our acceptance region. The calculated value of mean (–2) is inside this region. We should accept the null hypothesis. There is no significant difference in mean attitude score between group A and group B.

Example 7:

An interest test is administered to 10 staff nurses of medical ward and 6 staff nurses in intensive care unit. The mean interest scores are 30 and 24 respectively. The combined standard deviation ($s_{(Combn)}$) of difference is 5.00. Is the difference between the means significant at 0.05 level?

Null hypothesis: There is no significant difference in mean interest score between group A and group B, or the 2 samples are drawn from the same parent population with respect to the interest being measured.

Alternative hypothesis: There is a significant difference in mean interest score between group A and group B.

Level of significance (α) = 0.05

Choosing the distribution and finding the critical value: A two-tailed test is appropriate since we are interested to know whether the two groups are equal or are not equal. The significance level of 0.05 corresponds to 0.025 and the rejection area will be at both tails. Because the sample size is small, t distribution is used. On looking at the table of t distribution, the table value of t for 14 [(10 + 6 – 2 = 14) ($N_1 + N_2 - 2$)] degree of freedom is 2.14.

Standard error of difference between two means $= \sigma_{(Comb)} \times \sqrt{\frac{1}{N_1}+\frac{1}{N_2}}$

$$= 5 \times \sqrt{\frac{1}{10} + \frac{1}{6}} = 5 \times \sqrt{\frac{6+10}{60}} = 5 \times \sqrt{16/60} = 5 \times 0.52 = 2.6$$

Calculation of t $= \frac{\bar{x}_1 - \bar{x}_2}{SE} = \frac{30-24}{2.6} = \frac{6}{2.6} = 2.31$

Interpretation of the result: The table value of t for acceptance area is ± 2.14. This is our acceptance region. The calculated value of mean (2.31) is outside this region. We should reject the null hypothesis. There is significant difference in mean interest score between group A and group B, or the 2 samples are drawn from the same parent population with respect to the interest being measured.

Example 8:

In a study to measure the muscle condition, the investigators reported the following information on a measure of overall muscle condition scores made by the subjects.

Sample	n	Mean	Standard deviation
Exercise group	12	4.8	0.4
Sedentary group	15	3.5	1.2

Find, if the difference between mean is significant at 0.05 level of significance.

Null hypothesis: There is no significant difference in mean in exercise group and sedentary group.

Alternative hypothesis: There is a significant difference in mean in exercise group and sedentary group.

Level of significance (α) = 0.05

Choosing the distribution and finding the critical value: A two-tailed test is appropriate since we are interested to know whether the two groups are equal or are not equal. The significance level of 0.05 corresponds to 0.025 and the rejection area will be at both tails. Because the sample size is small, t distribution is used. On looking at the table of t distribution, the table value of t for 25 [(12 + 15 – 2 = 25) ($N_1 + N_2 - 2$)] degree of freedom is 2.064.

Standard error of difference between two means

$$= \sqrt{\frac{(N_1-1)\sigma_1^2 + (N_2-1)\sigma_2^2}{N_1+N_2-2}} \times \sqrt{\frac{1}{N_1} + \frac{1}{N_2}}$$

$$= \sqrt{\frac{(12-1)(0.4)^2 + (15-1)(1.2)^2}{12+15-2}} \times \sqrt{\frac{1}{12} + \frac{1}{15}}$$

$$= \sqrt{\frac{11 \times 0.16 + 14 \times 1.44}{25}} \times \sqrt{\frac{15+12}{180}} = \sqrt{\frac{1.76+20.16}{25}} \times \sqrt{\frac{27}{180}}$$

$$= \sqrt{\frac{21.92}{25}} \times \sqrt{0.15} = \sqrt{0.877} \times 0.39 = 0.94 \times 0.39 = 0.37$$

Calculation of t $= \frac{\bar{x}_1 - \bar{x}_2}{SE} = \frac{4.8-3.5}{0.37} = \frac{1.3}{0.37} = 3.51$

Interpretation of the result: The table value of t for acceptance area is ± 2.064. This is our acceptance region. The calculated value of mean (3.51) is outside this region. We should reject the null hypothesis. There is no significant difference in mean in exercise group and sedentary group.

PAIRED t-TEST

In the examples in the above section, the samples were chosen independently of each other. Sometimes, however, it makes sense to take samples that are not independent of each other, but are paired. Such pairing is generally considered appropriate in a before and after treatment study. For example, in a program of dietary supplementation for the treatment of anemia, for a group of adolescent girls hemoglobin were measured before and after the treatment. Here, we have 2 samples (before sample and after sample) that are clearly dependent on each other because the same individuals have been observed twice.

To apply this test, we first work out on the differences for each matched pair and then find out the average of such differences ($\bar{d}$) and the standard deviation of these differences. Assuming the said differences to be normally distributed, the standard error is $\frac{\sigma_{diff}}{\sqrt{N}}$. Next, we standardize the observed average difference by subtracting the hypothesized average difference, and dividing by the standard error. The test statistics is calculated as follows:

$$t = \frac{\bar{d} - \text{Hypothesized difference}}{\frac{\sigma_{diff}}{\sqrt{N}}} = \frac{\bar{d} - \text{Hypothesized difference}}{\text{Standard error}}$$

Example 9:

An IQ test was administered to 5 persons before and after training. The results are given below:

Candidates	1	2	3	4	5
IQ before training	108	110	116	132	126
IQ after training	120	120	122	130	120

Test whether any change in IQ has taken place after training at 1% level of significance.

Null hypothesis: There is no change in the IQ of the candidates after training. or the mean of the difference in the pre- and post-training scores of candidates is zero.

Alternative hypothesis: There is a change in the IQ of the candidates after training or the mean of the difference in the pre- and post-training scores of candidates is not zero.

Level of significance (α) = 0.01

Choosing the distribution and finding the critical value: A two-tailed test is appropriate since we are interested to know whether the training has brought change in IQ after training. The significance level of 0.01 corresponds to 0.005 and the rejection area will be at both tails. Because the sample size is small, t distribution is used. On looking at the table of t distribution, the table value of t for 4 (N – 1) degree of freedom is 4.604.

Candidate	Before training	After training	Difference	d^2
1	108	120	−12	144
2	110	120	−10	100
3	116	122	−6	36
4	132	130	2	4
5	126	120	6	36
N = 5			Sum of d = −20	Total = 320

Mean of difference $(\bar{d}) = \frac{\Sigma d}{N} = \frac{-20}{5} = -4$

Standard deviation of differences

$$= \sqrt{\frac{\Sigma d^2 - (\bar{d})^2 \times N}{N-1}} = \sqrt{\frac{320-(-4\times-4)\times 5}{5-1}} = \sqrt{\frac{320-80}{4}} = \sqrt{\frac{240}{4}} = \sqrt{60} = 7.75$$

Standard error (SE) $= \frac{\sigma_{diff}}{\sqrt{N}} = \frac{7.75}{\sqrt{5}} = \frac{7.75}{2.24} = 3.46$

Calculation of t

Hence, $t = \frac{\bar{d} - \text{Hypothesized difference}}{\frac{\sigma_{diff}}{\sqrt{N}}} = \frac{4-0}{3.46} = \frac{4}{3.46} = 1.16$

Interpretation of the result: The table value of t for acceptance area is ± 4.604. This is our acceptance region. The calculated value of t (1.16) is inside this region. We should accept the null hypothesis. There is no change in the IQ of the candidates after training, or the mean of the difference in the pre- and post-training scores of candidates is zero.

Example 10:

A faculty has measured the students' attitude towards risk behavior before and after a health education session. The results are given below. Test whether there is a significant change in their attitude at 0.05 level of significance.

Students	1	2	3	4	5	6	7	8
Before health education	60	64	62	66	58	60	68	70
After health education	62	62	60	68	60	58	64	66

Null hypothesis: There is no change in their attitude towards risk behavior after health education or the mean difference health education score of students is zero.

Alternative hypothesis: There is a change in their attitude towards risk behavior after health education or the mean difference health education score is not zero.

Level of significance = 0.01

Choosing the distribution and finding the critical value: A two tailed test is appropriate since we are interested to know whether the health education has brought the change in the attitude towards high risk behavior. The significance level of 0.01 corresponds to 0.005 at both tails. Because the sample size is small, t distribution is used. On looking at the table of t distribution, the table value of t for 7 (N-1) degrees of freedom is 3.499.

Students	Before health education	After health education	Difference (d)	d^2
1	60	62	-2	4
2	64	62	2	4
3	62	60	2	4
4	66	68	-2	4
5	58	60	-2	4
6	60	58	2	4
7	68	64	4	16
8	70	66	4	16
Total			8	56

Mean of difference $(\bar{d}) = \frac{\Sigma d}{N} = \frac{8}{8} = 1$

Standard deviation of differences

$$= \sqrt{\frac{\Sigma d^2 - (\bar{d})^2 \times N}{N-1}} = \sqrt{\frac{56 - 1 \times 8}{8-1}} \sqrt{\frac{440}{7}} = \sqrt{62.86} = 7.93$$

Standard error $= \frac{\sigma_{diff}}{\sqrt{N}} = \frac{7.93}{2.82} = 2.81$

Calculation of t $= \dfrac{\bar{d} - \text{Hypothesized difference}}{\frac{\sigma_{diff}}{\sqrt{N}}} = \frac{1-0}{2.81} = 0.35$

Interpretation of the result: The table value of t for acceptance area is ±3.499. The calculated value of t (0.35) is inside this region. We accept the null hypothesis. There is no change in their attitude towards risk behavior after health education or the mean difference health education score is zero.

Hypothesis Testing of r

Hypothesis testing of r differs in different situations as described hereunder:

Hypothesis testing of the difference between the Sample r and Zero Population r. For testing whether r differs significantly from zero, as already stated earlier, the standard error of the correlation coefficient $\left(1 - \frac{r^2}{\sqrt{N}}\right)$ should be used only when N is large (say not less than 100) and the value of r is small. In small samples, we can use student's method where:

$$t = r\sqrt{\frac{N-2}{1-r^2}}$$

Example 11:

From a sample of 20 observations on prices and quantities, the investigator has computed the correlation coefficient r = 0.82. Can he/she infer from this result (at 5% level of significance) that the sample comes from a population with zero correlation? The t value for 18 degrees of freedom at 5% level of significance is 2.101.

We set up the null hypothesis that there is zero correlation in the population or $H_0 = r_p = 0$.

Substituting the values in the above formula, we get:

$$t = r\sqrt{\frac{20-2}{1-(0.82)^2}} = 6.04$$

The table value of $t_{0.05}$ for 18 degree of freedom is 2.1 (two-tailed test). The calculated value being much higher, we reject the null hypothesis and conclude that there is significant relationship between the two variables. In other words, the sample does not come from a population with zero correlation.

SUMMARY

- The t distribution, also known as student's t distribution is a sampling distribution derived from the parent normal distribution, introduced by WS Gossett.
- The t distribution is also a symmetric distribution about its mean. The shape of the t distribution varies according to the size of the sample or according to the degrees of freedom. When the size of the sample is large, the t distribution closely approximates the normal distribution.
- t-test is based on t distribution and is considered an appropriate test for judging the significance of a sample mean or for judging the significance of difference between the means of two samples in case of small sample(s) when population variance is not known t-test was specifically designed to evaluate statistical differences for samples of 30 or less.
- If two samples are related, we can use paired t-test (or what is known as difference test) for judging the significance of the mean of difference between the two related samples. It can also be used for judging the significance of the coefficients of simple and partial correlations.
- The relevant test statistic, t, is calculated from the sample data and then compared with its probable value based on t distribution at a specified level of significance for concerning degree of freedom for accepting or rejecting the null hypothesis.
- There are one sample t-test, two sample t-test and paired t-test.

EXERCISE

One sample t-test

- In a hospital, the average daily outpatient turnover is 675 with the standard deviation of 75 for the past one year. A sample of 20 selected days reveals a daily average patient turnover as 625. Test the null hypothesis that the average daily patient turnover is less than 675.
- The national survey reports that the mean accident score is 40 in a nation in a year. To test this, 5 states were randomly selected and the mean accident score was 30 with

the standard deviation of 8. Test the null hypothesis that the average accident score is less than the national score at 0.05 level of significance.

- Sample mean = 56; Standard deviation = 6 and the hypothesized mean = 60. Test if there is any significant difference between the sample mean and the hypothesized mean at 0.05 level of significance.
- Sample mean =12.5; Standard deviation = 1.2 and the hypothesized mean = 14. Test if there is any significant difference between the sample mean and the hypothesized mean at 0.05 level of significance.

Two sample t-test

- The below mentioned details are collected by a researcher to compare the performance of staff nurses in two hospitals. Test the null hypothesis that the hospital A is better than the hospital B with regard to the performance of the staff nurses. Let alpha (α) = 0.05.

Hospital	N	Mean	Standard deviation
A	20	78	6
B	18	70	5

- In a study, stress level of mothers of children with autism and cerebral palsy were assessed by a researcher to compare whether the stress levels are the same. Test if there is any significant difference in the stress level of mothers of two groups at 95% confidence level.

Mothers of children	N	Mean stress	Standard deviation
with autism	12	70	6
with cerebral palsy	10	68	5

- Test the null hypothesis that the two groups are drawn from the same population having the same mean.

N	Mean	Standard deviation
14	11	2
16	10	4

Paired t-test

- In 5 cities, the incidence of accidents were collected before and after implementation of special traffic regulation. The details are as follows:

City	1	2	3	4	5
Before	50	60	48	70	60
After	40	50	38	72	56

Test if there is any significant change in the incidence of accidents after implementation of special traffic regulation at 5% level of significance.

- In a college, data of the number of days leaves taken by the students before and after implementation of leave regulation were collected. The details are as follows:

Students	1	2	3	4	5	6	7	8	9	10	11
Before	10	12	8	6	10	14	10	8	16	10	12
After	8	10	6	8	12	12	12	6	12	8	10

Test if there is any significant reduction in the number of days of leave taken by the students after implementation of leave regulation at 5% level of significance.

- In an organization, staff satisfaction was assessed before and after introduction of staff welfare program. Test if there is any significant increase in staff satisfaction after introduction of staff welfare program at 5% level of significance.

Staff	1	2	3	4	5	6	7	8	9	10
Before	60	80	72	76	68	74	78	70	68	66
After	64	76	70	74	70	72	76	72	70	70

24 F Distribution

OBJECTIVES

After reading this chapter, you will be able to:

- Understand the meaning of F Distribution
- List the purposes of F Distribution and F-Test
- Explain the application of F Distribution
- Compute the F statistics
- Test hypothesis using F-Test

INTRODUCTION

Earlier we have discussed Z and t test for assessing the significant difference between the means of two independent samples. Sometimes, it may be required to compare the means of more than two independent samples. This can either be tested by comparing all possible pairings of samples. Such a procedure is unwise and time consuming. Here we can use Analyais of Variance, by which we can test whether there are any significant differences between the means overall, without testing each pair separately.

MEANING OF F DISTRIBUTION

F distribution is a continuous probability distribution. It is also known as Snedecor's F distribution or the Fisher-Snedecor distribution. Suppose we take samples, of sizes N1 and N2 respectively from either a single population or two populations with the same variance. We calculate the variances for both samples (S_1^2 and S_2^2) and then find the ratio between these variances (S_1^2/S_2^2). If we do this for a very large number of pairs of samples, the ratios would form a distribution known as the F distribution, whose properties are known for various numbers of degrees of freedom, these being (N1-1) and (N2-1) for the two samples. In other words, tables of F, the ratio of S_1^2 to S_2^2 allows us to find the probability of obtaining F ratios above any given value, for two samples from the same population, or from two populations with the same variance. F-test is based on F distribution and is used to compare the variance of the two-independent samples.

Purposes of F-Test

F-test is used to estimate and test hypothesis about population variance and population means.

Z test or t test is used to find out the significant difference between the mean value of two samples whereas F-test is used to examine the mean value of more than two groups for its significant difference.

This test is also used in the context of analysis of variance (ANOVA) for judging the significance of more than two sample means at one and the same time.

It is also used for judging the significance of multiple correlation coefficients. Test statistic, F, is calculated and compared with its probable value for accepting or rejecting the null hypothesis.

F-test

The t test is used to compare two mean values or treatments. Many experiments involve more than two treatments, and for such experiments the F-test is used. The F-test is based on the ratio of two variances. It is used to determine whether two independent estimates of variance can be assumed to be estimates of the same variance. If treatments are significantly different, the variation in treatment means will be greater than the variation due to random differences among individuals. This ratio was called 'F' by George W. Snedecor in honor of Ronald A. Fisher, a pioneer in the use of mathematical statistics in agriculture.

In the ANOVA, the F-test is used to test equality of means; that is, to answer the question, can it reasonably be assumed that the treatment means resulted from sampling populations with equal means? The two variances are calculated from sample means and by pooling the variances from the samples. If estimates of F were calculated many times for a series of samples drawn from a population of normally distributed variates (therefore, no difference between the variances would be expected), and the frequency of the F values obtained were plotted, an F distribution would result. F distribution is not symmetrical as was the t distribution and that only positive values are considered.

What is Variance?

The variance is a measure of how far a set of numbers is spread out. It is one of the several descriptors of a probability distribution, describing how far the numbers lie from the mean. It is the average of the squared differences from the Mean.

What is the Difference between Variance and Standard Deviation?

The standard deviation is a measure of how spread out numbers are. It is the square root of the variance.

How to Calculate the Variance?

Example 1:

The hours of playing violent video games per week for 5 adolescent children is given below. Calculate the variance and standard Deviation.

Number	1	2	3	4	5
Hours	8	6	10	12	8

To calculate the variance, first work out the mean.

$$\text{Mean} = \frac{8+6+10+12+8}{5} = \frac{44}{5} = 8.8$$

Find the difference between the individual item from mean and square it.

Difference	Squared difference
8–8.8 = – 0.8	00.64
6–8.8 = – 2.8	07.84
10–8.8 = 1.2	01.44
12–8.8 = 3.2	10.24
8–8.8 = – 0.8	00.64
Total	20.8

Find out the average.

$$\text{Variance} = \frac{20.8}{5} = 4.16 = 4.16$$

Variance = 4.16

Standard Deviation = $\sqrt{4.16}$ = 2.04

Standard Deviation = 2.04

Testing for Homogeneity of Variance

We may be interested to know whether or not the variances of two samples differ sufficiently to test the null hypothesis that the variances of the population from which the two samples were drawn were equal. This is usually known as testing for 'homogeneity of vairance'. To test this, one must calculate the variance for each sample and take the ratio of the larger to the smaller variance, so that the F value obtained is never less than 1. We then have to check the critical value of F in table for the required significance level. We have to look along the top of the table for the number of degrees of freedom (N1-1) associated with the larger variance and then follow this column down until we find the row corresponding to the number of degrees of freedom (N2-1) associated with the smaller variance. The calculated value is compared with the table value to accept or reject the null hypothesis.

Analysis of Variance

Analysis of Variance is abbreviated as ANOVA which is a parametric test. Students would recall that for testing the hypothesis of equality of two sample means we had used the t-test in an earlier section. F-test (developed by RA Fisher) is used for testing the hypothesis of equality of more than two sample means. This test is based on the ratio of two variances. Hence, it is also known as the variance ratio test or analysis of variance.

The two variances which are used in F ratio are: (a) variance between samples and (b) variance within samples.

The rationale of this test is that if it should prove that the 'between sample variation' is significantly greater than the 'within sample variation' then we should suspect that the samples were not, in fact, drawn from the same population, but from populations whose average values differ so that on top of the 'within population variation' there exists also a 'between population variation.' In one-way ANOVA, the values of one dependent variable (always continuous) and exactly one-independent variable (always categorical) is analyzed. In multiple analysis of variance (MANOVA), the analysis are done with the multiple dependent variable and multiple independent variables.

Essentials of ANOVA

- Random Sampling
- Variable of study must have normal distribution
- The variance of a variable must be the same for each population or for each group of data.

For the sake of clarity the technique of computing F may be discussed separately for:

a. One-way ANOVA where data are classified according to only one criterion, (only one independent variable is involved) and
b. Two-way ANOVA where data are classified according to two criteria.

In ANOVA, an independent variable is called factor. The independent variable or factor may have different levels. For example, pain as an independent variable or factor may have different levels, such as mild, moderate and severe. Perceived difficulty as easy, moderate and high or low, moderate and high. The symbol for number of levels in a factor is k.

In ANOVA, a factor that is studied using independent samples in all conditions is called a between subject factor. For example, an independent variable or factor is knowledge.

The knowledge on infection control measures can be studied among DGNM, BSc (N), PBBSc (N) groups. The mean knowledge score of all these three groups can be compared.

A factor studied using dependent samples in all conditions is a within subject factor. For example, in a single group the effectiveness of various treatments, such as meditation, Yoga and moderate exercise on level of stress (independent variable or factor) can be assessed. Here the same group is exposed to meditation, Yoga and moderate exercise. The statistic that forms the basis for ANOVA is called F. The F statistic is used to determine whether two or more sample means represent different population means. The F we calculate is the F obtained. We compare the F obtained to the critical value of F.

When F obtained is not significant, it indicates that there are no significant differences between any of the sample means and that all means are likely to represent the same population mean.

If F obtained is significant, it indicates that atleast two means are different from population mean. But we may not know which two means are different. To indentify this, we can perform post hoc analysis (Post hoc means 'after the fact'). Post hoc comparisons are like t test in which we compare pairs of sample means from a factor, one pair at a time. By comparing all possible pairs, we determine which means differ significantly from eachg other. We perform post hoc comparisons only when F obtained is significant.

Steps in One-way Classification

- First of all, the null hypothesis is to be laid down thus - $H_0 : \mu_1 = \mu_2 = \mu_3 \ldots \mu_k$ that is, the arithmetic means of populations from which the k samples are randomly drawn are equal.
- Next, variance between the samples is to be calculated. The steps involved are:
  - Calculate the mean of each sample and the grand mean.
  - Replace each item by its own sample average and calculate the squares of the deviations of the new entries from their grand average.
  - Obtain the total which will give sum of squares between the samples.
  - Divide the above total by the relevant degrees of freedom (one less than the number of sample averages on which the computation is based). This will give variance between samples eliminating the within sample effect.
- Next, variance within the samples is to be calculated, The steps involved are:
  - Calculate the mean value of each sample.
  - Take the deviations of various items of each sample from its mean value.
  - Square the above deviations and obtain their total. This will give sum of squares within samples.
  - Divide the above total by the relevant degrees of freedom. For this purpose we argue as follows: For each sample the number of degrees of freedom within that sample are one less than the number of items within that sample. Hence for n samples having N items the degrees of freedom are $N - n$. This will give variance within samples.
- Last, calculate the ratio F as follows:

$$F = \frac{\text{Between} - \text{Sample variance}}{\text{Within} - \text{Sample variance}}$$

If there is a real difference between the samples, the between-sample variance will be significantly larger than the within-sample variance. The calculated value of F is compared with the table value for the given degrees of freedom both in respect of the numerator and the denominator at a certain level of significance. If the calculated value of F is greater than the table value, the difference is significant and the null hypothesis is rejected. If the calculated value is less than the table value of F, the difference is not significant and the null hypothesis of equality of sample averages is accepted.

Example 2:

The aggression level of children playing violent video games were measured in two groups. The data were as follows:

Group A	:	1	2	3	4	5	6	7	8	9	10
Aggression score	:	60	50	40	40	60	70	54	62	68	50
Group B	:	1	2	3	4	5	6	7	8	9	
Aggression score	:	50	40	60	70	56	64	40	48	56	

Find the variance and test the null hypothesis that the variance of the two groups are equal.

Null hypothesis: The group A and group B have the same variance and the variance of the two groups are equal.

Computation of variance for Group A

$\overline{X} = 554/10 = 55.4$

X	$(X - \overline{X})$	$(X - \overline{X})^2$
60	60 – 55.4 = 4.6	21.16
50	50 – 55.4 = – 5.4	29.16
40	40 – 55.4 = – 15.4	237.16
40	40 – 55.4 = – 15.4	237.16
60	60 – 55.4 = 4.6	21.16
70	70 – 55.4 = 14.6	213.16
54	54 – 55.4 = – 1.4	1.96
62	62 – 55.4 = 6.6	43.56
68	68 – 55.4 = 12.6	158.76
50	50 – 55.4 = – 5.4	29.16
		Total = 992.4

$$\text{Variance of group A} = \frac{992.4}{10} = 99.24 = 99.24$$

Computation of Variance for Group B

$\overline{X} = 484/9 = 53.8$

X	$(X - \overline{X})$	$(X - \overline{X})^2$
50	50 – 53.8 = – 3.8	14.44
40	40 – 53.8 = – 13.8	190.44
60	60 – 53.8 = 6.2	38.44
70	70 – 53.8 = 16.2	262.44
56	56 – 53.8 = 2.2	4.84
64	64 – 53.8 = 10.2	104.04
40	40 – 53.8 = – 13.8	190.44
48	48 – 53.8 = – 5.8	33.64
56	56 – 53.8 = 2.2	4.84
		Total = 843.56

$$\text{Variance of group B} = \frac{843.6}{9} = 93.7$$

$S_1^2 = 99.24$ for N = 10

$S_2^2 = 93.7$ for N = 9

Taking F as the ratio of the larger to the smaller variance

F = 99.24/93.7 = 1.06

There are (10–1) or 9 degrees of freedom for the calculation of larger variance and (9–1) or 8 degrees of freedom for the smaller variance. When we refer F table, the value for larger variance at 9 df and smaller variance at 8 df is 3.388 at 5% level and at 1% level is 5.91

Conclusion: The calculated value is less than the table value. So we accept the null hypothesis. The variance are the same. We are safe in assuming homogenity of variance.

Example 3:

The following table illustrates the adolescents weight at 3 major cities. Can we consider the weight of children in 3 cities to be equal at 5% level of significance.

Chennai (A)	45	48	51	55	46
Madurai (B)	48	52	38	42	55
Trichy (C)	44	50	40	52	54

Null Hypothesis: The mean weight of the adolescents children in the three cities are the same.

Calculate the mean of each sample.

$$\text{Children of Chennai (A) } \bar{X}_1 = \frac{45 + 48 + 51 + 55 + 46}{5} = 245/5 = 49$$

$$\text{Children of Madurai (B) } \bar{X}_2 = \frac{48 + 52 + 38 + 42 + 55}{5} = 235/5 = 47$$

$$\text{Children of Trichy (C) } \bar{X}_3 = \frac{44 + 50 + 40 + 52 + 54}{5} = 240/5 = 48$$

$$\text{Mean of the sample means (Grand mean } \bar{\bar{x}}) = \bar{\bar{x}} = \frac{49 + 47 + 48}{3} = 144/3 = 48$$

Now, we work out SS between and SS within samples.

$$\begin{aligned}
\text{SS between} &= n_1(\bar{X}_1 - \bar{\bar{x}})^2 + n_2(\bar{X}_2 - \bar{\bar{x}})^2 + n_3(\bar{X}_3 - \bar{\bar{x}})^2 \\
&= 5(49 - 48)^2 + 5(47 - 48)^2 + 5(48 - 48)^2 \\
&= 5(1)^2 + 5(-1)^2 + 5(0)^2 \\
&= 5 + 5 + 0 = 10 \\
\text{SS between} &= 10 \\
\text{SS within} &= S_1(\bar{X}_{1i} - \bar{x}_1)^2 + S_2(\bar{X}_{2i} - \bar{x}_2)^2 + S_3(\bar{X}_{3i} - \bar{x}_3)^2\ i = A, B, C \\
&= \{(45 - 49)^2 + (48 - 49)^2 + (51 - 49)^2 + (55 - 49)^2 + \\
&\quad (46 - 49)^2\} + \{(48 - 47)^2 + (52 - 47)^2 + (38 - 47)^2 + \\
&\quad (42 - 47)^2 + (55 - 47)^2\} + \{(44 - 48)^2 + (50 - 48)^2 + \\
&\quad (40 - 48)^2 + (52 - 48)^2 + (54 - 48)^2\} \\
&= \{(-4)^2 + (-1)^2 + (2)^2 + (6)^2 + (-3)^2\} + \{(1)^2 + (5)^2 + (-9)^2 + \\
&\quad (-5)^2 + (8)^2\} + \{(-4)^2 + (2)^2 + (-8)^2 + (4)^2 + (6)^2\} \\
&= (16 + 1 + 4 + 36 + 9) + (1 + 25 + 81 + 25 + 64) + \\
&\quad (16 + 4 + 64 + 16 + 36) \\
&= 66 + 196 + 136 = 398
\end{aligned}$$

SS within = 398

SS for total variance = SS between + SS within

= 10 + 398 = 408

Alternatively, SS for total variance can be calculated as follows:

SS for total variance

$= S(x_{ij} - \bar{\bar{x}})^2$ i = A, B, C and j = 1, 2, 3.....

$= [(45 - 48)^2 + (48 - 48)^2 + (51 - 48)^2 + (55 - 48)^2 + (46 - 48)^2] + [(48 - 48)^2 + (52 - 48)^2 + (38 - 48)^2 + (42 - 48)^2 + (55 - 48)^2] + [(44 - 48)^2 + (50 - 48)^2 + (40 - 48)^2 + (52 - 48)^2 + (54 - 48)^2]$

$= [(-3)^2 + (0)^2 + (3)^2 + (7)^2 + (-2)^2] + [(0)^2 + (4)^2 + (-10)^2 + (-6)^2 + (7)^2] + [(-4)^2 + (2)^2 + (-8)^2 + (4)^2 + (6)^2]$

= 9 + 0 + 9 + 49 + 4 + 0 + 16 + 100 + 36 + 49 + 16 + 4 + 64 + 16 + 36 = 408

Now we can set up the ANOVA table for this problem

Source of variation	SS	Degrees of freedom	MS	F ratio	5% F limit (From the table)
Between Sample	10	(3 – 1) = 2	10/2 = 5	5/33.17 = 0.15	3.89
Within sample	398	(15 – 3) = 12	398/12 = 33.17		

The table value for v1, 2 degrees of freedom and for v2, 12 degrees of freedom at 5% is 3.89.

Conclusion: The calculated value is less than the table value. So, we accept the null hypothesis. The mean weight of the adolescent children in the three cities are the same.

Solution through short cut method

In this case, we first take the total of all the individual values of n items and call it as T.

City	Weight of the adolescent children					Total
Chennai	45	48	51	55	46	245
Madurai	48	52	38	42	55	235
Trichy	44	50	40	52	54	240
Total	137	150	129	149	155	720

T in the given case = 720

Hence the correction factor = $(T)^2/n = (720)^2/15 = \dfrac{720 \times 720}{15}$ = 518400/15 = 34560

Now total SS, SS between and SS within can be worked out as under:

Total SS = $S(x^2_{ij} - \dfrac{T^2}{n})$ i = A,B,C.. j = 1,2,3.....

$= (45)^2 + (48)^2 + (51)^2 + (55)^2 + (46)^2 + (48)^2 + (52)^2 + (38)^2 + (42)^2 + (55)^2 + (44)^2 + (50)^2 + (40)^2 + (52)^2 + (54)^2 - (720)^2/15$

= 2025 + 2304 + 2601 + 3025 + 2116 + 2304 + 2704 + 1444 + 1764 + 3025 + 1936 + 2500 + 1600 + 2704 + 2916 – 34560

= 34968 – 34560 = 408

SS total = **408**

$$\text{SS between} = S\frac{(Tj)^2}{nj} - \frac{(T)^2}{n}$$

$$\text{SS between} = (245)^2/5 + (235)^2/5 + (240)^2/5 - (720)^2/15$$

$$= \frac{60025}{5} + \frac{55225}{5} + \frac{57600}{5} - 34560$$

$$= 12005 + 11045 + 11520 - 34560 = 34570 - 34560 = 10$$

SS between = 10

SS within

$$= \Sigma x_{ij}^2 - \Sigma\frac{(Tj)^2}{nj} = 34968 - 34570 = 398$$

SS within = 398

Example 4:

The general well-being score of nurses working in OT, ICU, and Emergency unit were as follows.

Nurses in ICU	70	60	65	55	60
Nurses in OT	55	65	65	60	60
Nurses in Emergency	65	55	55	70	70

Test whether the general well-being is the same in nurses working in these areas at 5% level of significance.

Null hypothesis: The general wellbeing of the nurses working in these three areas are the same.

Calculate the mean of each sample.

Nurses in ICU $\bar{X}_1 = \frac{70 + 60 + 65 + 55 + 60}{5} = 310/5 = 62$

Nurses in OT $\bar{X}_2 = \frac{55 + 65 + 65 + 60 + 60}{5} = 305/5 = 61$

Nurses in Emergency $\bar{X}_3 = \frac{65 + 55 + 55 + 70 + 70}{5} = 315/5 = 63$

Mean of the sample means (Grand mean) $\bar{\bar{x}} = \frac{62 + 61 + 63}{3} = 186/3 = 62$

Now we work out SS between and SS within samples.

$$\text{SS between} = n_1(\bar{X}_1 - \bar{\bar{x}})^2 + n_2(\bar{X}_2 - \bar{\bar{x}})^2 + n_3(\bar{X}_3 - \bar{\bar{x}})^2$$

$$= 5(62 - 62)^2 + 5(61 - 62)^2 + 5(63 - 62)^2 = 5(0)^2 + 5(-1)^2 + 5(1)^2$$

$$= 0 + 5 + 5 = 10$$

SS between = 10

$$\text{SS within} = S_1(\bar{X}_{1i} - \bar{x}_1)^2 + S_2(\bar{X}_{2i} - \bar{x}_2)^2 + S_3(\bar{X}_{3i} - \bar{x}_3)^2 \; i = A, B, C$$

$$= \{(70 - 62)^2 + (60 - 62)^2 + (65 - 62)^2 + (55 - 62)^2 + (60 - 62)^2\} + \{(55 - 61)^2 + (65 - 61)^2 + (65 - 61)^2 + (60 - 61)^2 + (60 - 61)^2\} + \{(65 - 63)^2 + (55 - 63)^2 + (55 - 63)^2 + (70 - 63)^2 + (70 - 63)^2\}$$

$$= \{(8)^2 + (-2)^2 + (3)^2 + (-7)^2 + (-2)^2\} + \{(-6)^2 + (4)^2 + (4)^2 + (-1)^2 + (-1)^2\} + \{(2)^2 + (-8)^2 + (-8)^2 + (7)^2 + (7)^2\}$$

$= (64 + 4 + 9 + 49 + 4) + (36 + 16 + 16 + 1 + 1) + (4 + 64 + 64 + 49 + 49)$

$= 130 + 70 + 230 = 430$

SS within $= 430$

SS for total variance = SS between + SS within

$= 10 + 430 = 440$

Alternatively, SS for total variance can be calculated as follows:-

SS for total variance = $S(x_{ij} - \bar{\bar{x}})^2$ i = A, B, C and j = 1, 2, 3.....

$= (70 - 62)^2 + (60 - 62)^2 + (65 - 62)^2 + (55 - 62)^2 + (60 - 62)^2 + (55 - 62)^2 + (65 - 62)^2 + (65 - 62)^2 + (60 - 62)^2 + (60 - 62)^2 + (65 - 62)^2 + (55 - 62)^2 + (55 - 62)^2 + (70 - 62)^2 + (70 - 62)^2$

$= [(8)^2 + (-2)^2 + (3)^2 + (-7)^2 + (-2)^2] + [(-7)^2 + (3)^2 + (3)^2 + (-2)^2 + (-2)^2] + [(3)^2 + (-7)^2 + (-7)^2 + (8)^2 + (8)^2]$

$= 64 + 4 + 9 + 49 + 4 + 49 + 9 + 9 + 4 + 4 + 9 + 49 + 49 + 64 + 64 = 440$

Now we can set-up the ANOVA table for this problem

Source of variation	SS	Degrees of freedom	MS	F ratio	5% F limit From the table
Between sample	10	(3 – 1) = 2	10/2 = 5	5/35.8 = 0.14	3.89
Within sample	430	(15 – 3) = 12	430/12 = 35.8		

The table value for v1, 2 degrees of freedom and for v2, 12 degrees of freedom at 5% is 3.89.

Conclusion: The calculated value is less than the table value. So we accept the null hypothesis. The general well-being of the nurses working in these three areas are the same.

Solution through short cut method

In this case, we first take the total of all the individual values of n items and call it as T.

Nurses in	General well-being score					Total
ICU	70	60	65	55	60	310
OT	55	65	65	60	60	305
Emergency	65	55	55	70	70	315
Total						930

T in the given case = 930

Hence, the correction factor = $(T)^2/n = (930)^2/15 = \frac{930 \times 930}{15}$ = 864900/15 = 57660

Now total SS, SS between and SS within can be worked out as under:

Total SS = $\Sigma(x_{ij}^2 - \frac{T^2}{n})$ i = A,B,C.. j = 1,2,3.....

$= (70)^2 + (60)^2 + (65)^2 + (55)^2 + (60)^2 + (55)^2 + (65)^2 + (65)^2 + (60)^2 + (60)^2 + (65)^2 + (55)^2 + (55)^2 + (70)^2 + (70)^2 - (930)^2/15$

$= 4900 + 3600 + 4225 + 3025 + 3600 + 3025 + 4225 + 4225 + 3600 + 3600 + 4225 + 3025 + 3025 + 4900 + 4900 - 57660$

$= 58100 - 57660 = 440$

SS total = 440

SS between = $\Sigma\frac{(Tj)^2}{nj} - \frac{(T)^2}{n}$

SS between $= (310)^2/5 + (305)^2/5 + (315)^2/5 - (930)^2/15$

$= \frac{96100}{5} + \frac{93025}{5} + \frac{99225}{5} - 57660$

$= 19220 + 18605 + 19845 - 57660 = 57670 - 57660 = 10$

SS between = 10

SS within $= \Sigma x^2_{ij} - \Sigma\frac{(Tj)^2}{nj}$

$= 58100 - 57670 = 430$

SS within = 430

Example 5:

The data on reduction of weight in kg in adults by 3 different interventions are given below. Test whether these three interventions bring the same effect or they differ in their effect.

	Intervention 1 (x_1)	Intervention 2 (x_2)	Intervention 3 (x_3)
	2	4	1
	3	2	2
	1	3	2
	4	2	3
	2	5	4
	1	4	0
	3	5	1
Total	16	25	13

Null Hypothesis: The effect of three interventions are same.

$16 + 25 + 13 = 54$

T in the given case = 54

Hence, the correction factor = $(T)^2/n = (54)^2/21 = \frac{54 \times 54}{21} = 2916/21 = 139$

Now, total SS, SS between and SS within can be worked out as under:

Total SS = $\Sigma(x^2_{ij} - \frac{T^2}{n})$ i = A,B,C.. j = 1,2,3.....

$= \{(2)^2 + (3)^2 + (1)^2 + (4)^2 + (2)^2 + (1)^2 + (3)^2\} + \{(4)^2 + (2)^2 + (3)^2 + (2)^2 + (5)^2 + (4)^2 + (5)^2\} + \{(1)^2 + (2)^2 + (2)^2 + (3)^2 + (4)^2 + (0)^2 + (1)^2\} - (54)^2/21$

$= \{4 + 9 + 1 + 16 + 4 + 1 + 9\} + \{16 + 4 + 9 + 4 + 25 + 16 + 25\} + \{1 + 4 + 4 + 9 + 16 + 0 + 1\} - 139$

$= (44 + 99 + 35) - 139 = 178 - 139 = 39$

SS total = 39

$$\text{SS between} = \Sigma\frac{(Tj)^2}{nj} - \frac{(T)^2}{n}$$

$$\text{SS between} = (16)^2/7 + (25)^2/7 + (13)^2/7 - (54)^2/21$$

$$= \frac{256}{7} + \frac{625}{7} + \frac{169}{7} - 139$$

$$= 36.6 + 89.3 + 24.1 - 139$$

$$= 150 - 139 = 11$$

SS between = 11

SS within

$$= \Sigma x^2_{ij} - \Sigma\frac{(Tj)^2}{nj}$$

$$= 178 - 150 = 28$$

SS within = 28

Other method

$\overline{X}_1 = 16/7 = 2.29$

$\overline{X}_2 = 25/7 = 3.57$

$\overline{X}_3 = 13/7 = 1.86$

Mean of the sample means (Grand mean) $= \frac{2.29 + 3.57 + 1.86}{3} = 7.72/3$ $= 2.6$

$$\text{SS between} = n_1(\overline{X}_1 - \overline{\overline{x}})^2 + n_2(\overline{X}_2 - \overline{\overline{x}})^2 + n_3(\overline{X}_3 - \overline{\overline{x}})^2$$

$$= 7(2.3 - 2.6)^2 + 7(3.6 - 2.6)^2 + 7(1.9 - 2.6)^2 = 7(-0.3)^2 + 7(1)^2 + 7(-0.7)^2$$

$$= 7(0.09) + 7(1) + 7(0.49) = 0.63 + 7 + 3.43 = 11.06$$

SS between = 11.06

$$\text{SS within} = \Sigma_1(\overline{X}_{1i} - \overline{x}_1)^2 + \Sigma_2(\overline{X}_{2i} - \overline{x}_2)^2 + \Sigma_3(\overline{X}_{3i} - \overline{x}_3)^2 \; i = A, B, C$$

$$= \{(2 - 2.3)^2 + (3 - 2.3)^2 + (1 - 2.3)^2 + (4 - 2.3)^2 + (2 - 2.3)^2 + (1 - 2.3)^2 + (3 - 2.3)^2\} + \{(4 - 3.6)^2 + (2 - 3.6)^2 + (3 - 3.6)^2 + (2 - 3.6)^2 + (5 - 3.6)^2 + (4 - 3.6)^2 + (5 - 3.6)^2\} + \{(1 - 1.9)^2 + (2 - 1.9)^2 + (2 - 1.9)^2 + (3 - 1.9)^2 + (4 - 1.9)^2 + (0 - 1.9)^2 + (1 - 1.9)^2\}$$

$$= \{(-0.3)^2 + (0.7)^2 + (-1.3)^2 + (1.7)^2 + (-0.3)^2 + (-1.3)^2 + (0.7)^2\} + \{(0.4)^2 + (-1.6)^2 + (-0.6)^2 + (-1.6)^2 + (1.4)^2 + (0.4)^2 + (1.4)^2\} + \{(-0.9)^2 + (0.1)^2 + (0.1)^2 + (1.1)^2 + (2.1)^2 + (-1.9)^2 + (-0.9)^2\}$$

$$= (0.09 + 0.49 + 1.69 + 2.89 + 0.09 + 1.69 + 0.49) + (0.16 + 2.56 + 0.36 + 2.56 + 1.96 + 0.16 + 1.96) + (0.81 + 0.01 + 0.01 + 1.21 + 4.41 + 3.61 + 0.81)$$

$$= 7.43 + 9.72 + 10.87 = 28.02$$

SS within = 28

Now, we can set-up the ANOVA table for this problem

Source of variation	SS	Degrees of freedom	MS	F ratio	5% F limit (From the table)
Between sample	11	(3 – 1) = 2	11/2 = 5.5	5.5/1.6 = 3.44	3.55
Within sample	28	(21 – 3) = 18	28/18 = 1.6		

The table value for v1, 2 degrees of freedom and for v2, 18 degrees of freedom at 5% is 3.55.

Conclusion: The calculated value is less than the table value. So we accept the null hypothesis.

The effect of three interventions are the same.

Two-Way ANOVA

In two-way ANOVA, we have two independent variables or factors. Each factor may contain any number of levels. One independent variable can be denoted as factor A and the other independent variable can be denoted as factor B. If factor A has two levels and factor B has two levels, it is a 2 × 2 design. If factor A has 3 levels and factor B has 2 levels, it is 3 × 2 design. If one factor has 4 levels and the other factor has 3 levels we have 4 × 3 ANOVA and so on.

For example, Independent variable or factor A is Yoga and the other independent variable or factor B is gender.

	Level A1(Yoga once a day)	Level A2 (Yoga twice a day)
Male	x	x
Female	x	x

Combining all levels of one factor with all levels of the other factor produces a complete factorial design.

Example 6:

The number of admissions for the month of April, May and June for three different hospitals were given below. Test whether there is a significant difference in admissions in three hospitals for three different months.

	April	May	June	Total
Hospital 1	20	15	10	45
Hospital 2	30	25	40	95
Hospital 3	15	20	30	65
Total	65	60	80	205

Null hypothesis: There is no significant difference in admission in these three hospitals and there is no significant difference in admission in these three months. Or the admissions into these three hospitals in three different months are the same.

T in the given case = 205

Hence, the correction factor = $(T)^2/n = (205)^2/9 = \frac{205 \times 205}{9} = 42025/9 = 4669.4$

SS between hospitals (rows)

$$= \frac{(\Sigma x1)^2}{N} + \frac{(\Sigma x2)^2}{N} + \frac{(\Sigma x3)^2}{N} - \frac{(T)^2}{N}$$

$$= \frac{(45)^2}{3} + \frac{(95)^2}{3} + \frac{(65)^2}{3} - \frac{(205)^2}{9}$$

$$= 2025/3 + 9025/3 + 4225/3 - 4669.4$$

$$= 675 + 3008.3 + 1408.3 - 4669.4$$
$$= 5091.6 - 4669.4 = 422.2$$

Between three hospitals there are two degrees of freedom.

SS between months (columns)

$$= \frac{(65)^2}{3} + \frac{(60)^2}{3} + \frac{(80)^2}{3} - \frac{(205)^2}{9}$$
$$= 4225/3 + 3600/3 + 6400/3 - 4669.4$$
$$= 1408.3 + 1200 + 2133.3 - 4669.4$$
$$= 4741.6 - 4669.4 = 72.2$$

Between three months there are two degrees of freedom.

Total Sum of Squares $= (20)^2 + (15)^2 + (10)^2 + (30)^2 + (25)^2 + (40)^2 + (15)^2 + (20)^2 + (30)^2 - 4669.4$

$$= 400 + 225 + 100 + 900 + 625 + 1600 + 225 + 400 + 900 - 4669.4$$
$$= 5375 - 4669.4 = 705.6$$

Between 9 items there are 8 degrees of freedom.

Source of variation	SS	Degrees of freedom	MS	F ratio	5% F limit (from the table)
Between hospitals	422.2	(3 – 1) = 2	422.2/2 = 211.1	F (Hospital) = 211.1/52.8 = 3.998 = 4	v1 = 2; v2 = 4 6.94
Between months	72.2	(3 – 1) = 2	72.2/2 = 36.1		
Residual	211.2	4	211.2/4 = 52.8	F (Months) = 36.1/52.8 = 0.6837	v1 = 2; v2 = 4 6.94
Total	705.6	(9 – 1) = 8			

Conclusion: For both hospitals and months, the calculated value is less than the table value. So, we accept the null hypothesis. There is no significant difference in admission in these three hospitals and there is no significant difference in admission in these three months.

Example 7:

The pulse rate of children of various age group was measured on various intervals after playing violent video games. Test whether there is a significant difference in pulse rate among children of various age groups. Also test whether the there is a significant difference in pulse rate measured at different interval.

	30 minutes	1 hour	2 hours	4 hours	Total
13 years	90	86	100	90	366
14 years	88	90	86	80	344
15 years	80	76	82	76	314
Total	258	252	268	246	1024

Null hypothesis: There is no significant difference in the pulse rate measured on various timings and there is no significant difference in pulse rate measured in various age groups.

T in the given case = 1024

Hence, the correction factor = $(T)^2/n = (1024)^2/12 = \frac{1024 \times 1024}{12}$ = 1048576/12

= 87381.3

SS between age (rows)

$$= \frac{(\Sigma x1)^2}{N} + \frac{(\Sigma x2)^2}{N} + \frac{(\Sigma x3)^2}{N} - \frac{(T)^2}{N}$$

$$= \frac{(366)^2}{4} + \frac{(344)^2}{4} + \frac{(314)^2}{4} - \frac{(1024)^2}{12}$$

= 133956/4 + 118336/4 + 98596/4 – 87381.3

33489 + 29584 + 24649 – 87381.3

= 87722 – 87381.3 = 340.7

Between three age groups there are two degrees of freedom.

SS between interval (columns)

$$= \frac{(258)^2}{3} + \frac{(252)^2}{3} + \frac{(268)^2}{3} + \frac{(246)^2}{3} - \frac{(1024)^2}{12}$$

= 66564/3 + 63504/3 + 71824/3 + 60516/3 – 87381.3

= 22188 + 21168 + 23941.3 + 20172 – 87381.3

= 87469.3 – 87381.3 = 88

Between four intervals there are three degrees of freedom.

Total Sum of Squares

= $(90)^2 + (86)^2 + (100)^2 + (90)^2 + (88)^2 + (90)^2 + (86)^2 +$
$(80)^2 + (80)^2 + (76)^2 + (82)^2 + (76)^2$ - 87381.3

= 8100 + 7396 + 10000 + 8100 + 7744 + 8100 + 7396 +
6400 + 6400 + 5776 + 6724 + 5776 – 87381.3

= 87912 – 87381.3 = 530.7

Between 12 items there are 11 degrees of freedom.

Source of variation	SS	Degrees of freedom	MS	F ratio	5% F limit (from the table)
Between age groups	340.7	(3 – 1) = 2	340.7/2 = 170.35	F (Age groups) = 170.35/17 = 10.02	V1 = 3; V2 = 6 4.76
Between time intervals	88	(4 – 1) = 3	88/3 = 29.33		
Residual	102	6	102/6 = 17	F (Intervals) = 29.33/17 = 1.72	v1 = 2; v2 = 6 5.14
Total	530.7	(12 – 1) = 11			

Conclusion: For pulse rate measured in different age groups the calculated value is more than the table value. We reject the null hypothesis. There is a significant difference in the pulse rate measured in different age groups.

For the pulse rate measured in various intervals, the calculated value is less than the table value. So, we accept the null hypothesis. There is no significant difference in pulse rate measured at various intervals.

SUMMARY

- F distribution is a continuous probability distribution. It is also known as Snedecor's F distribution or the Fisher-Snedecor distribution. F-test is based on F distribution and is used to compare the variance of the two-independent samples and is used to estimate and test hypothesis about population variance and population means.
- F-test otherwise known as ANOVA is used for testing the hypothesis of equality of more than two sample means. This test is based on the ratio of two variances. Hence, it is also known as the variance ratio test or analysis of variance. The two variances which are used in F ratio are (a) variance between samples and (b) variance within samples.
- In one-way ANOVA, the values of one dependent variable (always continuous) and exactly one independent variable (always categorical) is analyzed. In Multiple Analysis of Variance (MANOVA), the analysis are done with the multiple dependent variable and multiple independent variables.

EXERCISE

1. The general well-being score of nurses working in Government, private hospitals and community were as follows.

Nurses in government	72	58	70	55	66
Nurses in private	55	60	55	60	60
Nurses in community	65	60	68	70	80

Test whether the general well-being is the same in nurses working in these areas at 5% level of significance.

2. The following table illustrates the adolescent boys weight at 3 major cities. Can we consider the weight of children in 3 cities to be equal at 5% level of significance.

Coimbatore (A)	50	60	55	56	66
Madurai (B)	50	62	48	52	55
Salem (C)	44	60	40	50	54

3. The exam scores of nursing students studying in 3 nursing colleges were given as below. Can we consider the performance of students are the same in three colleges.

College A	80	90	72	68	58
College B	74	86	73	64	60
College C	78	62	74	80	58

4. The data on birth weight of newborn in 3 districts were collected to assess whether they are same. Test at 5% level of significance.

District 1	2.2	2.5	3.1	3.2	4.0	4.2
District 2	2.6	3.4	2.8	2.0	3.0	2.9
District 3	3.4	3.6	2.4	3.0	2.8	2.6

25 Chi Square Distribution

OBJECTIVES

After reading this chapter, you will be able to:

- Understand chi square distribution
- List the purposes of chi square distribution and $\mathcal{X}^2$ test
- Compute the chi square statistics
- Test hypothesis using $\mathcal{X}^2$ test
- Explain the application of $\mathcal{X}^2$ test in nursing research

INTRODUCTION

Chi square distribution is one of the most commonly used probability distribution in inferential statistics. It is a very versatile test used both as a parametric and non parametric measure. The chi square distribution is used in chi square test for goodness of fit and test for independence. Chi square test is one of the statistical test commonly used to compare observed data with the expected data. If it is expected that 2 out of 8 children should possess some feature, and if the observed number of children with some feature is 3 out of 8 children, the chi square test helps us to decide whether the difference between the observed and the expected is due to some factor or is the result of chance. That is, chi square is the sum of the squared difference between observed (o) and the expected (e) data (or the deviation, d), divided by the expected data in all possible categories.

CHI SQUARE DISTRIBUTION

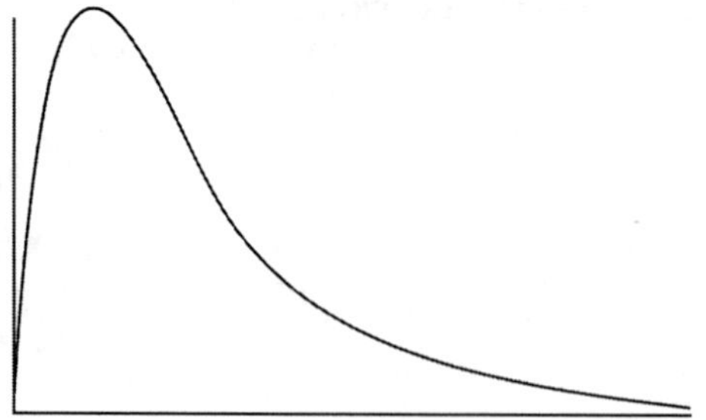

The chi square distribution is an asymmetric distribution. In chi square distribution, along the horizontal axis is the $\mathcal{X}^2$ value. The minimum possible value for a $\mathcal{X}^2$ variable is 0, but there is no maximum value. The vertical axis is the probability, or probability density, associated with each value of $\mathcal{X}^2$. The curve reaches a peak not far above 0 that is to the right of 0, and then gradually declines in height as the $\mathcal{X}^2$ value increases, so that the curve is asymmetric. As with the distributions introduced earlier, as larger $\mathcal{X}^2$ values are obtained, the curve is asymmetric to the horizontal axis, always approaching it, but never quite touching the axis. So, the curve comes closer to the horizontal axis but it never touches. Each $\mathcal{X}^2$ distribution has a degree of freedom associated with it, so that there are many different chi squared distributions.

The mean of the chi square distribution is the degree of freedom and the standard deviation is twice the degrees of freedom. This implies that the $\mathcal{X}^2$ distribution is more spread out, with a peak farther to the right, for larger degrees of freedom than smaller degrees of freedom. As a result, for any given level of significance, the critical region begins at a larger chi square value for the larger degree of freedom.

The chi square distribution has the following properties:

- The mean of the distribution is equal to the number of degrees of freedom: $\mu = v$.
- The variance is equal to two times the number of degrees of freedom: $\sigma^2 = 2 \times v$
- As the degrees of freedom increases, the chi square curve approaches a normal distribution.
- The smaller the number of degrees of freedom, the more skewed is the distribution.
- Since $\mathcal{X}^2$ is the sum of a set of squared values, it can never be negative. The minimum chi squared value would be 0. There is no upper limit to the $\mathcal{X}^2$ value.

Purposes of Chi Square Distribution and Chi Square Test

$\mathcal{X}^2$ test is based on chi square distribution. The chi square test can be used as a parametric and nonparametric test. As a parametric test, it is used to establish confidence interval for the variance of a population and also to compare a sample variance to a theoretical population variance. It is used to test the hypothesis that the population variance is the same as the sample variance. The deviations of the observed numbers from those specified by the hypothesis form the basis of the chi square. Each deviation is squared, each square is divided by the hypothetical or expected number or value and the results are added. As a non parametric measure it is used as a test of goodness of fit and the test of independence.

The Goodness of Fit Test

Many times we want to check how far a theoretical distribution fit to the observed data. The chi square test measures the actual difference between the expected and observed frequencies. The quantitative data used in the computation of the test statistics are the frequencies associated with each category of the one or more variables under study. The major concern in chi square test is the observed frequencies and the expected frequencies. The observed frequencies are the number of subjects in total sample that fall into the various categories of the variable of interest. For example, if we have a sample of 60 adults, we may observe that 45 are Hindus, 10 are Christians and 5 are Muslims. Expected frequencies are the number of subjects in the total sample that is expected to observe if some null hypothesis about the variable is true. For example, the null hypothesis might be that the three categories of religion are equally represented in the population from which the sample is drawn. In that case it is expected that the sample to contain 20 Hindus, 20 Christians and 20 Muslims. Here, the actual (observed) is different from the expected. Whether this difference is significant one or something which can be ignored, is decided by referring to the chi square table. In this, an observed frequency distribution is compared to find out whether its pattern is as good as a hypothetical or theoretical pattern. The key idea of the chi square test is a comparison of observed and expected values for estimating how closely an observed distribution matches an expected distribution (Goodness of Fit test). If there is a large discrepancy between the observed and the expected values, the x^2 statistic would be large, suggesting a significant difference between observed and expected values. If the calculated value is small when compared to the table value of chi square, it indicates that the difference is not significant and is the result of sampling fluctuations and can be ignored.

Testing Independence

The other primary use of the chi square test is to examine whether two variables are independent or not. What does it mean to be independent, in this sense? It means that the two factors are not related. The chi square test of independence allows the researcher to determine whether variables are independent of each other or whether there is a pattern of dependence between them. If there is a dependence, the researcher can claim that the two variables have a statistical relationship with each other. Typically, in nursing and social science research, we are interested in finding factors that are related such as education and income, occupation and income, age and attitude, education and knowledge, etc. and the chi square test can be used to assess whether two variables are related or not. It is important to keep in mind that the chi square test only tests whether two variables are independent. It cannot address questions of which is greater or less. For both the goodness of fit test and the test of independence, the chi square statistic is the same. The null and alternative hypotheses for each chi square test can be stated as

$$H_0 = O_i = E_i$$
$$H_1 = O_i \neq E_i$$

If the claim made in the null hypothesis is true, the observed and the expected values are close to each other and $O_i - E_i$ is small for each category. When the observed data does not conform to what has been expected on the basis of the null hypothesis, the difference between the observed and expected values, $O_i - E_i$, is large. The chi square statistic is thus small when the null hypothesis is true and large when the null hypothesis is not true. Exactly how large the $\mathcal{X}^2$ value must be in order to be considered large enough to reject the null hypothesis, can be determined from the level of significance and the chi square table. One should remember that the goodness of fit test examines only one variable, while the test of independence is concerned with the relationship between two variables.

The chi square test for independence is conducted by assuming that there is no relationship between the two variables being examined. The alternative hypothesis is that there is some relationship between the variables. The chi square test of independence begins with the hypothesis of no association, or no relationship, between the two variables. In intuitive terms this means that the two variables do not influence each other and are not connected in any way. If one variable changes in value, and this is not associated with changes in the other variable in a predictable manner, then there is no relationship between the two variables.

Test of Association

The chi square statistic is often thought of as a test of association (the opposite of independence) between variables. phi (φ) statistic is used to standardize a measure of association to values between 0 and 1 (with 0 indicating completely independent variables and a value close to 1 indicating a strong association between variables) phi statistic is a measure of strength of association between two categorical variables. It is calculated by using the below mentioned formula

$$(\varphi) = \sqrt{x^2/N}$$

Test of Homogeneity

Another use of x^2 test is in the testing of homogeneity or similarity between frequency distributions or groups.

Conditions for Application of X^2 test

- The total number of observations should be atleast 50 because our assumption in $\mathcal{X}^2$ test is that the differences will be normally distributed. With the small number of observations, this assumption will not hold good.
- No class should contain very few frequencies, i.e. less than 10. If so, two more adjoining classes should be grouped together before calculating the differene between the observed and expected frequencies.
- Chi square tests can only be used on actual numbers (number of events or frequencies) and not on percentages, proportions, means, etc.)

Computation of Chi Square Statistics

Chi square test is also classified as 1 way and 2 way test.

One way Chi Square Test

One way chi square test compares observed frequencies within groups to their expected frequencies. The null hypothesis in this type of test is as follows:

H_0 = 'observed' frequencies are not different from the 'expected' frequencies. Observed frequencies and the expected frequencies are the same.

Research hypothesis: They are different.

f_o = observed frequency

f_e = expected frequency

Chi square statistic can be calculated by using the formula:

$$X^2 = \Sigma \frac{(f_o - f_e)^2}{f_e}$$

Calculate the degrees of freedom.

Degrees of freedom = k – 1, where k is the number of categories.

Compare the calculated value to table value of $\mathcal{X}^2$. The general rule is that if the calculated value of chi square is less than the table value, accept or retain H_0. If the calculated chi square is greater than the table value, reject H_0.

Two way Chi Square

Two way chi square test ascertains that are the differences in responses of two groups statistically significantly different?

One way test checks the values of observed vs expected whereas two way test checks one set of observed frequencies with that of another set. Comparison between frequencies (rather than scores as in 't' or 'F' tests) are made to test the null hypothesis. So, null hypothesis is that the two or more populations do not differ with respect to frequency of occurrence.

Steps in Computation of Chi Square Statistic

- Formulate hypothesis.
- Calculate chi square statistic. To calculate this, one must know the number of observations, expected values and observed values.
- The formula to calculate the $\mathcal{X}^2$ value = $\Sigma \frac{(O-E)^2}{E}$

  O - observed value E - expected value
- Find the degrees of freedom. The formula to find the degrees of freedom is (row-1) (column-1).
- Compare the calculated value with the table value and assess significance level.
- Finally, decide whether to accept or reject the null hypothesis.

Uses of Chi Square Test

I. In Establishing Confidence Intervals

The equation used is

$\mathcal{X}^2 = \frac{\sigma_s^2}{\sigma_p^2}$ (N – 1) where N is the number of items in the sample; (N – 1) is the degrees of freedom; σ_s^2 is the variance of the sample and σ_p^2 is the variance of the population.

Example 1:

σ_s^2 = 50; N = 20. Construct a 95% and 99% confidence interval for the population variance.

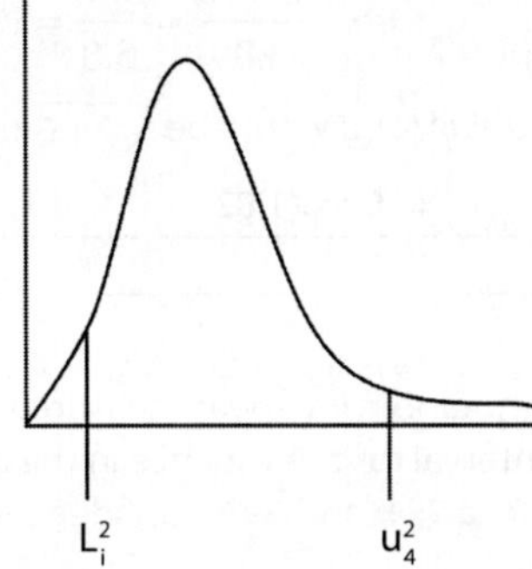

In case of 95% confidence interval, the upper and lower limit of chi square distribution is 0.025 of the area in the upper tail and 0.025 of the area in the lower tail. The values of the upper and lower limit of chi square value can be found in the chi square table.

In our problem, the degrees of freedom is 20 – 1 = 19; and the X_L^2 value is 8.907 and X_U^2 value is 32.852.

The confidence interval is given by:

For lower confidence limit $= \sigma_L^2 = \frac{\sigma_s^2}{X_u^2}$ (N – 1)

$$= \frac{50 \times 19}{32.85} = \frac{950}{32.85} = 28.9$$

For upper confidence limit $= \sigma_u^2 = \frac{\sigma_s^2}{X_L^2}$ (N – 1)

$$= \frac{50 \times 19}{8.9} = \frac{950}{8.9} = 106.74$$

So, a 95% confidence interval for σ would be $\sqrt{28.9} - \sqrt{106.74}$ = 5.4 – 10.33.

For 99% Confidence Interval

The upper and lower limit of chi square distribution is 0.005 of the area in the upper tail and 0.005 of the area in the lower tail. The values of the upper and lower limit of chi square value can be found in the chi square table.

In our problem, the degrees of freedom is 20 – 1 = 19; and the X_L^2 is 6.844 and X_u^2 value is 38.58.

The confidence interval is given by:

$$\text{For lower confidence limit} = \sigma_L^2 = \frac{\sigma_s^2}{X_u^2}(N-1)$$

$$= \frac{50 \times 19}{38.58} = \frac{950}{38.58} = 24.6$$

$$\text{For upper confidence limit} = \sigma_u^2 = \frac{\sigma_s^2}{X_L^2}(N-1)$$

$$= \frac{50 \times 19}{6.8} = \frac{950}{6.8} = 139.7$$

So a 99% confidence interval for σ would be $\sqrt{24.6}$ to $\sqrt{139.7}$

= 5 to 11.82

Example 2:

In 30 adolescent girls the hemoglobin level was measured and the sample variance is 0.8. Find a 95% confidence interval for the variance in the hemoglobin.

$\sigma_s^2 = 0.8$; N = 30. Construct a 95% and 99% confidence interval for the population variance.

In case of 95% confidence interval, the upper and lower limit of chi square distribution is 0.025 of the area in the upper tail and 0.025 of the area in the lower tail. The values of the upper and lower limit of chi square value can be found in the chi square table.

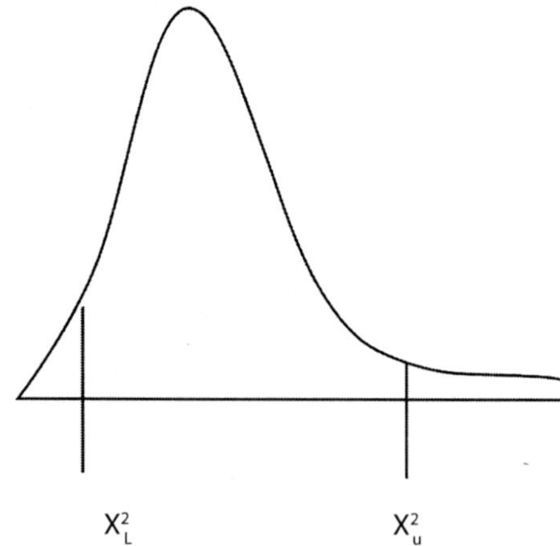

X_L^2 X_u^2

In our problem, the degrees of freedom is 30 – 1 = 29; and the X_L^2 value is 16.05 and X_u^2 value is 45.77.

The confidence interval is given by:

$$\text{For lower confidence limit} = \sigma_L^2 = \frac{\sigma_s^2}{X_u^2}(N-1)$$

$$= \frac{0.8 \times 29}{45.77} = \frac{23.2}{45.77} = 0.51$$

$$\text{For upper confidence limit} = \sigma_u^2 = \frac{\sigma_s^2}{X_L^2}(N-1)$$

$$= \frac{0.8 \times 29}{16.05} = \frac{23.2}{16.05} = 1.45$$

So a 95% confidence interval for the variance in hemoglobin would be 0.51 to 1.45.

For 99% Confidence Interval

The upper and lower limit of chi square distribution is 0.005 of the area in the upper tail and 0.005 of the area in the lower tail. The values of the upper and lower limit of chi square value can be found in the chi square table.

In our problem, the degrees of freedom is 30 – 1 = 29; and the X_L^2 value is 13.12 and X_4^2 value is 52.34.

The confidence interval is given by:

$$\text{For lower confidence limit} = \sigma_L^2 = \frac{\sigma_s^2}{X_u^2}(N-1)$$

$$= \frac{0.8 \times 29}{52.34} = \frac{23.2}{52.34} = 0.44$$

$$\text{For upper confidence limit} = \sigma_u^2 = \frac{\sigma_s^2}{X_L^2}(N-1)$$

$$= \frac{0.8 \times 29}{13.12} = \frac{23.2}{13.12} = 1.77$$

So, a 99% confidence interval for the variance in hemoglobin would be 0.44 to 1.77.

II. Hypothesis Testing for Population Variance

Example 3:

The variance of distribution of weight of infants is hypothesized to be 4 kgs. A sample of 20 infants gives the variance of 6 kgs. Do the 2 variances differ significantly at alpha = 0.05 level?

Null hypothesis: The variance of infants is equal to 4 kgs. or the two variances are the same.

Alternate hypothesis: The variance of infants is not equal to 4 kgs. The two variances differ significantly.

$$\mathcal{X}^2 = \frac{\sigma_s^2}{\sigma_p^2}(N-1) = \frac{6 \times 19}{4} = \frac{114}{4} = 28.5$$

$$\mathcal{X}^2 = 28.5$$

As per Chi square distribution table, for 19 degrees of freedom, the chi square value for lower limit is 8.907($\mathcal{X}^2$ value at 0.025) and for upper limit is 32.852 ($\mathcal{X}^2$ value at 0.975). The chi square value of 28.5 falls in the acceptance region.

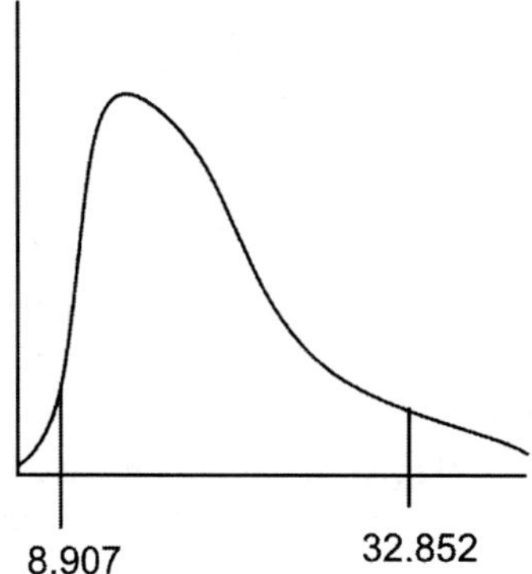

Conclusion: We accept the null hypothesis. The two variances are the same.

Example 4:

A random samples of 10 adolescents give their mean weight as 48 kgs and variance as 22. Test the null hypothesis that the population variance is 60kg against the alternative hypothesis that it is more than 60 kg. α = 0.05.

Null hypothesis: The population variance is 60 kg.

Alternative hypothesis: The population variance is more than 60 kg.

$$\mathcal{X}^2 = \frac{\sigma_s^2}{\sigma_p^2}(N-1) = \frac{22 \times 9}{60} = \frac{198}{60} = 3.3$$

Since population variance is more than the sample variance, this is one tailed test. The table value for $\mathcal{X}^2$ for (10 – 1) degrees of freedom that leaves an area of 0.05 in the upper tail is 16.92. (refer chi square table)

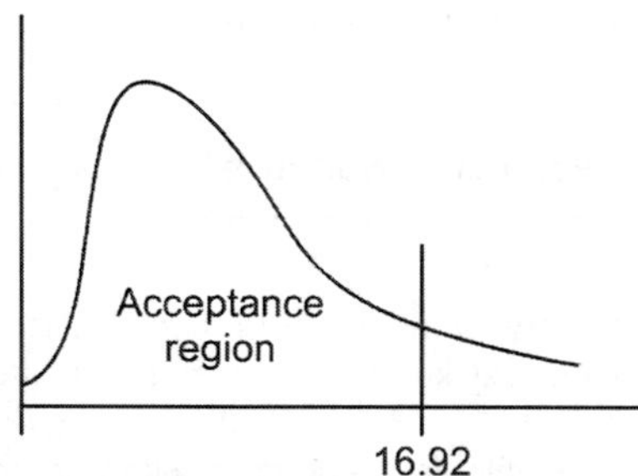

The region from this chi square value to the left tail is the acceptance region. Our calculated value falls within the acceptance region.

Conclusion: We accept the null hypothesis. The population variance is 60 kg.

Example 5:

A random samples of 22 children give their mean height as 110 cm and the variance as 80 cm. Test the null hypothesis that the population variance is 100 cm against the alternative hypothesis that is less than 100 cm. α = 0.05.

Null hypothesis: The population variance is 100 cm.

Alternative hypothesis: The population variance is less than 100 cm.

contd...

$$\mathcal{X}^2 = \frac{\sigma_s^2}{\sigma_p^2}(N-1) = \frac{80 \times 21}{100} = \frac{1680}{100} = 16.8$$

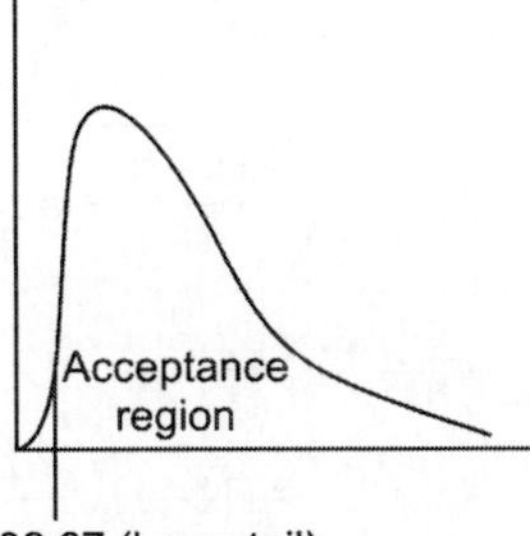

Since, the population variance is lower than the sample variance, this is one tailed test. The table value for $\mathcal{X}^2$ for (22 – 1) degrees of freedom that leaves an area of 0.05 in the lower tail is 32.67. The region from this chi square value to the right tail is the acceptance region. Our calculated value falls within the rejection region.

Conclusion: We reject the null hypothesis. The population variance is less than 100 cm.

Example 6:

The test score of 10 nursing students is as follows:

S. No.	1	2	3	4	5	6	7	8	9	10
Test score	80	78	60	72	56	66	78	62	74	66

Can we say that the variance of the distribution of test score of all students from which the above sample of 10 students was drawn is equal to 60? Test this at 5% and 1% level of significance.

Null hypothesis: The variance of the test score is equal to 60. The sample was drawn from the population with the variance of the test score 60.

Step 1

Calculate the variance of the sample.

Find out the mean test score

$$\bar{x} = \frac{80+78+60+72+56+66+78+62+74+66}{10}$$

$$= \frac{692}{10} = 69.2$$

S. No.	x (Test score)	$(x - \bar{x})$	$(x - \bar{x})^2$
1	80	80 – 69 = 11	121
2	78	78 – 69 = 9	81
3	60	60 – 69 = – 9	81
4	72	72 – 69 = 3	9
5	56	56 – 69 = – 13	169
6	66	66 – 69 = – 3	9

S. No.	x (Test score)	$(x - \bar{x})$	$(x - \bar{x})^2$
7	78	78 – 69 = 9	81
8	62	62 – 69 = – 7	49
9	74	74 – 69 = 5	25
10	66	66 – 69 = – 3	9
n = 10	$\Sigma x = 692$		$\Sigma (x - \bar{x})^2 = 634$

$$\sigma_s = \sqrt{\frac{\Sigma(x-\bar{x})^2}{n-1}} = \sqrt{\frac{634}{10-1}} = \sqrt{\frac{634}{9}} = \sqrt{70.44}$$

Sample variance $\sigma_s^2 = 70.44$

$$\mathcal{X}^2 = \frac{\sigma_s^2}{x_p^2}(N-1) = \frac{70.44 \times 9}{60} = \frac{633.96}{60} = 10.6$$

Degrees of freedom = (10 – 1) = 9

At 5% level of significance the table value for $\mathcal{X}^2 = 16.919$ and at 1% level of significance, the table value for $\mathcal{X}^2 = 21.67$.

The calculated value is less than the table value for chi square at 5% and 1% level of significance.

Conclusion: We accept the null hypothesis. The variance of the test score is equal to 60. The sample was drawn from the population with the variance of the test score 60.

III. Chi Square Test as a Nonparametric Test

Example 7:

A survey conducted among adolescents revealed the frequency of playing violent video games and the level of aggression. Calculate the chi square value and test its significance for the below mentioned data.

Frequency of Playing Violent Video Games	Level of Aggression		
	Low	Moderate	High
1 to 3 days in a week	114	72	6
4 to 6 days in a week	23	30	8
Daily	39	52	6

Null hypothesis: There is no association between the frequency of playing violent video games and the level of aggression in adolescents.

The formula to calculate the $\mathcal{X}^2$ value = $\Sigma \frac{(O-E)^2}{E}$

Observed value

114	72	6	192
23	30	8	61
39	52	6	97
176	154	20	350

Calculation of expected value

Frequency of playing violent video games	Low	Moderate	High
1 to 3 days in a week	$\frac{176 \times 192}{350} = 96.6$	$\frac{154 \times 192}{350} = 84.5$	$\frac{20 \times 192}{350} = 11$
4 to 6 days in a week	$\frac{176 \times 61}{350} = 30.7$	$\frac{154 \times 61}{350} = 26.8$	$\frac{20 \times 61}{350} = 3.5$
Daily	$\frac{176 \times 97}{350} = 48.8$	$\frac{154 \times 97}{350} = 42.7$	$\frac{20 \times 97}{350} = 5.5$

Calculation of chi square value

O	E	O – E	$(O - E)^2$	$(O - E)^2/E$
114	96.6	114 – 96.6 = 17.4	302.8	3.13
72	84.5	72 – 84.5 = – 12.5	156.3	1.9
6	11	6 – 11 = – 5	25	2.3
23	30.7	23 – 30.7 = – 7.7	59.3	1.9
30	26.8	30 – 26.8 = 3.2	10.2	0.4
8	3.5	8 – 3.5 = 4.5	20.3	5.8
39	48.8	39 – 48.8 = – 9.8	96	2.0
52	42.7	52 – 42.7 = 9.3	86.5	2.0
6	5.5	6 – 5.5 = 0.5	0.25	0.05
			Total	19.48

Degrees of freedom = (r – 1) (c – 1)
= (3 – 1) (3 – 1) = 2 × 2 = 4

The table value chi square for 4 degrees of freedom at 5% level of significance is 9.488.

The chi square value for 4 degrees of freedom at 1% level of significance is 13.277

The calculated value of $\mathcal{X}^2$ is much higher than this table value which means that the calculated value cannot be said to have arisen just because of chance. It is significant.

Conclusion: So the null hypothesis is rejected. There is an association between the frequency of playing violent video games and the level of aggression in adolescents.

Example 8:

A survey conducted among adolescents revealed the type of video games played and the level of aggression. Calculate the chi square value and test its significance for the below mentioned data.

Favorite Video Game	Level of Aggression		
	Low	Moderate	High
Racing game	10	40	22
Fighting game	10	71	22
Shooting game	5	70	50

Null hypothesis: There is no association between the type of video games played and the level of aggression in adolescents.

The formula to calculate the X^2 value = $\Sigma\frac{(O-E)^2}{E}$

Observed value

10	40	22	72
10	71	22	103
5	70	50	125
25	181	94	300

Calculation of expected value

Frequency of playing violent video games	Low	Moderate	High
Racing game	$\frac{25\times72}{300}=6$	$\frac{181\times72}{300}=43.4$	$\frac{94\times72}{300}=22.6$
Fighting game	$\frac{25\times103}{300}=8.6$	$\frac{181\times103}{300}=62.1$	$\frac{94\times103}{300}=32.3$
Shooting game	$\frac{25\times125}{300}=10.4$	$\frac{181\times125}{300}=75.4$	$\frac{94\times125}{300}=39.2$

Calculation of chi square value

O	E	O - E	(O - E)^2	(O - E)^2/E
10	06	10 – 6 = 4	16	2.7
40	43.4	40 – 43.4 = – 3.4	11.56	0.27
22	22.6	22 – 22.6 = – 0.6	0.36	0.02
10	08.6	10 – 8.6 = 1.4	1.96	0.23
71	62.1	71 – 62.1 = 8.9	79.21	1.28
22	32.3	22 – 32.3 = – 10.3	106.09	3.3
05	10.4	5 - 10.4 = – 5.4	29.16	2.8
70	75.4	70 – 75.4 = – 5.4	29.16	0.39
50	39.2	50 – 39.2 = 10.8	116.6	2.98
			Total	13.97

Degrees of freedom = (r – 1) (c – 1)
= (3 – 1) (3 – 1) = 2 × 2 = 4

The table value chi square for 4 degrees of freedom at 5% level of significance is 9.488.

The chi square value for 4 degrees of freedom at 1% level of significance is 13.277.

The calculated value of $\mathcal{X}^2$ is higher than this table value which means that the calculated value cannot be said to have arisen just because of chance. It is significant.
Conclusion: So, the null hypothesis is rejected. There is an association between the type of video game played and the level of aggression in adolescents.

Example 9:

A survey was conducted among 100 nursing students to know their choice of college for post graduate studies. The data were as follows:

College A	B	C	D
25	30	37	8

Use $\mathcal{X}^2$ test at 5% level of significance to know if students have any distinct preference towards college.
Null Hypothesis: The nursing students do not have any preference towards the college. Each college can equally attract students, i.e. 25.

Observed value	Expected value	O – E	(O – E)²	(O – E)²/E
25	25	0	0	0
30	25	5	25	1
37	25	12	144	5.76
8	25	–17	289	11.56
			Total	18.32

$$\Sigma\frac{(O-E)^2}{E} = 18.32$$

$$\text{Degrees of freedom} = 4 - 1 = 3$$

The table value of Chi square for 3 degrees of freedom at 5 % level of significance is 7.815.
Conclusion: Calculated value is more than the table value. So we reject the null hypothesis. The nursing students have preference towards the college for their post graduate studies.

Example 10:

The below mentioned data gives the number of students passed and failed after special coaching and regular coaching. Use $\mathcal{X}^2$ test at 5% level of significance to test whether the coaching caused any difference in the results.

	Passed	Failed	Total
Special coaching	30	10	40
Regular coaching	40	20	60
Total	70	30	100

Null hypothesis: There is no difference in the results of special coaching and regular coaching.

Observed value	Expected value	O – E	(O – E)²	(O – E)²/E
30	28	2	4	0.14
10	12	–2	4	0.33
40	42	2	4	0.09
20	18	–2	4	0.22
			Total	0.78

$$\Sigma\frac{(O-E)^2}{E} = 0.78$$

Degrees of freedom = (r – 1)(c – 1) = (2 – 1)(2 – 1) = 1

The table value of Chi square for 1 degree of freedom at 5% level of significance is 3.841.

Conclusion: Calculated value is less than the table value. So we accept the null hypothesis. There is no difference in the results of special coaching and regular coaching.

Example 11:

A sample of 500 college students participated in a study designed to evaluate the level of college students' knowledge of certain common diseases. The following table shows the students classified by major field of study and level of knowledge on diseases:

Major field of study	Adequate	Inadequate	Total
Science	31	91	122
Arts	19	359	378
Total	50	450	500

Do these data suggest that is there a relationship between knowledge on the diseases and major field of study? Let alpha = 0.5

Null hypothesis: There is no relationship between the major field of study and the level of knowledge among the students. The major field of studies and the knowledge levels are independent.

The formula to calculate the $\mathcal{X}^2$ value = $\Sigma\frac{(O-E)^2}{E}$

Observed value

31	91	122
19	359	378
50	450	500

Calculation of expected value

	Adequate	Inadequate
Science	$\frac{50 \times 122}{500} = 12.2$	$\frac{450 \times 122}{500} = 109.8$
Arts	$\frac{50 \times 378}{500} = 37.8$	$\frac{450 \times 378}{500} = 340.2$

Calculation of chi square statistics

Observed Value	Expected Value	O – E	(O – E)²	(O – E)²/E
31	12.2	31 – 12.2 = 18.8	353.44	28.97
91	109.8	91 – 109.8 = – 18.8	353.44	3.22
19	37.8	19 – 37.8 = – 18.8	353.44	9.35
359	340.8	359 – 340.8 = 18.2	331.24	0.97
			Total	42.51

$$\Sigma\frac{(O-E)^2}{E} = 42.51$$

Degrees of freedom = (r – 1) (c – 1) = (2 – 1) (2 – 1) = 1

The table value of Chi square for 1 degrees of freedom at 5% level of significance is 3.841.

Conclusion: Calculated value is more than the table value. So we reject the null hypothesis. There is a relationship between the major field of study and the level of knowledge among the students. They are dependent.

Example 12:

A survey was conducted to assess whether the education on menstrual hygiene was provided to the adolescents girls in their schools. The following results were reported:

Education on Menstrual Hygiene provided

Schools	Yes	No
Urban	58	12
Rural	44	20
Hilly areas	25	12

May we conclude that the education on menstrual hygiene is independent of the location of schools? Let alpha = 0.5.

Null hypothesis: There is no association between the type of school and the provision of education on menstrual hygiene or education on menstrual hygiene is independent of the location of schools.

Observed value

	Yes	No	Total
Urban	58	12	70
Rural	44	20	64
Hill	25	12	37
Total	127	44	171

Expected value

	Yes	No
Urban	$\frac{127 \times 70}{171} = 51.99$	$\frac{44 \times 70}{171} = 18.01$

Contd...

Contd...

	Yes	No
Rural	$\frac{127 \times 64}{171} = 47.5$	$\frac{44 \times 64}{171} = 16.47$
Hill	$\frac{127 \times 37}{171} = 27.48$	$\frac{44 \times 37}{171} = 9.5$

Calculation of chi square statistics

Observed Value	Expected Value	O – E	$(O - E)^2$	$(O - E)^2/E$
58	51.99	58 – 51.99 = 6.01	36.12	0.69
12	18.01	12 – 18.01 = – 6.01	36.12	2.00
44	47.5	44 – 47.5 = – 3.5	12.25	0.26
20	16.47	20 – 16.47 = 3.53	12.46	0.76
25	27.48	25 – 27.48 = – 2.48	6.15	0.22
12	9.5	12 – 9.5 = 2.5	6.25	0.66
Total				4.59

$$\Sigma\frac{(O-E)^2}{E} = 4.59$$

Degrees of freedom = (r – 1)(c – 1) = (3 – 1)(2 – 1) = 2

The table value of Chi square for 2 degrees of freedom at 5% level of significance is 5.991.

Conclusion: Calculated value is less than the table value. So we accept the null hypothesis. There is no association between the type of school and the provision of education on menstrual hygiene.

Example 13:

In a survey conducted among adolescent population, respondents were asked to indicate their level of agreement with the statement: 'Playing video games improve computer skills'. The results were as follows:

Level of agreement					
Gender	**Strongly agree**	**Agree**	**Uncertain**	**Disagree**	**Strongly disagree**
Male	32	48	12	25	15
Female	26	38	10	30	10

Can we conclude on the basis of these data that males and females differ with respect to their levels of agreement on the statement 'Playing violent video games improve computer skills'. Let alpha = 0.5.

Null hypothesis: There is no association between the gender and the level of agreement or males and females do not differ with respect to their levels of agreement on the statement.

Observed value

	Strongly agree	Agree	Uncertain	Disagree	Strongly disagree	Total
Male	32	48	12	25	15	132
Female	26	38	10	30	10	114
Total	58	86	22	55	25	246

Expected value

	Strongly agree	Agree	Uncertain	Disagree	Strongly disagree
Male	31.12	46.15	11.80	29.5	13.41
Female	26.88	39.85	10.20	25.49	11.59

Calculation of chi square statistics

Observed Value	Expected Value	O – E	$(O-E)^2$	$(O-E)^2/E$
32	31.12	32 – 31.12 = 0.88	0.77	0.02
48	46.15	48 – 46.15 = 1.85	3.42	0.07
12	11.8	12 – 11.8 = 0.2	0.04	0.003
25	29.5	25 – 29.5 = – 4.5	20.25	0.69
15	13.41	15 – 13.41 = 1.59	2.53	0.19
26	26.88	26 – 26.88 = – 0.88	0.77	0.03
38	39.85	38 – 39.85 = – 1.85	3.42	0.09
10	10.2	10 – 10.2 = – 0.2	0.04	0.004
30	25.49	30 – 25.49 = 4.51	20.34	0.8
10	11.59	10 – 11.59 = – 1.59	2.53	0.23
			Total	2.13

$$\Sigma\frac{(O-E)^2}{E} = 2.13$$

Degrees of freedom = (r – 1)(c – 1) = (2 – 1)(5 – 1) = 4

The table value of Chi square for 4 degrees of freedom at 5% level of significance is 9.488.

Conclusion: Calculated value is less than the table value. So we accept the null hypothesis. There is no association between the gender and the level of agreement or males and females do not differ with respect to their levels of agreement on the statement.

Example 14:

The hemoglobin level was assessed among adolescent girls of various income status. The results were as follows:

		Hemoglobin level (g/dL)	
Income status	10.0 or greater	9.0 – 9.9	<9.0
Upper income	50	32	10
Middle income	45	40	28
Low income	10	38	25

Do these data provide sufficient evidence to indicate, at the .05 level of significance, that the two variables are related?

Null hypothesis: There is no relationship between the income status and the hemoglobin level of the adolescent girls or the two variables are not related.

Observed value

	10.0 or greater	9.0 – 9.9	<9.0	Total
Upper income	50	32	10	92
Middle income	45	40	28	113
Low income	10	38	25	73
Total	105	110	63	278

Expected value

	10.0 or greater	9.0 – 9.9	<9.0
Upper income	34.75	36.4	20.85
Middle income	42.68	44.7	25.61
Low income	27.57	28.9	16.54

Calculation of chi square statistics

Observed Value	Expected Value	O – E	(O – E)²	(O – E)²/E
50	34.75	50 – 34.75 = 15.25	232.56	6.70
32	36.4	32 – 36.4 = – 4.4	19.36	0.53
10	20.85	10 – 20.85 = – 10.85	117.72	5.65
45	42.68	45 – 42.68 = 2.32	5.38	0.13
40	44.7	40 – 44.7 = – 4.7	22.09	0.49
28	25.61	28 – 25.61 = 2.39	5.71	0.22
10	27.57	10 – 27.57 = – 17.57	308.70	11.20
38	28.9	38 – 28.9 = 9.1	82.81	2.87
25	16.54	25 – 16.54 = 8.46	71.57	4.33
			Total	32.12

$$\Sigma\frac{(O-E)^2}{E} = 32.12$$

Degrees of freedom = (r – 1)(c – 1) = (3 – 1)(3 – 1) = 4

The table value of Chi square for 4 degrees of freedom at 5% level of significance is 9.488.

Conclusion: Calculated value is more than the table value. So we reject the null hypothesis. There is a relationship between the income status and the hemoglobin level of the adolescent girls or the two variables are related.

Example 15:

Symptom which;

Troubled them most	Primipara	Multipara
Vomiting	68	36
Heart burn	32	64

Do these data provide sufficient evidence to indicate that the two populations are not homogeneous with respect to major symptoms? Let alpha = 0.5.

Null hypothesis: The two populations are homogeneous or Primipara and Multipara are same/equal in experiencing in the symptoms.

Observed Value

	Primipara	Multipara	Total
Vomiting	68	36	104
Heartburn	32	64	96
Total	100	100	200

Expected Value

	Primipara	Multipara
Vomiting	52	52
Heartburn	48	48

Calculation of Chi Square Statistics

Observed Value	Expected Value	O – E	$(O-E)^2$	$(O-E)^2/E$
68	52	68 – 52 = 16	256	4.92
36	52	36 – 52 = – 16	256	4.92
32	48	32 – 48 = – 16	256	5.33
64	48	64 – 48 = 16	256	5.33
			Total	20.5

The other method

There is an alternative method of calculating the value of chi square in case of a (2x2) table.

The formula for calculating the value of chi square will be stated as follows:

a	b	a + b
c	d	c + d
(a + b)	(b + d)	N

$$\mathcal{X}^2 = \frac{N.(ad-bc)^2}{(a+c)(b+d)(a+b)(c+d)}$$

$$= \frac{[(68\times 64)-(32\times 36)]^2 \times 200}{100\times 100\times 104\times 96}$$

$$= \frac{200 \times (4352 - 1152)^2}{99840000}$$

$$= \frac{3200 \times 3200 \times 200}{99840000}$$

$$= 2048000000/99840000 = 20.51$$

$$\Sigma \frac{(O-E)^2}{E} = 20.5$$

Degrees of freedom = (r – 1)(c – 1) = (2 – 1)(2 – 1) = 1

The table value of Chi square for 1 degree of freedom at 5% level of significance is 3.841.

Conclusion: Calculated value is more than the table value. So we reject the null hypothesis. The two populations are not homogeneous.

Example 16:

Tests for effectiveness have been conducted on three nursing interventions on pain. The chi square results are as under. What conclusion about the effectiveness of nursing intervention can be drawn on the basis of three samples taken together?

Nursing Intervention	χ^2 Value	df
A	2.68	1
B	4.80	1
C	3.54	1
N = 3	$\chi^2 = 11.02$	3

Null hypothesis: The nursing intervention is not effective in reducing pain.

The table value of Chi square for 3 degrees of freedom at 5% level of significance is 7.815.

Conclusion: Calculated value is more than the table value. So, we reject the null hypothesis. The nursing intervention is effective in reducing the pain.

Example 17:

Using the data given below, test for association between smoking and cancer:

Group	Smoking	No Smoking
Cancer	40	20
No Cancer	10	30

Chi square (χ^2) with one degree of freedom (1df) 5% level = 3.84.

***Null hypothesis:* H_0** = There is no association between smoking and cancer.

Observed frequency tables

Group	Smoking	No Smoking	Total
Cancer	40	20	60
No Cancer	10	30	40
Total	50	50	100

Expected frequency Tables

Group	Smoking	No Smoking	Total
Cancer	$\frac{60 \times 50}{100} = 30$	$\frac{60 \times 50}{100} = 30$	60
No Cancer	$\frac{40 \times 50}{100} = 20$	$\frac{40 \times 50}{100} = 20$	40
Total	50	50	100

Chi square (χ^2) Table

O	E	(O – E)	(O – E)²	$\frac{(O-E)^2}{E}$
40	30	10	100	3.33
20	30	– 10	100	3.33
10	20	– 10	100	5
30	20	10	100	5
				16.66

$$\chi^2 = \Sigma\frac{(O-E)^2}{E}$$

$$\chi^2 = 16.66$$

Alternative method

$$= \frac{N(ad-bc)^2}{(a+b)(c+d)+(a+c)(b+d)}$$

$$= \frac{100[(40\times 30)-(10\times 20)]^2}{(40+20)(10+30)(40+10)(20+30)}$$

$$= \frac{100\times(1200-200)^2}{60\times 40\times 50\times 50} = \frac{100\times 1000\times 1000}{6000000}$$

$$= 100000000/6000000 = 16.66$$

No of degrees of freedom $= (r-1)(c-1)$

$= (2-1)(2-1)$

$= 1$

The table value of 1 degree of freedom at 5% level = 3.84.

Conclusion: H_0 is rejected. The calculated value is greater than the table value. There is an association between smoking and cancer.

Example 18:

A study revealed that among 30 Males , 10 were obese and 20 females, 10 were obese. Use chi square test to find whether gender and obesity are associated.

Null Hypothesis: There is no association between the gender and obesity.

Observed Frequency Table

Sex \ Weight	Obese	Normal weight	Total
Male	10	20	30
Female	10	10	20
Total	20	30	50

Expected Frequency Table

Sex \ Weight	Obese	Normal weight	Total
Male	12	18	30
Female	8	12	20
Total	20	30	50

Chi Square (χ^2) Table

O	E	(O – E)	$(O-E)^2$	$\frac{(O-E)^2}{E}$
10	12	–2	4	0.33
20	18	2	4	0.22
10	8	2	4	0.5
10	12	–2	4	0.33
				1.38

$$\chi^2 = \Sigma\frac{(O-E)^2}{E}$$

$$\chi^2 = 1.38$$

No of degree of freedom $= (r-1)(c-1)$

$= (2-1)(2-1)$

$= 1$

The table value of 1 degree of freedom at 5% level = 3.84.

Conclusion: The calculated value is lesser than the table value. We accept the null hypothesis. There is no association between gender and obesity.

Example 19:

In an epidemic of certain disease, 92 children contracted the disease, of these 41 received no treatment and of these 10 showed after effects. The remainder who did receive treatment, 17 showed after effects. Test the hypothesis that treatment was not effective.

Null Hypothesis: The treatment was not effective.

Observed Frequency Table

	Effects	No effects	Total
No treatment	10	31	41
Received treatment	17	34	51
Total	27	65	92

Expected Frequency Table

	Effects	No effects	Total
No treatment	12	29	41
Received treatment	15	36	51
Total	27	65	92

Chi Square (χ^2) Table

O	E	(O – E)	$(O-E)^2$	$\frac{(O-E)^2}{E}$
10	12	–2	4	0.33
31	29	2	4	0.13
17	15	2	4	0.26
34	36	–2	4	0.11
				0.83

$$\chi^2 = \Sigma\frac{(O-E)^2}{E}$$

$$\chi^2 = 0.83$$

No of degree of freedom $=(r-1)(c-1)$

$= (2-1)(2-1)$

$= 1$

The table value of 1 degree of freedom at 5% level = 3.84.

Conclusion: The calculated value is lesser than the table value. We accept the null hypothesis. The treatment was not effective.

Example 20:

A company manufactures white coats such as large, medium and small size in the ratio of 2:6:2. The sale of different size coats are 300, 500, 200 respectively. Do you think the purchase of coats is different from the earlier one? Alpha = 0.05.

Null hypothesis: The purchase of coats is not different from the earlier one.

$$300 + 500 + 200 = 1000/10 = 100$$

Size	O	E	O – E	$(O-E)^2$	$\frac{(O-E)^2}{E}$
Large	300	200	100	10000	50
Medium	500	600	– 100	10000	16.66
Small	200	200	0	0	0
				Total	66.66

$$\chi^2 = \Sigma\frac{(O-E)^2}{E} = 66.66$$

No of degree of freedom $= 3 - 1 = 2$

The table value of 2 degree of freedom at 5% level = 5.991.

Conclusion: The calculated value is very much higher than the table value. We reject the null hypothesis. The purchase of coat is different from the earlier one.

Application in Nursing Research

The chi square statistic is most appropriate for use with categorical variables, such as marital status whose values are categories like married, single, widowed and divorced. The calculated value of chi square will be small if the observed and expected frequencies are close together and will be large if the difference is large.

The important concern in the chi square test is the frequency in each cell. We can note that when we formulate cross table, there are one or more cells contain the smaller frequency. Many statisticians suggest that the lower limit of a frequency in a cell should be 10 whereas few others suggest a minimum frequency of 5 in a cell. In such case, adjacent categories may be combined to achieve the suggested minimum. Combining reduces the number of categories and therefore, the number of degrees of freedom.

In the use of chi square test for normality, it is not the most appropriate test to use when the hypothesized distribution is continuous. The Kolmogorov -Smirnov test can be used for goodness of fit tests involving continuous distributions.

The chi square test only explains the association or relationship between two variables. The strength and type of association will not be calculated by the chi square test. For example, if you test your null hypothesis that there is an association between smoking and lung cancer which simply states the association. But we cannot conclude smoking causes lung cancer as well as smoking increases the risk of developing lung cancer. Chi square test is not the suitable test to explain the cause and effect. But it gives an idea of association or relationship between two variables.

SUMMARY

- Chi square test is used both as a parametric and non parametric measure. The chi squared distribution is used in chi squared test for goodness of fit and test for independence. Chi squared test is one of the statistical test commonly used to compare observed data with the expected data.
- As a parametric test, it is used to establish confidence interval for the variance of a population and also to compare a sample variance to a theoretical population variance.
- As a non parametric measure it is used as a test of goodness of fit and the test of independence.
- In goodness of fit test, if there is a large discrepancy between the observed and the expected values, the x^2 statistic would be large, suggesting a significant difference between observed and expected values. If the calculated value is small when compared to the table value of chi square, it indicates that the difference is not significant and is the result of sampling fluctuations and can be ignored.
- The formula to calculate the χ^2 value = $\Sigma\frac{(O-E)^2}{E}$

EXERCISE

- In a research, data was collected on number of antenatal mothers who visited two health centers in one month. Find the association between the health center and parity.

Parity	Centre A	Centre B
Primipara	80	60
Multipara	40	28

- The following table given data on number of donors and the blood group. Find out the association between the gender and the blood group.

Gender	O	A	B	AB
Male	20	12	10	8
Female	16	10	8	6

- The data on perceived difficulties in adhering to dietary management and educational status are given. Test is there any statistically significant association.

Educational status	**Perceived difficulties**		
	Low	Medium	High
Nonliterate	9	12	12
School Education	10	10	8
Collegiate Education	8	12	10

- In a study, knowledge and attitude towards antenatal exercise was assessed among antenatal mothers. Calculate the chi square value and test for significance.

Attitude	Knowledge	
	Average	Good
Favorable	30	20
Unfavorable	40	10

- In a study, knowledge and compliance towards dietary management in Chronic Kidney Disease was assessed. Calculate the chi square value and test for significance.

Compliance	Knowledge	
	Inadequate	Adequate
Low	20	10
Moderate	14	8
High	10	12

- In a study, learning needs of parents of children with cerebral palsy was assessed. Find the association between their learning need and their educational status.

Educational status	Learning needs		
	Low	Moderate	High
Nonliterate	20	10	20
School Education	10	10	10
Collegiate Education	10	20	12

- In a research, psychosocial problems experienced by the parents of children with Mental Retardation was assessed. Calculate the chi square and interpret the findings.

Parents	Psychosocial problem		
	Low	Moderate	High
Father	8	20	20
Mother	6	20	12

- In a study, data on parenting style and literacy level of parents were collected to find if there is any association.

	Literacy of parents			
Parenting style	Urban	Urban	Rural	Rural
	Literate	Illiterate	Literate	Illiterate
Authoritarian	7	8	9	19
Permissive	18	22	20	8

- The below given table gives data on the type of family and level of support received by the breastfeeding mothers. Calculate the chi square value and interpret its findings.

Type of family	Level of support		
	Poor	Moderate	Good
Nuclear family	22	18	14
Joint family	16	12	20

- In a study, the data on employment of women and their perceived level of stress were collected to assess if there is any association.

Employment	Level of stres			
	No stress	Mild	Moderate	Severe
Homemaker	19	16	10	8
Self employed	12	12	12	10
Govt Job	11	8	10	6

26 Nonparametric Tests

OBJECTIVES

After reading this chapter, you will be able to:

- Explain the meaning of nonparametric tests
- List out the nonparametric tests
- Calculate various test statistic

INTRODUCTION

A parametric test is one that is based on certain parameters. Nonparametric tests procedure deals primarily with populations that are not normally distributed and considers how to conduct statistical tests if the assumptions of normality are violated. For data that are not normally distributed, the nonparametric tests use other statistical techniques to test hypotheses. These techniques may use the following for the calculation of values.

- Ranked values
- Single group tests of deviation from normality
- Comparisons of frequencies and
- Calculation of the frequency of values above or below a grand median to compare.

Nevertheless, for some kinds of data (such as nominal and ordinal) it would be unwise to assume anything like a normal distribution and in such cases, nonparametric tests should be used. These tests do not make any assumptions about the shape of the population from which the sample scores were drawn and are, therefore, known as ***distribution free*** tests. We may use them regardless of the shape of population. Further, these tests may be applied to data which are not accurately measured against any interval or ratio scale but are classified or ranked only, that is, the researcher is only able to say how much more or less.

Two other merits of these tests are:

- These tests are much easier to learn and to apply than parametric tests.
- These tests are particularly useful in case of small samples—a feature which should be helpful to the researcher collecting pilot study data and to the researcher whose samples must be small because of their very nature (e.g. samples of persons with a rare form of mental illness).

VARIOUS NONPARAMETRIC TESTS

A. One-sample and two-sample Tests
Appropriate for nominal data
1. Chi square test: $\mathcal{X}^2$
2. McNemar test

B. Appropriate for ordinal data
3. Kolmogorov-Smirnov Test : Dn
4. Sign test
5. Wilcoxon signed rank test: T
6. Median test
7. Ordinary one-sample runs test and two-sample runs test
8. Sum of ranks test
9. Mann-whitney test: U
10. Fisher-irwin test
11. Spearman's rank correlation coefficient: Rho

C. K-sample tests (K≥3)
1. Kruskal-Wallis test : H
2. Friedman test
3. Kendall's coefficient of concordance: W

In this unit, few tests are discussed in detail.

Chi Square Test: $\mathcal{X}^2$

Chi square is a very versatile test used both as a nonparametric and a parametric measure. Chi square, symbolically written as $\mathcal{X}^2$ (pronounced as Ki square), is a statistical technique used to compare the sample variance to the theoretical variance. As a nonparametric measure, it is used (i) as a test of goodness of fit, and (ii) as a test of independence. It can be used to determine if categorical data shows dependency or the two classifications are independent. As a parametric measure, it is used to establish confidence intervals for the variance of population. It is used to test the hypothesis that the population variance is the same as the sample. The other uses are explained below:

Use of Chi Square as a Test of Goodness of Fit

Many a time the researcher wants to know how well does the assumed theoretical distribution (such as normal, binomial or poisson or any other based on experience) fit to the observed data. The chi square test gives answer to this. The test measures the actual difference between the expected and observed frequencies and then ascertains whether the difference is so great that it could hardly have occurred accidentally due to sampling fluctuations. This is known by comparing the calculated value of $\mathcal{X}^2$ with the table value at different levels of significance. If the calculated value of $\mathcal{X}^2$ is very small as compared to its table value, it indicates that the difference is not significant. It is the result of sampling fluctuations and can be ignored. The theory adequately describes the fact and, consequently the fit is good. On the other hand, if the calculated value of $\mathcal{X}^2$ is very big as compared to its table value, it indicates that the difference is significant. It is not the result of sampling fluctuations and cannot be ignored. The theory does not adequately describe the fact and, therefore, the fit is not good. In the first case, the results support theory, in the second case, they do not.

Use of Chi Square as a Test of Independence

$\mathcal{X}^2$ test enables the researcher to explain whether or not two attributes are associated. For example, he may be interested in knowing whether a new medicine is effective in controlling fever or not. $\mathcal{X}^2$ test will help him in deciding this issue. In such a situation, he proceeds with the null hypothesis that the two attributes (viz. the new medicine and control of fever) are independent which means that the new medicine is not effective in controlling fever. On this basis he first calculates the expected frequencies and then works out the value of $\mathcal{X}^2$. If this calculated value of $\mathcal{X}^2$ is more than the table value at a predetermined level of significance he may reject the null hypothesis that the two attributes are independent. If it is less than the table value he may conclude that his hypothesis of independence is correct.

In order that we may apply the chi square test either as a test of goodness of fit or as a test to judge the significance of association between attributes, it is necessary that the observed as well as theoretical or expected frequencies must be grouped in the same way and the theoretical distribution must be adjusted to give the same total frequency as we find in case of observed distribution. Chi square is then calculated as follows:

$$\mathcal{X}^2 = \Sigma\frac{(O-E)^2}{E}$$

O = Observed frequency

E = Expected frequency

If two distributions (observed and theoretical) are exactly alike, $\mathcal{X}^2 = 0$. But generally due to sampling errors, chi square is not equal to zero and as such we must know the sampling distribution of $\mathcal{X}^2$ so that we may find the probability of an observed $\mathcal{X}^2$ being given by a random sample from the hypothetical universe. Instead of working out the probabilities, we can use ready table which gives probabilities for given values of $\mathcal{X}^2$. Whether the calculated value of chi square is significant or not can be checked by comparing the table value for a specific degrees of freedom at the specific level of significance. If the calculated value of chi square is more than the table value, the difference between the observed and expected frequencies is taken as significant, but if the calculated value is less than the table value then the difference is considered as insignificant, i.e. considered to have arisen as results of chance and such can be ignored.

For determining degrees of freedom, If there are 10 frequency classes and there is one independent constraint, then there are (10 – 1) = 9 degrees of freedom. Thus, if 'n' is the number of groups and one constraint is placed by making the totals of observed and expected frequencies equal, the df would be equal to (n – 1). In the case of a contingency table, the degrees of freedom is worked out as follows.

df – (r – 1) (c – 1) where 'c' means the number of columns and 'r' means the number of rows.

Points to be Remembered in Using Chi Square Test

- All the items in the sample must be independent.
- Chi square value must be calculated for frequencies and not for percentages or proportions.
- The chi square test is only a test of significance. It is not a measure of association.
- No group should contain very few items, say less than 10. In case where the frequencies are less than 10, regrouping is done by combining the frequencies of adjoining groups so that new frequencies become greater than 10. Some statisticians take this number as 5, but 10 is regarded as better by most of the statisticians. The combination of classes or grouping weakens the sensitivity of the chi square test. If more than one cell contains an expected number less than 1, the chi square test should not be applied.
- Wherever necessary Yates correction for continuity must be applied especially when number involved in the study are small.
- The overall number of items must also be reasonably large. It should normally be at least 50, however small the number of groups may be.
- Symbolically sometimes the degrees of freedom and a given probability level are shown as subscripts. Thus $\chi^2_{05, (8)}$ indicate the χ^2 values with 8 degrees of freedom and p = 0.05.

Alternative Formula

There is an alternative method of calculating the value of χ^2 in the case of a (2 × 2) table. If we write the cell frequencies and margianl totals in case of a (2 × 2) table, thus:

a	b	(a + b)
c	d	(c + d)
(a + c)	(b + d)	N

Then the formula for calculating the value of chi square will be stated as follows:

$$\chi^2 = \frac{N(ad-bc)^2}{(a+c)(b+d)(a+b)(c+d)}$$

Where N means the total frequency, ad means the larger cross product, bc means the smaller cross product and (a + c), (b + d), (a + b) and (c + d) are the marginal totals. The alternative formula is rarely used in finding out the value of chi square as it is not applicable uniformly in all cases but can be used only in a (2 × 2) contingency table.

Yates' Correction

F. Yates has suggested a correction for continuity in χ^2 value calculated in connection with a (2 × 2) table, particularly when cell frequencies are small, i.e. less than 5. But many prefer 10 is better. The correction suggested by Yates is popularly known as ***yates correction***. The rule for correction is to adjust the observed frequency in each cell of a (2 × 2) table in such a way as to reduce the deviation of the observed from expected frequency for that cell by 0.5. But this adjustment is made in all the cells without disturbing the marginal totals. The formula for finding the value of chi square after applying Yates correction can be stated thus:

$$\mathcal{X}^2 \text{(corrected)} = \frac{N(|ad-bc|-0.5N)^2}{(a+b)(c+d)(a+c)(b+d)}$$

In case we use the usual formula for calculating the value of chi square $\mathcal{X}^2 = \frac{\Sigma(O-E)^2}{E}$ then Yates' correction can be applied as under:

$$\mathcal{X}^2 \text{(corrected)} = \frac{\Sigma(|O1-E1|-0.5)^2}{E1} + \frac{(|O2-E2|-0.5)^2}{E2} + \ldots\ldots$$

It may again be emphasized that Yates' correction is made only in case of (2 × 2) table and that too when cell frequencies are small.

Additive Property of Chi Square

An important property of $\mathcal{X}^2$ is its additive nature. This means that several values of $\mathcal{X}^2$ can be added together and if the degrees of freedom are also added, this number gives the degrees of freedom of the total value of $\mathcal{X}^2$.

Important Characteristics of $\mathcal{X}^2$ Test

- This test as a nonparametric test is based on frequencies and not on the parameters like mean and standard deviation.
- This test is used for testing the hypothesis and is not useful for estimation.
- This test is also applied to complex contingency table.

Chi Square as a Test for Comparing Variance

When we want to ascertain that the sample variance is equal to population variance or to compare the sample variance with the population variance, we can calculate the $\mathcal{X}^2$ value by using this formula.

$$\mathcal{X}^2 = \frac{\sigma^2 s}{\sigma^2 p}(n-1) \text{ where}$$

σ^2_s = Variance of the sample

σ^2_p = Variance of the population

(n - 1) = degrees of freedom, n being the number of items in the sample

The calculated $\mathcal{X}^2$ value is compared with the table value for (n - 1) degrees of freedom at a given level of significance, we may either accept or reject the null hypothesis. If the calculated value is less than the table value, the null hypothesis is accepted, but if the calculated value is equal or greater than the table value, the hypothesis is rejected.

Example 1:

Weight of 10 students is as follows:

Sl. No.	1	2	3	4	5	6	7	8	9	10
Weight (kg)	40	38	46	40	43	44	42	50	52	45

Can we say that the variance of the distribution of weight of all students from which the above sample of 10 students was drawn is equal to 15 kgs? Test this at 5% and 1% level of significance?

S. No.	**Weight in Kgs**	**$(x - \bar{x})$**	**$(x - \bar{x})^2$**
1	40	–4	16
2	38	–6	36
3	46	2	4
4	40	–4	16
5	43	–1	1
6	44	0	0
7	42	–2	4
8	50	6	36
9	52	8	64
10	45	1	1
	440		178

$$\text{Mean} = \frac{440}{10} = 44$$

$$\text{Variance} = \frac{\Sigma(x-\bar{x})^2}{N-1} = \frac{178}{9} = 19.78$$

$$\text{Variance} = 19.8$$

Null hypothesis: There is no difference between sample variance and population variance or sample variance is equal to 15 kg.

$$\chi^2 = \frac{\sigma^2 s}{\sigma^2 p}(n-1)$$

$$\chi^2 = \frac{19.78}{15}(10-1) = 1.32 \times 9 = 11.88$$

The degrees of freedom is (n – 1) = 9.

At 5% level of significance, the table value of chi square is 16.92 and at 1% level of significance, it is 21.67 for 9 degrees of freedom. Both these values are greater than the calculated values of chi square that is 11.88. Hence we accept the null hypothesis and conclude that the variance of the given distribution can be taken as 15 kg. In other words, the sample can be said to have been taken from a population with variance of 15 kgs.

Example 2:

A sample of 8 is drawn from a population. The sum of squared deviations from the mean of the given sample is 40. Test the hypothesis that the variance of the population is 6 at 5% level of significance.

$$n = 8$$

$$\Sigma(x - \bar{x})^2 = 40$$

$$\sigma^2_s = \Sigma(x - \bar{x})^2/n - 1$$

$$40/7 = 5.7$$

$$\chi^2 = \frac{\sigma^2 s}{\sigma^2 p}(n-1) = 5.7/6 \times 7$$

$$= 0.95 \times 7 = 6.65$$

$$\text{Degrees of freedom} = (8 - 1) = 7$$

The table value of chi square at 5% level for 7 degrees of freedom is 14.067. The calculated value of chi square is less than the table value, so we accept the null hypothesis and conclude that the variance of population is 6 as given in the question.

MCNEMAR TEST

McNemar test is one of the important tests often used when data is nominal and two related samples. This test is useful with before-after measurement of the same subjects. The experiment is designed for the use of this test in such a way that the subjects initially are divided into equal groups as to their favorable and unfavorable views about something, practice or concept. After some treatment, the same numbers of subjects are asked to express their views about the given system whether they favour it or do not favor it. By using this test, we can assess any significant change in views of the same subjects before and after the treatment by developing a table in respect of the first and second measurement.

	After treatment	
Before treatment	Do not favor	Favor
Favor	A	B
Do not Favor	C	D

A indicates those who give positive response before treatment and negative response after treatment. D indicates those who give negative response before treatment and positive response after treatment. B and D indicate those who give the same response before and after treatment.

Since A + D indicates change in the people's responses, the expectation under null hypothesis is that (A + D)/2 cases change in one direction and the same proportion in other direction. The test statistic under McNemar test is worked out as under:

$$x^2 = \frac{(|A-D|-1)^2}{A+D} \text{ with df} = 1$$

The minus 1 in the above equation is a correction for continuity as the chi square test happens to be a continuous distribution, whereas the observed data represent a discrete distribution.

Example 3:

A survey was conducted among 200 adults to know their response towards smoking. Then the Structured Teaching Program on the health effect of smoking was given and their response towards smoking was reassessed. The details are as follows:

	After STP		
Before STP	No to smoking	Yes to smoking	
Yes to smoking	30	70	100
No to smoking	90	10	100
Total	120	80	200

Test is there any significant change in the people's response before and after Structured Teaching Programme.

Null hypothesis: There is no change in the people's response before and after Structured Teaching Programme.

$$x^2 = \frac{(|A-D|-1)^2}{A+D}$$

$$x^2 = \frac{(|30-10|-1)^2}{30+10} = \frac{(|20|-1)^2}{40} = \frac{19^2}{40} = \frac{361}{40} = 9.025$$

Degrees of Freedom = 1.

Interpretation: The table value for 1 degree of freedom at 5% level of significance is 3.84. The calculated value is more than the table value. Hence the null hypothesis is rejected. We conclude that the change in the people's response before and after structured teaching programme is significant.

Example 4:

In a sample size of 1000 adults, their response towards wearing helmet was assessed. Then they were given instruction regarding the importance of wearing helmet and their response was assessed. The data were as follows: Test whether the instruction is effective in changing the attitude of the adults.

	After Instruction		
Before instruction	Unfavorable	Favorable	Total
Favorable	60	440	500
Unfavorable	60	440	500
Total	120	880	1000

Null hypothesis: There is no change in their people's attitude before and after instruction on wearing helmet. The instruction is not effective.

$$x^2 = \frac{(|A-D|-1)^2}{A+D}$$

$$x^2 = \frac{(|60-440|-1)^2}{60+440} = \frac{(|380|-1)^2}{500} = \frac{(379)^2}{500} = \frac{143641}{500} = 287.28$$

Degrees of Freedom = 1.

Interpretation: The table value for 1 degree of freedom at 5% level of significance is 3.84. The calculated value is more than the table value. Hence the null hypothesis is rejected. We conclude that the change in the people's attitude before and after instruction on wearing helmet is significant. The instruction is effective.

Example 5:

In a certain before-after experiment the response obtained from 2000 respondents, when classified gave the following information. Test whether the distribution of pamphlets have changed their attitude towards alcohol.

	After giving pamphlet		
Before giving pamphlet	Do not favor	Favor	
Favor to alcohol	240	760	1000
Do not favor to alcohol	860	140	1000

Null hypothesis: There is no change in the people's attitude before and after giving pamphlet.

$$x^2 = \frac{(|A-D|-1)^2}{A+D}$$

$$x^2 = \frac{(|240-140|-1)^2}{240+140} = \frac{(|100|-1)^2}{380} = \frac{99^2}{380} = \frac{9801}{380} = 25.79$$

Degrees of Freedom = 1.

Interpretation: The table value for 1 degrees of freedom at 5% level of significance is 3.84. The calculated value is more than the table value. Hence the null hypothesis is rejected. We conclude that the change in the people's attitude before and after giving pamphlet is significant.

Example 6:

600 individuals were shown as advertisement film on a nursing college and their response were counted before and after showing the advertisement. Test at 5% level of significance whether there has been any significant change in the individual's attitude.

	After advertisement	
Before Advertisement	Do not favor	Favor
Favor	100	400
Do not favor	50	50

Null hypothesis: There is no change in the individual's attitude towards college before and after advertisement.

$$x^2 = \frac{(|A-D|-1)^2}{A+D}$$

$$x^2 = \frac{(|100-50|-1)^2}{100+50} = \frac{(|50|-1)^2}{150} = \frac{49^2}{150} = \frac{2401}{150} = 16$$

Degrees of Freedom = 1.

Interpretation: The table value for 1 degree of freedom at 5% level of significance is 3.84. The calculated value is more than the table value. Hence the null hypothesis is rejected. We conclude that the change in the individual's attitude towards college before and after advertisement is significant.

SIGN TEST

Assumption of Sign Test

Data is not normally distributed. This test makes no assumption about the shape of the population distribution, therefore this test can handle a data set that is nonsymmetric, that is skewed either to the left or the right.

A sign test is quite simple to do and applies to both one tailed and two-tailed tests. It is usually based on the binomial distribution. This test is used both in the study of single and paired samples. The sign test utilizes pairwise comparisons of two different distributions to identify which is larger than which and then from this information it determines if the two distributions differ significantly from each other. The sign test sums all the positives, negatives, and ties and then computes z score and a 'p' value associated with the frequency of the positives and negatives. In the former case the steps involved in its application are as under:

(a) First of all, the null hypothesis that there is no difference between the sample mean (or median) and the hypothesized mean (or median) is set up. It is assumed that the population from which the sample has been drawn is symmetrical and the probability of a sample item being greater or less than the hypothesized mean (or median) is equal.
(b) Next, differences between the sample items and the hypothesized mean (or median), i.e. $X - \mu_0$ or $X - Med_H$ are computed and expressed in terms of plus and minus signs. If any item happens to be exactly equal to the hypothesized value (resulting into zero difference), then it is simply ignored and the sample size is considered correspondingly reduced.
(c) Next, the number of times the less frequent sign (plus or minus) occurs among the differences is counted as success and denoted as *r*.
(d) Next, with *N* as the number of trails and $p = q = \frac{1}{2}$, the cumulative probability of r is either calculated or seen in Table in Appendix.
(e) Last, the computed value of probability is compared with the prefixed significance level (1% or 5%) and if the computed value is smaller than the alpha, the null hypothesis is rejected and if it is greater, the null hypothesis accepted.

Other Method

As already mentioned, calculate the + and - sign for the given distribution. Put a + sign for a value greater than the mean value, and put a - sign for a value less than the mean value. Put 0 as the value is equal to the mean value; pairs with 0 as the mean value are considered ties. Denote the total number of signs by 'n' (ignore the zero sign) and the number of less frequent signs by 'r.' Obtain the critical value (K) at .05 of the significance level by using the following formula in case of small samples:

$$\text{The critical value } K = \frac{n-1}{2} - 0.98\sqrt{n}$$

Sign test in case of large sample:

$$Z = \frac{S - np}{\sqrt{np(1-p)}}$$

Compare the value of 'r' with the critical value (K). If the value of r is greater than the value of K, then the null hypothesis is accepted. If the value of the r is less than the critical value of K, then the null hypothesis is rejected. In the case of large samples, S (Success) is compared with the Z value.

I. Sign Test for Single Samples

Example 7:

On 15 days, the number of patients attending skin OPD is as follows:

3, 6, 3, 8, 8, 5, 8, 7, 1, 8, 6, 6, 5, 8, and 5. Use sign test at 5% level of significance to verify that the average number of patients attending skin OPD is 5.

Null hypothesis: The average number of patients attending skin OPD is 5. In order to test this hypothesis, we first workout the difference between the observed values and the hypothesized value (μ = 5) and state the difference in plus or minus signs as under.

3	6	3	8	8	5	8	7	1	8	6	6	5	8	5
–	+	–	+	+	0	+	+	–	+	+	+	0	+	0

Total plus = 9

Total minus = 3

Total zero = 3

The sample size is reduced to 12.

One can find from the table, the cumulative binomial probability for N = 12, r = 3 and p = 0.5. It is 0.0729. that is (0.0002 + 0.0029 + 0.0161 + 0.0537). The rule is that if the computed value is smaller than the alpha, the null hypothesis is rejected and if it is greater, the null hypothesis accepted. Since this value is greater than the prefixed alpha level of 0.05, we accept the null hypothesis. We conclude that the average number of patient attending skin OPD is 5.

Other method: In the above example, total plus = 9; total minus=3; total zero = 3; the sample size is reduced to 12.

The critical value $K = \frac{n-1}{2} - 0.98\sqrt{n}$

The critical value $K = \frac{12-1}{2} - 0.98\sqrt{12} = 5.5 - 0.98 \times 3.46 = 5.5 - 3.39 = 2.11$

K = 2.11; r = 3.

The general rule is that if the value of k is lesser than the value of r, then the null hypothesis is accepted. If the value of the K is greater than the value of r, then the null hypothesis is rejected.

The null hypothesis is accepted. We conclude that the average number of patient attending skin OPD is 5.

Example 8:

The following data relate to the Hb level of 10 adolescent girls. 11, 10.5, 9.8, 12, 11.4, 11.6, 11, 10.8, 10.9 and 11.2. Use sign test to test the null hypothesis that the average Hb value of adolescent girls is 11.

Null hypothesis: The average Hb value of adolescent girls is 11.

11	10.5	9.8	12	11.4	11.6	11	10.8	10.9	11.2
0	–	–	+	+	+	0	–	–	+

Total plus = 4

Total minus = 4

Total zero = 2

The sample size is reduced to 8.

n = 8; r = 4; p = 0.5

One can find from the table, the cumulative binomial probability for N = 8, r = 4 and p = 0.5. It is 0.6367 that is (0.0039 + 0.0312 + 0.1094 + 0.2188 + 0.2734). The rule is that if the computed value is smaller than the alpha, the null hypothesis is rejected and if it is greater, the null hypothesis accepted. Since this value is greater than the prefixed alpha level of 0.05, we accept the null hypothesis. The average Hb value of adolescent girls is 11.

Other Method

$$\text{The critical value K} = \frac{n-1}{2} - 0.98\sqrt{8}$$

$$\text{The critical value K} = \frac{8-1}{2} - 0.98\sqrt{8} = 3.5 - 0.98 \times 2.83 = 3.5 - 2.77 = 0.73$$

K = 0.73; r = 4.

The general rule is that if the value of k is lesser than the value of r, then the null hypothesis is accepted. If the value of the K is greater than the value of r, then the null hypothesis is rejected.

K is lesser than r. We accept the null hypothesis. The average Hb value of adolescent girls is 11.

Example 9:

The number of students absented for 15 months is as follows:

Use sign test at 5% level of significance to verify that the average number of students absented per month is 5.

4	8	2	7	7	5	7	6	3	8	6	7	5	7	5

Null hypothesis: The average number of students absented per month is 5. In order to test this hypothesis, we first work out the difference between the observed values and the hypothesized value and state the difference is plus or minus signs as under.

4	8	2	7	7	5	7	6	3	8	6	7	5	7	5
–	+	–	+	+	0	+	+	–	+	+	+	0	+	0

Total plus – 9

Total minus – 3

Total zero – 3

The sample size is reduced to 12.

One can find from the table, the cumulative binomial probability for N = 12, r = 3 and p = 0.5. It is 0.0729 that is (0.0002 + 0.0029 + 0.0161 + 0.0537). The rule is that if the computed value is smaller than the alpha, the null hypothesis is rejected and if it is greater, the null hypothesis accepted. Since this value is greater than the prefixed alpha level of 0.05, we accept the null hypothesis. The average number of students absented per month is 5.

Other method: In the above example, Total plus = 9; Total minus=3; Total zero = 3; The sample size is reduced to 12.

$$\text{The critical value K} = \frac{n-1}{2} - 0.98\sqrt{n}$$

The critical value

$$K = \frac{12-1}{2} - 0.98\sqrt{12} = 5.5 - 0.98 \times 3.46 = 5.5 - 3.39 = 2.11$$

K = 2.11; r = 3.

The general rule is that if the value of k is lesser than the value of r, then the null hypothesis is accepted. If the value of the K is greater than the value of r, then the null hypothesis is rejected.

The null hypothesis is accepted. We conclude that the average number of students absented per month is 5.

Example 10:

The following data relate to the blood glucose level of a sample for 30 days. Use sign test to test the null hypothesis that the sample's average blood glucose level is 108 as against the alternative hypothesis $\mu < 108$ at 0.05 level of significance.

120	110	114	100	110	108	106	122	110	112	114	116	118
100	102	104	106	108	110	120	114	116	118	114	100	106
108	106	106	110									

Null hypothesis: The sample's average blood glucose level is 108.

Alternative hypothesis: The sample's average blood glucose level is less than 108.

We first work out the difference between the observed values and the hypothesized value and state the difference is plus or minus signs as under.

+	+	+	–	+	0	–	+	+	+	+	+	+	–
–	–	–	0	+	+	+	+	+	+	–	–	0	–
–	+												

Total plus – 17

Total minus – 10

Total zero – 3

The sample size is 27.

If N is more than 25, we can use the normal approximation to the binomial distribution.

$$\text{Standard error of proportion} = \sqrt{\frac{pq}{N}} = \sqrt{\frac{0.5 \times 0.5}{27}} = \sqrt{\frac{0.25}{27}} = \sqrt{0.009} = 0.096.$$

(assuming p = 0.5)

For testing the null hypothesis, a one tail test with critical region on the left is to be used. From the table of normal curve area, we find that Z value for 0.45 area of the curve is 1.64. Using this, we can work out the limit of acceptance region as under:

p – Z SE(prop)

0.5 – 1.64 × 0.096

0.5 – 0.16 = 0.34

The observed proportion of success is 17/27 = 0.63 which falls in the acceptance region. We accept the null hypothesis.

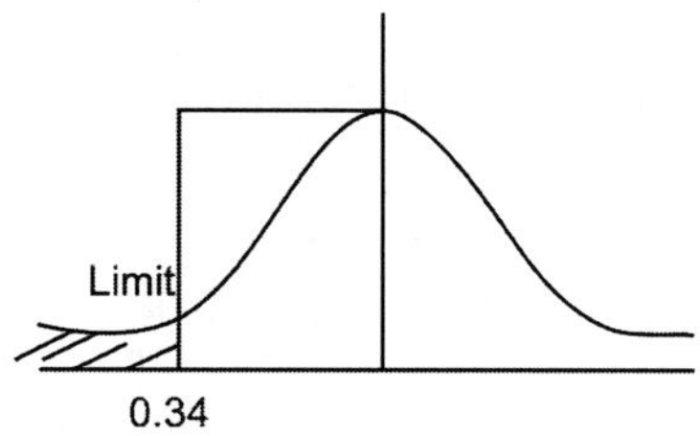

Other method: sign test in case of large sample

$$Z = \frac{S-np}{\sqrt{np-(1-p)}} = \frac{10-27\times 0.5}{\sqrt{27\times 0.5-(1-0.5)}} \frac{10-13.5}{\sqrt{(13.5-0.5)}} = \frac{3.5}{\sqrt{13}} = \frac{3.5}{3.61} = 0.96$$

S – No. of less frequent sign

n – No. of sample

p – Probability

The probability value is greater than prefixed alpha value, i.e. 0.05. We accept the null hypothesis.

Example 11:

The following are the marks of 9 MSc(N) students in the subject Nursing Research and Statistics. Test the null hypothesis that the average mark is 68.

64	70	72	69	80	78	74	62	66
–	+	+	+	+	+	+	–	–

Null hypothesis: The average mark is 68.

Total plus – 6

Total minus – 3

The sample size is 9

p – 0.5

One can find from the table, the cumulative binomial probability for N = 9, r = 3 and p = 0.5. It is 0.254 that is (0.0020 + 0.0176 + 0.0703 + 0.1641). The rule is that if the computed value is smaller than the alpha, the null hypothesis is rejected and if it is greater, the null hypothesis accepted. Since this value is greater than the prefixed alpha level of 0.05, we accept the null hypothesis. The average mark is 68.

Other method: In the above example, Total plus = 6; Total minus=3; The sample size is reduced to 9.

The critical value $K = \frac{n-1}{2} - 0.98\sqrt{n}$

The critical value $K = \frac{9-1}{2} - 0.98\sqrt{9} = 4 - 0.98 \times 3 = 4 - 2.94 = 1.06$

K = 1.06; r= 3.

The general rule is that if the value of k is lesser than the value of r, then the null hypothesis is accepted. If the value of the K is greater than the value of r, then the null hypothesis is rejected.

The null hypothesis is accepted. We conclude that the average mark is 68.

II. Sign Test for Paired Samples

Example 12:

Two nonpharmacologic techniques were used to reduce the pain during postoperative period in two groups of children. The pain was measured using 10 point pain scale in two groups after administering these techniques. The data were given below. Use sign test at 5% level of significance to test the null hypothesis that there is no difference in the pain score in using these techniques against the alternative hypothesis that there is significant difference.

Technique 1	6	4	6	8	2	4	4	6	4	6	8	4
Technique 2	4	6	8	8	4	4	2	4	2	4	6	4

Null hypothesis: There is no difference in the pain score in using these techniques.

Technique 1	6	4	6	8	2	4	4	6	4	6	8	4
Technique 2	4	6	8	8	4	4	2	4	2	4	6	4
difference	+	–	–	0	–	0	+	+	+	+	+	0

No. of plus 6
No. of minus 3
No. of Zero 3

One can find from the table, the cumulative binomial probability for N = 9, r = 3 and p = 0.5. It is 0.254 that is (0.0020 + 0.0176 + 0.0703 + 0.1641). The rule is that if the computed value is smaller than the alpha, the null hypothesis is rejected and if it is greater, the null hypothesis accepted. Since this value is greater than the prefixed alpha level of 0.05, we accept the null hypothesis. Their is no difference in the pain score in using these techniques.

Other method: In the above example, Total plus = 6; Total minus=3; Total zero = 3; The sample size is reduced to 9.

The critical value $K = \frac{n-1}{2} - 0.98\sqrt{n}$

The critical value $K = \frac{9-1}{2} - 0.98\sqrt{9} = 4 - 0.98 \times 3 = 4 - 2.94 = 1.06$

K = 1.06; r= 3.

The general rule is that if the value of k is lesser than the value of r, then the null hypothesis is accepted. If the value of the K is greater than the value of r, then the null hypothesis is rejected.

The null hypothesis is accepted. We conclude that there is no difference in the pain score in using these techniques.

Example 13:

The table below shows the duration of analgesic effect (in hours) provided by drug A and drug B. Is there any evidence that drug A provides longer relief than drug B?

Drug A	6	4	5	4	6.5	3.5	4	9	8	3	5
Drug B	4	4	4	2	4	4	4	6	5	3	4

Null hypothesis: Drug A and drug B are equal in pain relief duration.

Drug A	6	4	5	4	6.5	3.5	4	9	8	3	5
Drug B	4	4	4	2	4	4	4	6	5	3	4
Difference	+	0	+	+	+	–	0	+	+	0	+

Total pluses – 7
Total minuses – 1
Total Zero – 3
The sample size is reduced to 8

The critical value $K = \frac{n-1}{2} - 0.98\sqrt{n}$

The critical value $K = \frac{8-1}{2} - 0.98\sqrt{8} = 3.5 - 0.98 \times 2.83 = 3.5 - 2.77 = 0.73$

K = 0.73; r = 1.

The general rule is that if the value of k is lesser than the value of r, then the null hypothesis is accepted. If the value of the K is greater than the value of r, then the null hypothesis is rejected.

The null hypothesis is accepted. We conclude that drug A and drug B are equal in pain relief duration.

WILCOXON SIGNED RANK TEST: T

Unlike the Sign Test which is based on only the number of plus or minus signs, this test utilizes both the signs and magnitudes of the differences. This makes it more sensitive and powerful than the ordinary sign test.

Wilcoxon Signed Rank Test also applies both to single and paired samples. Following are the steps involved in applying this test to a single sample (Table 26.1).

1. Set up the H_0 that there is no difference between the sample mean or median and the hypothesized mean or median.
2. Find the differences (d) between the sample items and the hypothesized mean or median, i.e. $X - \mu_0$ or $X - Med_{H.}$
3. Assign the ranks to all differences (except zero differences) in increasing order of absolute magnitude disregarding signs. If 2 or more of the differences have the same value, give them a rank which is the average of the ranks they would have had if they had differed. Thus, if the two numerically lowest values of d happen to be '3' give 1.5 ranks (which is the mean of ranks 1 and 2) to each '3'.
4. Assign the same signs to the ranks which their original differences possessed.
5. Total the positive and negative ranks separately. The smaller of the 2 rank sums is our test statistic T.

6. Compare the calculated value of T with the critical value of T given in Table in the Appendix for the given number of matched pairs (dropping the number of pairs with difference = 0) at the desired level of significance. If the calculated T is equal to or less than the table value of T, reject the null hypothesis. Otherwise accept it.

Table gives values of T for numbers up to 25 only. For N larger than 25, the test statistic Z should be worked out as under:

$$Z = \frac{T - \text{Mean}}{\sigma} \text{ where Mean} = \frac{N(N+1)}{4} \text{ and } \sigma = \sqrt{\frac{N(N+1)(2N+1)}{24}}$$

While calculating the above mean and σ dropped out pairs should not be counted in *N*. The decision about H_0 should be taken in the same manner as described.

The test is applied to paired samples also in the same way as described above. The null hypothesis in such cases is that there is no difference in the means or medians of the two-paired samples.

Example 14:

The following are the scores obtained by the samples in experimental and control group. Test at 0.05 level of significance that experimental group performed better than the control group.

Experimental group	80	90	70	40	20	80	80	70	80
Control group	70	94	82	60	40	70	80	78	78

Null hypothesis: There is no significant difference in performance between experimental and control group.

Alternative hypothesis: Experimental group performed better than control group.

Experimental group	Control group	Difference(d)	Rank	Rank with signs	
80	70	10	4.5	4.5	
90	94	–4	2		–2
70	82	–12	6		–6
40	60	–20	7.5		–7.5
20	40	–20	7.5		–7.5
80	70	10	4.5	4.5	
80	80	0	0		
70	78	–8	3		–3
80	78	2	1	1	
				10	–26

Add here

N = Number of matched pairs – Number of dropped out pairs.

N = 9 – 1 = 8

T = Smaller of the two sums (negative ranks and the positive ranks).

N = 8; T = 10

The table value of T at 5% level of significance when N = 8 is 4. The calculated value is more than the table value. We accept the null hypothesis. There is no significant difference in experimental and control group.

Example 15:

16 preterm infants were fed a special diet from 7 months onwards. Their weight gain was as follows:

6.3	6.8	7.9	6.5	6.4	6.3	6.5	6.4	7.6	7.4	6.6	6.6	6.7	7.3	6.9	7.6

Can we conclude from these data that the diet results in a mean weight gain of less than 7.0 kg. Test at 0.05 level of significance.

Null hypothesis: The mean weight gain is equal to or more than 7 kg.

Alternative hypothesis: The diet results in mean weight gain of less than 7 kg.

Weight of Infants	Difference(d) D = x − 7	Rank	Rank with signs	
6.3	−0.7	15	−14.5	
6.8	−0.2	2	−2	
7.9	0.9	16		16
6.5	−0.5	9	−8.5	
6.4	−0.6	12	−11.5	
6.3	−0.7	14	−14.5	
6.5	−0.5	8	−8.5	
6.4	−0.6	11	−11.5	
7.6	0.6	10		11.5
7.4	0.4	7		6
6.6	−0.4	6	−6	
6.6	−0.4	5	−6	
6.7	−0.3	4	−3.5	
7.3	0.3	3		3.5
6.9	−0.1	1	−1	
7.6	0.6	13		11.5
		Total	−87.5	48.5

N = 16; T = 48.5

The calculated value (48.5) is greater than the table value 30 (when N=16, at 0.05 level of significance). We accept the null hypothesis. The mean weight gain is equal to or more than 7 kg.

Example 16:

The reduction of weight in kgs were given below. Can we conclude that the average weight reduction is not equal to 4 kg.

5	6	8	2	4	6	4	5	7	9

Null hypothesis: The average weight reduction is equal to 4 kg.

Alternate hypothesis: The average weight reduction is not equal to 4 kg.

Weight	Difference(d) D = x − 4	Rank	Rank with signs	
5	1	1.5	1.5	
6	2	4	4	
8	4	7	7	
2	−2	−4		−4
4	0			
6	2	4	4	
4	0			
5	1	1.5	1.5	
7	3	6	6	
9	5	8	8	
		Total	32	−4

N = 9; T = 4

The calculated value (4) is lesser than the table value 6 (when N = 9, at 0.05 level of significance). We reject the null hypothesis. The average weight reduction is not equal to 4 kg.

Example 17:

The mid arm circumference of under 5 children before and after dietary supplementation was measured. Can we conclude from these data that the dietary supplementation is effective? Test at 0.05 level of significance.

Before	12	13	14	11.5	12.5	13	11.5
After	12	13.5	14	12	13	12.5	12

Null hypothesis: Dietary supplementation is not effective.
Alternative hypothesis: Dietary supplementation is effective.

Before	After	Difference	Rank	Rank with signs	
12	12	0			
13	13.5	−0.5	3	−3	
14	14	0			
11.5	12	−0.5	3	−3	
12.5	13	−0.5	3	−3	
13	12.5	0.5	3		3
11.5	12	−0.5	3	−3	
			Total	−12	3

T = 3; N = 5

The calculated value (3) is greater than the table value zero (0) (when N = 5 at 0.05 level of significance). We reject null hypothesis. Dietary supplementation is effective.

Example 18:

The table below shows the duration of analgesic effect (in hours) provided by drug A and drug B. Is there any evidence that drug A provides longer relief than drug B. Use Wilcoxon signed rank test.

Drug A	6	4	5	4	6.5	3.5	4	9	8	3	5
Drug B	4	4	4	2	4	4	4	6	5	3	4

Null hypothesis: Drug A and drug B are equal in pain relief duration.
Alternative hypothesis: Drug A provides longer relief than drug B.

Drug A	Drug B	Difference	Rank	Rank with signs	
6	4	2	5.5	5.5	
4	4	0			
5	4	1	2.5	2.5	
4	2	2	5.5	5.5	
6.5	4	1.5	4	4	
3.5	4	–0.5	–1		–1
4	4	0			
9	6	3	7.5	7.5	
8	5	3	7.5	7.5	
3	3	0			
5	4	1	2.5	2.5	
			Total	35	–1

N = 8; T = 1

The calculated value 1 is lesser than the table value 4 (when N = 8 at 0.05 level of significance). We reject null hypothesis. We conclude that Drug A provides longer relief than drug B.

MEDIAN TEST

We have seen above that in 2-sample studies, both the ordinary Sign Test and the Wilcoxon Test require the samples to be paired. If the samples are unpaired, as is very often the case, the use of these tests should be avoided. Median Test should be preferred in such situations. This test can be used even when more than 2 samples are being studied.

Steps:

- Set up the null hypothesis that the given samples belong to populations with the same median and that there is no significant difference in their scores.
- Through together the scores of all samples and work out a common median.
- Find out sample wise the number of scores which are above and below the common median.

- Draw a 2 × k table. One side of this table will always consist of 'above' and 'below' the common median categories and the other side will consist of the different sample groups. Fill in the different cells of this table with numbers.
- Calculate Chi square and interpret the results.

Example 19:

Patient satisfaction on care given by staff A and B were assessed from 10 patients who received care from staff A and B.

Staff A	60	50	70	72	68	58	76	78	68	68
Staff B	62	58	60	70	70	65	76	76	68	76

Test at 0.05 level of significance that two population medians are different.

Null hypothesis: The two population medians are different.

Arrangement of the data in ascending order.

50, 58, 58, 60, 60, 62, 65, 68, 68, 68, 68, 70, 70, 70, 72, 76, 76, 76, 76, 78

Median = 69

	Above median	Below median
Staff A	4a	6b
Staff B	5c	5d

a + b = 10; c + d = 10; a + c = 9; b + d = 11

$$\mathcal{X}^2 = \frac{n(ad-bc)^2}{(a+c)(b+d)(a+b)(c+d)} = \frac{20(20-30)^2}{9\times 11\times 10\times 10}$$

$$= \frac{20(-10)^2}{99\times 100} = \frac{2000}{9900} = 0.202$$

Degrees of freedom = (Row – 1)(Column – 1)

= (2 – 1) (2 – 1) = 1

The table value for $\mathcal{X}^2$ for 1 degree of freedom at 5% level of confidence is 3.841. The computed value is lesser than the table value. We accept the null hypothesis.

Example 20:

A random sample of 15 adolescent children from school A was selected and their general well being was assessed. Another random samples of 18 students were selected from school B and their general well being was assessed. The score was as follows.

School A	78	62	66	70	65	80	58	56	60	50	62	76	54	64	66			
School B	62	66	70	78	76	60	58	64	68	72	74	76	78	80	56	58	60	66

Test whether students from school A and School B differ with respect to their level of general well being? Let alpha = 0.05 level.

Null hypothesis: The general well being of adolescent children from school A and school B is same.

Arrangement of data in ascending order

50	54	56	56	58	58	58	60	60	60	62	62
62	64	64	65	66	66	66	66	68	70	70	72
74	76	76	76	78	78	78	80	80			

$$\text{Median} = \left(\frac{N+1}{2}\right) \text{th item} = \frac{34}{2} = 17\text{th item.}$$

$$\text{Median} = 66$$

	Above median	Below median
School A	4a	9b
School B	9c	7d

$$a + b = 13; c + d = 16; a + c = 13; b + d = 16$$

$$\mathcal{X}^2 = \frac{n(ad-bc)^2}{(a+c)(b+d)(a+b)(c+d)} = \frac{33(28-81)^2}{13 \times 16 \times 13 \times 16}$$

$$= \frac{33(-53)^2}{43264} = \frac{92697}{43264} = 2.14$$

$$\text{Degrees of freedom} = (\text{Row} - 1)(\text{Column} - 1)$$
$$= (2 - 1)(2 - 1) = 1$$

The table value for $\mathcal{X}^2$ for 1 degree of freedom at 5% level of confidence is 3.841. The computed value is lesser than the table value. We accept the null hypothesis.

SUM OF RANKS TEST

This test is used to test the hypothesis that 2 independent groups of 8 or more observations have been drawn at random from the same population and hence there is no real difference between them.

1. Rank the entire set of scores of the 2 groups in ascending order from smallest to largest. Assign mean of the ranks to each of the tied observations.
2. Total the ranks separately for each group and check that these 2 totals denoted as $\Sigma(R_1)$ and $\Sigma(R_2)$ sum up to $\frac{N(N+1)}{2}$.
3. Compute σ scores (denoted as Z_1 and Z_2) for the 2 rank totals by the following formula:

$$\text{Sample 1: } Z_1 = \frac{2\Sigma(R_1) - N_1(N+1)}{\sqrt{\frac{N_1N_2(N+1)}{3}}}$$

$$\text{Sample 2: } Z_2 = \frac{2\Sigma(R_2) - N_2(N+1)}{\sqrt{\frac{N_1N_2(N+1)}{3}}}$$

4. Check that the two Zs equals each other with opposite sign.
5. Refer to the normal distribution table. If the computed values of Z at the given level of significance fall in the rejected region, reject the null hypothesis of 'no difference' between the 2 groups, otherwise accept the hypothesis.

Example 21:

Two groups of nursing college students, 8 in each group, earn the following scores:

A:	19	28	14	23	14	17	12	15
B:	25	23	29	15	27	21	24	20

Do the two groups differ significantly? Apply the sum of ranks test.

Null hypothesis: There is no difference between the two groups.

In our problem, following are the ranks assigned to various scores in the entire group of 16 students.

Group A:	19	28	14	23	14	17	12	15
Ranks:	7	15	2.5	10.5	2.5	6	1	4.5
Group B:	25	23	29	15	27	21	24	20
Ranks:	13	10.5	16	4.5	14	9	12	8

$N_1 = 8$; Sum of $R_1 = 49$; $N_2 = 8$; Sum of $R_2 = 87$; $N = 16$

$$R_1 + R_2 = \frac{N(N+1)}{2} = \frac{16(16+1)}{2} = \frac{16 \times 17}{2} = \frac{272}{2} = 136$$

$$Z_1\text{(Sample A)} = \frac{2\Sigma(R_1) - N_1(N+1)}{\sqrt{\frac{N_1 N_2 (N+1)}{3}}}$$

$$Z_1\text{(Sample A)} = \frac{2(49) - 8(16+1)}{\sqrt{\frac{8 \times 8(16+1)}{3}}} = \frac{98 - 136}{\sqrt{\frac{64 \times 17}{3}}}$$

$$= \frac{-38}{\sqrt{362.67}} = \frac{-38}{19.04} = -2$$

$$Z_2\text{(Sample B)} = \frac{2(87) - 8(16+1)}{\sqrt{\frac{8 \times 8(16+1)}{3}}} = \frac{174 - 136}{\sqrt{\frac{64 \times 17}{3}}}$$

$$= \frac{38}{\sqrt{362.67}} = \frac{38}{19.04} = 2$$

At 0.05 level of significance, the table value of $Z = \pm 1.96$. The computed values fall in the rejection regions. Therefore we reject the null hypothesis. We conclude that there is a significant difference between the two groups A and B.

ONE SAMPLE RUNS TEST

One Sample Runs Test is used to know whether the observations in a given series can be regarded as random. This is done by ascertaining the number of runs which are present in a series. A run is a sequence of like symbols which are followed and preceded by other kinds of symbols or no symbol on either side. A sequence of symbols exhibiting a pattern of symbols is usually indicative of lack of randomness. For instance, looking at a sequence of persons waiting for the bus at a bus stop, we observed the following sequence of males (M) and females (F);

M/F/M/F/M/F/M/F/M/F/M/F/M/F

This sequence shows a definite pattern, i.e. the males and females are standing alternatively. Look at the below mentioned sequence.

MMMMMMM/FFFFFFF

This shows clustering of males and females which indicates lack of randomness.

It is not always that we have sequence of symbols. Any data at hand can be converted into runs. Look into the below given sequence.

MM	FF	M	F	MM	FF	MMM
1	2	3	4	5	6	7

The above sequences have 7 runs.

n_1 = Number of occurrences of type one
n_2 = Number of occurrences of type two
r_1 = Number of runs of type one
r_2 = Number of runs of type two
r = Total number of runs.

We begin with the null hypothesis that the symbols occur in random order against the alternative hypothesis that they do not occur in random order.

Mean of r can be calculated by using the formula $\mu_r = \frac{2n_1n_2}{n_1+n_2}+1$ and standard error of r can be calculated as given below:

$$\text{Standard error r} = \sqrt{2n_1n_2\frac{(2n_1n_2-n_1-n_2)}{(n_1+n_2)^2(n_1+n_2-1)}}$$

Example 22:

The following were the arrangement of the MS(N) students of College of Nursing A(12) and B(16) based on their results in university examination. Test this sample for randomness at 1% level of significance.

FF PPP FF PP FF P F PPP FF PPP F PPPP FF

$n = 28; n_1 = 12; n_2 = 16$

$r = 13; r_1 = 7; r_2 = 6$

For this the normal curve approximation can be assumed.

$$\mu_r = \frac{2n_1n_2}{n_1+n_2}+1$$

$$\textbf{\textit{Standard error r}} = \sqrt{2n_1n_2\frac{(2n_1n_2-n_1-n_2)}{(n_1+n_2)^2(n_1+n_2-1)}}$$

$$\mu_r = \frac{2\times12\times16}{12+16}+1 = \frac{384}{28}+1 = 13.71 + 1 = 14.71$$

$$\textbf{\textit{Standard error r}} = \sqrt{2\times12\times16\times\frac{(2\times12\times16-12-16)}{(12+16)^2(12+16-1)}}$$

$$= \sqrt{384\times\frac{384-28}{(28)^2(27)}} = \sqrt{384\times\frac{356}{784\times27}}$$

$$= \sqrt{384\times\frac{356}{21168}} = \sqrt{384\times0.017} = \sqrt{6.528} = 2.55$$

By consulting the normal curves area table, we find the appropriate Z value for 0.495 of the area of the curve and it is 2.58. Hence, the limits of our acceptance region are:

Upper limit = μ_r + (2.58)(2.55) = 14.71 + 6.58 = 21.29

Lower limit = μ_r – (2.58)(2.55) = 14.71 – 6.58 = 8.13

The observed number of runs in our case is 13 which falls inside the acceptance region. Hence, we accept the null hypothesis at 1% level of significance. This means that the results are random.

RANK SUM TEST

Rank sum test are a whole family of test, but we shall describe only two such test which are commonly used. U test and H test popularly known as ***Wilcoxon-Mann-Whitney*** U test and ***Kruskal Wallis H test***.

MANN-WHITNEY TEST: U

This is a very popular test amongst the rank sum tests. This test is used to determine whether two independent samples have been drawn from the same population. It uses more information than the sign test or the Fisher Irwin test. This test applies under very general conditions and requires only that the populations sampled are continuous (Table 26.1).

Steps

1. Set up the null hypothesis that the 2 samples have been drawn from the same population and that there is no difference in their scores.
2. Throw together all the scores of the 2 samples and rank them in ascending or descending order indicating beside each symbol of the sample. In case 2 or more scores are equal, give average of ranks to all.
3. Sum up separately the ranks assigned to the scores of the 2 samples as $\Sigma(R_1)$ and $\Sigma(R_2)$.

4. Calculate the statistic U for any one of the two samples. U for the first sample (denoted as U_1) is equal to $(N_1N_2) + \frac{N(N+1)}{2} - \Sigma(R_1)$. Similarly, U for the second sample (denoted as U_2) is equal to $(N_1N_2) + \frac{N(N+1)}{2} - \Sigma(R_2)$.
   It is immaterial which sample is denoted as the first sample.
   If any one U(U_1 or U_2) has been calculated, the other can also be determined by the relationship $U_1 = (N_1 N_2) - U_2$.
5. If N_1 and N_2 lie between 9 and 20, the smaller of the calculated values of U_1 and U_2 should be compared with the critical value of U given in Table for $\sigma = 0.05$ for a two-tail test. If the calculated U is less than or equal to the table value of U, H_0 is rejected, otherwise not (This is because the smaller the U obtained, the more likely it is that the group represents a distribution of ranks that is different from the distribution represented by the other group).
   If N_1 and N_2 are so large that the critical values cannot be determined by table, a normal approximation can be made and Z value decided as under:

$$Z_\mu = \frac{U-\mu_u}{\sigma_u}, \text{ where } \mu_u = \frac{N_1 \times N_2}{2} \text{ and}$$

$$\sigma_\mu = \sqrt{\frac{(N_1 \times N_2)(N_1 + N_2 + 1)}{12}}$$

Thus,

$$Z\mu = \frac{U - |N_1 \times N_2 / 2|}{\sqrt{\frac{(N_1 \times N_2)(N_1 \times N_2 + 1)}{2}}}$$

This is interpreted in the same way as we have been doing previously in the case of normal deviate tests.

Example 23:

Following are the scores of 12 randomly selected students at the Model examination and University examination.

Model Exam:	55	57	72	90	57	74
University Exam:	80	76	63	58	56	37

Test the null hypothesis that the distribution of scores on the two examinations is the same.

Null hypothesis: The distribution of scores on the two examinations is the same.

Model Exam	R_1	University exam	R_2
55	2	80	11
57	4.5	76	10
72	8	63	7
90	12	58	6
57	4.5	56	3
74	9	37	1
Total	40	Total	38

$$u_1 = n_1 n_2 + \frac{n_1(n_1+1)}{2} - R_1$$

$$u_1 = 6\times 6 + \frac{6(6+1)}{2} - 40 = 36 + (21) - 40$$

$$= 57 - 40 = 17$$

$$u_2 = n_1 n_2 + \frac{n_2(n_2+1)}{2} - R_2$$

$$u_2 = 36 + \frac{6\times 7}{2} - 38 = 36 + (21) - 38 = 57 - 38 = 19$$

The critical value for Mann-Whitney U for $n_1 = 6$ and $n_2 = 6$ at the significance level alpha, 0.05 is 5. The computed value of U is 19. In a two tailed test, the value of U obtained equals the smaller of U_1 or U_2. This is greater than the table value. Hence we accept the null hypothesis. The distribution of scores on the two examinations is the same.

Example 24:

Calculate Mann Whitney U test value for following hemoglobin data and give your interpretation.

Study group:	6	9	10	11	14		
Control group:	9	12	8	10	11	12	14

Null hypothesis: There is no difference in two groups with regard to hemoglobin level. The hemoglobin levels in both groups are same.

Study group	R_1	Control group	R_2
6	1	10	5.5
8	2	11	7.5
9	3.5	11	7.5
9	3.5	12	9.5
10	5.5	12	9.5
		14	11.5
		14	11.5
	15.5		62.5

$$u_1 = n_1 n_2 + \frac{n_1(n_1+1)}{2} - R_1$$

$$u_2 = n_1 n_2 + \frac{n_2(n_2+1)}{2} - R_2$$

$$u_1 = 5\times 7 + \frac{5(5+1)}{2} - 15.5 = 35 + \frac{30}{2} - 15.5$$

$$u_1 = 35 + 15 - 15.5 = 34.5$$

$$u_2 = 5\times 7 + \frac{7(7+1)}{2} - 62.5 = 35 + \frac{56}{2} - 62.5$$

$$u_2 = 35 + 28 - 62.5 = 0.5$$

The critical value of 'U' for $n_1 = 5$ and $n_2 = 7$ at 0.05 level of significance is 5. Calculated value is 0.5. The calculated value is less than the table value. We reject the null hypothesis. There is a difference in two groups with regard to hemoglobin level. The hemoglobin levels in both groups are different.

Example 25:

A survey is conducted to test the difference between 2 alternative methods of teaching. A sample of 20 students is selected at random. Two groups of 10 students each of equal ability are formed and taught by different methods. A standardized test is then given to both the groups and the following marks (out of 100) are scored by the 10 students in each group.

Group A:	39	45	48	46	51	56	72	85	67	73
Group B:	41	68	45	63	85	78	87	62	84	88

Test the significance of difference between the performances of the 2 groups by using U test for alpha 0.05 level.

Null Hypothesis: The difference between the performances of the 2 groups is not significant.

Group A	Rank	Group B	Rank
39	1	41	2
45	3.5	68	12
48	6	45	3.5
46	5	63	10
51	7	85	16.5
56	8	78	15
72	13	87	19
85	16.5	62	9
67	11	84	18
73	14	88	20
Total	85	Total	125

$$u_1 = n_1 n_2 + \frac{n_1(n_1+1)}{2} - R_1$$

$$u_2 = n_1 n_2 + \frac{n_2(n_2+1)}{2} - R_2$$

$$u_1 = 10 \times 10 + \frac{10(10+1)}{2} - 85 = 100 + \frac{110}{2} - 85$$

$$u_1 = 100 + 55 - 85 = 70$$

$$u_2 = 10 \times 10 + \frac{10(10+1)}{2} - 125 = 100 + \frac{110}{2} - 125$$

$$u_2 = 100 + 55 - 125 = 30$$

The critical value of 'U' for $n_1 = 10$ and $n_2 = 10$ at 0.05 level of significance is 23. Calculated value is 30. The calculated value is greater than the table value. We accept the null hypothesis. The difference between the performances of the 2 groups is not significant.

The above problem can also be solved by applying normal approximation and calculating Z as under.

Thus $$Z_m = \frac{U - |N_1 \times N_2/2|}{\sqrt{\frac{(N_1 \times N_2)\ (N_1 + N_2 + 1)}{2}}}$$

$$Z_m = \frac{30 - \left|\frac{10 \times 10}{2}\right|}{\sqrt{\frac{(10 \times 10)(10 + 10 + 1)}{12}}} = \frac{30 - |50|}{\sqrt{\frac{100 \times 21}{12}}}$$

$$= \frac{20}{\sqrt{\frac{100 \times 21}{12}}} = \frac{20}{\sqrt{\frac{2100}{12}}} = \frac{20}{\sqrt{175}} = \frac{20}{13.23} = 1.5$$

Since the calculated value of 1.5 is less than 1.96, we accept the null hypothesis.

KRUSKAL-WALLIS H TEST

The Kruskal-Wallis H test is analogous to a one-way between subjects ANOVA for ranked data. It assumes that the study involves one independent variable and that there are three or more independent samples with at least five participants in each sample. The null hypothesis is that all conditions represent the same distribution of ranks in the population (Table 26.1).

Table 26.1: Parametric procedures and their nonparametric counterparts

Sl. No.	Type of design	Parametric test	Nonparametric test
1.	Two independent samples	Independent samples 't' test	Mann-Whitney U or Rank Sums test
2.	Two dependent samples	Dependent samples 't' test	Wilcoxon T test
3.	Three or more independent samples	Between subjects ANOVA	Kruskal-Wallis H test
4.	Three or more dependent samples	Within subject ANOVA	Friedman chi square test

The Steps in Computation of Kruskal-Wallis H Test

1. Assign ranks, using all scores in the experiment.
2. Compute the sum of the ranks in each condition.
3. Compute the sum of squares between groups.

   $$\text{SS between} = \frac{\Sigma R_1^2}{n_1} + \frac{\Sigma R_{21}^2}{n_2} + \ldots\ldots\ldots + \frac{\Sigma R_k^2}{n_k}$$. For each level, square the sum of the ranks and then divide that quantity by the n in the level. (There may be a different n in each level).

4. Compute the Hobt.

$$\text{Hobt.} = \left[\frac{12}{n(N+1)}\right] SS_{bn} - 3(N+1)$$ where N is the total N of the study.

5. Find the critical value of H in the chi square table. Values of H have the same sampling distribution as chi square. The degrees of freedom are df = k – 1, where k is the number of levels in the factor.
6. Compare the obtained value of H to the critical value of chi square.

If the computed value is greater than the table value, Ho is rejected. If it is less, Ho is acceptable.

Example 26:

A study explores the relationship between the year of study and the attitude towards nursing profession among nursing students. The data is as given below:

Year of study		
I	II	III
Score	Score	Score
10	24	68
28	27	71
26	35	57
39	44	60
6	58	62

***Null hypothesis*:** There is no relationship between the year of study and the students' attitude towards their profession.

1. ***Assign ranks, using all scores in the experiment.***

I year		II Year		III Year	
Score	Rank	Score	Rank	Score	Rank
10	2	24	3	68	14
28	6	27	5	71	15
26	4	35	7	57	10
39	8	44	9	60	12
6	1	58	11	62	13
Sum of R	21	Sum of R	35	Sum of R	64

Compute the sum of the ranks in each condition.

Sum of R_1 = 21; Sum of R_2 = 35; Sum of R_3 = 64

Compute the sum of squares between groups.

$$\text{SS between} = \frac{\Sigma R_1^2}{n_1} + \frac{\Sigma R_{21}^2}{n_2} + \ldots\ldots\ldots + \frac{\Sigma R_k^2}{n_k}$$

$$\text{SS between} = \frac{(21)^2}{5} + \frac{(35)^2}{5} + \ldots\ldots\ldots + \frac{(64)^2}{5}$$

$$\text{SS between} = \frac{441}{5} + \frac{1225}{5} + \ldots\ldots\ldots + \frac{4096}{5} = 88.2 + 245 + 819.2 = 1152.4$$

Compute the Hobt.

$$H_{obt.} = \left[\frac{12}{N(N+1)}\right] SS_{bn} - 3(N+1) \text{ where N is the total N of the study.}$$

$$H_{obt.} = \left[\frac{12}{15(15+1)}\right] 1152.4 - 3(15+1)$$

$$H_{obt.} = \left[\frac{12}{15 \times 16}\right] 1152.4 - 3 \times 16 = \left[\frac{12}{240}\right] 1152.4 - 48$$

$H_{obt.} = 0.05 \times 1152.4 - 48$

57.62 – 48 = 9.62

Find the critical value of H in the chi square table. Values of H have the same sampling distribution as chi square. The degrees of freedom are df = k – 1, where k is the number of levels in the factor.

k = 3; in the chi square table for alpha at 0.05 and df = 2, the critical value is 5.99.

Compare the obtained value of H to the critical value of chi square.

H obtained is larger than table value of chi square. We reject the null hypothesis. So it is significant. There is a relationship between the year of study and the students' attitude towards their profession.

Example 27:

A major city hospital established OPD services at 3 different locations. The number of patients attended the OPD on 10 days is given below:

Location A	Location B	Location C
99	83	89
64	102	98
101	125	56
85	61	105
79	91	87
88	96	90
97	94	87
95	89	101
90	93	76
100	75	89

Using H test, can you say at 5% level of significance that the OPD services have the same number of patients.

Null Hypothesis: The number of patients attending OPD services at 3 locations are not same.

1. ***Assign ranks, using all scores in the experiment.***

Location A		Location B		Location C	
Score	**Rank**	**Score**	**Rank**	**Score**	**Rank**
99	24	83	7	89	13
64	3	102	28	98	23
101	26.5	125	30	56	1
85	8	61	2	105	29

Contd...

Contd...

Location A		Location B		Location C	
Score	**Rank**	**Score**	**Rank**	**Score**	**Rank**
79	6	91	17	87	9.5
88	11	96	21	90	15.5
97	22	94	19	87	9.5
95	20	89	13	101	26.5
90	15.5	93	18	76	5
100	25	75	4	89	13
Sum of R	161	Sum of R	159	Sum of R	145

Compute the sum of the ranks in each condition.

Sum of R_1 = 161; Sum of R_2= 159; Sum of R_3 = 145

Compute the sum of squares between groups.

$$\text{SS between} = \frac{\Sigma R_1^2}{n_1} + \frac{\Sigma R_{21}^2}{n_2} + \ldots\ldots\ldots + \frac{\Sigma R_k^2}{n_k}$$

$$\text{SS between} = \frac{(161)^2}{10} + \frac{(159)^2}{10} + \ldots\ldots\ldots + \frac{(145)^2}{10}$$

$$\text{SS between} = \frac{25921}{10} + \frac{25281}{10} + \ldots\ldots\ldots + \frac{21025}{10}$$

$$= 2592.1 + 2528.1 + 2102.5 = 7222.7$$

Compute the Hobt.

$$H_{obt.} = \left[\frac{12}{N(n+1)}\right] SS_{bn} - 3(N+1) \text{ where N is the total N of the study.}$$

$$H_{obt.} = \left[\frac{12}{30(30+1)}\right] 7222.7 - 3(30+1)$$

$$H_{obt.} = \left[\frac{12}{30 \times 31}\right] 7222.7 - 3 \times 31 = \left[\frac{12}{930}\right] 7222.7 - 93$$

$H_{obt.} = 0.013 \times 7222.7 - 93$

$93.9 - 93 = 0.9$

Find the critical value of H in the chi square table. Values of H have the same sampling distribution as chi square. The degrees of freedom are df = k – 1, where k is the number of levels in the factor.

k = 3; in the chi square table for alpha at 0.05 and df = 2, the critical value is 5.99.

Compare the obtained value of H to the critical value of chi square.

H obtained is lesser than table value of chi square. We accept the null hypothesis. The number of patients attending OPD services at 3 locations are not same.

SUMMARY

- A parametric test is one that is based on certain parameters. Nonparametric tests procedure deals primarily with populations that are not normally distributed and considers how to conduct statistical tests if the assumptions of normality are violated.

- Nonparametric tests are much easier to learn and to apply than parametric tests. These tests are particularly useful in case of small samples.
- Chi square is a very versatile test used both as a nonparametric and a parametric measure. Chi square, symbolically written as $\mathcal{X}^2$ (pronounced as Ki square), is a statistical technique used to compare the sample variance to the theoretical variance. As a nonparametric measure, it is used as a test of goodness of fit, and as a test of independence. It can be used to determine if categorical data shows dependency or the two classifications are independent.
- McNemar test is often used when data is nominal and two related samples. This test is useful with before-after measurement of the same subjects.
- A sign test is quite simple to do and applies to both one-tailed and two-tailed tests. It is usually based on the binomial distribution. This test is used both in the study of single and paired samples.
- Wilcoxon Signed Rank Test, unlike the sign test which is based on only the number of plus or minus signs, this test utilizes both the signs and magnitudes of the differences. This makes it more sensitive and powerful than the ordinary sign test. It also applies both to single and paired samples.
- Mann-Whitney U test is a very popular test amongst the rank sum tests. This test is used to determine whether two independent samples have been drawn from the same population. It uses more information than the sign test or the Fisher-Irwin test. This test applies under very general conditions and requires only that the populations sampled are continuous.
- The Kruskal-Wallis H test is analogous to a one-way between subjects ANOVA for ranked data. It assumes that the study involves one independent variable and that there are three or more independent samples with at least five participants in each sample. The null hypothesis is that all conditions represent the same distribution of ranks in the population.

EXERCISE

McNemar test

- Use McNemar test and state at 5% level of significance whether there is any significant change in the people's attitude before and after intervention.

	After reading	
Before reading	Do not recommend	Recommend
Recommend	12	88
Do not recommend	10	6

- Use McNemar test and state at 5% level of significance whether there is any significant change in the people's attitude towards yoga.

	After Yoga	
Before yoga	Do not favor	Favor
Favor	80	400
Do not favor	50	100

- Use McNemar test and state at 5% level of significance whether there is any significant change in the people's attitude before and after health education.

	After health education	
Before health education	Do not favor	Favor
Favor	10	24
Do not favor	10	30

Sign test

- The weight of 8 newborn babies are as follows: Test the null hypothesis that the average birth weight of babies is 2.9 kg.

2.5	2.9	3.0	3.2	2.0	2.7	2.8	2.9

- The calories intake of a adolescent girls were as follows: Test the null hypothesis that the average calorie intake was more than 1800.

Sample No.	1	2	3	4	5	6	7	8
Calorie intake	1750	1850	1900	1700	1850	1900	1700	1750

- The number of students admitted into 12 nursing colleges were as follows. Test the null hypothesis that the average number of students admitted are less than 40 for BSc(N) programme.

College	11	2	3	4	5	6	7	8	9	10	11	12
No. admitted	45	48	30	35	36	37	38	40	45	46	44	40

- The following data show the rating of faculty performance before and after a change in the wage plan. Use the sign test to see whether the change in wage plan has increased the performance. Test at 0.05 level of significance.

Before	6	5	8	4	7	6	7	8	5	6
After	8	8	8	6	8	7	6	8	6	7

- Use Sign test to see whether there is a difference between the number of days leave taken by the students after leave regulation.

Before	6	11	4	8	7	2	10	4	6	1	2
After	5	10	2	12	5	0	12	3	2	1	0

- A student satisfaction rating survey was conducted before and after introduction of curriculum change. Use the sign test to see whether the change in curriculum has increased the student's satisfaction. Test at 0.05 level of significance.

Before	3	5	8	4	5	3	4	4	5	7	6	4	2	7	6	6	5	5	4	4	5	8
After	7	6	9	7	8	6	8	7	8	9	8	8	7	8	8	7	7	7	5	6	7	4

Wilcoxon Signed Rank test

- A psychologist assessed the mental health of 15 adolescent children and the data were as follows:

60	70	80	78	60	50	72	76	80	82	62	74	66	84	68

Can we conclude that the mean score of mental health is equal to 70? Let alpha = 0.05.

- The hemoglobin values of 12 adolescent girls were as follows:

10.5	11	10.2	9.5	8.8	7.5	12	11.6	12.5	13	11	10.8

Can we say that the mean hemoglobin level is less than 10 gm/dL? Let alpha 0.05.

- A researcher assessed the well being score before and after selected psychological intervention among adolescent girls. The data were as follows:

Before	15	11	10	14	16	18	12	10	8	18	12	14
After	18	13	14	15	15	16	16	16	12	15	15	16

Can we conclude that the intervention is effective in increasing the well being?

- A researcher assessed the effectiveness of foot reflexology on pain? The data were as follows:

Pain before	8	6	4	5	7	6	5	3	6	7	8
Pain after	6	5	4	6	6	5	4	3	4	6	6

Can we conclude that foot reflexology is effective in reducing pain. Let alpha = 0.05.

Median test

- The following random blood glucose levels were obtained from random samples of 16 adults from community and 14 adults from the hospital. Would you conclude at 0.05 level of significance that the medians of the two population samples are different?

Community:	90	96	100	102	88	78	86	80	130	140	200	200	150	160	130	146
Hospital:	88	140	160	180	200	78	86	98	100	110	106	182	190	88		

- The following were the marks obtained by the students from two nursing colleges in the University exam in the subject Nursing Education. Can we conclude at 0.05 level of significance that the median marks obtained in the Nursing education subject is same?

College A:	70	72	75	68	52	58	80	82	74	76	70	66	60
College B:	80	78	76	70	56	50	58	70	74	78	68	66	62

- 16 nursing colleges from each of two districts were given score to measure their performance. The scores were as follows:

District 1:	80	78	90	96	70	88	76	70	82	84	80	90	88	86	78	70
District 2:	72	74	80	78	82	86	84	80	90	92	80	88	76	76	70	72

Test whether colleges from two districts differ with respect to their median score of performance? Let alpha = 0.05 level.

Mann-Whitney U test

- The days of hospital stay of cholera in two hospitals H1 and H2 during an outbreak were as given below:

H1:	10	14	12	13	16	9	4	7	18	12	7	11
H2:	15	11	16	16	18	13	18	9	17	18	13	15

Do this data prove that treatment of Cholera is better at H1 given that the better the treatment the shorter the hospital stay?

- A large hospital recruits most of its nurses from the two popular nursing colleges in the area. Over the last year, they have been giving a test to the newly graduated nurses entering the hospital to determine which college, if either seems to educate its nurses better. Based on the following scores, help the personnel office of the hospital determine whether the colleges differ in quality. Use the Mann-Whitney U test with 5% level of significance.

College A:	97	69	73	84	76	92	90	88	84	87
College B:	88	99	65	69	97	84	85	89	91	90

Kruskal-Wallis H test

- Nurses working in three hospitals A, B, and C scored on job satisfaction. The data were as given below:
  Test the hypothesis that the nurses working in the 3 hospitals have identical distribution of scores at significance level alpha = 0.1. Apply H test.

No. of staffs	Hospitals		
	A	B	C
1	33	32	55
2	38	15	68
3	39	87	27
4	48	32	88
5	58	22	46
6	70	63	52
7	61	56	76
8	41	57	–
9	45	44	–
10	49	–	–

- The following are the marks obtained by students studying in 3 colleges on a same test. Use the Kruskal-Wallis test at the 0.05 level of significance to test the null hypothesis that there is no difference in the average marks obtained by the students studying in 3 different colleges.

No. of Students	College		
	A	B	C
1	30	39	29
2	41	28	41
3	34	39	26
4	43	29	36
5	33	30	41
6	34	31	43
7	38	44	38
8	26	43	38
9	29	40	35
10	39	33	40

27 Application of Statistics in Psychology and Education

OBJECTIVES

After reading this chapter, you will be able to:

- Understand interpretation of test scores
- Explain T scoring
- Explain Z scoring
- Understand validity and reliability.

INTRODUCTION

In the field of psychology and education, we conduct many tests and are interpreted for various purposes. There are intelligence test, attitude test, aptitude test, personality test, etc. These tests are conducted to see the individual's performance in those areas as well as to compare and interpret how far is his performance with the standard values. Basically, the interpretation of test scores is based on two concepts. They are norms and reliability. In the process of interpretation, the raw scores obtained from the individuals are standardized since the raw score does not make any sense. The standardized scores help in comparison of individuals and communities.

NORMS

In most cases, scores on psychological tests are interpreted by reference to norms that are based upon the distribution of scores obtained by a representative sample of examinees, i.e. the process of standardizing a test against an appropriate norm group so that test users can make sense out of individual test scores. A norm group consists of a sample of examinees that are representative of the population for whom the test is intended. The very objective of test standardization is to determine the distribution of raw scores in the norm group, which helps the test developer to establish norms; for example norm like age and grade equivalent, percentile rank, i.e. the performance of other person from the same age, grade, sex and so on.

Age Norm

Age norm is used to depict the level of test performance for each separate age group in the normative sample. The purpose of age norm is to compare same age group as per the age norms. The performance of an examinee is interpreted in relation to standardization subjects of the same age.

Grade Norms

Grade norms are widely used with standardized achievement test. Grade norms depict the level of test performance for each grade in the normative sample. These are much useful in school achievement where the grade-wise curriculum is similar to all the children and it is compared with the standard normative sample. Here, grade is more appropriate when compared to age. The raw scores of a particular grade sample are converted into grade equivalent.

Percentile Rank

Percentile rank or percentile score indicates a student's relative position in a group in terms of the percentage of students scoring lower. For instance, if a student gests a raw score of 50 and his percentile rank is 70, that means 70% of the students in the group who appeared for the same test have obtained a score below 50 marks.

Calculation of percentile rank:

$$100 - \frac{100R - 50}{N}$$

For instance, Devaki ranks 7th in her class of 50 students. Six students rank above her, 43 students below her. Her percentile rank is

$$100 - \frac{100R - 50}{N} = 100 - \frac{100 \times 7 - 50}{50} = 100 - \frac{700 - 50}{50} = 100 - \frac{650}{50}$$

$$= 100 - 13 = 87$$

Devaki got 87th percentile rank in her class.

If Kalpana ranks 22nd in her class of 40 students, the percentile rank is calculated as follows:-

$$100 - \frac{100 \times 22 - 50}{40} = 100 - \frac{2200 - 50}{40} = 100 - \frac{2150}{40}$$

$$= 100 - 53.75 = 46.25$$

Kalpana secured 46.25th percentile rank in her class.

Standard Scores

This is also another method of indicating a student's relative position in a group by showing how far this raw score is above or below average. The standard scores are the expression of test performance in standard deviation units from the mean. As we all know, mean is the arithmetic average, and standard deviation is a measure of the spread of scores in a group. These standard scores are mostly explained in terms of normal probability curve.

A standard score uses the standard deviation of the total distribution of raw scores as the fundamental unit of measurement. Standard score expresses the distance from the mean in standard deviation units.

Some of the important standard scores, which are popularly used are:

- Z score
- T score
- Stanines (Stay-nine).

Z SCORE

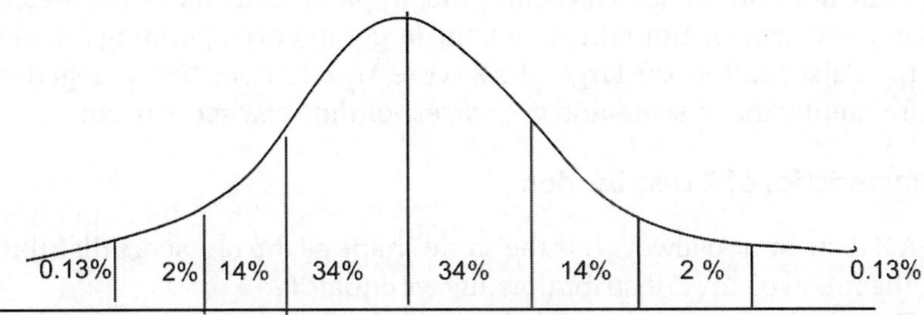

Fig. 27.1: Z distribution

Z score is the distance a raw score deviates from the mean when measured in standard deviations. It is a single number that summarizes a raw score's relative standing. A Z score describes a raw score's location in terms of the number of standard deviations the score is from the mean.

The symbol of a Z score is Z. The formula for transforming a raw score of a sample into a Z score is

$$Z = \frac{x - \bar{x}}{s_x} = \frac{\text{Raw score} - \text{Mean}}{\text{Standard deviation}}$$

For example, if x = 68; mean = 60; and standard deviation = 3.5, the Z score is calculated as follows:

$$Z = \frac{x - \bar{x}}{s_x} = \frac{68 - 60}{3.5} = \frac{8}{3.5} = 2.28$$

For example, if x = 52; mean = 56; and standard deviation = 4, the Z score is calculated as follows:

$$Z = \frac{x - \bar{x}}{s_x} = \frac{52 - 56}{4} = \frac{-4}{4} = -1$$

Here, Z score is –1 which indicates that the sample's score is below mean. Z score is for describing the relative standing of a score within a sample.

Computing a Raw Score when Z is known

$$X = (Z)(Sx) + \bar{x}$$

In the above example, we know that the Z score is 2.28; standard deviation is 3.5 and the mean value is 60

$$X = 2.28 \times 3.5 + 60$$

$$X = 7.98 + 60 = 67.98 = 68.$$

Interpreting Z Scores and Z Distribution

The Z score of Zero corresponds to the mean raw score. A person having the mean score is Zero distance from the mean. In Z score, we have to note two things, the number and the sign in front of it. The number indicates the distance the score is from the mean, measured in standard deviations.

The sign indicates the direction the score lies relative to the mean. A '+' indicates that the score is above and graphed to the right of the mean. A '–' sign indicates that the score is below and graphed to the left of the mean. The farther a raw score is from the mean, the larger its corresponding Z score. On a normal distribution, the larger the Z score, whether positive or negative, the less frequently that Z score and the corresponding raw score occur.

Characteristics of Z Distribution

- A Z distribution always has the same shape as the raw score distribution.
- The mean of any Z distribution always equals 0.
- The standard deviation of any Z distribution always equals 1. For example, one standard deviation is one Z score unit.

Application in the Field of Education and Psychology

- Each Z score indicates an individual's relative standing in any particular subject when compared with other students.
- The same method can be used to compare a relative standing in different subjects.
- Z transformation equates or standardizes the distributions and so Z scores are often referred to as standard scores.
- Z scores help us to describe the nature of the relative frequency of the score which ultimately leads to performance analysis of the faculty and students.
- For example, if you have many scores below the mean and the direction is negative which will indicate that the performance is less than average.
- Relative frequency is the proportion of the time that a score occurs.
- On any normal Z distribution, the relative frequency of Z scores between $\pm$ 1 is approximately 0.68.

Z Score and its Percentile

–2	2nd percentile
–1	16th percentile (2 + 14)
0	50th percentile (2 + 14 + 34 = 50)
+1	84th percentile (50 + 34 = 84)
+ 2	98th percentile (84 + 14 = 98)

34% of the samples or cases fall between the mean and +1 standard deviation, 14% between +1 SD and +2 SD and 2% between +2 and +3 standard deviation. Only 0.13% of the cases fall below –3 or above +3 SD (Fig. 27.1).

T SCORE

It is one of the standard score that has a mean of 50 and a standard deviation of 10. Thus, T score can be calculated as follows:

T score = 50 + 10 (Z)

The formula will provide T scores only when the original distribution of raw scores is normal. One reason that T scores are preferred to Z scores for reporting test results is that only positive integers are produced. If we apply either positive or negative of Z score to the formula, T score obtained will be only positive value; T score of 33 and a Z score of –1.7 are equivalent.

Conversion of Z score into T score. We can use the same value of Z given in the above example;

If Z = 2.28, the T score is calculated as follows:

T score = 50 + 10 (2.28) = 50 + 22.8 = 72.8

If Z = –1, the T score is calculated as follows:

T score = 50 + 10 (–1) = 50 – 10 = 40.

STANINES (STAY-NINES)

Here, the term ***stanines*** is derived from the way the scores have been divided into nine parts (standard nine). Stanine '5' is in the center like the average and 1 is lowest and 9 is highest which cover the tails of the distribution; 40–60 percentiles of rank which fall on stanine '5' which is 1/4th of the standard deviation on either side of the mean. In this the standard score has a mean of 5 and standard deviation of 2.

These scores are very much useful to explain to parents and students. The test performance is distributed into nine parts. It would be easy to compare in 2 tests as for instance, if the child gets stanine of 7 in English and 5 in Maths, it clearly shows the superior performance in English.

USE OF NORMAL CURVE IN GRADING

These are the relative grades assigned to the students in a single classroom group or the combined distribution of several classroom groups taking the same course. It is essentially a matter of ranking the students in terms of overall achievement. The grade is normally assigned in view of the distribution pattern of normal curve. Here, the grades are equally distributed regardless of the group's level of ability (Fig. 27.2).

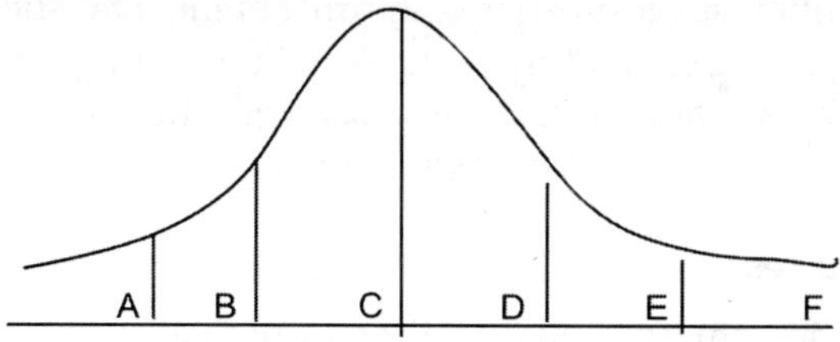

Fig. 27.2: Normal curve

CONSTRUCTION AND STANDARDIZATION OF TEST/SCALES

Scale construction is a complex procedure that should not be undertaken lightly. It requires careful work. The steps in constructing the scales are as follows:

Defining the Concept

A scale cannot be constructed to measure a concept until the nature of the concept has been delineated. The more clearly the concept is defined, the easier it is to write items to measure it (Spector, 1992). Concept analysis helps in defining the concept clearly.

Design the Scale

Items should be constructed to reflect the concept as fully as possible. The process of construction will differ somewhat depending on whether the scale is a rating scale, likert scale or semantic differential scale. A blue print can be prepared to ensure coverage of all elements of the concept. Items should be constructed keeping in mind the potential respondents. It should be clearly stated and express only one idea. The number of items constructed needs to be considerably larger than planned for the completed instrument because items will be discarded during the item analysis step of scale construction. Nunnally (1978) suggests developing an item pool at least twice the size of that desired for the final scale.

Seek Item Review

As items are constructed, it is advisable to ask qualified individuals to review them. Feedback can be obtained in relation to accuracy, appropriateness or relevance to test specifications; technical flaws in item construction; grammar; appearance of bias and level of readability. Based on the critique and suggestion of the expert, items can be revised.

Conduct Preliminary Item Tryouts

Items can be tested on a limited number of subjects (15–30) representatives of the target population. It is good to observe the reactions of respondents during testing to note behavior such as long pauses, answer changing or other indications of confusion about specific items. After testing, a debriefing session needs to be held during which respondents are invited to comment on items and offer suggestions for improvement. Statistical analysis are performed on data from these tryouts while noting means, response distributions, items left blank and outliers. Revise these items on the basis of this analysis and comments from respondents.

Perform a Field Test

Administer all the items in their final draft form to a large sample of subjects representative of the target population. Spector (1992) recommends a sample size of 100–200 subjects. However, the sample size needed for the statistical analysis to follow is somewhat dependent on the number of items. Some recommend including 10 subjects for each item being tested. If the final instrument was expected to have 20 items and 20 items were constructed for the field test, as many as 400 subjects could be required.

Conduct Item Analyses

The purpose of item analysis is to form an internally consistent scale and eliminate items that do not meet this criterion. Internal consistency implies that all the items measure the same concept. Before these analyses negatively worded items need to be reverse scored. Some statistical computer program such as SPSS performs item analysis. This package performs item-item correlations and item-total correlation. In some cases, the value of the item being examined is subtracted from the total score and an item remainder coefficient is calculated. The latter coefficient is most useful in evaluating items for retention in the scale.

Select Items to Retain

Depending on the number of items desired in the final scale, items with the highest coefficients are retained. Alternatively, a criterion value for the coefficient can be set and all items greater than this value retained. The greater the number of items retained, the smaller the item remainder coefficients can be and still have an internally consistent scale. After this selection process, coefficient alpha or Cronbach's alpha can be calculated for the scale. This value is a direct function of the number of items and the magnitude of inter correlation, thus one can increase the value of coefficient alpha by increasing the number of items or raise the intercorrelations through inclusion of more highly intercorrelated items. The value of coefficient alpha varies from 0 to 1. The alpha value should be at least 0.70 to indicate sufficient internal consistency. An iterative process of removing or replacing items, or both, recalculating item remainder coefficients and recalculating the alpha coefficient is repeated until a satisfactory alpha coefficient is obtained. Deleting poorly correlated items will raise the alpha coefficient, but decreasing the number of items will lower it. The initial attempt at scale development may not achieve a sufficiently high coefficient alpha. In this case, additional items will need to be written, more data collected, and the item analysis redone. This scenario is most likely to occur when too few items were developed initially or when many of the initial items were poorly written. It may also be a consequence of attempts to operationalize an inadequately defined concept.

Conduct Validity Studies

When scale development is judged to be satisfactory, studies must be performed to evaluate the validity of the scale. These studies require the collection of additional data from large samples. As part of this process, scale scores need to be correlated with scores on other variables proposed to be related to the concept being put into operation. Hypothesis need to be generated regarding variations in mean values of the scale in different groups.

Exploratory and then confirmatory factor analysis is usually performed as part of establishing validity of the instrument.

Evaluate the Reliability of the Scale

Various statistical procedures need to be performed to determine the reliability of the scale.

Compile Norms on the Scale

Determination of norms requires administration of the scale to a large sample representative of the groups to which the scale is likely to be given. Norms should be acquired for as many diverse groups as possible. Data acquired during validity and reliability studies can be included for this analysis. To obtain the large samples needed for this purpose, many researchers give permission to others to use their scale with the condition that data from these studies be provided for compiling norms.

Publish the Results of Development of the Scale

Scales are often not published for a number of years after the initial development because of the length of time required to validate the instrument. Some researchers never publish the results of this work. Studies using this scale are published, but the instrument development process may not be available except by writing to the author. This information needs to be added to the body of the knowledge, and instrument developers need to be encouraged by their colleagues to complete the work and submit it.

VALIDITY

Validity is concerned with the soundness and the effectiveness of the measuring instrument (Leedy 1993). Validity is the accuracy with which a test measures whatever it is intended to/supposed to measure. Validity is regarded as the absolutely indispensable property of any measuring instrument. Without validity, the instrument has no value. Validity is concerned with the general question: 'To what extent will this assessment information help us make an appropriate decision?'. It is a matter of degree; it does not exist on an all or nothing basis. It should be considered in terms of categories—highly valid, moderately valid, and invalid.

Nature of Validity

- Validity is a matter of degree. It does not exist on an all-or-none basis. It is not valid or invalid. Validity is best considered in terms of categories that specify degree, such as high validity, moderate validity and low validity.
- Validity involves an overall evaluative judgment.
- Validity is always specific to some particular use or interpretation.

Types of Validity

Face Validity

It is the validity of a test at face value. A test can be said to have face validity if it 'looks like'; it is going to measure what it is supposed to measure and is concerned with how a measure or procedure appears. A measure has face validity to the extent that it appears to measure what it sets out to measure. A measure may only appear to be a valid index of some characteristic under study but may really lack it. Conversely, a measure may lack face validity but be an excellent index of some characteristics. This is the least scientific method of validity as it is not quantified using statistical methods.

Content Validity

Face validity of a measure is the most superficial type. A more systematic type is content validity. It is a non-statistical type of validity and is qualitative in nature. Content validity refers to whether we actually and only measure an intended variable. Content validity deals with the accuracy with which an instrument measures the factors or content of the course or situations, under study. It refers to the content in the tool whether does it measure whatever it is intended to measure? Whether the content is appropriate to measure what is supposed to measure. A measure has content validity to the extent that it is representative of the subject matter or topic being measured. Content validity suffers when the measure contains items which measure subject matter or topic outside the domain of interest. For example, a tool which intends to measure the knowledge of the samples on prevention and management of anemia in adolescent girls supposed to measure the knowledge on anemia only. It should include the questions relevant to prevention and management of anemia in adolescent girls. Content validity suffers when the items in a measure under represent the relevant domain. Content validation is basically a judgmental. The content validity of the tool is ensured by showing the content of the tool to the experts in the field and getting approval for its appropriateness and relevance, etc. Their suggestions and recommendations for improvising and modification of the tool can be taken for improving content validity.

Criterion Validity

The question of criterion related validity arises when the scores obtained by an individual on one measure (called ***predictor***) are used to infer his standing on some other variable (called ***criterion***). The criterion may be either a behavior or attitude. Criterion related validity is a measure of how well the test performance reflects either concurrent performance of the same behavior based on some other measuring instrument or future performance obtained by another test given at some future time. The accuracy of a measure is demonstrated by comparing it with a measure that has been demonstrated to be valid (to a known standard). It is otherwise known as ***convergent validity***. Convergent validity is the extent to which the scores obtained from one procedure are positively correlated with scores obtained from another procedure that is already accepted as valid. In other words, correlations with other measures that have known validity. To measure the criterion validity of a test, researchers must calibrate it against a known standard or against itself.

Criterion related validity may be of two different types depending upon when the predictor and criterion variables are measured: Comparison of test scores with other scores obtained by other measuring instruments at the same time is called ***concurrent validity*** and comparison with subsequent scores obtained in future is called ***predictive validity***.

Comparing the test with an established measure is known as ***concurrent validity***; testing it over a period of time is known as ***predictive validity***.

Predictive validity involves testing a group of subjects for a certain construct, and then comparing them with results obtained at some point in the future.

Construct Validity

Construct validity refers to whether a variable actually and only reflects the intended hypothetical construct. Abstract variables which cannot be directly observed (e.g. motivation, morale, beauty, etc) are known as constructs. The values of such variables cannot be directly observed but can only be inferred from other observable variables. These other observable variables then become our operational definitions of these constructs. By construct validity of a measure is meant the appropriateness of the operational definition of the construct. Construct validity is interested in the degree to which the construct is actually measured. Construct validity is really a comparison of the test scores with scores obtained by other measuring instruments which measure a related ability which is usually associated with that tested by the current measuring instrument.

Discriminant validity is the extent to which the scores obtained from one procedure are not correlated with the scores from another procedure that measures other variables or constructs.

Reliability

Reliability refers to the consistency of the measurement. Reliability of measurement is needed to obtain valid results, but we can have reliability without validity. That is, we can have consistent measures that provide the wrong information or are interpreted inappropriately. Reliability is a necessary but not sufficient condition for validity.

Reliability is the degree to which measurements are consistent and do not contain measurement error. Reliability is defined as the extent to which on repeated measures, an instrument yields similar results. Measurements should be stable over time and across situations. For example, if we use a weighing scale to measure the weight of a group of adults, then the weighing scale should show the similar results when it is used to measure the weight for the same adults in different time periods or when it is used by the different investigator for the same adults. When the three attributes of acceptability, practicability and reliability have been established, validity can be investigated. In simple terms, any tool or instrument should be stable, that is on repeated usage or administration it should produce the similar findings or no variation between administration. Terms such as dependability, consistency, stability and accuracy are often used interchangeably to refer to reliability. The first three terms refer to the instrument's ability to produce the same results on repeated measures. The fourth term, accuracy, reflects a different dimension of reliability; the measurement tool's ability to reflect the true value being measured. Reliability is the term used to deal with accuracy.

True value is the value that would be obtained if the measurement tool is perfect. In other words, the true value is free of random measurement error. Few, if any, instruments or measurement tools are totally free of measurement error.

A scale measurement is considered reliable if it measures what it is supposed to measure. Further refining of the term ***reliable*** is that when a test is repeated by the same researcher, i.e. with a different group representing the original group, the same results should be obtained.

Reliability refers to the stability or consistency of the measurement. Reliability is a measure of reproducibility of the test. In other words, if the same or an equivalent test is given to the students, the scores obtained by individual students and the group as a whole would be similar. Reliability refers to the results of the test, not to the instrument itself. A reliable test does not indicate a valid one since the test can consistently measure something but not necessarily what is intended to be measured.

Reliability is a relative term. It exists in degrees and is usually expressed as a form of correlation coefficient, with 1.00 indicates perfect reliability and 0.00 indicating an absence of reliability. Nunnally (1978) suggests that reliability coefficients of 0.70 or above for new instruments and 0.80 or above for established instruments are acceptable.

Stability

Stability is concerned with the consistency of the results with repeated measures. Perhaps, the easiest way to assess stability is to repeat a question that has been posed. The idea of test-retest is whether the respondent is able to understand the question on both occasions on identical terms and have and infer similar meaning. So that the variable measured would be the same on two occasions. This type of reliability is most important in repeated measures design, especially the one with the pretest and post-test design of single and two groups (Table 27.1).

Table 27.1: Validity tests and its measures

Method	Type of reliability measure
Test-retest	Measure of stability
Equivalent forms	Measure of equivalence
Test retest with equivalent forms	Measure of stability and measure of equivalence
Split half	Measure of internal consistency
Kuder-Richardson and coefficient alpha	Measure of internal consistency
Interrater	Measure of consistency of ratings

Test-Retest Method

Two observations (measurements) are made using same instrument (either on different time period or by different persons) and calculating the correlations coefficient (r) is a method of establishing reliability. 'r' value closer to 1 indicates the high reliability and low value indicates the low reliability.

Internal Consistency

It refers to the ability of the items in an instrument to measure the same variable. Homogeneity is often used to refer to the internal consistency of an instrument. A homogenous instrument means which contains items that are strongly correlated with each other. The higher the correlations among the items, the greater the internal consistency of the instrument. Homogenous instruments are unidimensional; that is the items taken together measure one construct. Because all the items reflect the same underlying construct, the researcher can sum the individual item scores to get total score that reflects the construct. Methods available to test the internal consistency of a measure include the Kuder-Richardson coefficient, item total correlations, split half reliability and Cronbach's alpha.

Split-Half Method

The values of the Odd number and Even number questions can be computed for each sample and with the resultant values the correlation coefficient can be calculated. Or else, the values of the first half and the second half of the questions can be computed for each individual and with the values the correlation coefficient value can be calculated. Also, the items in a tool can be randomly divided into two groups, and correlation coefficient is calculated for the resulting two scores. The advantage of this method is that it allows the researchers to assess the test-retest reliability without administering the instrument twice. The Spearman-Brown correlation is usually used in this procedure.

Another procedure to assess homogeneity is to compare an individual item's correlation with the total index score. If an item is consistent with the total score, it will correlate with it. This technique is known as the internal consistency approach to reliability.

The item total correlations represent a group of correlations between each item and total score for an instrument. Item total correlations are useful in instrument development. They are helpful in retaining which items to retain and which one to discard in creating a final index. The item total correlations should be high enough to indicate internal consistency but low enough that they are not redundant. Nunnally (1978) suggests that uncorrected item total correlations above 0.25 and below 0.70 are typically acceptable for item retention when developing a new index.

The most common method used by nurse researchers for assessing internal consistency is Cronbach's alpha. This test is based on the strength of the inter correlations of all the items in the instrument as well as the number of items used. The alpha value ranges from 0 to 1, with 1 indicating perfect internal consistency and '0' no internal consistency.

Equivalence

Equivalence refers to the degree of agreement among two or more different observers using the same measurement tool or the agreement between two or more alternate forms of an instrument.

Measures to Improve Reliability

Reliability can be increased by increasing the length of a test or questionnaire to optimum level, ensuring objectivity of scoring and ensuring validity of the instrument used.

SUMMARY

- In most cases, scores on psychological tests are interpreted by reference to norms that are based upon the distribution of scores obtained by a representative sample of examinees, i.e. the process of standardizing a test against an appropriate norm group so that test users can make sense out of individual test scores. A norm group consists of a sample of examinees that are representative of the population for whom the test is intended.
- Age norm is used to depict the level of test performance for each separate age group in the normative sample. Grade norms depict the level of test performance for each grade in the normative sample. These are much useful in school achievement.
- The standard scores are the expression of test performance in standard deviation units from the mean. A standard score uses the standard deviation of the total distribution of raw scores as the fundamental unit of measurement. Standard score expresses the distance from the mean in standard deviation units.
- Z score is the distance a raw score deviates from the mean when measured in standard deviations. T score is one of the standard score that has a mean of 50 and a standard deviation of 10.
- Validity is the accuracy with which a test measures whatever it is intended to/supposed to measure. Validity is regarded as the absolutely indispensable property of any measuring instrument.
- Reliability refers to the consistency of the measurement. Reliability of measurement is needed to obtain valid results, but we can have reliability without validity.

EXERCISES

- I. Calculate the Z score for the following:

S. No.	Raw score (x)	Mean	Standard deviation
1	40	35	2
2	55	40	6
3	60	70	4
4	58	60	2
5	70	75	3
6	62	67	4
7	22	30	4.5
8	15	22	4

- II. Calculate the T score for the following Z scores.

S. No.	Z score
1	−1
2	−1.5
3	−1.8
4	−2
5	−2.1
6	1
7	1.3
8	1.7

28 Vital Health Statistics

OBJECTIVES

After reading this chapter, you will be able to:

- Define terms
- Explain the collection of vital statistics
- Explain the basic measurement tools
- Describe the measures of morbidity and mortality
- Explain the measures of fertility
- Calculate the various measures.

INTRODUCTION

Vital statistics is the statistical study of population. They provide information on causes of morbidity, mortality, fertility and its trend over a period of time. It gives information on the incidence and prevalence of various diseases and its distribution in population. It is a useful tool in estimating the population trend and growth. Information on vital health statistics are used in deciding public health priorities, planning and implementation of various health programmes for the population. Registration of births and deaths is an important source for demographic data for socioeconomic development and population control in developing countries. The data on population growth, fertility and mortality serves as the starting point for population projections. Apart from these vital indicators, an adequate evaluation of a number of programs in the health sector, including family planning, maternal and reproductive health, immunization programs, is dependent upon the availability of accurate, up-to-date fertility and mortality data. Epidemiological investigation helps in collection of data which provides vital information on public health. Epidemiology focuses on the measurement of health, morbidity, mortality and fertility.

Epidemiology is defined as "the study of the distribution and determinants of health-related states or events in specified populations, and the application of this study to the prevention and control of health problems". The word "epidemiology" is derived from the Greek words: epi "upon", demos "people" and logos "study". This broad definition of epidemiology can be further elaborated as follows: Study includes surveillance, observation, hypothesis testing, analytic research and experiments. Distribution refers to analysis of times, persons, places and classes of people affected. Determinants include factors that influence health, biological, chemical, physical, social, cultural, economic, genetic and behavioral. Health-related states and events refer to diseases, causes of death, behaviors such as use of tobacco, positive health states, reactions to preventive regimes and provision and use of health services. Specified populations include those with identifiable characteristics, such as occupational groups. Application to prevention and control is the aim of public health—to promote, protect, and restore health (Last JM, 2001).

VITAL STATISTICS

The vital statistical system deals with the individual's entrance into and departure from the world and with change in the marital status. The concerned events are birth, death, marriage and divorce. Data which gives quantitative information on vital events such as birth, death, marriage, divorce, etc. are called vital statistics.

Importance of Collecting Vital Statistics

- To calculate indices that measures levels of health and morbidity in a population
- To describe level of public health and illness
- To compare mortality and morbidity of different places, times, communities and professions
- To monitor the progress made in health and family welfare programme.
- To fix up priorities in adoption of future health interventions
- To determine survival, population growth and population explosion
- To plan and control fertility, morbidity and mortality
- To decide on administrative action
- To improve health standard.

In India, vital statistics are obtained from the following sources or ways. They are as follows:

- Population census
- Civil Registration system
- Sample Registration system
- National population register
- National Sample surveys
- Community surveys
- Institutional records.

Population Census

Census means the enumeration of the total population of the people in a country at a given point of time. It is defined by the United Nations as ' the total process of collecting, compiling and publishing demographic, economic and social data pertaining at a specified time or times to all persons in a country or a delimited territory'. Census is normally conducted at fixed intervals. In India, it is carried out once in every 10 years. The first All India census was carried out in 1881. The last census was performed in 2011.

The census provides useful demographic and social data about age, sex, marital status, language, education, occupation, economic status, place of birth, number of children born alive to a woman, etc. Such data are useful for planning of health and family welfare services, analyzing the growth rate of the population and calculation of indices like, birth, death and morbidity rates.

The latest and 15th Indian census was conducted in two phases, house listing and population enumeration. House listing phase began on 1 April 2010 and involved collection of information about all buildings. Information for National Population Register was also collected in the first phase. The second population enumeration phase was conducted from 9 to 28 February 2011. Census has been conducted in India since 1872 and 2011 marks the first time biometric information was collected. According to the provisional reports released on 31 March 2011, the Indian population increased to 1.21 billion with a decadal growth of 17.64%. Adult literacy rate increased to 74.04% with a decadal growth of 9.21%. The motto of census 2011 was 'Our census, Our future'. The 2011 census covered 28 states and 7 union territories which included 640 districts, 5,767 tehsils, 7,933 towns and more than 600,000 villages. A total of 2.7 million officials visited households in 7,933 towns and 600,000 villages, classifying the population according to gender, religion, education and occupation. Census data was collected in 16 languages and training manual was prepared in 18 languages.

The House listing schedule contained 35 questions, such as building number, census house number, predominant material of floor, wall and roof of the census house, use of actual house, condition of the census house, household number, total number of persons in the household, name of the head of the household, sex of the head, caste status (SC or ST or others), ownership status of the house, number of dwelling rooms, number of married couple in the household, main source of drinking water, availability of drinking water source, main source of lighting, latrine within the premises, type of latrine facility, waste water outlet connection, bathing facility within the premises, availability of kitchen, fuel used for cooking, radio/transistor, television, computer/laptop, telephone/mobile phone, bicycle, scooter/motorcycle/moped, car/jeep/van, availing banking services.

The Population enumeration schedule contained 30 questions such as name of the person, relationship to head, sex, date of birth and age, current marital status, age at marriage, religion, Scheduled Caste/Scheduled Tribe, disability, mother tongue, other languages known, Literacy status, status of attendance (Education), highest educational level attained, working any time during last year, category of economic activity, occupation nature of industry, trade or service, class of worker, non economic activity, seeking or available for work, travel to place of work, birthplace, place of last residence, Reason for migration, duration of stay in the place of migration, children surviving, children ever born, number of children born alive during the last one year.

Civil Registration System

It is a Continuous, Permanent and Systematic recording of births and deaths obtained under the Registration of Births and Deaths (RBD) Act, 1969 is called the Civil Registration System. The registration of births, deaths and still births are compulsory under the provisions of Registration of Births and Deaths (RBD) Act, 1969 in all parts of the country. The normal period of 21 days (from the date of occurrence) has been prescribed for reporting the birth, death and stillbirth events. If event of a birth or death is reported for registration to the prescribed authority within the normal period of 21days, no fee would be charged. If any event of birth or death is not reported for registration within the 21 days, the same can be reported any time under the Delayed Registration provisions prescribed under Section 13 of the Act with payment of fee prescribed. In respect of birth or death occurred in a house, it is the duty of the Head of the house/household or nearest relative of the head present in the house or in the absence of any such person, the oldest male person present therin during the said period is responsible to report the event to the concerned Registrar/sub registrar. These events can also be reported through the prescribed notifiers such as Anaganwadi Workers, ANM's, ASHA's and others. In respect of birth or death occurred in a hospital, health center, maternity or nursing home or other such institutions, the medical officer incharge or any person authorized by him in this behalf is responsible for reporting. Under the provision of Section 7 of the RBD Act, the Registrars of Births and Deaths are appointed for each local area comprising the area within the jurisdiction of the Municipality, Panchayat or other local authority. The Subregistrars are also appointed under Section 7(5) of the Act and assigned them any or all powers of Registrars. The Registrars/ Subregistrars are deemed to be the public servant under section 21 of the Indian Penal Code. The Registrars/Subregistrars are separately appointed for Rural and Urban areas.

Sample Registration System

In India, the need for dependable demographic data was felt soon after independence. The registration of births and deaths started on voluntary basis and there was no uniformity in statistical returns resulting in both under-registration and incomplete coverage. In order to unify the civil registration activities, the Registration of Births and Deaths Act, 1969 was enacted. Despite having the registration of birth and death compulsory under the statute, the level of registration of births and deaths under the Act has continued to be far from satisfactory in several states/UTs. With a view to generate reliable and continuous data on these indicators, the Office of the Registrar General, India, initiated the scheme of sample registration of births and deaths in India popularly known as Sample Registration System (SRS) in 1964-65 on a pilot basis and on full scale from 1969-70. The SRS since then has been providing data on regular basis. The SRS in India is based on a dual record system. The field investigation under Sample Registration System consists of continuous enumeration of births and deaths in a sample of villages/urban blocks by a resident part time enumerator, and an independent six monthly retrospective survey by a full time supervisor. The data obtained through these two sources are matched. The unmatched and partially matched events are reverified in the field to get an unduplicated count of correct events. The revision of SRS sampling frame is undertaken in every ten years based on the results of latest census. While changing the sample, modifications in the sampling design; wider representation of population; overcoming the limitations in the existing scheme; meeting the additional requirements are taken into account. The first replacement was carried out in 1977–78 and the last being in 2004. Whereas the replacement of samples in earlier years was undertaken in phases spread over 2–3 years, the replacement in 2004 was done in one go within a year.

The main objective of SRS is to provide reliable estimates of birth rate, death rate and infant mortality rate at the natural division level for the rural areas and at the state level for the urban areas. Natural divisions are National Sample Survey (NSS) classified group of contiguous administrative districts with distinct geographical and other natural characteristics. It also provides data for other measures of fertility and mortality including total fertility, infant and child mortality rate at higher geographical levels. To give more impetus covering both rural and urban areas and wider representation of sample villages and urban blocks for Causes of Death; the Survey of Causes of Deaths (Rural) has been merged with Sample Registration System from 1st January 1999. The primary objective of the survey is to build up statistics on 'Most Probable Causes of Death' for rural and urban areas using 'lay diagnosis reporting (Post Death Verbal Autopsy)' method through post death enquiry based on symptoms, conditions, duration and anatomical site of the disease as observed by family members of the deceased at the time of death.

The component of the sample registration system is as follows:

- Conduction of the baseline surveys of the sample units to obtain resident population of the sample areas
- Continuous enumeration of vital events in this specified population by the enumerator
- Conduction of independent retrospective half yearly surveys for recording births and deaths and updating the house lists, and list of women in the reproductive age group along with their pregnancy status
- Matching of events recorded during continuous enumeration and those listed in the half yearly survey
- Field verification of unmatched and partially matched events
- Filling of Verbal Autopsy Forms for finalized deaths.

Under sample registration system, baseline survey is conducted prior to the start of continuous enumeration. This involves preparation of a notional map of the area to be surveyed, house numbering and house listing and filling in of a household schedule. Then an appointed enumerator records the residential status and demographic particulars of each individual residing in the household viz. name, sex, age, educational/marital status and relation to head of household, etc. The inmates of public institutions like hotels, inns, schools and hospitals are excluded, but households living permanently within the compound of such institutions are covered. A list of pregnant women is also prepared at the time of the base line survey.

In case of continuous enumeration, the enumerator maintains a Birth Record and a Death Record in respect of his area. The enumerator is expected to record all births and deaths occurring within the sample unit, as well as those of the usual residents occurring outside the sample unit. The events in respect of visitors occurring within the sample unit are also listed, but these are not taken into account while calculating rates. Thus the events to be enumerated by the enumerator are those pertaining to: (i) usual residents inside the sample unit; (ii) usual residents outside the sample unit; (iii) immigrants present; (iv) immigrants absent; (v) visitors inside the sample unit. The enumerator takes help of the village priest, barber, village headman, midwife and such other functionaries. The enumerators maintain contact with these informants at frequent intervals and collects information about the occurrence of births and deaths. He also keeps in touch with other socially important persons and visits local or nearby hospitals, nursing homes, cremation or burial grounds, at frequent intervals to keep himself updated about the occurrence of events. Despite all these efforts, the enumerator may miss out information about some of the events. Therefore, he is required to visit all the households once in each quarter (in rural areas) and once a month (in urban areas) so as to ensure that all the events have been recorded.

Half yearly survey is carried out independently in each sample unit by a fulltime supervisor. The supervisor belonging to the statistical cadre of the State Census Directorates (either a Compiler or a Sr Compiler or Statistical Investigator or any suitable official) visits each household in the sample unit and records the particulars of births and deaths in respect of all the usual residents and visitors (only those occurring within the sample unit) which had occurred during the halfyearly period (January-June or July-December) under reference. Simultaneously, he updates the house-list, the household schedule and the pregnancy status of women by making entries of changes, if any. While carrying out this survey he does not have access to the birth and death records of the enumerator for the same periods which are withdrawn from the field before the supervisor's visit for the half yearly survey.

On completion of the half yearly survey, the forms filled in by the supervisors are compared with those in the forms filled in by the enumerators. This is done at the office of Directorate of Census Operations for all states except for rural areas of Kerala and Maharashtra, where it is done at the office of Directorate of Economics and Statistics of the respective states. Selected important entries in the enumerator's and supervisor's record are matched item by item and events are classified as fully matched, partially matched and unmatched. The items generally considered for matching are: Identification code of the head of Household and mother, relationship of the mother to head, date of live birth, month in case of stillbirth/abortion, sex in case of live birth/stillbirth (for birth) and identification code of the head of household and mother in infant death, relationship of the deceased to head, date of death and sex.

Every unmatched or partially matched event is verified by a visit to the concerned household. This is done either by a third period or jointly by the supervisor and the enumerator, depending upon the availability of staff.

The sample design adopted for SRS is a uni stage stratified simple random sampling technique. In rural areas, both strata and sub-strata was decided. The number of sample villages in each state was allocated to the substrata proportionally to their size (population). The sample villages within each substratum were selected at random with equal probability. In urban areas, the categories of towns/cities have been divided into four strata based on the size classes in contrast to the six strata in the earlier sampling frame. Towns with population less than one lakh have been placed under stratum I, towns/cities with population one lakh or more but less than 5 lakhs under stratum II, towns/cities with population 5 lakh or more under stratum III and four metro cities of Delhi, Mumbai, Chennai and Kolkata as separate strata, viz. stratum IV. The sampling unit in urban area is a Census Enumeration Block. The sample Census Enumeration Block within each substratum was selected at random with equal probability. A simple random sample of these enumeration blocks have been selected within each sub-strata without replacement from each of the size classes of towns/cities in each State/Union Territory.

National Population Register

The National Population Register (NPR) is a register of usual residents of the country. It is being prepared at the local (Village level), sub district (Tehsil/taluk level), district, state and national level under provisions of the citizenship act 1955 and the citizenship (registration of citizens and issue of national identity cards) rules, 2003. The objective of the NPR is to create a comprehensive identity database in the country with full identification and other details by registering each and every usual resident in the country. This would help in better targeting the benefits and services under the Government schemes/programs, improve planning and prevent identity fraud.

The national population register household schedule contained 9 questions such as name of the person and resident status, name of the person as should appear in the population register, relationship to head, gender, date of birth, marital status, educational qualification, occupation/activity, names of father, mother and spouse.

National Sample Surveys and Community Surveys

The National Sample Survey is a continuous activity undertaken by the Central Government on all India basis to collect data relating to social, economic and demographic aspects. Apart from this, health, nutrition and morbidity surveys are conducted in certain communities from time to time. These surveys provide useful information. They provide information on incidence and prevalence of specific disease conditions such as tuberculosis, leprosy, malaria, protein energy malnutrition and goiter.

Institutional Records

Hospitals, primary health centers and maternity homes prepare monthly returns of inpatient and outpatient census to the State Health Authorities. These data gives information on the disease prevalence in the institutional catchment area and often used to assess the needs of the local public.

RATES AND RATIOS; THE BASIC MEASUREMENT TOOLS

The most ambitious definition of health is that proposed by WHO in 1948: 'health is a state of complete physical, mental, and social well-being and not merely the absence of disease or infirmity'. The World Health Assembly resolved in 1977 that all people should attain a level of health permitting them to lead socially and economically productive lives by the year 2000. This commitment to the 'health for all' strategy was renewed in 1998 and again in 2003. The WHO definition of health is not an operational definition, i.e. it does not lend itself to direct measurement. In the epidemiological studies, the cases are defined clearly in order to measure the outcome. In a simple term, presence or absence of a disease is measured in a person. Presence of a disease is established by observing and identifying the diagnostic criteria in the person. The epidemiologists measured the health status of an individual as well as community by using various measurement tools. The basic tools of measurement are:

- Rate
- Ratios
- Proportions

Rate

A rate measures the occurrence of some particular event (development of disease or the occurrence of death) in a population during a given period. It is the statement of the risk of developing a condition. For example, death rate is calculated as follows:

$$\text{Death rate} = \frac{\text{Number of deaths in one year}}{\text{Mid-year population}} \times 1000$$

In calculation of rates, one must look for the elements such as numerator, denominator, time specification and multiplier. The time dimension is usually a calendar year. The various rates are crude rates, specific rates and standardized rates. Crude rates are actual observed rates such as the birth and death rates. They are also known as unstandardized rates. Specific rates are the actual observed rates due to specific causes (e.g. Malaria); or occurring in specific groups (e.g. age-gender groups) or during specific time periods (e.g. annual, monthly or weekly rates). The standardized rates are obtained by direct or indirect method of standardization or adjustment, e.g. age and sex standardized rates. Calculations of various rates are discussed under various headings.

Ratio

Ratio is one of the measures of disease frequency. It states the relationship between the numerator and denominator. It is expressed in the form of x:y or $\frac{x}{y}$.

The examples of ratio include sex ratio, i.e. male-female ratio, nurse-patient ratio, doctor population ratio etc. For example, the ratios are calculated as follows:

Male-Female ratio in a school

$$\frac{\text{The number of male children studying in a school at a certain time}}{\text{The number of female children studying in a school at a certain time}}$$

Proportion

A proportion is a ratio which indicates the relation in magnitude of a part of the whole. The numerator is always included in the denominator. A proportion is usually expressed as a percentage. For example, proportion is calculated as follows:

$$\frac{\text{The number of children with malnutrition at a certain time}}{\text{The total number of children in the village at the same time}} \times 100$$

$$\frac{\text{The number of adolescent girls with anemia at a certain time}}{\text{The total number of adolescent girls in the village at the same time}} \times 100$$

MEASUREMENT OF MORBIDITY

Death rates are particularly useful for investigating diseases with a high case fatality. However, many diseases have low case fatality, for example, most mental illnesses, musculoskeletal diseases, rheumatoid arthritis, chickenpox and mumps. In this situation, data on morbidity (illness) are more useful than mortality rates.

Morbidity is any deviation from the well-being which may be either subjective or objective. The synonyms for morbidity is sickness, illness, disability, etc. Morbidity data are often helpful in clarifying the reasons for particular trends in mortality. Changes in death rates could be due to changes in morbidity rates or in case-fatality. For example, the recent decline in cardiovascular disease mortality rates in many developed countries could be due to a fall in either incidence (suggesting improvements in primary prevention) or in case-fatality (suggesting improvements in treatment).

Because population age structures change with time, time-trend analyses should be based on age-standardized morbidity and mortality rates.

Other sources of morbidity data include:

- Hospital admissions and discharges
- Outpatient and primary health care consultations
- Specialist services (such as injury treatment)
- Registers of disease events (such as cancer and congenital malformations).

Incidence and prevalence are two important measures of morbidity. The incidence of disease represents the rate of occurrence of new cases arising in a given period in a specified population, while prevalence is the frequency of existing cases in a defined population at a given point in time. These are fundamentally different ways of measuring occurrence and the relation between incidence and prevalence varies among diseases. There may be low incidence and a high prevalence—as for diabetes—or a high incidence and a low prevalence—as for the common cold. Colds occur more frequently than diabetes but last only a short time, whereas diabetes is essentially lifelong.

INCIDENCE

Incidence refers to the rate at which new events occur in a population. Incidence takes into account the variable time periods during which individuals are disease free and thus 'at risk' of developing the disease.

In the calculation of incidence, the numerator is the number of new events that occur in a defined time period, and the denominator is the population at risk of experiencing the event during this period.

Incidence rate is defined as 'the number of new cases occurring in a defined population during a specified period of time'. It is given by the formula:

$$\text{Incidence} = \frac{\text{Number of new cases of specific disease during a given time period}}{\text{Population at risk during that period}} \times 1000$$

Example 1:

If there are 300 new cases of an illness in a population of 20,000 in a year, the incidence rate would be calculated as follows:

$$\text{Incidence} = \frac{300}{20000} \times 1000 = 15$$

It should be expressed as 15 per 1000 per year.

The most accurate way of calculating incidence is to calculate what last calls the 'person-time incidence rate.' Each person in the study population contributes one person—year to the denominator for each year (or day, week, month) of observation before disease develops, or the person is lost to follow-up.

The numerator strictly refers only to first events of disease. The units of incidence rate must always include a unit of time (cases per 10n and per day, week, month, year, etc.) For each individual in the population, the time of observation is the period that the person remains disease-free. The denominator used for the calculation of incidence is therefore the sum of all the disease—free person—time periods during the period of observation of the population at risk.

Example 2:

If the number of cases of dengue fever in a population of 10000 during the months of June and July were 102 and 120 respectively, compute the incidence rate of two months and compare.

$$\text{Incidence rate in June} = \frac{102}{10000} \times 1000 = 10.2 \text{ per } 1000$$

$$\text{Incidence rate in July} = \frac{120}{10000} \times 1000 = 12 \text{ per } 1000.$$

The incidence rate in July is increased.

Example 3:

There were 45 motor accidents in a town with population of 90000 in a year. Calculate the incidence rate.

$$\text{Incidence rate} = \frac{45}{90000} \times 1000 = 0.5 \text{ per } 1000 \text{ per year}$$

Cumulative incidence is a simpler measure of the occurrence of a disease or health status. Unlike incidence, it measures the denominator only at the beginning of a study. The cumulative incidence can be calculated as follows:

Cumulative Incidence

$$= \frac{\text{Number of people who get a disease during a specified period}}{\text{Number of people free of the disease in the population at risk at the beginning of the period}} \times 1000$$

Cumulative incidence is often presented as cases per 1000 population. In a statistical sense, the cumulative incidence is the probability that individuals in the population get the disease during the specified period.

The period can be of any length but is usually several years, or even the whole lifetime. The cumulative incidence rate therefore is similar to the 'risk of death' concept used in life-table calculations. The simplicity of cumulative incidence rates makes them useful when communicating health information to the general public.

Prevalence

The term 'prevalence' refers to all current cases (old and new) existing at a given point in time, or over a period of time in a given population. Prevalence (P) of a disease is calculated as follows:

$$P = \frac{\text{Number of people with the disease or condition at a specified time}}{\text{Number of people in the population at risk at the specified time}}$$

Prevalence is often expressed as cases per 100 (percentage), or per 1000 population. In this case, P has to be multiplied by the appropriate factor: 10n.

Prevalence of two types:

1. Point prevalence
2. Period prevalence

Point Prevalence

If the data have been collected for one point in time, P is the "point prevalence rate." Point prevalence of a disease is defined as the number of all old and new cases of a disease at one point of time, in relation to a defined population. The "point" in point prevalence refers to a day, or several days, or even few weeks, depending upon the time it takes to examine the population sample.

Point prevalence is given by the formula:

$$\frac{\text{Number of all current cases (old and new) of a specified disease existing at a given point in time}}{\text{Estimated population at the same point in time}} \times 100$$

Example 4:

Tuberculosis survey was done in a town with 20,000 population. It was found that 40 cases were radiologically positive while 10 were sputum positive. Calculate the point prevalence of sputum positive cases at the time of survey.

$$\text{Point prevalence of sputum positive cases} = \frac{10}{20000} \times 1000 = 0.5 \text{ per } 1000.$$

Period Prevalence

It is sometimes more convenient to use the 'period prevalence rate,' calculated as the total number of cases at any time during a specified period, divided by the population at risk midway through the period. It measures the frequency of all current cases (old and new) existing during a defined period of time (e.g. annual prevalence) expressed in relation to a defined population. Period prevalence is given by the formula:

$$\frac{\text{Number of existing cases (old and new) of a specified disease during a given period of time interval}}{\text{Estimated mid-interval population at risk}} \times 100$$

Similarly, a 'lifetime prevalence' is the total number of persons known to have had the disease for at least some part of their lives. Refer Table 28.1 for the differences between incidence and prevalence.

Example 5:

If 12 cases of diabetes mellitus were found in 15,000 population in a particular year, calculate the prevalence rate.

$$\text{Prevalence Rate} = \frac{12}{15000} \times 1000 = 0.8 \text{ per } 1000.$$

Table 28.1: Differences between incidence and prevalence

	Incidence	Prevalence
Numerator	Number of **new** cases of disease during a specified period of time	Number of **existing** cases of disease at a given point of time
Denominator	Population at risk	Population at risk
Focus	Whether the event is a new case Time of onset of the disease	Presence or absence of a disease Time period is arbitrary; rather a "snapshot" in time
Uses	Expresses the risk of becoming ill The main measure of acute diseases or conditions, but also used for chronic diseases More useful for studies of causation	Estimates the probability of the population being ill at the period of time being studied Useful in the study of the burden of chronic diseases and implication for health services

Measuring prevalence and incidence involves the counting of cases in defined population at risk. Reporting the number of cases without reference to the population at risk can be used to give an impression of the overall magnitude of a health problem, or of short-term trends in a population, for instance, during an epidemic. The term 'attack rate' is often used instead of incidence during a disease outbreak in a narrowly-defined population over a short period of time. The attack rate can be calculated as the number of people affected divided by the number exposed. For example, in the case of a food borne disease outbreak, the attack rate can be calculated for each type of food eaten, and then these rates compared to identify the source of the infection.

Data on prevalence and incidence become much more useful if converted into rates. A rate is calculated by dividing the number of cases by the corresponding number of people in the population at risk and is expressed as cases per 10n people. Some epidemiologists use the term 'rate' only for measurements of disease occurrence per time unit (week, year, etc.). Apart from age, several factors determine prevalence. In particular:

- The severity of illness (if many people who develop a disease die within a short time, its prevalence is decreased)
- The duration of illness (if a disease lasts a short time its prevalence is lower than if it lasts a long time)
- The number of new cases (if many people develop a disease, its prevalence is higher than if few people do so).

Prevalence can be increased by:

- Longer duration of the disease
- Prolongation of life of patients without cure
- Increase in new cases (increase in incidence)

- In-migration of cases
- Out-migration of healthy people
- In-migration of susceptible people
- Improved diagnostic facilities (better reporting).

Prevalence can be decreased by:

- Shorter duration of the disease
- High case-fatality rate from disease
- Decrease in new cases (decrease in incidence)
- In-migration of healthy people
- Out-migration of cases
- Improved cure rate of cases.

Since, prevalence can be influenced by many factors unrelated to the cause of the disease, prevalence studies do not usually provide strong evidence of causality. Measures of prevalence are, however, helpful in assessing the need for preventive action, healthcare and the planning of health services. Prevalence is a useful measure of the occurrence of conditions for which the onset of disease may be gradual, such as maturity-onset diabetes or rheumatoid arthritis.

Relationship between Prevalence and Incidence

Prevalence depends upon 2 factors, the incidence and duration of illness. The realtionship between incidence and prevalence can be expressed as:

$$P = I \times D$$

$$P = \text{Incidence} \times \text{Mean duration}$$

Example 6:

Incidence = 8 per 1000 population; mean duration of disease is 4 years.

Prevalence = 8 × 4 = 32 per 1000 population.

The above equation (P = I × D) shows that the longer the duration of the disease, the greater its prevalence.

MEASUREMENT OF MORTALITY

Crude Death Rate

It is defined as 'the number of deaths (from all causes) per 1000 estimated mid-year population in one year, in a given place'. The crude death rate is calculated from the formula:

$$\frac{\text{Number of deaths during the year}}{\text{Mid-year population}} \times 1000$$

Example 7:

In a town with 18000 populations, 520 deaths were recorded in 2010. Find the crude death rate.

$$\text{Crude death rate} = \frac{520}{18000} \times 1000 = 28.88$$

Specific Death Rates

Specific death rates are the actual observed rates due to specific causes (e.g. AIDS, Malaria); or occurring in specific groups (e.g. age – gender groups) or during specific time periods (e.g. annual, monthly or weekly rates).

Specific death rate for females

$$= \frac{\text{Number of deaths among females during the year}}{\text{Mid-year population of females}} \times 1000$$

Specific death rate for the month of April

$$= \frac{\text{Number of deaths in the month of April} \times 12}{\text{Mid-year population}} \times 1000$$

Specific death rate due to Dengue Fever

$$= \frac{\text{Number of deaths from dengue fever during the year}}{\text{Mid-year population}} \times 1000$$

Example 8:

In a place, out of 5 lakh population, 2000 died of Tuberculosis, 500 died of cancer and 3000 died of coronary heart disease in a year. Calculate the cause specific mortality rates per 1,00,000 population.

$$\text{Mortality due to Tuberculosis} = \frac{2000}{500000} \times 100000 = 400 \text{ per } 1{,}00{,}000$$

$$\text{Mortality due to Cancer} = \frac{500}{500000} \times 100000 = 100 \text{ per } 1{,}00{,}000$$

$$\text{Mortality due to Coronary heart disease} = \frac{3000}{500000} \times 100000 = 600 \text{ per } 1{,}00{,}000$$

Age-specific Mortality Rate (ASMR)

$$= \frac{\text{Number of deaths in a particular age-group}}{\text{Mid-year population of the same age-group}} \times 1000$$

Case Fatality Rate

Case fatality is a measure of disease severity and is defined as the proportion of cases with a specified disease or condition who die within a specified time. It is usually expressed as a percentage.

$$\textit{Case fatality } (\%) = \frac{\text{Number of deaths from diagnosed cases in a given period}}{\text{Number of diagnosed cases of the disease in the same period}} \times 100$$

Example 9:

If 20 out of 110 cases died in a dengue fever, find the case fatality rate.

$$\textit{Case fatality } (\%) = \frac{20}{110} \times 100 = 18.18\%$$

Example 10:

In a place, during cholera epidemic, 34 cases died out of 200 attacks while in dengue fever 20 died out of 102 attacks. Find the case fatality rates of both and compare.

$$\text{Case fatality rate due to cholera} = \frac{34}{200} \times 100 = 17\%$$

$$\text{Case fatality rate due to dengue fever} = \frac{20}{102} \times 100 = 19.6\%$$

Case fatality due to dengue fever is higher than cholera. Dengue fever is more fatal than cholera.

Proportional Mortality Rate

It expresses the 'number of deaths due to a particular cause (or in a specific age-group) per 100 (or 1000) total deaths.'

Proportional mortality rate from a specific disease

$$= \frac{\text{Number of deaths from the specific disease in a year}}{\text{Total deaths from all causes in that year}} \times 100$$

Example 11:

In a place, in the year 2000, out of 500 total deaths that occurred 60 were due to accidents. What is the proportional death rate due to accidents?

$$\text{Proportional death rates due to accidents} = \frac{60}{500} \times 100 = 12\%$$

Example 12:

In a place, in a year 2012, the total numbers of deaths were 800. In which death in children less than 2 years was 60. Calculate < 2 Age Proportional Mortality Rate.

$$\text{Less than 2 age Proportional Mortality Rate} = \frac{60}{800} \times 100 = 7.5\%$$

Infant Mortality Rate

The infant mortality rate is commonly used as an indicator of the level of health in a community. It measures the rate of death in children during the first year of life, the denominator being the number of live births in the same year.

The infant mortality rate is calculated as follows:

$$\textbf{\textit{Infant mortality rate}} = \frac{\text{Number of deaths in a year of children less than 1 year of age}}{\text{Number of live births in the same year}} \times 1000$$

Infant mortality rate comprises of two parts, viz. Neonatal mortality rate and Postneonatal mortality rate. The neonatal mortality rate also comprises of two parts viz. early neonatal mortality rate and late neonatal mortality rate. These are defined as:

***Neonatal mortality rate* (NMR)**

$$= \frac{\text{Number of infant deaths of < than 29 days during the year}}{\text{Number of live births during the year}} \times 1000$$

Early neonatal mortality rate

$$= \frac{\text{Number of infant deaths of < than 7 days during the year}}{\text{Number of live births during the year}} \times 1000$$

Late neonatal mortality rate

$$= \frac{\text{Number of infant deaths of 7 days to < than 29 days during the year}}{\text{Number of live births during the year}} \times 1000$$

***Postneonatal mortality rate* (PNMR)**

$$= \frac{\text{Number of infant deaths of 29 days to < than one year during the year}}{\text{Number of live births during the year}} \times 1000$$

Example 13:

In a town with a population of 80,000, there were 3200 births and 180 infant deaths in the year 2008. Eighty infants died in the first month of life while 42 of them died in the first week of life. There were 120 still births in the same year. Calculate the infant mortality rate, neonatal mortality rate and perinatal and postneonatal mortality rates.

Infant Mortality Rate $= \frac{180}{3200} \times 1000 = 56.25$ per 1000

Neonatal Mortality Rate (NMR) $= \frac{80}{3200} \times 1000 = 25$ per 1000.

Perinatal Mortality Rate (PMR)

$$= \frac{120+42}{3200+120} \times 1000 = \frac{162}{3320} \times 1000 = 48.80 \text{ per } 1000.$$

Postneonatal Mortality Rate

$$= \frac{180-80}{3200} \times 1000 = \frac{100}{3200} \times 1000 = 31.25 \text{ per } 1000.$$

Child Mortality Rate or Under-5 Mortality Rate

The child mortality rate (under-5 mortality rate) is based on deaths of children aged 1–4 years, and is frequently used as a basic health indicator. Injuries, malnutrition and infectious diseases are common causes of death in this age group. The under-5 mortality rate describes the probability (expressed per 1000 live births) of a child dying before reaching 5 years of age.

$$\text{Under-5 mortality rate} = \frac{\text{Deaths under 5 years of age}}{\text{Live births}} \times 1000$$

Maternal Mortality Rate

The maternal mortality rate refers to the risk of mothers dying from causes associated with delivering babies, complications of pregnancy or childbirth. The maternal mortality rate is given by:

Maternal Mortality Rate

$$= \frac{\begin{array}{c}\text{Total no. of female deaths due to complications of}\\ \text{pregnancy, child birth or within 42 days of delivery}\\ \text{from puperperal causes in an area during a given year}\end{array}}{\text{Total no. of live births in the same area and year}} \times 1000$$

Maternal Mortality Ratio

$$= \frac{\begin{array}{c}\text{Number of maternal deaths in a given}\\ \text{geographic area in a given year}\end{array}}{\begin{array}{c}\text{Total number of live births}\\ \text{during the same year}\end{array}} \times 1000$$

Perinatal mortality Rate (PMR)

$$= \frac{\begin{array}{c}\text{Number of stillbirths and infant deaths}\\ \text{of < than 7 days during the year}\end{array}}{\text{Number of live births and still-births during the year}}$$

Stillbirth Rate

$$= \frac{\text{Number of stillbirths during the year}}{\text{Number of live births and stillbirths during the year}} \times 1000$$

Stillbirth is a death of a fetus weighing 1000 g (this is equivalent to 28 weeks of gestation) or more.

Fetal Death: Fetal death is death prior to the complete expulsion or extraction from its mother of a product of conception, irrespective of the duration of pregnancy; the death is indicated by the fact that after such separation the fetus does not breathe or show any other evidence of life, such as beating of the heart, pulsation of the umbilical cord, or definite movement of voluntary muscles.

Adult Mortality Rate

The adult mortality rate is defined as the probability of dying between the ages of 15 and 60 years per 1000 population. The adult mortality rate offers a way to analyze health gaps between countries in the main working age groups. The probability of dying in adulthood is greater for men than for women in almost all countries, but the variation between countries is very large.

Age-standardized Death Rate

An age-standardized death rate (also referred to as an age-adjusted rate) is a summary measure of the death rate that a population would have if it had a standard age structure. The standardization of rates can be done either directly or indirectly. Age-standardized rates enable comparisons to be made between populations that have different age structures.

Standardization can also be done for variables other than age. This is necessary when comparing two or more populations that have different basic characteristics that independently influence the risk of death (such as age, race, socioeconomic status, etc.).

The direct method of standardization is more frequently used, and is done by applying the disease rates of the populations being compared to a standard population. This method yields the number of cases that would be expected if the age-specific rates in the standard population were true for the study population. Standardized rates are used, whenever relevant, for morbidity as well as mortality. The choice of a standard population is arbitrary, but can be problematic when comparing rates of low-income and high-income countries.

$$\text{Standardized Mortality Rate} = \frac{\text{Observed deaths}}{\text{Expected deaths}} \times 100$$

Example 14:

Calculate the standardized death rates for the data given below.

The age-specific death rates and crude death rates of two places A and B for the year 2010 are shown in the following table:

Age-specific death rate per 1000	A	B
0 – 2	22	20
2 – 6	12	10
6 – 16	5	5
16 – 46	7	6
46 – 61	10	12
61 and above	25	20
Crude death rate	16/1000	12/1000

The age wise composition of the selected standard population is given below.

Age-group	No. of persons
0 – 2	2000
2 – 6	12000
Age-group	No. of persons

Contd...

Contd...

6 – 16	10000
16 – 46	20000
46 – 61	12000
61 and above	2000
Total	58000

Calculate the standardized death of the two places and comment.
Standardized Death Rates of place 'A' is calculated as follows:

Age-group	Age specific death rate/1000	Persons in the standard population	Expected death
0 – 2	22	2000	$\frac{22}{1000}\times 2000 = 44$
2 – 6	12	12000	$\frac{12}{1000}\times 12000 = 144$
6 – 16	5	10000	$\frac{5}{1000}\times 10000 = 50$
16 – 46	7	20000	$\frac{7}{1000}\times 20000 = 140$
46 – 61	10	12000	$\frac{10}{1000}\times 12000 = 120$
61 and above	25	2000	$\frac{25}{1000}\times 2000 = 50$
	Total	58000	548

$$\text{Standardized Death Rate of A} = \frac{548}{58000}\times 1000 = 9.45/1000 \text{ population}$$

Next the Standardized Death Rate of "B" is calculated as follows:

Age-group	Age-specific death rate/1000	Persons in the standard population	Expected deaths
0 – 2	20	2000	$\frac{20}{1000}\times 2000 = 40$
2 – 6	10	12000	$\frac{10}{1000}\times 12000 = 120$
6 – 16	5	10000	$\frac{5}{1000}\times 10000 = 50$

Age-group	Age-specific death rate/1000	Persons in the standard population	Expected deaths
16 – 46	6	20000	$\frac{6}{1000} \times 20000 = 120$
46 – 61	12	12000	$\frac{12}{1000} \times 12000 = 144$
61 and above	20	2000	$\frac{20}{1000} \times 2000 = 40$
	Total	58000	514

$$\text{Standardized Death Rate of B} = \frac{514}{58000} \times 1000 = 8.86/1000 \text{ population}$$

As per the Standardized Death Rates, mortality experience of "A" is worse off than that of "B". The Crude Death Rates are also showing the same.

Survival Rate

It is the proportion of survivors in a group, studied and followed over a period.

$$\text{Survival rate} = \frac{\text{Total number of patients alive after 5 years}}{\text{Total number of patients diagnosed or treated}} \times 100$$

MEASUREMENT OF FERTILITY

Fertility may be measured by a number of indicators, as given below:

Live Birth

Live Birth is the complete expulsion or extraction from its mother of a product of conception, irrespective of the duration of pregnancy, which after such separation, breathes or shows any other evidence of life, such as beating of the heart, pulsation of the umbilical cord, or definite movement of voluntary muscles.

Crude Birth Rate

It is the number of live births per 1000 estimated mid-year population, in a given year. It is given by the formula:

$$\text{Crude birth rate} = \frac{\text{Number of live births during the year}}{\text{Estimated mid-year population}} \times 1000$$

Example 15:

The mid year population in a city in a year was 4,50,000 and the number of live births during that year was 22000. Find the crude birth rate.

$$\text{Crude birth rate} = \frac{22{,}000}{4{,}50{,}000} \times 1000 = 45.88 \text{ per } 1000.$$

Example 16:

In a country, the mid year population was 700 million and 22 million births took place in a year. Calculate the crude birth rate.

$$\text{Crude birth rate} = \frac{22{,}000000}{700000{,}000} \times 1000 = 31.4 \text{ per } 1000.$$

Example 17:

Birth rate in India in 2003 was 24.8 and death rate was 8 per 1000 population. Find the natural increase.
Natural increase = 24.8 – 8 = 16.8 per 1000 population or 1.68%

General Fertility Rate (GFR)

It is the number of live births per 1000 women in the reproductive age group (15–44 or 49) in a given year.

$$\text{GFR} = \frac{\text{Number of live births in an area during the year}}{\text{Mid-year female population age 15–44 or 49 in the same area in same year}} \times 1000$$

General Marital Fertility Rate (GMFR)

It is the number of live births per 1000 married women in the reproductive age group (15 – 44 or 49) in a given year.

$$\text{GMFR} = \frac{\text{Number of live births in a area}}{\text{Mid-year married female population in the age group 15–44 or 49 years}} \times 1000$$

Age-specific Fertility Rate (ASFR)

It is defined as the number of live births in a year to 1000 women in any specified age group.

$$\text{ASFR} = \frac{\text{Number of live births in a particular age group}}{\text{Mid-year female population of the same age group}} \times 1000$$

Age-specific Marital Fertility Rate (ASMFR)

It is the number of live births in a year to 1000 married women in any specified age group.

$$\text{ASMFR} = \frac{\text{Number of live births in a particular age group}}{\text{Mid-year married female population of the same age group}} \times 1000$$

Total Fertility Rate

Total fertility rate represents the average number of children a woman would have, if she were to pass through her reproductive years bearing children at the same rates as the women now in each age group. It is computed by summing the age specific fertility rates for all ages; if 5 year age groups are used, the sum of the rates is multiplied by 5.

Total Marital Fertility Rate

It is the average number of children that would be born to a married woman if she experiences the current fertility pattern throughout her reproductive span.

Gross Reproduction Rate (GRR)

It is the average number of girls that would be born to a women if she experiences the current fertility pattern throughout her reproductive span (15 – 44 or 49 years), assuming no mortality.

Example 18:

The total fertility rate of a place in 2013 was 3. The sex ratio of the population of that place that year was 956. Calculate Gross Reproductive Rate.

The proportion of women in the total population = 956 + 1000 = 1956

That is $\frac{956}{1956}$

$$\text{Gross Reproductive Rate} = \frac{3 \times 956}{1956} = \frac{2868}{1956} = 1.466 = 1.5$$

Example 19:

Compute the Specific Fertility Rate, General Fertility Rate, Total Fertility Rate and Gross Reproduction Rate from the data given below:

Age-group	No. of women per 1000	Number of women	No. of live births
15–19	22	22000	600
20–24	20	20000	2000
25–29	16	16000	1500

Contd...

Contd...

Age-group	No. of women per 1000	Number of women	No. of live births
30–34	12	12000	1000
35–39	10	10000	500
40–44	6	6000	130
45–49	4	4000	5
	Total	90000	5735

It is given that out of 5735, the number of female birth was 3000.

$$\text{Specific Fertility Rate (SFR)} = \frac{\text{No. of live births}}{\text{No. of women}} \times 1000$$

$$\text{SFR in 15–19 years} = \frac{600}{22000} \times 1000 = 27.27$$

$$\text{SFR in 20–24 years} = \frac{2000}{20000} \times 1000 = 100$$

$$\text{SFR in 25–29 years} = \frac{1500}{16000} \times 1000 = 93.75$$

$$\text{SFR in 30–34 years} = \frac{1000}{12000} \times 1000 = 83.33$$

$$\text{SFR in 35–39 years} = \frac{500}{10000} \times 1000 = 50$$

$$\text{SFR in 40–44 years} = \frac{130}{6000} \times 1000 = 21.66$$

$$\text{SFR in 45–49 years} = \frac{5}{4000} \times 1000 = 1.25$$

$$\text{General Fertility Rate} = \frac{\text{No. of live births}}{\text{Mid year female population of ages}} \times 1000$$

$$\text{General Fertility Rate} = \frac{5735}{90000} \times 1000 = 63.72$$

Total Fertility Rate = $\sum$SFR × t where 't' is the magnitude of the class.

= (27.27 + 100 + 93.75 + 83.33 + 50 + 21.66 + 1.25) × 5 = 377.26 × 5 = 1886.3

Age in years	SFR × 5 = TFR	Total births
15	0	0
20	27.27 × 5 = 136.35	136.4
25	100 × 5 = 500	636.4
30	93.75 × 5 = 468.75	1105.2
35	83.33 × 5 = 416.65	1521.9
40	50 × 5 = 250	1771.9
45	21.66 × 5 = 108.3	1880.2
50	1.25 × 5 = 6.25	1886.45

$$\text{Gross Reproduction Rate} = \frac{\text{No. of female births}}{\text{Total births}} \times \text{Total fertility rate}$$

$$\text{Gross Reproduction Rate} = \frac{3000}{5735} \times 1886.5 = 986.8 = 987$$

Net Reproduction Rate

Net reproduction rate is defined as the number of daughters a newborn girls will bear during her lifetime assuming fixed age specific fertility and mortality rates.

Child-Woman Ratio

It is the number of children 0–4 years of age per 1000 women of child-bearing age.

Pregnancy Rate

It is the ratio of number of pregnancies in a year to married women in the ages 15–44 or 49 years. The number of pregnancies includes all pregnancies whether these had terminated as live births, still births or abortions or had not yet terminated.

This is number of times women in child bearing age have become pregnant since their marriage divided by the total years they were at risk of becoming pregnant and multiplied with 100.

Example 20:

If 80 women are married for the last 8 years and give history of 200 pregnancies in the same period, find the pregnancy rate.

$$\text{Pregnancy rate} = \frac{200}{80 \times 8} \times 100 = \frac{200}{640} \times 100 = 31.25\%$$

Example 21:

A survey was conducted in a village. The results were as follows:

Women in child-bearing age = 120

Number of pregnancies since their marriage = 380

Length of married life for:

12 women	5 years
30 women	10 years
40 women	15 years
20 women	20 years
18 women	25 years

Calculate the pregnancy rate of the village.

The total years at risk = (12 × 5) + (30 × 10) + (40 × 15) + (20 × 20) + (18 × 25) = 60 + 300 + 600 + 400 + 450 = 1810 women years.

$$\text{Pregnancy rate} = \frac{380}{1810} \times 100 = 20.99 = 21 \text{ per } 100 \text{ women years of age.}$$

Abortion Rate

The annual number of all types of abortions, usually per 1000 women of child bearing age.

Abortion Ratio

This is calculated by dividing the number of abortions performed during a particular time period by the number of live births over the same period.

Marriage Rate

It is the number of marriages in the year per 1000 population:

$$\text{Crude Marriage Rate} = \frac{\text{Number of marriages in the year}}{\text{Mid-year population}} \times 1000$$

$$\text{General Marriage Rate} = \frac{\text{Number of marriages within one year}}{\text{Number of unmarried persons aged 15–49 years}} \times 1000$$

Life Expectancy Rate

Life expectancy is another summary measure of the health status of a population. It is defined as the average number of years an individual of a given age is expected to live if current mortality rates continue.

SUMMARY

- Vital statistics is the statistical study of population. They provide information on causes of morbidity, mortality, fertility and its trend over a period of time.
- Epidemiology is defined as 'the study of the distribution and determinants of health-related states or events in specified populations, and the application of this study to the prevention and control of health problems.
- The vital statistical system deals with the individual's entrance into and departure from the world and with change in the marital status. The concerned events are birth, death , marriage and divorce.
- In India, vital statistics are obtained from the sources such as population census, civil registration system, sample registration system, national population register, national sample surveys, community surveys and from institutional records.
- Census means the enumeration of the total population of the people in a country at a given point of time. In India, it is carried out once in every 10 years. The first All India census was carried out in 1881. The last census was performed in 2011.

- Civil Registration System is a continuous, permanent and systematic recording of births and deaths obtained under the Registration of Births and Deaths (RBD) Act, 1969. The National Population Register (NPR) is a register of usual residents of the country.
- The epidemiologists measured the health status of an individual as well as community by using various measurement tools. The basic tools of measurement are rate, ratios and proportions.
- Incidence and prevalence are two important measures of morbidity. The incidence of disease represents the rate of occurrence of new cases arising in a given period in a specified population, while prevalence is the frequency of existing cases in a defined population at a given point in time.
- There are various measures of mortality, morbidity and fertility. These indicators provide useful information for health planning and implementation.

EXERCISE

- The following annual data were reported for a certain geographic area:

	Total	Urban	Rural
Estimated population as of July 1	597500	361700	235800
Total live births	12400	6400	6000
Preterm births	1240	640	600
Fetal deaths	600	365	235
Deaths total all ages	6200	3600	2600
Under one year	260	140	120
Under 28 days	200	110	90
Maternal deaths	4	2	2
Causes of death			
Cardiac diseases	1680	1100	580
Communicable diseases	800	450	350

From these data compute the following rates and ratios: Crude death rate, Specific death rates for urban and rural population, maternal mortality rate, infant mortality rate neonatal mortality rate, fetal death ratios, disease specific death rate.

- The following table shows the estimated population and deaths in a city for 2012. Use these data to compute the age adjusted standard death rate. The standard population is also given.

Age-group	Population	No. of deaths	Standard population
0–10	18,000	300	22,000
10–30	45,000	200	38,000
30–55	25,000	180	40,000
55–80	48,000	210	24,000
Above 80	20,000	230	8,000

- In a village with a population of 3000, 4 new cases of diabetes occurred in April 2012. Calculate the morbidity rate.

- Midyear population of a place is 50000 and the total number of deaths is 800, calculate the crude death rate.
- Out of 50 women questioned 18 were married 5 years ago and 32 were married 10 years ago. They gave history of 200 pregnancies. Calculate pregnancy rate.
- In 2013, crude birth rate of a village was 28 per 1000 population and death rate was 14 per 1000 population. Calculate its growth rate for 2013.
- During 2008, there were 200 deaths in town A and 350 deaths in town B. The estimated midyear population for 2008 in towns A and B were 35,900 and 32,800 respectively. Calculate crude death rate for both the towns.
- The number of live birth in a place during 2000 was 3580. The number of infant deaths during the same year was 280. Calculate Infant Mortality Rate.
- In a town, with a population of 60,000, there were 2500 births and 300 infant deaths in a year 2000. Of these 60 infants died in the first 28 days of life and 20 of them died in the first week of life. There were 100 still births in the same year. Calculate IMR, Perinatal, Neonatal and Post neonatal mortality rate.
- In a country having a population of 280 million, 2,80,000 people died of Tuberculosis, 80,000 died of accidents and 20,000 died out of cancer. Calculate cause specific mortality rate per 1,00,000 population.
- In a town with a population of 80,000, there were 1500 births and 300 infant deaths in a year. Of these, 80 infants died in the first 28 days of life and 40 of them died in the first week of life. There were 140 still births in the same year. Calculate IMR, Perinatal Mortality rate, Neonatal Mortality rate and Post neonatal mortality rate.
- Calculate Specific Fertility Rate for the following data.

Age-group	Female population in 1000s	Births
15–19	40	600
20–24	36	2500
25–29	30	3000
30–34	34	3200
35–39	28	2000
40–44	24	100
45–49	20	40

Appendices

Table A1: Descriptive and inferential statistical tests and its application

	Terms	Meaning	Application
Measures of Central Tendency	Mean	The arithmetic average of a distribution. An important estimate of a parameter.	A pediatric nurse wants to know the average weight of the children in her ward. A nursing faculty wants to know the average marks scored by the students in the subject Nursing Research and Biostatistics.
	Median	The middle value when arranged in ascending or descending order. 50% of distribution is below median and 50% is above median.	A teacher may want to know the median height of children in a class. She can make the students to stand in ascending order of their height. The middle student's height is the median height.
	Mode	The most frequently occurring value or repeated value. When all scores are different, no mode exists.	A nursing faculty may want to know the modal value of leave taken by the students. If 3 and 4 days are repeated frequently and equally, we can say that it has two modes.
Measures of Dispersion	Range	The difference between the maximum value and the minimum value in a series. The values are extreme.	A teacher may want to know the range of marks scored by the students, that is the difference between the top score and the least score.
	Quartile deviation	The values between the 25th and 75th percentile. Not often used. It can be calculated by finding the median and then first quartile (the middle value below the median) and third quartile (the middle value above the median).	A nursing faculty wants to identify the highest and lowest quartiles of a group of students based on their marks in the university examination.
	Mean deviation	The sum of the deviation of each value from the mean value ignoring the signs (+ or –).	A teacher may wish to calculate how far each student's weight deviates from the average weight of the student group. A teacher may wish to note how far each student deviates from the average score in a test.

contd...

contd...

	Variance	The summed squared deviations from the mean.	Not used often; gives a general picture of variability. Most often the standard deviation is used.
	Standard Deviation	Most commonly used measure of variability. The square root of summed squared deviations from mean divided by the size of the sample (N). It tells the dispersion around the mean. An important estimate of a parameter.	A teacher may like to know how far the students are dispersed in relation to the average weight in a group of students.
	Coefficient of Variation	The Coefficient of Variation is the standard deviation expressed as a percentage of the arithmetic mean. When we want to compare the dispersion in two sets of data which are measured in different units, the coefficient of variation is used.	A teacher may wish to measure and compare the dispersion of height and weight in samples. The height and weight are measured in different units.
Measures of Relationship	Correlation Coefficient	It is a measure of relationship between two variables. It tells the direction and the strength of relationship.	A teacher may find the correlation between the intelligence and test performance. A nurse researcher may wish to assess the correlation between knowledge and attitude towards safety behavior in adolescents.
	Regression	It is used to examine the predictive ability of one variable for another variable.	A nurse researcher may determine the predictive ability of years of experience on nursing competencies. A nurse researcher may determine the predictive ability of years of playing violent video games on aggression in children.
Parametric test (Interval and Ratio level data)	T test (Independent)	To compare the mean value of two different groups.	A faculty may compare the academic performance of the groups of male and female nursing students; or attitude of male and female students towards nursing.
	T test (Dependent)	To compare the mean value of the same group measured in two different times (tested twice).	A nursing faculty may assess the attitude of students towards nursing at the beginning and the end of the course. Testing and comparing the mean knowledge score of students before and after a structured education program.
	One way ANOVA	To compare the mean value of more than two different groups.	A nurse researcher can compare the mean attitude score of I, II, III and IV year BSc (N) students towards nursing.

contd...

contd...

	Two way ANOVA	To compare the groups' mean value when there are more than one independent variable and only one dependent variable.	A nurse researcher may wish to assess the gender difference in attitude towards nursing profession.
	Multivariate analysis of variance	To test the difference between more than two group means when there are more than one dependent variable and more than one independent variable.	A nurse researcher may wish to assess the effect of video assisted teaching program and demonstration on gain in knowledge among UG and PG nursing students.
	Analysis of Covariance	Combines ANOVA with regression; allows researcher to measure group differences when certain variables are controlled; reduces variability and error.	Nurse researcher wants to compare the competencies of the staff nurses with diploma, BSc (N) and PBBSc (N) qualification; the covariate will be their level of educational preparation and experience.
	Repeated measures analysis of variance (within subjects design)	Testing the response or effect of a group of samples on various treatment. A repeated measures design is one in which measurements of the same variable are made on each subject on two or more different occasions. The different occasions during which measurements are taken may be either points in time or different conditions such as different treatments.	A researcher may want to see the effect of yoga versus moderate walking on weight reduction in participants. In case of repeated measures design, the samples have to be exposed first to the yoga for a specific duration say example, two weeks and their weight before and after should be measured. The same sample can be asked to go for moderate walking for two weeks and their weight before and after can be measured.
Nonparametric test (Nominal and Ordinal level data)	Chi square	This test compares the expected frequencies with the actual frequencies.	A nurse researcher can see the difference between the expected frequencies of aggression and the actual frequencies of aggression among children playing violet video games. Based on the differences, it is concluded whether the difference is by chance or a significant difference.
	Mann-Whitney U	It is parallel to the independent t test; allows the researcher to compare the ranked scores two different groups. This test is used to determine whether two independent samples have been drawn from the same population.	If sample size is very small instead of 't' test Mann-Whitney U is used. A survey is conducted to test the difference between 2 alternative methods of teaching. A sample of 10 students is selected at random. Two groups of 5 students each of equal ability are formed and taught by different methods. A standardized test is then given to both the groups and the scores are obtained. This test is used to assess the significant difference between the performances of two groups.

contd...

contd...

	Kruskal Wallis H test	The Kruskal Wallis H test is analogous to a one-way between subjects ANOVA for ranked data. It assumes that the study involves one independent variable and that there three or more independent samples with at least five participants in each sample. The null hypothesis is that all conditions represent the same distribution of ranks in the population.	A major city hospital established OPD services at 3 different locations. When the number of patients attended the OPD on 10 days is given, we can test whether it is same in all three locations.
	Wilcoxon Matched pairs rank test	The test is equal to the dependent (paired T test) T test; used with ordinal level data.	The mid arm circumference of under 5 children before and after dietary supplementation was measured. This test is used to conclude whether the dietary supplementation is effective.
	Spearman rank correlation	The nonparametric equivalent of the pearson's correlation coefficient uses ordinal data; compares the ranked responses of two groups and tells the strength and nature of a relationship between two variables.	Two teacher can rank the students performance and the correlation can be found out.

Table A2: Types of data and various measures of descriptive statistics

Type of data	Individual scores	Measures of central tendency	Measures of dispersion	Measures of relationship
Nominal data	Frequency and percentage	Mode	Range	Phi coefficient
Ordinal data	Frequency and percentage	Median	Range	Spearman rank correlation
Interval or ratio data (skewed distribution)	Frequency and percentage	Median	Range or inter-quartile range	None
Interval or ratio data (normal distribution)	Frequency and percentage	Mean	Standard deviation or variance	Pearson 'r' and regression analysis

Table A3: Research designs and its suitable parametric and nonparametric tests

Research design	Parametric test	Nonparametric test
Two independent groups: To compare the mean value.	Independent samples t test	Mann-Whitney U or Rank sums test
Two dependent groups of samples: To compare the means before and after or measured at two different times for the same samples.	Dependent samples t test	Wilcoxon T test

contd...

contd...

Three or more groups of independent samples: To compare the means.	Between subjects ANOVA	Kruskal Wallis H test
Three or more dependent samples: To compare the means.	Within subjects ANOVA	Friedman Chi Square test

Table A4: Types of reliability and validity and its procedure

Criteria	Types	Procedure
Reliability	Inter-rater reliability	Checked by obtaining the rating from two different raters and checking for positive correlation.
	Test-retest	Checked by testing first and retesting again and both scores are checked for positive correlation.
	Split-half	Subjects scores for first half and the second half or the scores of odd number and even number items are computed and checked for positive correlation.
Validity	Face validity	Checked whether the items appears to be valid.
	Convergent validity	Procedure correlates with other accepted measures.
	Discriminant validity	Procedure does not correlate with other unintended measures.
	Criterion-Concurrent validity	Procedure correlates with a present behavior
	Predictive validity	Procedure correlates with a future behavior.

Table A5: Comparison of types of validity

Aspects	Face validity	Content validity	Criterion validity	Construct validity
Nature	This is the least scientific method of validity as it is not quantified using statistical methods.	It is a non-statistical type of validity and is qualitative in nature.	Criterion validity is regarded as a very strong measure of statistical validity.	A whole battery of statistical tools and coefficients are used to prove strong construct validity, and researchers continue until they feel that they have found the balance between providing validity and practicality. Construct validity can be evaluated by statistical methods that show whether a common factor can be shown to exist underlying several measurements using different observable indicators.

contd...

contd...

Meaning	It is the validity of a test at face value. A test can be said to have face validity if it 'looks like'; it is going to measure what it is supposed to measure and is concerned with how a measure or procedure appears.	It refers to the extent to which a measure represents all facets of a given construct. Content validity refers to whether we actually and only measure an intended variable. Content validity deals with the accuracy with which an instrument measures the factors or content of the course or situations, under study.	It is used to demonstrate the accuracy of a measure or procedure by comparing it with another measure or procedure which has been demonstrated to be valid. Criterion-related validity is a measure of how well the test performance reflects either concurrent performance of the same behavior based on some other measuring instrument or future performance obtained by another test given at some future time. It is of two types. Comparison of test scores with other scores obtained by other measuring instruments at the same time is called ***concurrent validity*** and comparison with subsequent scores obtained in future is called ***predictive validity***.	Construct validity defines how well a test or experiment measures up to its claims. It refers to whether the operational definition of a variable actually reflect the true theoretical meaning of a concept. Construct validity refers to whether a variable actually and only reflects the intended hypothetical construct.
Other name	-	It is also known as logical validity or rational validity.	It is also referred to as instrumental validity or concrete validity.	-
Process	Face validity assesses whether the test 'looks valid' to the examinees who take it.	It is the systematic examination of the test content to determine whether it covers a representative sample of the behavior domain to be measured.	Concurrent validity is a measure of how well a particular test correlates with a previously validated measure. The tests are for the same, or very closely related, constructs and allow a researcher to validate new methods against a tried and tested one. One common way of looking at concurrent validity is measuring a new test or procedure against a gold-standard benchmark.	A construct represents a collection of behaviors that are associated in a meaningful way to create an image or an idea invented for a research purpose.

contd...

contd...

Adequacy	It is never sufficient to rely on face judgments alone and more quantifiable methods of validity are necessary in order to draw acceptable conclusions.	It is adequate in terms of content coverage.	Concurrent validity is regarded as a fairly weak type of validity, and is rarely accepted on its own.	Establishing good construct validity is a matter of experience and judgment, building up as much supporting evidence as possible.
Reliability	Face validity should never be trusted on its own merits since it refers not to what the test actually measures, but to what it superficially appears to measure.	It may be said to be reliable since this involves the systematic examination by the panelists of each item in a test or tool to verify whether each item is essential. It is often seen as a prerequisite to criterion validity because it is a good indicator of whether the desired trait is measured. If elements of the test are irrelevant to the main construct, then they are measuring something else completely, creating potential bias.	It is not reliable. The problem is that the benchmark test may have some inaccuracies and, if the new test shows a correlation, it merely shows that the new test contains the same problems.	Construct validity is all about semantics and labeling. Defining a construct in too broad or too narrow terms can invalidate the entire research.
Methods of obtaining	By showing it to others and checking whether does it look or appears to be valid? It requires a personal judgment, such as asking participants whether they thought that a test was well-constructed and useful.	It is essentially a method for gauging agreement among raters or judges regarding how essential a particular item is. A tool can be given to a group of panelists and can be asked to rate each item on a rating scale. According to Lawshe (1975), if more than half the panelists indicate that an item is essential that item has at least some content validity.	The accuracy of a measure is demonstrated by comparing it with a measure that has been demonstrated to be valid (to a known standard). In other words, correlations with other measures that have known validity. To measure the criterion validity of a test, researchers must calibrate it against a known standard or against itself. Comparing the test with an established measure is known as ***concurrent***	Construct validity is the degree to which inferences can be made from operationalizations (connecting concepts to observations) in a study to the constructs on which those operationalizations' are based. To establish construct validity, one must first provide evidence that their data supports the theoretical structure. Researcher must also show that he can control the operationalization of the construct, in other words, show that the

contd...

contd...

		Greater levels of content validity exist as larger numbers of panelists agree that a particular item is essential. It can be calculated by a formula Content Validity Ratio (CVR) = $(n_e - N/2)/(N/2)$ where n_e = number of panelists indicating 'essential' and N= total number of panelists. This formula yields values which range from +1 to −1; positive values indicate that at least half the panelists rated the item as essential. The mean CVR across items may be used as an indicator of overall test content validity.	validity; testing it over a period of time is known as ***predictive validity***. Predictive validity involves testing a group of subjects for a certain construct, and then comparing them with results obtained at some point in the future. A new intelligence test, for example, could be statistically analyzed against a standard IQ test; if there is a high correlation between the two data sets, then the criterion validity is high.	theory chosen has some correspondence with reality. For major and extensive research, especially in education and language studies, most researchers test the construct validity before the main research. These pilot studies establish the strength of their research and allow them to make any adjustments. Using an educational example, such a pre-test might involve a differential groups study, where researchers obtain test results for two different groups, one with the construct and one without. The other option is an intervention study, where a group with low scores in the construct is tested, taught the construct, and then remeasured. If there is a significant difference pre and post-test, usually analyzed with simple statistical tests, then this proves good construct validity.
Example	Does a tool appear to measure the IQ of the student?	Does an IQ questionnaire have items covering all areas of intelligence discussed in the scientific literature?	Testing a group of students for intelligence, with an IQ test, and then performing the new intelligence test a couple of days later would be perfectly acceptable for checking concurrent validity. How far does a new IQ test correlate with the standard IQ test? If the test takes place a considerable amount of time after the initial test, then it is regarded as predictive validity.	Does the theoretical concept match up with a specific measurement/scale used in research? Construct validity refers to whether a scale or test measures the construct adequately.

STATISTICAL TABLES

Table A6: Cumulative binomial probability distribution

		θ										
n	x	0.001	0.005	0.01	0.02	0.03	0.04	0.05	0.06	0.07	0.08	0.09
1	0	0.9990	0.9950	0.9900	0.9800	0.9700	0.9600	0.9500	0.9400	0.9300	0.9200	0.9100
	1	1.0000	1.0000	1.0000	1.0000	1.0000	1.0000	1.0000	1.0000	1.0000	1.0000	1.0000
2	0	0.9980	0.9900	0.9801	0.9604	0.9409	0.9216	0.9025	0.8836	0.8649	0.8464	0.8281
	1	1.0000	1.0000	0.9999	0.9996	0.9991	0.9984	0.9975	0.9964	0.9951	0.9936	0.9919
	2	1.0000	1.0000	1.0000	1.0000	1.0000	1.0000	1.0000	1.0000	1.0000	1.0000	1.0000
3	0	0.9970	0.9851	0.9703	0.9412	0.9127	0.8847	0.8574	0.8306	0.8044	0.7787	0.7536
	1	1.0000	0.9999	0.9997	0.9988	0.9974	0.9953	0.9928	0.9896	0.9860	0.9818	0.9772
	2	1.0000	1.0000	1.0000	1.0000	1.0000	0.9999	0.9999	0.9998	0.9997	0.9995	0.9993
	3	1.0000	1.0000	1.0000	1.0000	1.0000	1.0000	1.0000	1.0000	1.0000	1.0000	1.0000
4	0	0.9960	0.9801	0.9606	0.9224	0.8853	0.8493	0.8145	0.7807	0.7481	0.7164	0.6857
	1	1.0000	0.9999	0.9994	0.9977	0.9948	0.9909	0.9860	0.9801	0.9733	0.9656	0.9570
	2	1.0000	1.0000	1.0000	1.0000	0.9999	0.9998	0.9995	0.9992	0.9987	0.9981	0.9973
	3	1.0000	1.0000	1.0000	1.0000	1.0000	1.0000	1.0000	1.0000	1.0000	1.0000	1.9999
	4	1.0000	1.0000	1.0000	1.0000	1.0000	1.0000	1.0000	1.0000	1.0000	1.0000	1.0000
5	0	0.9950	0.9752	0.9510	0.9039	0.8587	0.8154	0.7738	0.7339	0.6957	0.6591	0.6240
	1	1.0000	0.9998	0.9990	0.9962	0.9915	0.9852	0.9774	0.9681	0.9575	0.9456	0.9326
	2	1.0000	1.0000	1.0000	0.9999	0.9997	0.9994	0.9988	0.9980	0.9969	0.9955	0.9937
	3	1.0000	1.0000	1.0000	1.0000	1.0000	1.0000	1.0000	0.9999	0.9999	0.9998	0.9997
	4	1.0000	1.0000	1.0000	1.0000	1.0000	1.0000	1.0000	1.0000	1.0000	1.0000	1.0000
6	0	0.9940	0.9704	0.9415	0.8858	0.8330	0.7828	0.7351	0.6899	0.6470	0.6064	0.5679
	1	1.0000	0.9996	0.9985	0.9943	0.9875	0.9784	0.9672	0.9541	0.9392	0.9227	0.9048
	2	1.0000	1.0000	1.0000	0.9998	0.9995	0.9988	0.9978	0.9962	0.9942	0.9915	0.9882
	3	1.0000	1.0000	1.0000	1.0000	1.0000	1.0000	0.9999	0.9998	0.9997	0.9995	0.9992
	4	1.0000	1.0000	1.0000	1.0000	1.0000	1.0000	1.0000	1.0000	1.0000	1.0000	1.0000
7	0	0.9930	0.9655	0.9321	0.8681	0.8080	0.7514	0.6983	0.6485	0.6017	0.5578	0.5168
	1	1.0000	0.9995	0.9980	0.9921	0.9829	0.9706	0.9556	0.9382	0.9187	0.8974	0.8745
	2	1.0000	1.0000	1.0000	0.9997	0.9991	0.9980	0.9962	0.9937	0.9903	0.9860	0.9807
	3	1.0000	1.0000	1.0000	1.0000	1.0000	0.9999	0.9998	0.9996	0.9993	0.9988	0.9982
	4	1.0000	1.0000	1.0000	1.0000	1.0000	1.0000	1.0000	1.0000	1.0000	0.9999	0.9999
	5	1.0000	1.0000	1.0000	1.0000	1.0000	1.0000	1.0000	1.0000	1.0000	1.0000	1.0000
8	0	0.9920	0.9607	0.9227	0.8508	0.7837	0.7214	0.6634	0.6096	0.5596	0.5132	0.4703
	1	1.0000	0.9993	0.9973	0.9897	0.9777	0.9619	0.9428	0.9208	0.8965	0.8702	0.8423
	2	1.0000	1.0000	0.9999	0.9996	0.9987	0.9969	0.9942	0.9904	0.9853	0.9789	0.9711
	3	1.0000	1.0000	1.0000	1.0000	0.9999	0.9998	0.9996	0.9993	0.9987	0.9978	0.9966
	4	1.0000	1.0000	1.0000	1.0000	1.0000	1.0000	1.0000	1.0000	0.9999	0.5168	0.9997
	5	1.0000	1.0000	1.0000	1.0000	1.0000	1.0000	1.0000	1.0000	1.0000	1.0000	1.0000
9	0	0.9910	0.9559	0.9135	0.8337	0.7602	0.6925	0.6302	0.5730	0.5204	0.4722	0.4279
	1	1.0000	0.9991	0.9966	0.9869	0.9718	0.9522	0.9288	0.9022	0.8729	0.8417	0.8088
	2	1.0000	1.0000	0.9999	0.9994	0.9980	0.9955	0.9916	0.9862	0.9791	0.9702	0.9595
	3	1.0000	1.0000	1.0000	1.0000	0.9999	0.9997	0.9994	0.9987	0.9977	0.9963	0.9943
	4	1.0000	1.0000	1.0000	1.0000	1.0000	1.0000	1.0000	0.9999	0.9998	0.9997	0.9995
	5	1.0000	1.0000	1.0000	1.0000	1.0000	1.0000	1.0000	1.0000	1.0000	1.0000	1.0000
10	0	0.9900	0.9511	0.9044	0.8171	0.7374	0.6648	0.5987	0.5386	0.4840	0.4344	0.3894
	1	1.0000	0.9989	0.9957	0.9838	0.9655	0.9418	0.9139	0.8824	0.8483	0.8121	0.7746
	2	1.0000	1.0000	0.9999	0.9991	0.9972	0.9938	0.9885	0.9812	0.9717	0.9599	0.9460
	3	1.0000	1.0000	1.0000	1.0000	0.9999	0.9996	0.9990	0.9980	0.9964	0.9942	0.9912
	4	1.0000	1.0000	1.0000	1.0000	1.0000	1.0000	0.9999	0.9998	0.9997	0.9994	0.9990
	5	1.0000	1.0000	1.0000	1.0000	1.0000	1.0000	1.0000	1.0000	1.0000	1.0000	0.9999
	6	1.0000	1.0000	1.0000	1.0000	1.0000	1.0000	1.0000	1.0000	1.0000	1.0000	1.0000

contd...

contd...

		θ										
n	x	0.001	0.005	0.01	0.02	0.03	0.04	0.05	0.06	0.07	0.08	0.09
11	0	0.9891	0.9464	0.8953	0.8007	0.7153	0.6382	0.5688	0.5063	0.4501	0.3996	0.3544
	1	0.9999	0.9987	0.9948	0.9805	0.9587	0.9308	0.8981	0.8618	0.8228	0.7819	0.7399
	2	1.0000	1.0000	0.9998	0.9988	0.9963	0.9917	0.9848	0.9752	0.9630	0.9481	0.9305
	3	1.0000	1.0000	1.0000	1.0000	0.9998	0.9993	0.9984	0.9970	0.9947	0.9915	0.9871
	4	1.0000	1.0000	1.0000	1.0000	1.0000	1.0000	0.9999	0.9997	0.9995	0.9990	0.9983
	5	1.0000	1.0000	1.0000	1.0000	1.0000	1.0000	1.0000	1.0000	1.0000	0.9999	0.9998
	6	1.0000	1.0000	1.0000	1.0000	1.0000	1.0000	1.0000	1.0000	1.0000	1.0000	1.0000
12	0	0.9881	0.9416	0.8864	0.7847	0.6938	0.6127	0.5404	0.4759	0.4186	0.3677	0.3225
	1	0.9999	0.9984	0.9938	0.9769	0.9514	0.9191	0.8816	0.8405	0.7967	0.7513	0.7052
	2	1.0000	1.0000	0.9998	0.9985	0.9952	0.9893	0.9804	0.9684	0.9532	0.9348	0.9134
	3	1.0000	1.0000	1.0000	0.9999	0.9997	0.9990	0.9978	0.9957	0.9925	0.9880	0.9820
	4	1.0000	1.0000	1.0000	1.0000	1.0000	0.9999	0.9998	0.9996	0.9991	0.9984	0.9973
	5	1.0000	1.0000	1.0000	1.0000	1.0000	1.0000	1.0000	1.0000	0.9999	0.9998	0.9997
	6	1.0000	1.0000	1.0000	1.0000	1.0000	1.0000	1.0000	1.0000	1.0000	1.0000	1.0000
13	0	0.9871	0.9369	0.8775	0.7690	0.6730	0.5882	0.5133	0.4474	0.3893	0.3383	0.2935
	1	0.9999	0.9981	0.9928	0.9730	0.9436	0.9068	0.8646	0.8186	0.7702	0.7206	0.6707
	2	1.0000	1.0000	0.9997	0.9980	0.9938	0.9865	0.9755	0.9608	0.9422	0.9201	0.8946
	3	1.0000	1.0000	1.0000	0.9999	0.9995	0.9986	0.9969	0.9940	0.9897	0.9837	0.9758
	4	1.0000	1.0000	1.0000	1.0000	1.0000	0.9999	0.9997	0.9993	0.9987	0.9976	0.9959
	5	1.0000	1.0000	1.0000	1.0000	1.0000	1.0000	1.0000	0.9999	0.9999	0.9997	0.9995
	6	1.0000	1.0000	1.0000	1.0000	1.0000	1.0000	1.0000	1.0000	1.0000	1.0000	0.9999
	7	1.0000	1.0000	1.0000	1.0000	1.0000	1.0000	1.0000	1.0000	1.0000	1.0000	1.0000
14	0	0.9861	0.9322	0.8687	0.7536	0.6528	0.5647	0.4877	0.4205	0.3620	0.3112	0.2670
	1	0.9999	0.9978	0.9916	0.9690	0.9355	0.8941	0.8470	0.7963	0.7436	0.6900	0.6368
	2	1.0000	1.0000	0.9997	0.9975	0.9923	0.9833	0.9699	0.9522	0.9302	0.9042	0.8745
	3	1.0000	1.0000	1.0000	0.9999	0.9994	0.9981	0.9958	0.9920	0.9864	0.9786	0.9685
	4	1.0000	1.0000	1.0000	1.0000	1.0000	0.9998	0.9996	0.9990	0.9980	0.9965	0.9941
	5	1.0000	1.0000	1.0000	1.0000	1.0000	1.0000	1.0000	0.9999	0.9998	0.9996	0.9992
	6	1.0000	1.0000	1.0000	1.0000	1.0000	1.0000	1.0000	1.0000	1.0000	1.0000	0.9999
	7	1.0000	1.0000	1.0000	1.0000	1.0000	1.0000	1.0000	1.0000	1.0000	1.0000	1.0000
15	0	0.9851	0.9276	0.8601	0.7386	0.6333	0.5421	0.4633	0.3953	0.3367	0.2863	0.2430
	1	0.9999	0.9975	0.9904	0.9647	0.9270	0.8809	0.8290	0.7738	0.7168	0.6597	0.6035
	2	1.0000	0.9999	0.9996	0.9970	0.9906	0.9797	0.9638	0.9429	0.9171	0.8870	0.8531
	3	1.0000	1.0000	1.0000	0.9998	0.9992	0.9976	0.9945	0.9896	0.9825	0.9727	0.9601
	4	1.0000	1.0000	1.0000	1.0000	0.9999	0.9998	0.9994	0.9986	0.9972	0.9950	0.9918
	5	1.0000	1.0000	1.0000	1.0000	1.0000	1.0000	0.9999	0.9999	0.9997	0.9993	0.9987
	6	1.0000	1.0000	1.0000	1.0000	1.0000	1.0000	1.0000	1.0000	1.0000	0.9999	0.9998
	7	1.0000	1.0000	1.0000	1.0000	1.0000	1.0000	1.0000	1.0000	1.0000	1.0000	1.0000
16	0	0.9841	0.9229	0.8515	0.7238	0.6143	0.5204	0.4401	0.3716	0.3131	0.2634	0.2211
	1	0.9999	0.9971	0.9891	0.9601	0.9182	0.8673	0.8108	0.7511	0.6902	0.6299	0.5711
	2	1.0000	0.9999	0.9995	0.9963	0.9887	0.9758	0.9571	0.9327	0.9031	0.8689	0.8306
	3	1.0000	1.0000	1.0000	0.9998	0.9989	0.9968	0.9930	0.9868	0.9779	0.9658	0.9504
	4	1.0000	1.0000	1.0000	1.0000	0.9999	0.9997	0.9991	0.9981	0.9962	0.9932	0.9889
	5	1.0000	1.0000	1.0000	1.0000	1.0000	1.0000	0.9999	0.9998	0.9995	0.9990	0.9981
	6	1.0000	1.0000	1.0000	1.0000	1.0000	1.0000	1.0000	1.0000	0.9999	0.9999	0.9997
	7	1.0000	1.0000	1.0000	1.0000	1.0000	1.0000	1.0000	1.0000	1.0000	1.0000	1.0000
17	0	0.9831	0.9183	0.8429	0.7093	0.5958	0.4996	0.4181	0.3493	0.2912	0.2423	0.2012
	1	0.9999	0.9968	0.9877	0.9554	0.9091	0.8535	0.7922	0.7283	0.6638	0.6005	0.5396
	2	1.0000	0.9999	0.9994	0.9956	0.9866	0.9714	0.9497	0.9218	0.8882	0.8497	0.8073
	3	1.0000	1.0000	1.0000	0.9997	0.9986	0.9960	0.9912	0.9836	0.9727	0.9581	0.9397
	4	1.0000	1.0000	1.0000	1.0000	0.9999	0.9996	0.9988	0.9974	0.9949	0.9911	0.9855
	5	1.0000	1.0000	1.0000	1.0000	1.0000	1.0000	0.9999	0.9997	0.9993	0.9985	0.9973
	6	1.0000	1.0000	1.0000	1.0000	1.0000	1.0000	1.0000	1.0000	0.9999	0.9998	0.9996
	7	1.0000	1.0000	1.0000	1.0000	1.0000	1.0000	1.0000	1.0000	1.0000	1.0000	1.0000

contd...

contd...

n	x	0.001	0.005	0.01	0.02	0.03	0.04	0.05	0.06	0.07	0.08	0.09
		θ										
18	0	0.9822	0.9137	0.8345	0.6951	0.5780	0.4796	0.3972	0.3283	0.2708	0.2229	0.1831
	1	0.9998	0.9964	0.9862	0.9505	0.8997	0.8393	0.7735	0.7055	0.6378	0.5719	0.5091
	2	1.0000	0.9999	0.9993	0.9948	0.9843	0.9667	0.9419	0.9102	0.8725	0.8298	0.7832
	3	1.0000	1.0000	1.0000	0.9996	0.9982	0.9950	0.9891	0.9799	0.9667	0.9494	0.9277
	4	1.0000	1.0000	1.0000	1.0000	0.9998	0.9994	0.9985	0.9966	0.9933	0.9884	0.9814
	5	1.0000	1.0000	1.0000	1.0000	1.0000	0.9999	0.9998	0.9995	0.9990	0.9979	0.9962
	6	1.0000	1.0000	1.0000	1.0000	1.0000	1.0000	1.0000	1.0000	0.9999	0.9997	0.9994
	7	1.0000	1.0000	1.0000	1.0000	1.0000	1.0000	1.0000	1.0000	1.0000	1.0000	0.9999
	8	1.0000	1.0000	1.0000	1.0000	1.0000	1.0000	1.0000	1.0000	1.0000	1.0000	1.0000
19	0	0.9812	0.9092	0.8262	0.6812	0.5606	0.4604	0.3774	0.3086	0.2519	0.2051	0.1666
	1	0.9998	0.9960	0.9847	0.9454	0.8900	0.8249	0.7547	0.6829	0.6121	0.5440	0.4798
	2	1.0000	0.9999	0.9991	0.9939	0.9817	0.9616	0.9335	0.8979	0.8561	0.8092	0.7585
	3	1.0000	1.0000	1.0000	0.9995	0.9978	0.9939	0.9868	0.9757	0.9602	0.9398	0.9147
	4	1.0000	1.0000	1.0000	1.0000	0.9998	0.9993	0.9980	0.9956	0.9915	0.9853	0.9765
	5	1.0000	1.0000	1.0000	1.0000	1.0000	0.9999	0.9998	0.9994	0.9986	0.9971	0.9949
	6	1.0000	1.0000	1.0000	1.0000	1.0000	1.0000	1.0000	0.9999	0.9998	0.9996	0.9991
	7	1.0000	1.0000	1.0000	1.0000	1.0000	1.0000	1.0000	1.0000	1.0000	0.9999	0.9999
	8	1.0000	1.0000	1.0000	1.0000	1.0000	1.0000	1.0000	1.0000	1.0000	1.0000	1.0000
20	0	0.9802	0.9046	0.8179	0.6676	0.5438	0.4420	0.3585	0.2901	0.2342	0.1887	0.1516
	1	0.9998	0.9955	0.9831	0.9401	0.8802	0.8103	0.7358	0.6605	0.5869	0.5169	0.4516
	2	1.0000	0.9999	0.9990	0.9929	0.9790	0.9561	0.9245	0.8850	0.8390	0.7879	0.7334
	3	1.0000	1.0000	1.0000	0.9994	0.9973	0.9926	0.9841	0.9710	0.9529	0.9294	0.9007
	4	1.0000	1.0000	1.0000	1.0000	0.9997	0.9990	0.9974	0.9944	0.9893	0.9817	0.9710
	5	1.0000	1.0000	1.0000	1.0000	1.0000	0.9999	0.9997	0.9991	0.9981	0.9962	0.9932
	6	1.0000	1.0000	1.0000	1.0000	1.0000	1.0000	1.0000	0.9999	0.9997	0.9994	0.9987
	7	1.0000	1.0000	1.0000	1.0000	1.0000	1.0000	1.0000	1.0000	1.0000	0.9999	0.9998
	8	1.0000	1.0000	1.0000	1.0000	1.0000	1.0000	1.0000	1.0000	1.0000	1.0000	1.0000

Cumulative distribution function for $0.1 \leq \theta \leq 0.5$

n	x	0.1	0.125	0.15	0.2	0.25	0.3	0.3333	0.35	0.4	0.45	0.5
		θ										
1	0	0.9000	0.8750	0.8500	0.8000	0.7500	0.7000	0.6667	0.6500	0.6000	0.5500	0.5000
	1	1.0000	1.0000	1.0000	1.0000	1.0000	1.0000	1.0000	1.0000	1.0000	1.0000	1.0000
2	0	0.8100	0.7656	0.7225	0.6400	0.5625	0.4900	0.4444	0.4225	0.3600	0.3025	0.2500
	1	0.9900	0.9844	0.9775	0.9600	0.9375	0.9100	0.8889	0.8775	0.8400	0.7975	0.7500
	2	1.0000	1.0000	1.0000	1.0000	1.0000	1.0000	1.0000	1.0000	1.0000	1.0000	1.0000
3	0	0.7290	0.6699	0.6141	0.5120	0.4219	0.3430	0.2963	0.2746	0.2160	0.1664	0.1250
	1	0.9720	0.9570	0.9392	0.8960	0.8438	0.7840	0.7407	0.7183	0.6480	0.5748	0.5000
	2	0.9990	0.9980	0.9966	0.9920	0.9844	0.9730	0.9630	0.9571	0.9360	0.9089	0.8750
	3	1.0000	1.0000	1.0000	1.0000	1.0000	1.0000	1.0000	1.0000	1.0000	1.0000	1.0000
4	0	0.6561	0.5862	0.5220	0.4096	0.3164	0.2401	0.1975	0.1785	0.1296	0.0915	0.0625
	1	0.9477	0.9211	0.8905	0.8192	0.7383	0.6517	0.5926	0.5630	0.4752	0.3910	0.3125
	2	0.9963	0.9929	0.9880	0.9728	0.9492	0.9163	0.8889	0.8735	0.8208	0.7585	0.6875
	3	0.9999	0.9998	0.9995	0.9984	0.9961	0.9919	0.9877	0.9850	0.9744	0.9590	0.9375
	4	1.0000	1.0000	1.0000	1.0000	1.0000	1.0000	1.0000	1.0000	1.0000	1.0000	1.0000
5	0	0.5905	0.5129	0.4437	0.3277	0.2373	0.1681	0.1317	0.1160	0.0778	0.0503	0.0312
	1	0.9185	0.8793	0.8352	0.7373	0.6328	0.5282	0.4609	0.4284	0.3370	0.2562	0.1875
	2	0.9914	0.9839	0.9734	0.9421	0.8965	0.8369	0.7901	0.7648	0.6826	0.5931	0.5000
	3	0.9995	0.9989	0.9978	0.9933	0.9844	0.9692	0.9547	0.9460	0.9130	0.8688	0.8125
	4	1.0000	1.0000	0.9999	0.9997	0.9990	0.9976	0.9959	0.9847	0.9998	0.9815	0.9688
	5	1.0000	1.0000	1.0000	1.0000	1.0000	1.0000	1.0000	1.0000	1.0000	1.0000	1.0000

contd...

contd...

		θ										
n	x	0.1	0.125	0.15	0.2	0.25	0.3	0.3333	0.35	0.4	0.45	0.5
6	0	0.5314	0.4488	0.3771	0.2621	0.1780	0.1176	0.0878	0.0754	0.0467	0.0277	0.0156
	1	0.8857	0.8335	0.7765	0.6554	0.5339	0.4202	0.3512	0.3191	0.2333	0.1636	0.1094
	2	0.9842	0.9709	0.9527	0.9011	0.8306	0.7443	0.6804	0.6471	0.5443	0.4415	0.3437
	3	0.9987	0.9970	0.9941	0.9830	0.9624	0.9295	0.8999	0.8826	0.8208	0.7447	0.6562
	4	0.9999	0.9998	0.9996	0.9984	0.9954	0.9891	0.9822	0.9777	0.9590	0.9308	0.8906
	5	1.0000	1.0000	1.0000	0.9999	0.9998	0.9993	0.9986	0.9982	0.9959	0.9917	0.9844
	6	1.0000	1.0000	1.0000	1.0000	1.0000	1.0000	1.0000	1.0000	1.0000	1.0000	1.0000
7	0	0.4783	0.3927	0.3206	0.2097	0.1335	0.0824	0.0585	0.0490	0.0280	0.0152	0.0078
	1	0.8503	0.7854	0.7166	0.5767	0.4449	0.3294	0.2634	0.2338	0.1586	0.1024	0.0625
	2	0.9743	0.9537	0.9262	0.8520	0.7564	0.6471	0.5706	0.5323	0.4199	0.3164	0.2266
	3	0.9973	0.9938	0.9879	0.9667	0.9294	0.8740	0.8267	0.8002	0.7102	0.6083	0.5000
	4	0.9998	0.9995	0.9988	0.9953	0.9871	0.9712	0.9547	0.9444	0.9037	0.8471	0.7734
	5	1.0000	1.0000	0.9999	0.9996	0.9987	0.9962	0.9931	0.9910	0.9812	0.9643	0.9375
	6	1.0000	1.0000	1.0000	1.0000	0.9999	0.9998	0.9995	0.9994	0.9984	0.9963	0.9922
	7	1.0000	1.0000	1.0000	1.0000	1.0000	1.0000	1.0000	1.0000	1.0000	1.0000	1.0000
8	0	0.4305	0.3436	0.2725	0.1678	0.1001	0.0576	0.0390	0.0319	0.0168	0.0084	0.0039
	1	0.8131	0.7363	0.6572	0.5033	0.3671	0.2553	0.1951	0.1691	0.1064	0.0632	0.0352
	2	0.9619	0.9327	0.8948	0.7969	0.6785	0.5518	0.4682	0.4278	0.3154	0.2201	0.1445
	3	0.9950	0.9888	0.9786	0.9437	0.8862	0.8059	0.7414	0.7064	0.5941	0.4770	0.3633
	4	0.9996	0.9988	0.9971	0.9896	0.9727	0.9420	0.9121	0.8939	0.8263	0.7396	0.6367
	5	1.0000	0.9999	0.9998	0.9988	0.9958	0.9887	0.9803	0.9747	0.9502	0.9115	0.8555
	6	1.0000	1.0000	1.0000	0.9999	0.9996	0.9987	0.9974	0.9964	0.9915	0.9819	0.9648
	7	1.0000	1.0000	1.0000	1.0000	1.0000	0.9999	0.9998	0.9998	0.9993	0.9983	0.9961
	8	1.0000	1.0000	1.0000	1.0000	1.0000	1.0000	1.0000	1.0000	1.0000	1.0000	1.0000
9	0	0.3874	0.3007	0.2316	0.1342	0.0751	0.0404	0.0260	0.0207	0.0101	0.0046	0.0020
	1	0.7748	0.6872	0.5995	0.4362	0.3003	0.1960	0.1431	0.1211	0.0705	0.0385	0.0195
	2	0.9470	0.9081	0.8591	0.7382	0.6007	0.4628	0.3772	0.3373	0.2318	0.1495	0.0898
	3	0.9917	0.9817	0.9661	0.9144	0.8343	0.7297	0.6503	0.6089	0.4826	0.3614	0.2539
	4	0.9991	0.9975	0.9944	0.9804	0.9511	0.9012	0.8552	0.8283	0.7334	0.6214	0.5000
	5	0.9999	0.9998	0.9994	0.9969	0.9900	0.9747	0.9576	0.9464	0.9006	0.8342	0.7461
	6	1.0000	1.0000	1.0000	0.9997	0.9987	0.9957	0.9917	0.9888	0.9750	0.9502	0.9102
	7	1.0000	1.0000	1.0000	1.0000	0.9999	0.9996	0.9990	0.9986	0.9962	0.9909	0.9805
	8	1.0000	1.0000	1.0000	1.0000	1.0000	1.0000	0.9999	0.9999	0.9997	0.9992	0.9980
	9	1.0000	1.0000	1.0000	1.0000	1.0000	1.0000	1.0000	1.0000	1.0000	1.0000	1.0000
10	0	0.3487	0.2631	0.1969	0.1074	0.0563	0.0282	0.0173	0.0135	0.0060	0.0025	0.0010
	1	0.7361	0.6389	0.5443	0.3758	0.2440	0.1493	0.1040	0.0860	0.0464	0.0233	0.0107
	2	0.9298	0.8805	0.8202	0.6778	0.5256	0.3828	0.2991	0.2616	0.1673	0.0996	0.0547
	3	0.9872	0.9725	0.9500	0.8791	0.7759	0.6496	0.5593	0.5138	0.3823	0.2660	0.1719
	4	0.9984	0.9955	0.9901	0.9672	0.9219	0.8497	0.7869	0.7515	0.6331	0.5044	0.3770
	5	0.9999	0.9995	0.9986	0.9936	0.9803	0.9527	0.9234	0.9051	0.8338	0.7384	0.6230
	6	1.0000	1.0000	0.9999	0.9991	0.9965	0.9894	0.9803	0.9740	0.9452	0.8980	0.8281
	7	1.0000	1.0000	1.0000	0.9999	0.9996	0.9984	0.9966	0.9952	0.9877	0.9726	0.9453
	8	1.0000	1.0000	1.0000	1.0000	1.0000	0.9999	0.9996	0.9995	0.9983	0.9955	0.9893
	9	1.0000	1.0000	1.0000	1.0000	1.0000	1.0000	1.0000	1.0000	0.9999	0.9997	0.9990
	10	1.0000	1.0000	1.0000	1.0000	1.0000	1.0000	1.0000	1.0000	1.0000	1.0000	1.0000
11	0	0.3138	0.2302	0.1673	0.0859	0.0422	0.0198	0.0116	0.0088	0.0036	0.0014	0.0005
	1	0.6974	0.5919	0.4922	0.3221	0.1971	0.1130	0.0751	0.0606	0.0302	0.0139	0.0059
	2	0.9104	0.8503	0.7788	0.6174	0.4552	0.3127	0.2341	0.2001	0.1189	0.0652	0.0327
	3	0.9815	0.9610	0.9306	0.8389	0.7133	0.5696	0.4726	0.4256	0.2963	0.1911	0.1133
	4	0.9972	0.9927	0.9841	0.9496	0.8854	0.7897	0.7110	0.6683	0.5328	0.3971	0.2744
	5	0.9997	0.9990	0.9973	0.9883	0.9657	0.9218	0.8779	0.8513	0.7535	0.6331	0.5000
	6	1.0000	0.9999	0.9997	0.9980	0.9924	0.9784	0.9614	0.9499	0.9006	0.8262	0.7256

contd...

contd...

		θ										
n	x	0.1	0.125	0.15	0.2	0.25	0.3	0.3333	0.35	0.4	0.45	0.5
	7	1.0000	1.0000	1.0000	0.9998	0.9988	0.9957	0.9912	0.9878	0.9707	0.9390	0.8867
	8	1.0000	1.0000	1.0000	1.0000	0.9999	0.9994	0.9986	0.9980	0.9941	0.9852	0.9673
	9	1.0000	1.0000	1.0000	1.0000	1.0000	1.0000	0.9999	0.9998	0.9993	0.9978	0.9941
	10	1.0000	1.0000	1.0000	1.0000	1.0000	1.0000	1.0000	1.0000	1.0000	0.9998	0.9995
	11	1.0000	1.0000	1.0000	1.0000	1.0000	1.0000	1.0000	1.0000	1.0000	1.0000	1.0000
12	0	0.2824	0.2014	0.1422	0.0687	0.0317	0.0138	0.0077	0.0057	0.0022	0.0008	0.0002
	1	0.6590	0.5467	0.4435	0.2749	0.1584	0.0850	0.0540	0.0424	0.0196	0.0083	0.0032
	2	0.8891	0.8180	0.7358	0.5583	0.3907	0.2528	0.1811	0.1513	0.0834	0.0421	0.0193
	3	0.9744	0.9472	0.9078	0.7946	0.6488	0.4925	0.3931	0.3467	0.2253	0.1345	0.0730
	4	0.9957	0.9887	0.9761	0.9274	0.8424	0.7237	0.6315	0.5833	0.4382	0.3044	0.1938
	5	0.9995	0.9982	0.9954	0.9806	0.9456	0.8822	0.8223	0.7873	0.6652	0.5269	0.3872
	6	0.9999	0.9998	0.9993	0.9961	0.9857	0.9614	0.9336	0.9154	0.8418	0.7393	0.6128
	7	1.0000	1.0000	0.9999	0.9994	0.9972	0.9905	0.9812	0.9745	0.9427	0.8883	0.8062
	8	1.0000	1.0000	1.0000	0.9999	0.9996	0.9983	0.9961	0.9944	0.9847	0.9644	0.9270
	9	1.0000	1.0000	1.0000	1.0000	1.0000	0.9998	0.9995	0.9992	0.9972	0.9921	0.9807
	10	1.0000	1.0000	1.0000	1.0000	1.0000	1.0000	1.0000	0.9999	0.9997	0.9989	0.9968
	11	1.0000	1.0000	1.0000	1.0000	1.0000	1.0000	1.0000	1.0000	1.0000	0.9999	0.9998
	12	1.0000	1.0000	1.0000	1.0000	1.0000	1.0000	1.0000	1.0000	1.0000	1.0000	1.0000
13	0	0.2542	0.1762	0.1209	0.0550	0.0238	0.0097	0.0051	0.0037	0.0013	0.0004	0.0001
	1	0.6213	0.5035	0.3983	0.2336	0.1267	0.0637	0.0385	0.0296	0.0126	0.0049	0.0017
	2	0.8661	0.7841	0.6920	0.5017	0.3326	0.2025	0.1387	0.1132	0.0579	0.0269	0.0112
	3	0.9658	0.9310	0.8820	0.7473	0.5843	0.4206	0.3224	0.2783	0.1686	0.0929	0.0461
	4	0.9935	0.9835	0.9658	0.9009	0.7940	0.6543	0.5520	0.5005	0.3530	0.2279	0.1334
	5	0.9991	0.9970	0.9925	0.9700	0.9198	0.8346	0.7587	0.7159	0.5744	0.4268	0.2905
	6	0.9999	0.9996	0.9987	0.9930	0.9757	0.9376	0.8965	0.8705	0.7712	0.6437	0.5000
	7	1.0000	1.0000	0.9998	0.9988	0.9944	0.9818	0.9653	0.9538	0.9023	0.8212	0.7095
	8	1.0000	1.0000	1.0000	0.9998	0.9990	0.9960	0.9912	0.9874	0.9679	0.9302	0.8666
	9	1.0000	1.0000	1.0000	1.0000	0.9999	0.9993	0.9984	0.9975	0.9922	0.9797	0.9539
	10	1.0000	1.0000	1.0000	1.0000	1.0000	0.9999	0.9998	0.9997	0.9987	0.9959	0.9888
	11	1.0000	1.0000	1.0000	1.0000	1.0000	1.0000	1.0000	1.0000	0.9999	0.9995	0.9983
	12	1.0000	1.0000	1.0000	1.0000	1.0000	1.0000	1.0000	1.0000	1.0000	1.0000	0.9999
	13	1.0000	1.0000	1.0000	1.0000	1.0000	1.0000	1.0000	1.0000	1.0000	1.0000	1.0000
14	0	0.2288	0.1542	0.1028	0.0440	0.0178	0.0068	0.0034	0.0024	0.0008	0.0002	0.0001
	1	0.5846	0.4626	0.3567	0.1979	0.1010	0.0475	0.0274	0.0205	0.0081	0.0029	0.0009
	2	0.8416	0.7490	0.6479	0.4481	0.2811	0.1608	0.1053	0.0839	0.0398	0.0170	0.0065
	3	0.9559	0.9127	0.8535	0.6982	0.5213	0.3552	0.2612	0.2205	0.1243	0.0632	0.0287
	4	0.9908	0.9770	0.9533	0.8702	0.7415	0.5842	0.4755	0.4227	0.2793	0.1672	0.0898
	5	0.9985	0.9953	0.9885	0.9561	0.8883	0.7805	0.6898	0.6405	0.4859	0.3373	0.2120
	6	0.9998	0.9993	0.9978	0.9884	0.9617	0.9067	0.8505	0.8164	0.6925	0.5461	0.3953
	7	1.0000	0.9999	0.9997	0.9976	0.9897	0.9685	0.9424	0.9247	0.8499	0.7414	0.6047
	8	1.0000	1.0000	1.0000	0.9996	0.9978	0.9917	0.9826	0.9757	0.9417	0.8811	0.7880
	9	1.0000	1.0000	1.0000	1.0000	0.9997	0.9983	0.9960	0.9940	0.9825	0.9574	0.9102
	10	1.0000	1.0000	1.0000	1.0000	1.0000	0.9998	0.9993	0.9989	0.9961	0.9886	0.9713
	11	1.0000	1.0000	1.0000	1.0000	1.0000	1.0000	0.9999	0.9999	0.9994	0.9978	0.9935
	12	1.0000	1.0000	1.0000	1.0000	1.0000	1.0000	1.0000	1.0000	0.9999	0.9997	0.9991
	13	1.0000	1.0000	1.0000	1.0000	1.0000	1.0000	1.0000	1.0000	1.0000	1.0000	0.9999
	14	1.0000	1.0000	1.0000	1.0000	1.0000	1.0000	1.0000	1.0000	1.0000	1.0000	1.0000
15	0	0.2059	0.1349	0.0874	0.0352	0.0134	0.0047	0.0023	0.0016	0.0005	0.0001	0.0000
	1	0.5490	0.4241	0.3186	0.1671	0.0802	0.0353	0.0194	0.0142	0.0052	0.0017	0.0005
	2	0.8159	0.7132	0.6042	0.3980	0.2361	0.1268	0.0794	0.0617	0.0271	0.0107	0.0037
	3	0.9444	0.8922	0.8227	0.6482	0.4613	0.2969	0.2092	0.1727	0.0905	0.0424	0.0176
	4	0.9873	0.9689	0.9383	0.8358	0.6865	0.5155	0.4041	0.3519	0.2173	0.1204	0.0592

contd...

contd...

		θ										
n	x	0.1	0.125	0.15	0.2	0.25	0.3	0.3333	0.35	0.4	0.45	0.5
	5	0.9978	0.9930	0.9832	0.9389	0.8516	0.7216	0.6184	0.5643	0.4032	0.2608	0.1509
	6	0.9997	0.9988	0.9964	0.9819	0.9434	0.8689	0.7970	0.7548	0.6098	0.4522	0.3036
	7	1.0000	0.9998	0.9994	0.9958	0.9827	0.9500	0.9118	0.8868	0.7869	0.6535	0.5000
	8	1.0000	1.0000	0.9999	0.9992	0.9958	0.9848	0.9692	0.9578	0.9050	0.8182	0.6964
	9	1.0000	1.0000	1.0000	0.9999	0.9992	0.9963	0.9915	0.9876	0.9662	0.9231	0.8491
	10	1.0000	1.0000	1.0000	1.0000	0.9999	0.9993	0.9982	0.9972	0.9907	0.9745	0.9408
	11	1.0000	1.0000	1.0000	1.0000	1.0000	0.9999	0.9997	0.9995	0.9981	0.9937	0.9824
	12	1.0000	1.0000	1.0000	1.0000	1.0000	1.0000	1.0000	0.9999	0.9997	0.9989	0.9963
	13	1.0000	1.0000	1.0000	1.0000	1.0000	1.0000	1.0000	1.0000	1.0000	0.9999	0.9995
	14	1.0000	1.0000	1.0000	1.0000	1.0000	1.0000	1.0000	1.0000	1.0000	1.0000	1.0000
16	0	0.1853	0.1181	0.0743	0.0281	0.0100	0.0033	0.0015	0.0010	0.0003	0.0001	0.0000
	1	0.5147	0.3879	0.2839	0.1407	0.0635	0.0261	0.0137	0.0098	0.0033	0.0010	0.0003
	2	0.7892	0.6771	0.5614	0.3518	0.1971	0.0994	0.0594	0.0451	0.0183	0.0066	0.0021
	3	0.9316	0.8698	0.7899	0.5981	0.4050	0.2459	0.1659	0.1339	0.0651	0.0281	0.0106
	4	0.9830	0.9593	0.9209	0.7982	0.6302	0.4499	0.3391	0.2892	0.1666	0.0853	0.0384
	5	0.9967	0.9900	0.9765	0.9183	0.8103	0.6598	0.5469	0.4900	0.3288	0.1976	0.1051
	6	0.9995	0.9981	0.9944	0.9733	0.9204	0.8247	0.7374	0.6881	0.5272	0.3660	0.2272
	7	0.9999	0.9997	0.9989	0.9930	0.9729	0.9256	0.8735	0.8406	0.7161	0.5629	0.4018
	8	1.0000	1.0000	0.9998	0.9985	0.9925	0.9743	0.9500	0.9329	0.8577	0.7441	0.5982
	9	1.0000	1.0000	1.0000	0.9998	0.9984	0.9929	0.9841	0.9771	0.9417	0.8759	0.7728
	10	1.0000	1.0000	1.0000	1.0000	0.9997	0.9984	0.9960	0.9938	0.9809	0.9514	0.8949
	11	1.0000	1.0000	1.0000	1.0000	1.0000	0.9997	0.9992	0.9987	0.9951	0.9851	0.9616
	12	1.0000	1.0000	1.0000	1.0000	1.0000	1.0000	0.9999	0.9998	0.9991	0.9965	0.9894
	13	1.0000	1.0000	1.0000	1.0000	1.0000	1.0000	1.0000	1.0000	0.9999	0.9994	0.9979
	14	1.0000	1.0000	1.0000	1.0000	1.0000	1.0000	1.0000	1.0000	1.0000	0.9999	0.9997
	15	1.0000	1.0000	1.0000	1.0000	1.0000	1.0000	1.0000	1.0000	1.0000	1.0000	1.0000
17	0	0.1668	0.1033	0.0631	0.0225	0.0075	0.0023	0.0010	0.0007	0.0002	0.0000	0.0000
	1	0.4818	0.3542	0.2525	0.1182	0.0501	0.0193	0.0096	0.0067	0.0021	0.0006	0.0001
	2	0.7618	0.6409	0.5198	0.3096	0.1637	0.0774	0.0442	0.0327	0.0123	0.0041	0.0012
	3	0.9174	0.8457	0.7556	0.5489	0.3530	0.2019	0.1304	0.1028	0.0464	0.0184	0.0064
	4	0.9779	0.9482	0.9013	0.7582	0.5739	0.3887	0.2814	0.2348	0.1260	0.0596	0.0245
	5	0.9953	0.9862	0.9681	0.8943	0.7653	0.5968	0.4777	0.4197	0.2639	0.1471	0.0717
	6	0.9992	0.9971	0.9917	0.9623	0.8929	0.7752	0.6739	0.6188	0.4478	0.2902	0.1662
	7	0.9999	0.9995	0.9983	0.9891	0.9598	0.8954	0.8281	0.7872	0.6405	0.4743	0.3145
	8	1.0000	0.9999	0.9997	0.9974	0.9876	0.9597	0.9245	0.9006	0.8011	0.6626	0.5000
	9	1.0000	1.0000	1.0000	0.9995	0.9969	0.9873	0.9727	0.9617	0.9081	0.8166	0.6855
	10	1.0000	1.0000	1.0000	0.9999	0.9994	0.9968	0.9920	0.9880	0.9652	0.9174	0.8338
	11	1.0000	1.0000	1.0000	1.0000	0.9999	0.9993	0.9981	0.9970	0.9894	0.9699	0.9283
	12	1.0000	1.0000	1.0000	1.0000	1.0000	0.9999	0.9997	0.9994	0.9975	0.9914	0.9755
	13	1.0000	1.0000	1.0000	1.0000	1.0000	1.0000	1.0000	0.9999	0.9995	0.9981	0.9936
	14	1.0000	1.0000	1.0000	1.0000	1.0000	1.0000	1.0000	1.0000	0.9999	0.9997	0.9988
	15	1.0000	1.0000	1.0000	1.0000	1.0000	1.0000	1.0000	1.0000	1.0000	1.0000	0.9999
	16	1.0000	1.0000	1.0000	1.0000	1.0000	1.0000	1.0000	1.0000	1.0000	1.0000	1.0000
18	0	0.1501	0.0904	0.0536	0.0180	0.0056	0.0016	0.0007	0.0004	0.0001	0.0000	0.0000
	1	0.4503	0.3228	0.2241	0.0991	0.0395	0.0142	0.0068	0.0046	0.0013	0.0003	0.0001
	2	0.7338	0.6051	0.4797	0.2713	0.1353	0.0600	0.0326	0.0236	0.0082	0.0025	0.0007
	3	0.9018	0.8201	0.7202	0.5010	0.3057	0.1646	0.1017	0.0783	0.0328	0.0120	0.0038
	4	0.9718	0.9354	0.8794	0.7164	0.5187	0.3327	0.2311	0.1886	0.0942	0.0411	0.0154
	5	0.9936	0.9814	0.9581	0.8671	0.7175	0.5344	0.4122	0.3550	0.2088	0.1077	0.0481
	6	0.9988	0.9957	0.9882	0.9487	0.8610	0.7217	0.6085	0.5491	0.3743	0.2258	0.1189
	7	0.9998	0.9992	0.9973	0.9837	0.9431	0.8593	0.7767	0.7283	0.5634	0.3915	0.2403
	8	1.0000	0.9999	0.9995	0.9957	0.9807	0.9404	0.8924	0.8609	0.7368	0.5778	0.4073
	9	1.0000	1.0000	0.9999	0.9991	0.9946	0.9790	0.9567	0.9403	0.8653	0.7473	0.5927

contd...

contd...

		θ										
n	x	0.1	0.125	0.15	0.2	0.25	0.3	0.3333	0.35	0.4	0.45	0.5
	10	1.0000	1.0000	1.0000	0.9998	0.9988	0.9939	0.9856	0.9788	0.9424	0.8720	0.7597
	11	1.0000	1.0000	1.0000	1.0000	0.9998	0.9986	0.9961	0.9938	0.9797	0.9463	0.8811
	12	1.0000	1.0000	1.0000	1.0000	1.0000	0.9997	0.9991	0.9986	0.9942	0.9817	0.9519
	13	1.0000	1.0000	1.0000	1.0000	1.0000	1.0000	0.9999	0.9997	0.9987	0.9951	0.9846
	14	1.0000	1.0000	1.0000	1.0000	1.0000	1.0000	1.0000	1.0000	0.9998	0.9990	0.9962
	15	1.0000	1.0000	1.0000	1.0000	1.0000	1.0000	1.0000	1.0000	1.0000	0.9999	0.9993
	16	1.0000	1.0000	1.0000	1.0000	1.0000	1.0000	1.0000	1.0000	1.0000	1.0000	0.9999
	17	1.0000	1.0000	1.0000	1.0000	1.0000	1.0000	1.0000	1.0000	1.0000	1.0000	1.0000
19	0	0.1351	0.0791	0.0456	0.0144	0.0042	0.0011	0.0005	0.0003	0.0001	0.0000	0.0000
	1	0.4203	0.2938	0.1985	0.0829	0.0310	0.0104	0.0047	0.0031	0.0008	0.0002	0.0000
	2	0.7054	0.5698	0.4413	0.2369	0.1113	0.0462	0.0240	0.0170	0.0055	0.0015	0.0004
	3	0.8850	0.7933	0.6841	0.4551	0.2631	0.1332	0.0787	0.0591	0.0230	0.0077	0.0022
	4	0.9648	0.9209	0.8556	0.6733	0.4654	0.2822	0.1879	0.1500	0.0696	0.0280	0.0096
	5	0.9914	0.9757	0.9463	0.8369	0.6678	0.4739	0.3519	0.2968	0.1629	0.0777	0.0318
	6	0.9983	0.9939	0.9837	0.9324	0.8251	0.6655	0.5431	0.4812	0.3081	0.1727	0.0835
	7	0.9997	0.9988	0.9959	0.9767	0.9225	0.8180	0.7207	0.6656	0.4878	0.3169	0.1796
	8	1.0000	0.9998	0.9992	0.9933	0.9713	0.9161	0.8538	0.8145	0.6675	0.4940	0.3238
	9	1.0000	1.0000	0.9999	0.9984	0.9911	0.9674	0.9352	0.9125	0.8139	0.6710	0.5000
	10	1.0000	1.0000	1.0000	0.9997	0.9977	0.9895	0.9759	0.9653	0.9115	0.8159	0.6762
	11	1.0000	1.0000	1.0000	1.0000	0.9995	0.9972	0.9926	0.9886	0.9648	0.9129	0.8204
	12	1.0000	1.0000	1.0000	1.0000	0.9999	0.9994	0.9981	0.9969	0.9884	0.9658	0.9165
	13	1.0000	1.0000	1.0000	1.0000	1.0000	0.9999	0.9996	0.9993	0.9969	0.9891	0.9682
	14	1.0000	1.0000	1.0000	1.0000	1.0000	1.0000	0.9999	0.9999	0.9994	0.9972	0.9904
	15	1.0000	1.0000	1.0000	1.0000	1.0000	1.0000	1.0000	1.0000	0.9999	0.9995	0.9978
	16	1.0000	1.0000	1.0000	1.0000	1.0000	1.0000	1.0000	1.0000	1.0000	0.9999	0.9996
	17	1.0000	1.0000	1.0000	1.0000	1.0000	1.0000	1.0000	1.0000	1.0000	1.0000	1.0000
20	0	0.1216	0.0692	0.0388	0.0115	0.0032	0.0008	0.0003	0.0002	0.0000	0.0000	0.0000
	1	0.3917	0.2669	0.1756	0.0692	0.0243	0.0076	0.0033	0.0021	0.0005	0.0001	0.0000
	2	0.6769	0.5353	0.4049	0.2061	0.0913	0.0355	0.0176	0.0121	0.0036	0.0009	0.0002
	3	0.8670	0.7653	0.6477	0.4114	0.2252	0.1071	0.0604	0.0444	0.0160	0.0049	0.0013
	4	0.9568	0.9050	0.8298	0.6296	0.4148	0.2375	0.1515	0.1182	0.0510	0.0189	0.0059
	5	0.9887	0.9688	0.9327	0.8042	0.6172	0.4164	0.2972	0.2454	0.1256	0.0553	0.0207
	6	0.9976	0.9916	0.9781	0.9133	0.7858	0.6080	0.4793	0.4166	0.2500	0.1299	0.0577
	7	0.9996	0.9981	0.9941	0.9679	0.8982	0.7723	0.6615	0.6010	0.4159	0.2520	0.1316
	8	0.9999	0.9997	0.9987	0.9900	0.9591	0.8867	0.8095	0.7624	0.5956	0.4143	0.2517
	9	1.0000	0.9999	0.9998	0.9974	0.9861	0.9520	0.9081	0.8782	0.7553	0.5914	0.4119
	10	1.0000	1.0000	1.0000	0.9994	0.9961	0.9829	0.9624	0.9468	0.8725	0.7507	0.5881
	11	1.0000	1.0000	1.0000	0.9999	0.9991	0.9949	0.9870	0.9804	0.9435	0.8692	0.7483
	12	1.0000	1.0000	1.0000	1.0000	0.9998	0.9987	0.9963	0.9940	0.9790	0.9420	0.8684
	13	1.0000	1.0000	1.0000	1.0000	1.0000	0.9997	0.9991	0.9985	0.9935	0.9786	0.9423
	14	1.0000	1.0000	1.0000	1.0000	1.0000	1.0000	0.9998	0.9997	0.9984	0.9936	0.9793
	15	1.0000	1.0000	1.0000	1.0000	1.0000	1.0000	1.0000	1.0000	0.9997	0.9985	0.9941
	16	1.0000	1.0000	1.0000	1.0000	1.0000	1.0000	1.0000	1.0000	1.0000	0.9997	0.9987
	17	1.0000	1.0000	1.0000	1.0000	1.0000	1.0000	1.0000	1.0000	1.0000	1.0000	0.9998
	18	1.0000	1.0000	1.0000	1.0000	1.0000	1.0000	1.0000	1.0000	1.0000	1.0000	1.0000

Table A7: Cumulative Poisson distribution

	λ												
x	0.02	0.04	0.06	0.08	0.1	0.15	0.2	0.25	0.3	0.35	0.4	0.45	0.5
0	0.9802	0.9608	0.9418	0.9231	0.9048	0.8607	0.8187	0.7788	0.7408	0.7047	0.6703	0.6376	0.6065
1	0.9998	0.9992	0.9983	0.9970	0.9953	0.9898	0.9825	0.9735	0.9631	0.9513	0.9384	0.9246	0.9098
2	1.0000	1.0000	1.0000	0.9999	0.9998	0.9995	0.9989	0.9978	0.9964	0.9945	0.9921	0.9891	0.9856
3	1.0000	1.0000	1.0000	1.0000	1.0000	1.0000	0.9999	0.9999	0.9997	0.9995	0.9992	0.9988	0.9982
4	1.0000	1.0000	1.0000	1.0000	1.0000	1.0000	1.0000	1.0000	1.0000	1.0000	0.9999	0.9999	0.9998
5	1.0000	1.0000	1.0000	1.0000	1.0000	1.0000	1.0000	1.0000	1.0000	1.0000	1.0000	1.0000	1.0000

	λ												
x	0.55	0.6	0.65	0.7	0.75	0.8	0.85	0.9	0.95	1	1.1	1.2	1.3
0	0.5769	0.5488	0.5220	0.4966	0.4724	0.4493	0.4274	0.4066	0.3867	0.3679	0.3329	0.3012	0.3012
1	0.8943	0.8781	0.8614	0.8442	0.8266	0.8088	0.7907	0.7725	0.7541	0.7358	0.6990	0.6626	0.6626
2	0.9815	0.9769	0.9717	0.9659	0.9595	0.9526	0.9451	0.9371	0.9287	0.9197	0.9004	0.8795	0.8795
3	0.9975	0.9966	0.9956	0.9942	0.9927	0.9909	0.9889	0.9865	0.9839	0.9810	0.9743	0.9662	0.9662
4	0.9997	0.9996	0.9994	0.9992	0.9989	0.9986	0.9982	0.9977	0.9971	0.9963	0.9946	0.9923	0.9923
5	1.0000	1.0000	0.9999	0.9999	0.9999	0.9998	0.9997	0.9997	0.9995	0.9994	0.9990	0.9985	0.9985
6	1.0000	1.0000	1.0000	1.0000	1.0000	1.0000	1.0000	1.0000	0.9999	0.9999	0.9999	0.9997	0.9997
7	1.0000	1.0000	1.0000	1.0000	1.0000	1.0000	1.0000	1.0000	1.0000	1.0000	1.0000	1.0000	1.0000
8	1.0000	1.0000	1.0000	1.0000	1.0000	1.0000	1.0000	1.0000	1.0000	1.0000	1.0000	1.0000	1.0000

	λ												
x	1.4	1.5	1.6	1.7	1.8	1.9	2	2.2	2.4	2.6	2.8	3	3.2
0	0.2466	0.2231	0.2019	0.1827	0.1653	0.1496	0.1353	0.1108	0.0907	0.0743	0.0608	0.0498	0.0408
1	0.5918	0.5578	0.5249	0.4932	0.4628	0.4337	0.4060	0.3546	0.3084	0.2674	0.2311	0.1991	0.1712
2	0.8335	0.8088	0.7834	0.7572	0.7306	0.7037	0.6767	0.6227	0.5697	0.5184	0.4695	0.4232	0.3799
3	0.9463	0.9344	0.9212	0.9068	0.8913	0.8747	0.8571	0.8194	0.7787	0.7360	0.6919	0.6472	0.6025
4	0.9857	0.9814	0.9763	0.9704	0.9636	0.9559	0.9473	0.9275	0.9041	0.8774	0.8477	0.8153	0.7806
5	0.9968	0.9955	0.9940	0.9920	0.9896	0.9868	0.9834	0.9751	0.9643	0.9510	0.9349	0.9161	0.8946
6	0.9994	0.9991	0.9987	0.9981	0.9974	0.9966	0.9955	0.9925	0.9884	0.9828	0.9756	0.9665	0.9554
7	0.9999	0.9998	0.9997	0.9996	0.9994	0.9992	0.9989	0.9980	0.9967	0.9947	0.9919	0.9881	0.9832
8	1.0000	1.0000	1.0000	0.9999	0.9999	0.9998	0.9998	0.9995	0.9991	0.9985	0.9976	0.9962	0.9943
9	1.0000	1.0000	1.0000	1.0000	1.0000	1.0000	1.0000	0.9999	0.9998	0.9996	0.9993	0.9989	0.9982
10	1.0000	1.0000	1.0000	1.0000	1.0000	1.0000	1.0000	1.0000	1.0000	0.9999	0.9998	0.9997	0.9995
11	1.0000	1.0000	1.0000	1.0000	1.0000	1.0000	1.0000	1.0000	1.0000	1.0000	1.0000	0.9999	0.9999
12	1.0000	1.0000	1.0000	1.0000	1.0000	1.0000	1.0000	1.0000	1.0000	1.0000	1.0000	1.0000	1.0000

	λ												
x	3.4	3.6	3.8	4	4.2	4.4	4.6	4.8	5	5.2	5.4	5.6	5.8
0	0.0334	0.0273	0.0224	0.0183	0.0150	0.0123	0.0101	0.0082	0.0067	0.0055	0.0045	0.0037	0.0030
1	0.1468	0.1257	0.1074	0.0916	0.0780	0.0663	0.0563	0.0477	0.0404	0.0342	0.0289	0.0244	0.0206
2	0.3397	0.3027	0.2689	0.2381	0.2102	0.1851	0.1626	0.1425	0.1247	0.1088	0.0948	0.0824	0.0715
3	0.5584	0.5152	0.4735	0.4335	0.3954	0.3594	0.3257	0.2942	0.2650	0.2381	0.2133	0.1906	0.1700
4	0.7442	0.7064	0.6678	0.6288	0.5898	0.5512	0.5132	0.4763	0.4405	0.4061	0.3733	0.3422	0.3127
5	0.8705	0.8441	0.8156	0.7851	0.7531	0.7199	0.6858	0.6510	0.6160	0.5809	0.5461	0.5119	0.4783
6	0.9421	0.9267	0.9091	0.8893	0.8675	0.8436	0.8180	0.7908	0.7622	0.7324	0.7017	0.6703	0.6384
7	0.9769	0.9692	0.9599	0.9489	0.9361	0.9214	0.9049	0.8867	0.8666	0.8449	0.8217	0.7970	0.7710
8	0.9917	0.9883	0.9840	0.9786	0.9721	0.9642	0.9549	0.9442	0.9319	0.9181	0.9027	0.8857	0.8672
9	0.9973	0.9960	0.9942	0.9919	0.9889	0.9851	0.9805	0.9749	0.9682	0.9603	0.9512	0.9409	0.9292
10	0.9992	0.9987	0.9981	0.9972	0.9959	0.9943	0.9922	0.9896	0.9863	0.9823	0.9775	0.9718	0.9651
11	0.9998	0.9996	0.9994	0.9991	0.9986	0.9980	0.9971	0.9960	0.9945	0.9927	0.9904	0.9875	0.9841

contd...

contd...

	λ												
x	3.4	3.6	3.8	4	4.2	4.4	4.6	4.8	5	5.2	5.4	5.6	5.8
12	0.9999	0.9999	0.9998	0.9997	0.9996	0.9993	0.9990	0.9986	0.9980	0.9972	0.9962	0.9949	0.9932
13	1.0000	1.0000	1.0000	0.9999	0.9999	0.9998	0.9997	0.9995	0.9993	0.9990	0.9986	0.9980	0.9973
14	1.0000	1.0000	1.0000	1.0000	1.0000	0.9999	0.9999	0.9999	0.9998	0.9997	0.9995	0.9993	0.9990
15	1.0000	1.0000	1.0000	1.0000	1.0000	1.0000	1.0000	1.0000	0.9999	0.9999	0.9998	0.9998	0.9996
16	1.0000	1.0000	1.0000	1.0000	1.0000	1.0000	1.0000	1.0000	1.0000	1.0000	0.9999	0.9999	0.9999
17	1.0000	1.0000	1.0000	1.0000	1.0000	1.0000	1.0000	1.0000	1.0000	1.0000	1.0000	1.0000	1.0000

	λ												
x	6	6.2	6.4	6.6	6.8	7	7.2	7.4	7.6	7.8	8	8.5	9
0	0.0025	0.0020	0.0017	0.0014	0.0011	0.0009	0.0007	0.0006	0.0005	0.0004	0.0003	0.0002	0.0001
1	0.0174	0.0146	0.0123	0.0103	0.0087	0.0073	0.0061	0.0051	0.0043	0.0036	0.0030	0.0019	0.0012
2	0.0620	0.0536	0.0463	0.0400	0.0344	0.0296	0.0255	0.0219	0.0188	0.0161	0.0138	0.0093	0.0062
3	0.1512	0.1342	0.1189	0.1052	0.0928	0.0818	0.0719	0.0632	0.0554	0.0485	0.0424	0.0301	0.0212
4	0.2851	0.2592	0.2351	0.2127	0.1920	0.1730	0.1555	0.1395	0.1249	0.1117	0.0996	0.0744	0.0550
5	0.4457	0.4141	0.3837	0.3547	0.3270	0.3007	0.2759	0.2526	0.2307	0.2103	0.1912	0.1496	0.1157
6	0.6063	0.5742	0.5423	0.5108	0.4799	0.4497	0.4204	0.3920	0.3646	0.3384	0.3134	0.2562	0.2068
7	0.7440	0.7160	0.6873	0.6581	0.6285	0.5987	0.5689	0.5393	0.5100	0.4812	0.4530	0.3856	0.3239
8	0.8472	0.8259	0.8033	0.7796	0.7548	0.7291	0.7027	0.6757	0.6482	0.6204	0.5925	0.5231	0.4557
9	0.9161	0.9016	0.8858	0.8686	0.8502	0.8305	0.8096	0.7877	0.7649	0.7411	0.7166	0.6530	0.5874
10	0.9574	0.9486	0.9386	0.9274	0.9151	0.9015	0.8867	0.8707	0.8535	0.8352	0.8159	0.7634	0.7060
11	0.9799	0.9750	0.9693	0.9627	0.9552	0.9467	0.9371	0.9265	0.9148	0.9020	0.8881	0.8487	0.8030
12	0.9912	0.9887	0.9857	0.9821	0.9779	0.9730	0.9673	0.9609	0.9536	0.9454	0.9362	0.9091	0.8758
13	0.9964	0.9952	0.9937	0.9920	0.9898	0.9872	0.9841	0.9805	0.9762	0.9714	0.9658	0.9486	0.9261
14	0.9986	0.9981	0.9974	0.9966	0.9956	0.9943	0.9927	0.9908	0.9886	0.9859	0.9827	0.9726	0.9585
15	0.9995	0.9993	0.9990	0.9986	0.9982	0.9976	0.9969	0.9959	0.9948	0.9934	0.9918	0.9862	0.9780
16	0.9998	0.9997	0.9996	0.9995	0.9993	0.9990	0.9987	0.9983	0.9978	0.9971	0.9963	0.9934	0.9889
17	0.9999	0.9999	0.9999	0.9998	0.9997	0.9996	0.9995	0.9993	0.9991	0.9988	0.9984	0.9970	0.9947
18	1.0000	1.0000	1.0000	0.9999	0.9999	0.9999	0.9998	0.9997	0.9996	0.9995	0.9993	0.9987	0.9976
19	1.0000	1.0000	1.0000	1.0000	1.0000	1.0000	0.9999	0.9999	0.9999	0.9998	0.9997	0.9995	0.9989
20	1.0000	1.0000	1.0000	1.0000	1.0000	1.0000	1.0000	1.0000	1.0000	0.9999	0.9999	0.9998	0.9996
21	1.0000	1.0000	1.0000	1.0000	1.0000	1.0000	1.0000	1.0000	1.0000	1.0000	1.0000	0.9999	0.9998
22	1.0000	1.0000	1.0000	1.0000	1.0000	1.0000	1.0000	1.0000	1.0000	1.0000	1.0000	1.0000	0.9999
23	1.0000	1.0000	1.0000	1.0000	1.0000	1.0000	1.0000	1.0000	1.0000	1.0000	1.0000	1.0000	1.0000

	λ												
x	9.5	10	10.5	11	11.5	12	12.5	13	13.5	14	14.5	15	15.5
0	0.0001	0.0000	0.0000	0.0000	0.0000	0.0000	0.0000	0.0000	0.0000	0.0000	0.0000	0.0000	0.0000
1	0.0008	0.0005	0.0003	0.0002	0.0001	0.0001	0.0001	0.0000	0.0000	0.0000	0.0000	0.0000	0.0000
2	0.0042	0.0028	0.0018	0.0012	0.0008	0.0005	0.0003	0.0002	0.0001	0.0001	0.0001	0.0000	0.0000
3	0.0149	0.0103	0.0071	0.0049	0.0034	0.0023	0.0016	0.0011	0.0007	0.0005	0.0003	0.0002	0.0001
4	0.0403	0.0293	0.0211	0.0151	0.0107	0.0076	0.0053	0.0037	0.0026	0.0018	0.0012	0.0009	0.0006
5	0.0885	0.0671	0.0504	0.0375	0.0277	0.0203	0.0148	0.0107	0.0077	0.0055	0.0039	0.0028	0.0020
6	0.1649	0.1301	0.1016	0.0786	0.0603	0.0458	0.0346	0.0259	0.0193	0.0142	0.0105	0.0076	0.0055
7	0.2687	0.2202	0.1785	0.1432	0.1137	0.0895	0.0698	0.0540	0.0415	0.0316	0.0239	0.0180	0.0135
8	0.3918	0.3328	0.2794	0.2320	0.1906	0.1550	0.1249	0.0998	0.0790	0.0621	0.0484	0.0374	0.0288
9	0.5218	0.4579	0.3971	0.3405	0.2888	0.2424	0.2014	0.1658	0.1353	0.1094	0.0878	0.0699	0.0552
10	0.6453	0.5830	0.5207	0.4599	0.4017	0.3472	0.2971	0.2517	0.2112	0.1757	0.1449	0.1185	0.0961
11	0.7520	0.6968	0.6387	0.5793	0.5198	0.4616	0.4058	0.3532	0.3045	0.2600	0.2201	0.1848	0.1538
12	0.8364	0.7916	0.7420	0.6887	0.6329	0.5760	0.5190	0.4631	0.4093	0.3585	0.3111	0.2676	0.2283
13	0.8981	0.8645	0.8253	0.7813	0.7330	0.6815	0.6278	0.5730	0.5182	0.4644	0.4125	0.3632	0.3171
14	0.9400	0.9165	0.8879	0.8540	0.8153	0.7720	0.7250	0.6751	0.6233	0.5704	0.5176	0.4657	0.4154
15	0.9665	0.9513	0.9317	0.9074	0.8783	0.8444	0.8060	0.7636	0.7178	0.6694	0.6192	0.5681	0.5170
16	0.9823	0.9730	0.9604	0.9441	0.9236	0.8987	0.8693	0.8355	0.7975	0.7559	0.7112	0.6641	0.6154
17	0.9911	0.9857	0.9781	0.9678	0.9542	0.9370	0.9158	0.8905	0.8609	0.8272	0.7897	0.7489	0.7052
18	0.9957	0.9928	0.9885	0.9823	0.9738	0.9626	0.9481	0.9302	0.9084	0.8826	0.8530	0.8195	0.7825

contd...

contd...

	λ												
x	9.5	10	10.5	11	11.5	12	12.5	13	13.5	14	14.5	15	15.5
19	0.9980	0.9965	0.9942	0.9907	0.9857	0.9787	0.9694	0.9573	0.9421	0.9235	0.9012	0.8752	0.8455
20	0.9991	0.9984	0.9972	0.9953	0.9925	0.9884	0.9827	0.9750	0.9649	0.9521	0.9362	0.9170	0.8944
21	0.9996	0.9993	0.9987	0.9977	0.9962	0.9939	0.9906	0.9859	0.9796	0.9712	0.9604	0.9469	0.9304
22	0.9999	0.9997	0.9994	0.9990	0.9982	0.9970	0.9951	0.9924	0.9885	0.9833	0.9763	0.9673	0.9558
23	0.9999	0.9999	0.9998	0.9995	0.9992	0.9985	0.9975	0.9960	0.9938	0.9907	0.9863	0.9805	0.9730
24	1.0000	1.0000	0.9999	0.9998	0.9996	0.9993	0.9988	0.9980	0.9968	0.9950	0.9924	0.9888	0.9840
25	1.0000	1.0000	1.0000	0.9999	0.9998	0.9997	0.9994	0.9990	0.9984	0.9974	0.9959	0.9938	0.9909
26	1.0000	1.0000	1.0000	1.0000	0.9999	0.9999	0.9997	0.9995	0.9992	0.9987	0.9979	0.9967	0.9950
27	1.0000	1.0000	1.0000	1.0000	1.0000	0.9999	0.9999	0.9998	0.9996	0.9994	0.9989	0.9983	0.9973
28	1.0000	1.0000	1.0000	1.0000	1.0000	1.0000	1.0000	0.9999	0.9998	0.9997	0.9995	0.9991	0.9986
29	1.0000	1.0000	1.0000	1.0000	1.0000	1.0000	1.0000	1.0000	0.9999	0.9999	0.9998	0.9996	0.9993
30	1.0000	1.0000	1.0000	1.0000	1.0000	1.0000	1.0000	1.0000	1.0000	0.9999	0.9999	0.9998	0.9997
31	1.0000	1.0000	1.0000	1.0000	1.0000	1.0000	1.0000	1.0000	1.0000	1.0000	1.0000	0.9999	0.9998
32	1.0000	1.0000	1.0000	1.0000	1.0000	1.0000	1.0000	1.0000	1.0000	1.0000	1.0000	1.0000	0.9999
33	1.0000	1.0000	1.0000	1.0000	1.0000	1.0000	1.0000	1.0000	1.0000	1.0000	1.0000	1.0000	1.0000

	λ												
x	16	17	18	19	20	21	22	23	24	25	30	35	40
2	0.0000	0.0000	0.0000	0.0000	0.0000	0.0000	0.0000	0.0000	0.0000	0.0000	0.0000	0.0000	0.0000
3	0.0001	0.0000	0.0000	0.0000	0.0000	0.0000	0.0000	0.0000	0.0000	0.0000	0.0000	0.0000	0.0000
4	0.0004	0.0002	0.0001	0.0000	0.0000	0.0000	0.0000	0.0000	0.0000	0.0000	0.0000	0.0000	0.0000
5	0.0014	0.0007	0.0003	0.0002	0.0001	0.0000	0.0000	0.0000	0.0000	0.0000	0.0000	0.0000	0.0000
6	0.0040	0.0021	0.0010	0.0005	0.0003	0.0001	0.0001	0.0000	0.0000	0.0000	0.0000	0.0000	0.0000
7	0.0100	0.0054	0.0029	0.0015	0.0008	0.0004	0.0002	0.0001	0.0000	0.0000	0.0000	0.0000	0.0000
8	0.0220	0.0126	0.0071	0.0039	0.0021	0.0011	0.0006	0.0003	0.0002	0.0001	0.0000	0.0000	0.0000
9	0.0433	0.0261	0.0154	0.0089	0.0050	0.0028	0.0015	0.0008	0.0004	0.0002	0.0000	0.0000	0.0000
10	0.0774	0.0491	0.0304	0.0183	0.0108	0.0063	0.0035	0.0020	0.0011	0.0006	0.0000	0.0000	0.0000
11	0.1270	0.0847	0.0549	0.0347	0.0214	0.0129	0.0076	0.0044	0.0025	0.0014	0.0001	0.0000	0.0000
12	0.1931	0.1350	0.0917	0.0606	0.0390	0.0245	0.0151	0.0091	0.0054	0.0031	0.0002	0.0000	0.0000
13	0.2745	0.2009	0.1426	0.0984	0.0661	0.0434	0.0278	0.0174	0.0107	0.0065	0.0004	0.0000	0.0000
14	0.3675	0.2808	0.2081	0.1497	0.1049	0.0716	0.0477	0.0311	0.0198	0.0124	0.0009	0.0000	0.0000
15	0.4667	0.3715	0.2867	0.2148	0.1565	0.1111	0.0769	0.0520	0.0344	0.0223	0.0019	0.0001	0.0000
16	0.5660	0.4677	0.3751	0.2920	0.2211	0.1629	0.1170	0.0821	0.0563	0.0377	0.0039	0.0003	0.0000
17	0.6593	0.5640	0.4686	0.3784	0.2970	0.2270	0.1690	0.1228	0.0871	0.0605	0.0073	0.0006	0.0000
18	0.7423	0.6550	0.5622	0.4695	0.3814	0.3017	0.2325	0.1748	0.1283	0.0920	0.0129	0.0012	0.0001
19	0.8122	0.7363	0.6509	0.5606	0.4703	0.3843	0.3060	0.2377	0.1803	0.1336	0.0219	0.0023	0.0002
20	0.8682	0.8055	0.7307	0.6472	0.5591	0.4710	0.3869	0.3101	0.2426	0.1855	0.0353	0.0043	0.0004
21	0.9108	0.8615	0.7991	0.7255	0.6437	0.5577	0.4716	0.3894	0.3139	0.2473	0.0544	0.0076	0.0007
22	0.9418	0.9047	0.8551	0.7931	0.7206	0.6405	0.5564	0.4723	0.3917	0.3175	0.0806	0.0128	0.0014
23	0.9633	0.9367	0.8989	0.8490	0.7875	0.7160	0.6374	0.5551	0.4728	0.3939	0.1146	0.0208	0.0026
24	0.9777	0.9594	0.9317	0.8933	0.8432	0.7822	0.7117	0.6346	0.5540	0.4734	0.1572	0.0324	0.0045
25	0.9869	0.9748	0.9554	0.9269	0.8878	0.8377	0.7771	0.7077	0.6319	0.5529	0.2084	0.0486	0.0076
26	0.9925	0.9848	0.9718	0.9514	0.9221	0.8826	0.8324	0.7723	0.7038	0.6294	0.2673	0.0705	0.0123
27	0.9959	0.9912	0.9827	0.9687	0.9475	0.9175	0.8775	0.8274	0.7677	0.7002	0.3329	0.0988	0.0193
28	0.9978	0.9950	0.9897	0.9805	0.9657	0.9436	0.9129	0.8726	0.8225	0.7634	0.4031	0.1343	0.0294
29	0.9989	0.9973	0.9941	0.9882	0.9782	0.9626	0.9398	0.9085	0.8679	0.8179	0.4757	0.1770	0.0432
30	0.9994	0.9986	0.9967	0.9930	0.9865	0.9758	0.9595	0.9360	0.9042	0.8633	0.5484	0.2269	0.0617
31	0.9997	0.9993	0.9982	0.9960	0.9919	0.9848	0.9735	0.9564	0.9322	0.8999	0.6186	0.2833	0.0855
32	0.9999	0.9996	0.9990	0.9978	0.9953	0.9907	0.9831	0.9711	0.9533	0.9285	0.6845	0.3449	0.1153
33	0.9999	0.9998	0.9995	0.9988	0.9973	0.9945	0.9895	0.9813	0.9686	0.9502	0.7444	0.4102	0.1514
34	1.0000	0.9999	0.9998	0.9994	0.9985	0.9968	0.9936	0.9882	0.9794	0.9662	0.7973	0.4775	0.1939
35	1.0000	1.0000	0.9999	0.9997	0.9992	0.9982	0.9962	0.9927	0.9868	0.9775	0.8426	0.5448	0.2424
36	1.0000	1.0000	0.9999	0.9998	0.9996	0.9990	0.9978	0.9956	0.9918	0.9854	0.8804	0.6102	0.2963
37	1.0000	1.0000	1.0000	0.9999	0.9998	0.9995	0.9988	0.9974	0.9950	0.9908	0.9110	0.6721	0.3547

contd...

contd...

	λ												
x	16	17	18	19	20	21	22	23	24	25	30	35	40
38	1.0000	1.0000	1.0000	1.0000	0.9999	0.9997	0.9993	0.9985	0.9970	0.9943	0.9352	0.7291	0.4160
39	1.0000	1.0000	1.0000	1.0000	0.9999	0.9999	0.9996	0.9992	0.9983	0.9966	0.9537	0.7802	0.4790
40	1.0000	1.0000	1.0000	1.0000	1.0000	0.9999	0.9998	0.9996	0.9990	0.9980	0.9677	0.8249	0.5419
41	1.0000	1.0000	1.0000	1.0000	1.0000	1.0000	0.9999	0.9998	0.9995	0.9988	0.9779	0.8631	0.6033
42	1.0000	1.0000	1.0000	1.0000	1.0000	1.0000	1.0000	0.9999	0.9997	0.9993	0.9852	0.8950	0.6618
43	1.0000	1.0000	1.0000	1.0000	1.0000	1.0000	1.0000	0.9999	0.9998	0.9996	0.9903	0.9209	0.7162
44	1.0000	1.0000	1.0000	1.0000	1.0000	1.0000	1.0000	1.0000	0.9999	0.9998	0.9937	0.9415	0.7657
45	1.0000	1.0000	1.0000	1.0000	1.0000	1.0000	1.0000	1.0000	1.0000	0.9999	0.9960	0.9575	0.8097
46	1.0000	1.0000	1.0000	1.0000	1.0000	1.0000	1.0000	1.0000	1.0000	0.9999	0.9975	0.9697	0.8479
47	1.0000	1.0000	1.0000	1.0000	1.0000	1.0000	1.0000	1.0000	1.0000	1.0000	0.9985	0.9788	0.8804
48	1.0000	1.0000	1.0000	1.0000	1.0000	1.0000	1.0000	1.0000	1.0000	1.0000	0.9991	0.9854	0.9075
49	1.0000	1.0000	1.0000	1.0000	1.0000	1.0000	1.0000	1.0000	1.0000	1.0000	0.9995	0.9902	0.9297
50	1.0000	1.0000	1.0000	1.0000	1.0000	1.0000	1.0000	1.0000	1.0000	1.0000	0.9997	0.9935	0.9474
51	1.0000	1.0000	1.0000	1.0000	1.0000	1.0000	1.0000	1.0000	1.0000	1.0000	0.9998	0.9957	0.9613
52	1.0000	1.0000	1.0000	1.0000	1.0000	1.0000	1.0000	1.0000	1.0000	1.0000	0.9999	0.9973	0.9719
53	1.0000	1.0000	1.0000	1.0000	1.0000	1.0000	1.0000	1.0000	1.0000	1.0000	0.9999	0.9983	0.9800
54	1.0000	1.0000	1.0000	1.0000	1.0000	1.0000	1.0000	1.0000	1.0000	1.0000	1.0000	0.9989	0.9860
55	1.0000	1.0000	1.0000	1.0000	1.0000	1.0000	1.0000	1.0000	1.0000	1.0000	1.0000	0.9993	0.9903
56	1.0000	1.0000	1.0000	1.0000	1.0000	1.0000	1.0000	1.0000	1.0000	1.0000	1.0000	0.9996	0.9934
57	1.0000	1.0000	1.0000	1.0000	1.0000	1.0000	1.0000	1.0000	1.0000	1.0000	1.0000	0.9998	0.9956
58	1.0000	1.0000	1.0000	1.0000	1.0000	1.0000	1.0000	1.0000	1.0000	1.0000	1.0000	0.9999	0.9971
59	1.0000	1.0000	1.0000	1.0000	1.0000	1.0000	1.0000	1.0000	1.0000	1.0000	1.0000	0.9999	0.9981
60	1.0000	1.0000	1.0000	1.0000	1.0000	1.0000	1.0000	1.0000	1.0000	1.0000	1.0000	1.0000	0.9988
61	1.0000	1.0000	1.0000	1.0000	1.0000	1.0000	1.0000	1.0000	1.0000	1.0000	1.0000	1.0000	0.9992
62	1.0000	1.0000	1.0000	1.0000	1.0000	1.0000	1.0000	1.0000	1.0000	1.0000	1.0000	1.0000	0.9995
63	1.0000	1.0000	1.0000	1.0000	1.0000	1.0000	1.0000	1.0000	1.0000	1.0000	1.0000	1.0000	0.9997
64	1.0000	1.0000	1.0000	1.0000	1.0000	1.0000	1.0000	1.0000	1.0000	1.0000	1.0000	1.0000	0.9998
65	1.0000	1.0000	1.0000	1.0000	1.0000	1.0000	1.0000	1.0000	1.0000	1.0000	1.0000	1.0000	0.9999
66	1.0000	1.0000	1.0000	1.0000	1.0000	1.0000	1.0000	1.0000	1.0000	1.0000	1.0000	1.0000	0.9999
67	1.0000	1.0000	1.0000	1.0000	1.0000	1.0000	1.0000	1.0000	1.0000	1.0000	1.0000	1.0000	1.0000

Table A8: Normal distribution

z

Probability content from –00 to z

z	0.00	0.01	0.02	0.03	0.04	0.05	0.06	0.07	0.08	0.09
0.0	0.5000	0.5040	0.5080	0.5120	0.5160	0.5199	0.5239	0.5279	0.5319	0.5359
0.1	0.5398	0.5438	0.5478	0.5517	0.5557	0.5596	0.5636	0.5675	0.5714	0.5753
0.2	0.5793	0.5832	0.5871	0.5910	0.5948	0.5987	0.6026	0.6064	0.6103	0.6141
0.3	0.6179	0.6217	0.6255	0.6293	0.6331	0.6368	0.6406	0.6443	0.6480	0.6517
0.4	0.6554	0.6591	0.6628	0.6664	0.6700	0.6736	0.6772	0.6808	0.6844	0.6879
0.5	0.6915	0.6950	0.6985	0.7019	0.7054	0.7088	0.7123	0.7157	0.7190	0.7224
0.6	0.7257	0.7291	0.7324	0.7357	0.7389	0.7422	0.7454	0.7486	0.7517	0.7549
0.7	0.7580	0.7611	0.7642	0.7673	0.7704	0.7734	0.7764	0.7794	0.7823	0.7852
0.8	0.7881	0.7910	0.7939	0.7967	0.7995	0.8023	0.8051	0.8078	0.8106	0.8133
0.9	0.8159	0.8186	0.8212	0.8238	0.8264	0.8289	0.8315	0.8340	0.8365	0.8389
1.0	0.8413	0.8438	0.8461	0.8485	0.8508	0.8531	0.8554	0.8577	0.8599	0.8621
1.1	0.8643	0.8665	0.8686	0.8708	0.8729	0.8749	0.8770	0.8790	0.8810	0.8830
1.2	0.8849	0.8869	0.8888	0.8907	0.8925	0.8944	0.8962	0.8980	0.8997	0.9015
1.3	0.9032	0.9049	0.9066	0.9082	0.9099	0.9115	0.9131	0.9147	0.9162	0.9177
1.4	0.9192	0.9207	0.9222	0.9236	0.9251	0.9265	0.9279	0.9292	0.9306	0.9319
1.5	0.9332	0.9345	0.9357	0.9370	0.9382	0.9394	0.9406	0.9418	0.9429	0.9441
1.6	0.9452	0.9463	0.9474	0.9484	0.9495	0.9505	0.9515	0.9525	0.9535	0.9545
1.7	0.9554	0.9564	0.9573	0.9582	0.9591	0.9599	0.9608	0.9616	0.9625	0.9633
1.8	0.9641	0.9649	0.9656	0.9664	0.9671	0.9678	0.9686	0.9693	0.9699	0.9706
1.9	0.9713	0.9719	0.9726	0.9732	0.9738	0.9744	0.9750	0.9756	0.9761	0.9767
2.0	0.9772	0.9778	0.9783	0.9788	0.9793	0.9798	0.9803	0.9808	0.9812	0.9817
2.1	0.9821	0.9826	0.9830	0.9834	0.9838	0.9842	0.9846	0.9850	0.9854	0.9857
2.2	0.9861	0.9864	0.9868	0.9871	0.9875	0.9878	0.9881	0.9884	0.9887	0.9890
2.3	0.9893	0.9896	0.9898	0.9901	0.9904	0.9906	0.9909	0.9911	0.9913	0.9916
2.4	0.9918	0.9920	0.9922	0.9925	0.9927	0.9929	0.9931	0.9932	0.9934	0.9936
2.5	0.9938	0.9940	0.9941	0.9943	0.9945	0.9946	0.9948	0.9949	0.9951	0.9952
2.6	0.9953	0.9955	0.9956	0.9957	0.9959	0.9960	0.9961	0.9962	0.9963	0.9964
2.7	0.9965	0.9966	0.9967	0.9968	0.9969	0.9970	0.9971	0.9972	0.9973	0.9974
2.8	0.9974	0.9975	0.9976	0.9977	0.9977	0.9978	0.9979	0.9979	0.9980	0.9981
2.9	0.9981	0.9982	0.9982	0.9983	0.9984	0.9984	0.9985	0.9985	0.9986	0.9986
3.0	0.9987	0.9987	0.9987	0.9988	0.9988	0.9989	0.9989	0.9989	0.9990	0.9990
3.1	0.9990	0.9991	0.9991	0.9991	0.9992	0.9992	0.9992	0.9992	0.9993	0.9993
3.2	0.9993	0.9993	0.9994	0.9994	0.9994	0.9994	0.9994	0.9995	0.9995	0.9995
3.3	0.9995	0.9995	0.9995	0.9996	0.9996	0.9996	0.9996	0.9996	0.9996	0.9997
3.4	0.9997	0.9997	0.9997	0.9997	0.9997	0.9997	0.9997	0.9997	0.9997	0.9998
3.5	0.9998	0.9998	0.9998	0.9998	0.9998	0.9998	0.9998	0.9998	0.9998	0.9998
3.6	0.9998	0.9998	0.9999	0.9999	0.9999	0.9999	0.9999	0.9999	0.9999	0.9999
3.7	0.9999	0.9999	0.9999	0.9999	0.9999	0.9999	0.9999	0.9999	0.9999	0.9999
3.8	0.9999	0.9999	0.9999	0.9999	0.9999	0.9999	0.9999	0.9999	0.9999	0.9999
3.9	1.0000	1.0000	1.0000	1.0000	1.0000	1.0000	1.0000	1.0000	1.0000	1.0000

Table A9: Student's t distribution

The table below contains the quartiles of student's t distribution with *v* degrees of freedom.

	p											
v	0.6	0.7	0.75	0.8	0.85	0.9	0.95	0.975	0.99	0.995	0.999	0.9995
1	0.3249	0.7265	1.0000	1.3764	1.9626	3.0777	6.3138	12.706	31.821	63.657	318.31	636.62
2	0.2887	0.6172	0.8165	1.0607	1.3862	1.8856	2.9200	4.3027	6.9646	9.9248	22.327	31.599
3	0.2767	0.5844	0.7649	0.9785	1.2498	1.6377	2.3534	3.1824	4.5407	5.8409	10.215	12.924
4	0.2707	0.5686	0.7407	0.9410	1.1896	1.5332	2.1318	2.7764	3.7469	4.6041	7.1732	8.6103
5	0.2672	0.5594	0.7267	0.9195	1.1558	1.4759	2.0150	2.5706	3.3649	4.0321	5.8934	6.8688
6	0.2648	0.5534	0.7176	0.9057	1.1342	1.4398	1.9432	2.4469	3.1427	3.7074	5.2076	5.9588
7	0.2632	0.5491	0.7111	0.8960	1.1192	1.4149	1.8946	2.3646	2.9980	3.4995	4.7853	5.4079
8	0.2619	0.5459	0.7064	0.8889	1.1081	1.3968	1.8595	2.3060	2.8965	3.3554	4.5008	5.0413
9	0.2610	0.5435	0.7027	0.8834	1.0997	1.3830	1.8331	2.2622	2.8214	3.2498	4.2968	4.7809
10	0.2602	0.5415	0.6998	0.8791	1.0931	1.3722	1.8125	2.2281	2.7638	3.1693	4.1437	4.5869
11	0.2596	0.5399	0.6974	0.8755	1.0877	1.3634	1.7959	2.2010	2.7181	3.1058	4.0247	4.4370
12	0.2590	0.5386	0.6955	0.8726	1.0832	1.3562	1.7823	2.1788	2.6810	3.0545	3.9296	4.3178
13	0.2586	0.5375	0.6938	0.8702	1.0795	1.3502	1.7709	2.1604	2.6503	3.0123	3.8520	4.2208
14	0.2582	0.5366	0.6924	0.8681	1.0763	1.3450	1.7613	2.1448	2.6245	2.9768	3.7874	4.1405
15	0.2579	0.5357	0.6912	0.8662	1.0735	1.3406	1.7531	2.1314	2.6025	2.9467	3.7328	4.0728
16	0.2576	0.5350	0.6901	0.8647	1.0711	1.3368	1.7459	2.1199	2.5835	2.9208	3.6862	4.0150
17	0.2573	0.5344	0.6892	0.8633	1.0690	1.3334	1.7396	2.1098	2.5669	2.8982	3.6458	3.9651
18	0.2571	0.5338	0.6884	0.8620	1.0672	1.3304	1.7341	2.1009	2.5524	2.8784	3.6105	3.9216
19	0.2569	0.5333	0.6876	0.8610	1.0655	1.3277	1.7291	2.0930	2.5395	2.8609	3.5794	3.8834
20	0.2567	0.5329	0.6870	0.8600	1.0640	1.3253	1.7247	2.0860	2.5280	2.8453	3.5518	3.8495
21	0.2566	0.5325	0.6864	0.8591	1.0627	1.3232	1.7207	2.0796	2.5176	2.8314	3.5272	3.8193
22	0.2564	0.5321	0.6858	0.8583	1.0614	1.3212	1.7171	2.0739	2.5083	2.8188	3.5050	3.7921
23	0.2563	0.5317	0.6853	0.8575	1.0603	1.3195	1.7139	2.0687	2.4999	2.8073	3.4850	3.7676
24	0.2562	0.5314	0.6848	0.8569	1.0593	1.3178	1.7109	2.0639	2.4922	2.7969	3.4668	3.7454
25	0.2561	0.5312	0.6844	0.8562	1.0584	1.3163	1.7081	2.0595	2.4851	2.7874	3.4502	3.7251
26	0.2560	0.5309	0.6840	0.8557	1.0575	1.3150	1.7056	2.0555	2.4786	2.7787	3.4350	3.7066
27	0.2559	0.5306	0.6837	0.8551	1.0567	1.3137	1.7033	2.0518	2.4727	2.7707	3.4210	3.6896
28	0.2558	0.5304	0.6834	0.8546	1.0560	1.3125	1.7011	2.0484	2.4671	2.7633	3.4082	3.6739
29	0.2557	0.5302	0.6830	0.8542	1.0553	1.3114	1.6991	2.0452	2.4620	2.7564	3.3962	3.6594
30	0.2556	0.5300	0.6828	0.8538	1.0547	1.3104	1.6973	2.0423	2.4573	2.7500	3.3852	3.6460
31	0.2555	0.5298	0.6825	0.8534	1.0541	1.3095	1.6955	2.0395	2.4528	2.7440	3.3749	3.6335
32	0.2555	0.5297	0.6822	0.8530	1.0535	1.3086	1.6939	2.0369	2.4487	2.7385	3.3653	3.6218
33	0.2554	0.5295	0.6820	0.8526	1.0530	1.3077	1.6924	2.0345	2.4448	2.7333	3.3563	3.6109
34	0.2553	0.5294	0.6818	0.8523	1.0525	1.3070	1.6909	2.0322	2.4411	2.7284	3.3479	3.6007
35	0.2553	0.5292	0.6816	0.8520	1.0520	1.3062	1.6896	2.0301	2.4377	2.7238	3.3400	3.5911
36	0.2552	0.5291	0.6814	0.8517	1.0516	1.3055	1.6883	2.0281	2.4345	2.7195	3.3326	3.5821
37	0.2552	0.5289	0.6812	0.8514	1.0512	1.3049	1.6871	2.0262	2.4314	2.7154	3.3256	3.5737
38	0.2551	0.5288	0.6810	0.8512	1.0508	1.3042	1.6860	2.0244	2.4286	2.7116	3.3190	3.5657
39	0.2551	0.5287	0.6808	0.8509	1.0504	1.3036	1.6849	2.0227	2.4258	2.7079	3.3128	3.5581
40	0.2550	0.5286	0.6807	0.8507	1.0500	1.3031	1.6839	2.0211	2.4233	2.7045	3.3069	3.5510
41	0.2550	0.5285	0.6805	0.8505	1.0497	1.3025	1.6829	2.0195	2.4208	2.7012	3.3013	3.5442
42	0.2550	0.5284	0.6804	0.8503	1.0494	1.3020	1.6820	2.0181	2.4185	2.6981	3.2960	3.5377
43	0.2549	0.5283	0.6802	0.8501	1.0491	1.3016	1.6811	2.0167	2.4163	2.6951	3.2909	3.5316
44	0.2549	0.5282	0.6801	0.8499	1.0488	1.3011	1.6802	2.0154	2.4141	2.6923	3.2861	3.5258
45	0.2549	0.5281	0.6800	0.8497	1.0485	1.3006	1.6794	2.0141	2.4121	2.6896	3.2815	3.5203
46	0.2548	0.5281	0.6799	0.8495	1.0483	1.3002	1.6787	2.0129	2.4102	2.6870	3.2771	3.5150
47	0.2548	0.5280	0.6797	0.8493	1.0480	1.2998	1.6779	2.0117	2.4083	2.6846	3.2729	3.5099
48	0.2548	0.5279	0.6796	0.8492	1.0478	1.2994	1.6772	2.0106	2.4066	2.6822	3.2689	3.5051
49	0.2547	0.5278	0.6795	0.8490	1.0475	1.2991	1.6766	2.0096	2.4049	2.6800	3.2651	3.5004

contd...

contd...

	p											
v	0.6	0.7	0.75	0.8	0.85	0.9	0.95	0.975	0.99	0.995	0.999	0.9995
50	0.2547	0.5278	0.6794	0.8489	1.0473	1.2987	1.6759	2.0086	2.4033	2.6778	3.2614	3.4960
51	0.2547	0.5277	0.6793	0.8487	1.0471	1.2984	1.6753	2.0076	2.4017	2.6757	3.2579	3.4918
52	0.2546	0.5276	0.6792	0.8486	1.0469	1.2980	1.6747	2.0066	2.4002	2.6737	3.2545	3.4877
53	0.2546	0.5276	0.6791	0.8485	1.0467	1.2977	1.6741	2.0057	2.3988	2.6718	3.2513	3.4838
54	0.2546	0.5275	0.6791	0.8483	1.0465	1.2974	1.6736	2.0049	2.3974	2.6700	3.2481	3.4800
55	0.2546	0.5275	0.6790	0.8482	1.0463	1.2971	1.6730	2.0040	2.3961	2.6682	3.2451	3.4764
56	0.2546	0.5274	0.6789	0.8481	1.0461	1.2969	1.6725	2.0032	2.3948	2.6665	3.2423	3.4729
57	0.2545	0.5273	0.6788	0.8480	1.0459	1.2966	1.6720	2.0025	2.3936	2.6649	3.2395	3.4696
58	0.2545	0.5273	0.6787	0.8479	1.0458	1.2963	1.6716	2.0017	2.3924	2.6633	3.2368	3.4663
59	0.2545	0.5272	0.6787	0.8478	1.0456	1.2961	1.6711	2.0010	2.3912	2.6618	3.2342	3.4632
60	0.2545	0.5272	0.6786	0.8477	1.0455	1.2958	1.6706	2.0003	2.3901	2.6603	3.2317	3.4602
61	0.2545	0.5272	0.6785	0.8476	1.0453	1.2956	1.6702	1.9996	2.3890	2.6589	3.2293	3.4573
62	0.2544	0.5271	0.6785	0.8475	1.0452	1.2954	1.6698	1.9990	2.3880	2.6575	3.2270	3.4545
63	0.2544	0.5271	0.6784	0.8474	1.0450	1.2951	1.6694	1.9983	2.3870	2.6561	3.2247	3.4518
64	0.2544	0.5270	0.6783	0.8473	1.0449	1.2949	1.6690	1.9977	2.3860	2.6549	3.2225	3.4491
65	0.2544	0.5270	0.6783	0.8472	1.0448	1.2947	1.6686	1.9971	2.3851	2.6536	3.2204	3.4466
66	0.2544	0.5269	0.6782	0.8471	1.0446	1.2945	1.6683	1.9966	2.3842	2.6524	3.2184	3.4441
67	0.2544	0.5269	0.6782	0.8470	1.0445	1.2943	1.6679	1.9960	2.3833	2.6512	3.2164	3.4417
68	0.2543	0.5269	0.6781	0.8469	1.0444	1.2941	1.6676	1.9955	2.3824	2.6501	3.2145	3.4394
69	0.2543	0.5268	0.6781	0.8469	1.0443	1.2939	1.6672	1.9949	2.3816	2.6490	3.2126	3.4372
70	0.2543	0.5268	0.6780	0.8468	1.0442	1.2938	1.6669	1.9944	2.3808	2.6479	3.2108	3.4350
71	0.2543	0.5268	0.6780	0.8467	1.0441	1.2936	1.6666	1.9939	2.3800	2.6469	3.2090	3.4329
72	0.2543	0.5267	0.6779	0.8466	1.0440	1.2934	1.6663	1.9935	2.3793	2.6459	3.2073	3.4308
73	0.2543	0.5267	0.6779	0.8466	1.0438	1.2933	1.6660	1.9930	2.3785	2.6449	3.2057	3.4289
74	0.2543	0.5267	0.6778	0.8465	1.0437	1.2931	1.6657	1.9925	2.3778	2.6439	3.2041	3.4269
75	0.2542	0.5266	0.6778	0.8464	1.0436	1.2929	1.6654	1.9921	2.3771	2.6430	3.2025	3.4250
76	0.2542	0.5266	0.6777	0.8464	1.0436	1.2928	1.6652	1.9917	2.3764	2.6421	3.2010	3.4232
77	0.2542	0.5266	0.6777	0.8463	1.0435	1.2926	1.6649	1.9913	2.3758	2.6412	3.1995	3.4214
78	0.2542	0.5266	0.6776	0.8463	1.0434	1.2925	1.6646	1.9908	2.3751	2.6403	3.1980	3.4197
79	0.2542	0.5265	0.6776	0.8462	1.0433	1.2924	1.6644	1.9905	2.3745	2.6395	3.1966	3.4180
80	0.2542	0.5265	0.6776	0.8461	1.0432	1.2922	1.6641	1.9901	2.3739	2.6387	3.1953	3.4163
81	0.2542	0.5265	0.6775	0.8461	1.0431	1.2921	1.6639	1.9897	2.3733	2.6379	3.1939	3.4147
82	0.2542	0.5264	0.6775	0.8460	1.0430	1.2920	1.6636	1.9893	2.3727	2.6371	3.1926	3.4132
83	0.2542	0.5264	0.6775	0.8460	1.0429	1.2918	1.6634	1.9890	2.3721	2.6364	3.1913	3.4116
84	0.2542	0.5264	0.6774	0.8459	1.0429	1.2917	1.6632	1.9886	2.3716	2.6356	3.1901	3.4102
85	0.2541	0.5264	0.6774	0.8459	1.0428	1.2916	1.6630	1.9883	2.3710	2.6349	3.1889	3.4087
86	0.2541	0.5263	0.6774	0.8458	1.0427	1.2915	1.6628	1.9879	2.3705	2.6342	3.1877	3.4073
87	0.2541	0.5263	0.6773	0.8458	1.0426	1.2914	1.6626	1.9876	2.3700	2.6335	3.1866	3.4059
88	0.2541	0.5263	0.6773	0.8457	1.0426	1.2912	1.6624	1.9873	2.3695	2.6329	3.1854	3.4045
89	0.2541	0.5263	0.6773	0.8457	1.0425	1.2911	1.6622	1.9870	2.3690	2.6322	3.1843	3.4032
90	0.2541	0.5263	0.6772	0.8456	1.0424	1.2910	1.6620	1.9867	2.3685	2.6316	3.1833	3.4019
91	0.2541	0.5262	0.6772	0.8456	1.0424	1.2909	1.6618	1.9864	2.3680	2.6309	3.1822	3.4007
92	0.2541	0.5262	0.6772	0.8455	1.0423	1.2908	1.6616	1.9861	2.3676	2.6303	3.1812	3.3994
93	0.2541	0.5262	0.6771	0.8455	1.0422	1.2907	1.6614	1.9858	2.3671	2.6297	3.1802	3.3982
94	0.2541	0.5262	0.6771	0.8455	1.0422	1.2906	1.6612	1.9855	2.3667	2.6291	3.1792	3.3971
95	0.2541	0.5262	0.6771	0.8454	1.0421	1.2905	1.6611	1.9853	2.3662	2.6286	3.1782	3.3959
96	0.2541	0.5261	0.6771	0.8454	1.0421	1.2904	1.6609	1.9850	2.3658	2.6280	3.1773	3.3948
97	0.2541	0.5261	0.6770	0.8453	1.0420	1.2903	1.6607	1.9847	2.3654	2.6275	3.1764	3.3937
98	0.2540	0.5261	0.6770	0.8453	1.0419	1.2902	1.6606	1.9845	2.3650	2.6269	3.1755	3.3926
99	0.2540	0.5261	0.6770	0.8453	1.0419	1.2902	1.6604	1.9842	2.3646	2.6264	3.1746	3.3915
100	0.2540	0.5261	0.6770	0.8452	1.0418	1.2901	1.6602	1.9840	2.3642	2.6259	3.1737	3.3905
110	0.2540	0.5259	0.6767	0.8449	1.0413	1.2893	1.6588	1.9818	2.3607	2.6213	3.1660	3.3812
120	0.2539	0.5258	0.6765	0.8446	1.0409	1.2886	1.6577	1.9799	2.3578	2.6174	3.1595	3.3735
150	0.2538	0.5255	0.6761	0.8440	1.0400	1.2872	1.6551	1.9759	2.3515	2.6090	3.1455	3.3566
200	0.2537	0.5252	0.6757	0.8434	1.0391	1.2858	1.6525	1.9719	2.3451	2.6006	3.1315	3.3398
500	0.2535	0.5247	0.6750	0.8423	1.0375	1.2832	1.6479	1.9647	2.3338	2.5857	3.1066	3.3101

Table A10: Chi-Square distribution

The table below contains the quartiles of the χ^2 (Chi-squared) distribution with v degrees of freedom.

	p											
v	0.005	0.01	0.025	0.05	0.1	0.5	0.9	0.95	0.975	0.99	0.995	0.999
1	0.0000	0.0002	0.0010	0.0039	0.0158	0.4549	2.7055	3.8415	5.0239	6.6349	7.8794	10.828
2	0.0100	0.0201	0.0506	0.1026	0.2107	1.3863	4.6052	5.9915	7.3778	9.2103	10.597	13.816
3	0.0717	0.1148	0.2158	0.3518	0.5844	2.3660	6.2514	7.8147	9.3484	11.345	12.838	16.266
4	0.2070	0.2971	0.4844	0.7107	1.0636	3.3567	7.7794	9.4877	11.143	13.277	14.860	18.467
5	0.4117	0.5543	0.8312	1.1455	1.6103	4.3515	9.2364	11.070	12.833	15.086	16.750	20.515
6	0.6757	0.8721	1.2373	1.6354	2.2041	5.3481	10.645	12.592	14.449	16.812	18.548	22.458
7	0.9893	1.2390	1.6899	2.1673	2.8331	6.3458	12.017	14.067	16.013	18.475	20.278	24.322
8	1.3444	1.6465	2.1797	2.7326	3.4895	7.3441	13.362	15.507	17.535	20.090	21.955	26.124
9	1.7349	2.0879	2.7004	3.3251	4.1682	8.3428	14.684	16.919	19.023	21.666	23.589	27.877
10	2.1559	2.5582	3.2470	3.9403	4.8652	9.3418	15.987	18.307	20.483	23.209	25.188	29.588
11	2.6032	3.0535	3.8157	4.5748	5.5778	10.341	17.275	19.675	21.920	24.725	26.757	31.264
12	3.0738	3.5706	4.4038	5.2260	6.3038	11.340	18.549	21.026	23.337	26.217	28.300	32.909
13	3.5650	4.1069	5.0088	5.8919	7.0415	12.340	19.812	22.362	24.736	27.688	29.819	34.528
14	4.0747	4.6604	5.6287	6.5706	7.7895	13.339	21.064	23.685	26.119	29.141	31.319	36.123
15	4.6009	5.2293	6.2621	7.2609	8.5468	14.339	22.307	24.996	27.488	30.578	32.801	37.697
16	5.1422	5.8122	6.9077	7.9616	9.3122	15.338	23.542	26.296	28.845	32.000	34.267	39.252
17	5.6972	6.4078	7.5642	8.6718	10.085	16.338	24.769	27.587	30.191	33.409	35.718	40.790
18	6.2648	7.0149	8.2307	9.3905	10.865	17.338	25.989	28.869	31.526	34.805	37.156	42.312
19	6.8440	7.6327	8.9065	10.117	11.651	18.338	27.204	30.144	32.852	36.191	38.582	43.820
20	7.4338	8.2604	9.5908	10.851	12.443	19.337	28.412	31.410	34.170	37.566	39.997	45.315
21	8.0337	8.8972	10.283	11.591	13.240	20.337	29.615	32.671	35.479	38.932	41.401	46.797
22	8.6427	9.5425	10.982	12.338	14.041	21.337	30.813	33.924	36.781	40.289	42.796	48.268
23	9.2604	10.196	11.689	13.091	14.848	22.337	32.007	35.172	38.076	41.638	44.181	49.728
24	9.8862	10.856	12.401	13.848	15.659	23.337	33.196	36.415	39.364	42.980	45.559	51.179
25	10.520	11.524	13.120	14.611	16.473	24.337	34.382	37.652	40.646	44.314	46.928	52.620
26	11.160	12.198	13.844	15.379	17.292	25.336	35.563	38.885	41.923	45.642	48.290	54.052
27	11.808	12.879	14.573	16.151	18.114	26.336	36.741	40.113	43.195	46.963	49.645	55.476
28	12.461	13.565	15.308	16.928	18.939	27.336	37.916	41.337	44.461	48.278	50.993	56.892
29	13.121	14.256	16.047	17.708	19.768	28.336	39.087	42.557	45.722	49.588	52.336	58.301
30	13.787	14.953	16.791	18.493	20.599	29.336	40.256	43.773	46.979	50.892	53.672	59.703
31	14.458	15.655	17.539	19.281	21.434	30.336	41.422	44.985	48.232	52.191	55.003	61.098
32	15.134	16.362	18.291	20.072	22.271	31.336	42.585	46.194	49.480	53.486	56.328	62.487
33	15.815	17.074	19.047	20.867	23.110	32.336	43.745	47.400	50.725	54.776	57.648	63.870
34	16.501	17.789	19.806	21.664	23.952	33.336	44.903	48.602	51.966	56.061	58.964	65.247
35	17.192	18.509	20.569	22.465	24.797	34.336	46.059	49.802	53.203	57.342	60.275	66.619
36	17.887	19.233	21.336	23.269	25.643	35.336	47.212	50.998	54.437	58.619	61.581	67.985
37	18.586	19.960	22.106	24.075	26.492	36.336	48.363	52.192	55.668	59.893	62.883	69.346
38	19.289	20.691	22.878	24.884	27.343	37.335	49.513	53.384	56.896	61.162	64.181	70.703
39	19.996	21.426	23.654	25.695	28.196	38.335	50.660	54.572	58.120	62.428	65.476	72.055
40	20.707	22.164	24.433	26.509	29.051	39.335	51.805	55.758	59.342	63.691	66.766	73.402
41	21.421	22.906	25.215	27.326	29.907	40.335	52.949	56.942	60.561	64.950	68.053	74.745
42	22.138	23.650	25.999	28.144	30.765	41.335	54.090	58.124	61.777	66.206	69.336	76.084
43	22.859	24.398	26.785	28.965	31.625	42.335	55.230	59.304	62.990	67.459	70.616	77.419
44	23.584	25.148	27.575	29.787	32.487	43.335	56.369	60.481	64.201	68.710	71.893	78.750
45	24.311	25.901	28.366	30.612	33.350	44.335	57.505	61.656	65.410	69.957	73.166	80.077
46	25.041	26.657	29.160	31.439	34.215	45.335	58.641	62.830	66.617	71.201	74.437	81.400
47	25.775	27.416	29.956	32.268	35.081	46.335	59.774	64.001	67.821	72.443	75.704	82.720
48	26.511	28.177	30.755	33.098	35.949	47.335	60.907	65.171	69.023	73.683	76.969	84.037
49	27.249	28.941	31.555	33.930	36.818	48.335	62.038	66.339	70.222	74.919	78.231	85.351

contd...

contd...

	p											
v	0.005	0.01	0.025	0.05	0.1	0.5	0.9	0.95	0.975	0.99	0.995	0.999
50	27.991	29.707	32.357	34.764	37.689	49.335	63.167	67.505	71.420	76.154	79.490	86.661
51	28.735	30.475	33.162	35.600	38.560	50.335	64.295	68.669	72.616	77.386	80.747	87.968
52	29.481	31.246	33.968	36.437	39.433	51.335	65.422	69.832	73.810	78.616	82.001	89.272
53	30.230	32.018	34.776	37.276	40.308	52.335	66.548	70.993	75.002	79.843	83.253	90.573
54	30.981	32.793	35.586	38.116	41.183	53.335	67.673	72.153	76.192	81.069	84.502	91.872
55	31.735	33.570	36.398	38.958	42.060	54.335	68.796	73.311	77.380	82.292	85.749	93.168
56	32.490	34.350	37.212	39.801	42.937	55.335	69.919	74.468	78.567	83.513	86.994	94.461
57	33.248	35.131	38.027	40.646	43.816	56.335	71.040	75.624	79.752	84.733	88.236	95.751
58	34.008	35.913	38.844	41.492	44.696	57.335	72.160	76.778	80.936	85.950	89.477	97.039
59	34.770	36.698	39.662	42.339	45.577	58.335	73.279	77.931	82.117	87.166	90.715	98.324
60	35.534	37.485	40.482	43.188	46.459	59.335	74.397	79.082	83.298	88.379	91.952	99.607
61	36.301	38.273	41.303	44.038	47.342	60.335	75.514	80.232	84.476	89.591	93.186	100.89
62	37.068	39.063	42.126	44.889	48.226	61.335	76.630	81.381	85.654	90.802	94.419	102.17
63	37.838	39.855	42.950	45.741	49.111	62.335	77.745	82.529	86.830	92.010	95.649	103.44
64	38.610	40.649	43.776	46.595	49.996	63.335	78.860	83.675	88.004	93.217	96.878	104.72
65	39.383	41.444	44.603	47.450	50.883	64.335	79.973	84.821	89.177	94.422	98.105	105.99
66	40.158	42.240	45.431	48.305	51.770	65.335	81.085	85.965	90.349	95.626	99.330	107.26
67	40.935	43.038	46.261	49.162	52.659	66.335	82.197	87.108	91.519	96.828	100.55	108.53
68	41.713	43.838	47.092	50.020	53.548	67.335	83.308	88.250	92.689	98.028	101.78	109.79
69	42.494	44.639	47.924	50.879	54.438	68.334	84.418	89.391	93.856	99.228	103.00	111.06
70	43.275	45.442	48.758	51.739	55.329	69.334	85.527	90.531	95.023	100.43	104.21	112.32
71	44.058	46.246	49.592	52.600	56.221	70.334	86.635	91.670	96.189	101.62	105.43	113.58
72	44.843	47.051	50.428	53.462	57.113	71.334	87.743	92.808	97.353	102.82	106.65	114.84
73	45.629	47.858	51.265	54.325	58.006	72.334	88.850	93.945	98.516	104.01	107.86	116.09
74	46.417	48.666	52.103	55.189	58.900	73.334	89.956	95.081	99.678	105.20	109.07	117.35
75	47.206	49.475	52.942	56.054	59.795	74.334	91.061	96.217	100.84	106.39	110.29	118.60
76	47.997	50.286	53.782	56.920	60.690	75.334	92.166	97.351	102.00	107.58	111.50	119.85
77	48.788	51.097	54.623	57.786	61.586	76.334	93.270	98.484	103.16	108.77	112.70	121.10
78	49.582	51.910	55.466	58.654	62.483	77.334	94.374	99.617	104.32	109.96	113.91	122.35
79	50.376	52.725	56.309	59.522	63.380	78.334	95.476	100.75	105.47	111.14	115.12	123.59
80	51.172	53.540	57.153	60.391	64.278	79.334	96.578	101.88	106.63	112.33	116.32	124.84
81	51.969	54.357	57.998	61.261	65.176	80.334	97.680	103.01	107.78	113.51	117.52	126.08
82	52.767	55.174	58.845	62.132	66.076	81.334	98.780	104.14	108.94	114.69	118.73	127.32
83	53.567	55.993	59.692	63.004	66.976	82.334	99.880	105.27	110.09	115.88	119.93	128.56
84	54.368	56.813	60.540	63.876	67.876	83.334	100.98	106.39	111.24	117.06	121.13	129.80
85	55.170	57.634	61.389	64.749	68.777	84.334	102.08	107.52	112.39	118.24	122.32	131.04
86	55.973	58.456	62.239	65.623	69.679	85.334	103.18	108.65	113.54	119.41	123.52	132.28
87	56.777	59.279	63.089	66.498	70.581	86.334	104.28	109.77	114.69	120.59	124.72	133.51
88	57.582	60.103	63.941	67.373	71.484	87.334	105.37	110.90	115.84	121.77	125.91	134.75
89	58.389	60.928	64.793	68.249	72.387	88.334	106.47	112.02	116.99	122.94	127.11	135.98
90	59.196	61.754	65.647	69.126	73.291	89.334	107.57	113.15	118.14	124.12	128.30	137.21
91	60.005	62.581	66.501	70.003	74.196	90.334	108.66	114.27	119.28	125.29	129.49	138.44
92	60.815	63.409	67.356	70.882	75.100	91.334	109.76	115.39	120.43	126.46	130.68	139.67
93	61.625	64.238	68.211	71.760	76.006	92.334	110.85	116.51	121.57	127.63	131.87	140.89
94	62.437	65.068	69.068	72.640	76.912	93.334	111.94	117.63	122.72	128.80	133.06	142.12
95	63.250	65.898	69.925	73.520	77.818	94.334	113.04	118.75	123.86	129.97	134.25	143.34
96	64.063	66.730	70.783	74.401	78.725	95.334	114.13	119.87	125.00	131.14	135.43	144.57
97	64.878	67.562	71.642	75.282	79.633	96.334	115.22	120.99	126.14	132.31	136.62	145.79
98	65.694	68.396	72.501	76.164	80.541	97.334	116.32	122.11	127.28	133.48	137.80	147.01
99	66.510	69.230	73.361	77.046	81.449	98.334	117.41	123.23	128.42	134.64	138.99	148.23
100	67.328	70.065	74.222	77.929	82.358	99.334	118.50	124.34	129.56	135.81	140.17	149.45
110	75.550	78.458	82.867	86.792	91.471	109.33	129.39	135.48	140.92	147.41	151.95	161.58
120	83.852	86.923	91.573	95.705	100.62	119.33	140.23	146.57	152.21	158.95	163.65	173.62
150	109.14	112.67	117.98	122.69	128.28	149.33	172.58	179.58	185.80	193.21	198.36	209.26
200	152.24	156.43	162.73	168.28	174.84	199.33	226.02	233.99	241.06	249.45	255.26	267.54
500	422.30	429.39	439.94	449.15	459.93	499.33	540.93	553.13	563.85	576.49	585.21	603.45

Table A11: F distribution

The table below contains the quartiles of the F distribution with *v*1 and *v*2 degrees of freedom.

		p				
v_1	v_2	0.9	0.95	0.975	0.99	0.995
1	1	39.863	161.45	647.79	4052.2	16211
	2	8.5263	18.513	38.506	98.503	198.50
	3	5.5383	10.128	17.443	34.116	55.552
	4	4.5448	7.7086	12.218	21.198	31.333
	5	4.0604	6.6079	10.007	16.258	22.785
	6	3.7759	5.9874	8.8131	13.745	18.635
	7	3.5894	5.5914	8.0727	12.246	16.236
	8	3.4579	5.3177	7.5709	11.259	14.688
	9	3.3603	5.1174	7.2093	10.561	13.614
	10	3.2850	4.9646	6.9367	10.044	12.826
	11	3.2252	4.8443	6.7241	9.6460	12.226
	12	3.1765	4.7472	6.5538	9.3302	11.754
	13	3.1362	4.6672	6.4143	9.0738	11.374
	14	3.1022	4.6001	6.2979	8.8616	11.060
	15	3.0732	4.5431	6.1995	8.6831	10.798
	16	3.0481	4.4940	6.1151	8.5310	10.575
	17	3.0262	4.4513	6.0420	8.3997	10.384
	18	3.0070	4.4139	5.9781	8.2854	10.218
	19	2.9899	4.3807	5.9216	8.1849	10.073
	20	2.9747	4.3512	5.8715	8.0960	9.9439
	21	2.9610	4.3248	5.8266	8.0166	9.8295
	22	2.9486	4.3009	5.7863	7.9454	9.7271
	23	2.9374	4.2793	5.7498	7.8811	9.6348
	24	2.9271	4.2597	5.7166	7.8229	9.5513
	25	2.9177	4.2417	5.6864	7.7698	9.4753
	30	2.8807	4.1709	5.5675	7.5625	9.1797
	35	2.8547	4.1213	5.4848	7.4191	8.9763
	40	2.8354	4.0847	5.4239	7.3141	8.8279
	45	2.8205	4.0566	5.3773	7.2339	8.7148
	50	2.8087	4.0343	5.3403	7.1706	8.6258
	60	2.7911	4.0012	5.2856	7.0771	8.4946
	70	2.7786	3.9778	5.2470	7.0114	8.4027
	80	2.7693	3.9604	5.2184	6.9627	8.3346
	100	2.7564	3.9361	5.1786	6.8953	8.2406
	120	2.7478	3.9201	5.1523	6.8509	8.1788
	150	2.7393	3.9042	5.1263	6.8069	8.1177
	200	2.7308	3.8884	5.1004	6.7633	8.0572
	500	2.7156	3.8601	5.0543	6.6858	7.9498
	+∞	2.7055	3.8415	5.0239	6.6349	7.8794
2	1	49.500	199.50	799.50	4999.5	19999
	2	9.0000	19.000	39.000	99.000	199.00
	3	5.4624	9.5521	16.044	30.817	49.799
	4	4.3246	6.9443	10.649	18.000	26.284
	5	3.7797	5.7861	8.4336	13.274	18.314
	6	3.4633	5.1433	7.2599	10.925	14.544
	7	3.2574	4.7374	6.5415	9.5466	12.404
	8	3.1131	4.4590	6.0595	8.6491	11.042
	9	3.0065	4.2565	5.7147	8.0215	10.107
	10	2.9245	4.1028	5.4564	7.5594	9.4270
	11	2.8595	3.9823	5.2559	7.2057	8.9122
	12	2.8068	3.8853	5.0959	6.9266	8.5096
	13	2.7632	3.8056	4.9653	6.7010	8.1865
	14	2.7265	3.7389	4.8567	6.5149	7.9216
	15	2.6952	3.6823	4.7650	6.3589	7.7008
	16	2.6682	3.6337	4.6867	6.2262	7.5138
	17	2.6446	3.5915	4.6189	6.1121	7.3536
	18	2.6239	3.5546	4.5597	6.0129	7.2148
	19	2.6056	3.5219	4.5075	5.9259	7.0935
	20	2.5893	3.4928	4.4613	5.8489	6.9865
	21	2.5746	3.4668	4.4199	5.7804	6.8914
	22	2.5613	3.4434	4.3828	5.7190	6.8064
	23	2.5493	3.4221	4.3492	5.6637	6.7300
	24	2.5383	3.4028	4.3187	5.6136	6.6609
	25	2.5283	3.3852	4.2909	5.5680	6.5982
	30	2.4887	3.3158	4.1821	5.3903	6.3547
	35	2.4609	3.2674	4.1065	5.2679	6.1878
	40	2.4404	3.2317	4.0510	5.1785	6.0664
	45	2.4245	3.2043	4.0085	5.1103	5.9741
	50	2.4120	3.1826	3.9749	5.0566	5.9016
	60	2.3933	3.1504	3.9253	4.9774	5.7950
	70	2.3800	3.1277	3.8903	4.9219	5.7204
	80	2.3701	3.1108	3.8643	4.8807	5.6652
	100	2.3564	3.0873	3.8284	4.8239	5.5892
	120	2.3473	3.0718	3.8046	4.7865	5.5393
	150	2.3383	3.0564	3.7811	4.7495	5.4900
	200	2.3293	3.0411	3.7578	4.7129	5.4412
	500	2.3132	3.0138	3.7162	4.6478	5.3549
	+∞	2.3026	2.9957	3.6889	4.6052	5.2983
3	1	53.593	215.71	864.16	5403.4	21615
	2	9.1618	19.164	39.165	99.166	199.17
	3	5.3908	9.2766	15.439	29.457	47.467
	4	4.1909	6.5914	9.9792	16.694	24.259
	5	3.6195	5.4095	7.7636	12.060	16.530
	6	3.2888	4.7571	6.5988	9.7795	12.917
	7	3.0741	4.3468	5.8898	8.4513	10.882
	8	2.9238	4.0662	5.4160	7.5910	9.5965
	9	2.8129	3.8625	5.0781	6.9919	8.7171
	10	2.7277	3.7083	4.8256	6.5523	8.0807
	11	2.6602	3.5874	4.6300	6.2167	7.6004
	12	2.6055	3.4903	4.4742	5.9525	7.2258
	13	2.5603	3.4105	4.3472	5.7394	6.9258
	14	2.5222	3.3439	4.2417	5.5639	6.6804
	15	2.4898	3.2874	4.1528	5.4170	6.4760
	16	2.4618	3.2389	4.0768	5.2922	6.3034
	17	2.4374	3.1968	4.0112	5.1850	6.1556
	18	2.4160	3.1599	3.9539	5.0919	6.0278
	19	2.3970	3.1274	3.9034	5.0103	5.9161

contd...

contd...

v_1	v_2	0.9	0.95	0.975	0.99	0.995
	20	2.3801	3.0984	3.8587	4.9382	5.8177
	21	2.3649	3.0725	3.8188	4.8740	5.7304
	22	2.3512	3.0491	3.7829	4.8166	5.6524
	23	2.3387	3.0280	3.7505	4.7649	5.5823
	24	2.3274	3.0088	3.7211	4.7181	5.5190
	25	2.3170	2.9912	3.6943	4.6755	5.4615
	30	2.2761	2.9223	3.5894	4.5097	5.2388
	35	2.2474	2.8742	3.5166	4.3957	5.0865
	40	2.2261	2.8387	3.4633	4.3126	4.9758
	45	2.2097	2.8115	3.4224	4.2492	4.8918
	50	2.1967	2.7900	3.3902	4.1993	4.8259
	60	2.1774	2.7581	3.3425	4.1259	4.7290
	70	2.1637	2.7355	3.3090	4.0744	4.6613
	80	2.1535	2.7188	3.2841	4.0363	4.6113
	100	2.1394	2.6955	3.2496	3.9837	4.5424
	120	2.1300	2.6802	3.2269	3.9491	4.4972
	150	2.1207	2.6649	3.2044	3.9149	4.4525
	200	2.1114	2.6498	3.1820	3.8810	4.4084
	500	2.0948	2.6227	3.1423	3.8210	4.3304
	+∞	2.0838	2.6049	3.1161	3.7816	4.2794
4	1	55.833	224.58	899.58	5624.6	22500
	2	9.2434	19.247	39.248	99.249	199.25
	3	5.3426	9.1172	15.101	28.710	46.195
	4	4.1072	6.3882	9.6045	15.977	23.155
	5	3.5202	5.1922	7.3879	11.392	15.556
	6	3.1808	4.5337	6.2272	9.1483	12.028
	7	2.9605	4.1203	5.5226	7.8466	10.050
	8	2.8064	3.8379	5.0526	7.0061	8.8051
	9	2.6927	3.6331	4.7181	6.4221	7.9559
	10	2.6053	3.4780	4.4683	5.9943	7.3428
	11	2.5362	3.3567	4.2751	5.6683	6.8809
	12	2.4801	3.2592	4.1212	5.4120	6.5211
	13	2.4337	3.1791	3.9959	5.2053	6.2335
	14	2.3947	3.1122	3.8919	5.0354	5.9984
	15	2.3614	3.0556	3.8043	4.8932	5.8029
	16	2.3327	3.0069	3.7294	4.7726	5.6378
	17	2.3077	2.9647	3.6648	4.6690	5.4967
	18	2.2858	2.9277	3.6083	4.5790	5.3746
	19	2.2663	2.8951	3.5587	4.5003	5.2681
	20	2.2489	2.8661	3.5147	4.4307	5.1743
	21	2.2333	2.8401	3.4754	4.3688	5.0911
	22	2.2193	2.8167	3.4401	4.3134	5.0168
	23	2.2065	2.7955	3.4083	4.2636	4.9500
	24	2.1949	2.7763	3.3794	4.2184	4.8898
	25	2.1842	2.7587	3.3530	4.1774	4.8351
	30	2.1422	2.6896	3.2499	4.0179	4.6234
	35	2.1128	2.6415	3.1785	3.9082	4.4788
	40	2.0909	2.6060	3.1261	3.8283	4.3738
	45	2.0742	2.5787	3.0860	3.7674	4.2941
	50	2.0608	2.5572	3.0544	3.7195	4.2316
	60	2.0410	2.5252	3.0077	3.6490	4.1399
	70	2.0269	2.5027	2.9748	3.5996	4.0758
	80	2.0165	2.4859	2.9504	3.5631	4.0285

v_1	v_2	0.9	0.95	0.975	0.99	0.995
	100	2.0019	2.4626	2.9166	3.5127	3.9634
	120	1.9923	2.4472	2.8943	3.4795	3.9207
	150	1.9827	2.4320	2.8722	3.4467	3.8785
	200	1.9732	2.4168	2.8503	3.4143	3.8368
	500	1.9561	2.3898	2.8114	3.3569	3.7632
	+∞	1.9449	2.3719	2.7858	3.3192	3.7151
5	1	57.240	230.16	921.85	5763.6	23056
	2	9.2926	19.296	39.298	99.299	199.30
	3	5.3092	9.0135	14.885	28.237	45.392
	4	4.0506	6.2561	9.3645	15.522	22.456
	5	3.4530	5.0503	7.1464	10.967	14.940
	6	3.1075	4.3874	5.9876	8.7459	11.464
	7	2.8833	3.9715	5.2852	7.4604	9.5221
	8	2.7264	3.6875	4.8173	6.6318	8.3018
	9	2.6106	3.4817	4.4844	6.0569	7.4712
	10	2.5216	3.3258	4.2361	5.6363	6.8724
	11	2.4512	3.2039	4.0440	5.3160	6.4217
	12	2.3940	3.1059	3.8911	5.0643	6.0711
	13	2.3467	3.0254	3.7667	4.8616	5.7910
	14	2.3069	2.9582	3.6634	4.6950	5.5623
	15	2.2730	2.9013	3.5764	4.5556	5.3721
	16	2.2438	2.8524	3.5021	4.4374	5.2117
	17	2.2183	2.8100	3.4379	4.3359	5.0746
	18	2.1958	2.7729	3.3820	4.2479	4.9560
	19	2.1760	2.7401	3.3327	4.1708	4.8526
	20	2.1582	2.7109	3.2891	4.1027	4.7616
	21	2.1423	2.6848	3.2501	4.0421	4.6809
	22	2.1279	2.6613	3.2151	3.9880	4.6088
	23	2.1149	2.6400	3.1835	3.9392	4.5441
	24	2.1030	2.6207	3.1548	3.8951	4.4857
	25	2.0922	2.6030	3.1287	3.8550	4.4327
	30	2.0492	2.5336	3.0265	3.6990	4.2276
	35	2.0191	2.4851	2.9557	3.5919	4.0876
	40	1.9968	2.4495	2.9037	3.5138	3.9860
	45	1.9796	2.4221	2.8640	3.4544	3.9090
	50	1.9660	2.4004	2.8327	3.4077	3.8486
	60	1.9457	2.3683	2.7863	3.3389	3.7599
	70	1.9313	2.3456	2.7537	3.2907	3.6980
	80	1.9206	2.3287	2.7295	3.2550	3.6524
	100	1.9057	2.3053	2.6961	3.2059	3.5895
	120	1.8959	2.2899	2.6740	3.1735	3.5482
	150	1.8861	2.2745	2.6521	3.1416	3.5075
	200	1.8763	2.2592	2.6304	3.1100	3.4674
	500	1.8588	2.2320	2.5919	3.0540	3.3963
	+∞	1.8473	2.2141	2.5665	3.0173	3.3499
6	1	58.204	233.99	937.11	5859.0	23437
	2	9.3255	19.330	39.331	99.333	199.33
	3	5.2847	8.9406	14.735	27.911	44.838
	4	4.0097	6.1631	9.1973	15.207	21.975
	5	3.4045	4.9503	6.9777	10.672	14.513
	6	3.0546	4.2839	5.8198	8.4661	11.073
	7	2.8274	3.8660	5.1186	7.1914	9.1553
	8	2.6683	3.5806	4.6517	6.3707	7.9520
	9	2.5509	3.3738	4.3197	5.8018	7.1339
	10	2.4606	3.2172	4.0721	5.3858	6.5446

contd...

contd...

v_1	v_2	0.9	0.95	0.975	0.99	0.995
	11	2.3891	3.0946	3.8807	5.0692	6.1016
	12	2.3310	2.9961	3.7283	4.8206	5.7570
	13	2.2830	2.9153	3.6043	4.6204	5.4819
	14	2.2426	2.8477	3.5014	4.4558	5.2574
	15	2.2081	2.7905	3.4147	4.3183	5.0708
	16	2.1783	2.7413	3.3406	4.2016	4.9134
	17	2.1524	2.6987	3.2767	4.1015	4.7789
	18	2.1296	2.6613	3.2209	4.0146	4.6627
	19	2.1094	2.6283	3.1718	3.9386	4.5614
	20	2.0913	2.5990	3.1283	3.8714	4.4721
	21	2.0751	2.5727	3.0895	3.8117	4.3931
	22	2.0472	2.5491	3.0546	3.7583	4.3225
	23	2.0472	2.5277	3.0232	3.7102	4.2591
	24	2.0351	2.5082	2.9946	3.6667	4.2019
	25	2.0241	2.4904	2.9685	3.6272	4.1500
	30	1.9803	2.4205	2.8667	3.4735	3.9492
	35	1.9496	2.3718	2.7961	3.3679	3.8123
	40	1.9269	2.3359	2.7444	3.2910	3.7129
	45	1.9269	2.3083	2.7048	3.2326	3.6376
	50	1.8954	2.2864	2.6736	3.1864	3.5785
	60	1.8747	2.2541	2.6274	3.1187	3.4918
	70	1.8600	2.2312	2.6949	3.0712	3.4313
	80	1.8491	2.2142	2.5708	3.0361	3.3867
	100	1.8339	2.1906	2.5374	2.9877	3.3252
	120	1.8238	2.1750	2.5154	2.9559	3.2849
	150	1.8138	2.1595	2.4936	2.9244	3.2452
	200	1.8038	2.1441	2.4720	2.8933	3.2059
	500	1.7859	2.1167	2.4335	2.8381	3.1366
	+∞	1.7741	2.0986	2.4082	2.8020	3.0913
7	1	58.906	236.77	948.22	5928.4	23715
	2	9.3491	19.353	39.355	99.356	199.36
	3	5.2662	8.8867	14.624	27.672	44.434
	4	3.9790	6.0942	9.0741	14.976	21.622
	5	3.3679	4.8759	6.8531	10.456	14.200
	6	3.0145	4.2067	5.6955	8.2600	10.786
	7	2.7849	3.7870	4.9949	6.9928	8.8854
	8	2.6241	3.5005	4.5286	6.1776	7.6941
	9	2.5051	3.2927	4.1970	5.6129	6.8849
	10	2.4140	3.1355	3.9498	5.2001	6.3025
	11	2.3416	3.0123	3.7586	4.8861	5.8648
	12	2.2828	2.9134	3.6065	4.6395	5.5245
	13	2.2341	2.8321	3.4827	4.4410	5.2529
	14	2.1931	2.7642	3.3799	4.2779	5.0313
	15	2.1582	2.7066	3.2934	4.1415	4.8473
	16	2.1280	2.6572	3.2194	4.0259	4.6920
	17	2.1017	2.6143	3.1556	3.9267	4.5594
	18	2.0785	2.5767	3.0999	3.8406	4.4448
	19	2.0580	2.5435	3.0509	3.7653	4.3448
	20	2.0397	2.5140	3.0074	3.6987	4.2569
	21	2.0233	2.4876	2.9686	3.6396	4.1789
	22	2.0084	2.4638	2.9338	3.5867	4.1094
	23	1.9949	2.4422	2.9023	3.5390	4.0469
	24	1.9826	2.4226	2.8738	3.4959	3.9905
	25	1.9714	2.4047	2.8478	3.4568	3.9394
	30	1.9269	2.3343	2.7460	3.3045	3.7416
	35	1.8957	2.2852	2.6755	3.2000	3.6066
	40	1.8725	2.2490	2.6238	3.1238	3.5088
	45	1.854.7	2.2212	2.5842	3.0658	3.4346
	50	1.8405	2.1992	2.5530	3.0202	3.3765
	60	1.8194	2.1665	2.5068	2.9530	3.2911
	70	1.8044	2.1435	2.4743	2.9060	3.2315
	80	1.793:3	2.1263	2.4502	2.8713	3.1876
	100	1.7778	2.1025	2.4168	2.8233	3.1271
	120	1.7675	2.0868	2.3948	2.7918	3.0874
	150	1.7571	2.0711	2.3730	2.7606	3.0483
	200	1.7470	2.0556	2.3513	2.7298	3.0097
	500	1.7288	2.0279	2.3129	2.6751	2.9414
	+∞	1.7167	2.0096	2.2875	2.6393	2.8968
8	1	59.439	238.88	956.66	5981.1	23925
	2	9.3668	19.371	39.373	99.374	199.37
	3	5.2517	8.8452	14.540	27.489	44.126
	4	3.9549	6.0410	8.9796	14.799	21.352
	5	3.3393	4.8183	6.7572	10.289	13.961
	6	2.9830	4.1468	5.5996	8.1017	10.566
	7	2.7516	3.7257	4.8993	6.8400	8.6781
	8	2.5893	3.4381	4.4333	6.0289	7.4959
	9	2.4694	3.2296	4.1020	5.4671	6.6933
	10	2.3772	3.0717	3.8549	5.0567	6.1159
	11	2.3040	2.9480	3.6638	4.7445	5.6821
	12	2.2446	2.8486	3.5118	4.4994	5.3461
	13	2.1953	2.7669	3.3880	4.3021	5.0761
	14	2.1539	2.6987	3.2853	4.1399	4.8566
	15	2.1186	2.6408	3.1987	4.0045	4.6744
	16	2.0880	2.5911	3.1248	3.8896	4.5207
	17	2.0613	2.5480	3.0610	3.7910	4.3894
	18	2.0379	2.5102	3.0053	3.7054	4.2759
	19	2.0171	2.4768	2.9563	3.6305	4.1770
	20	1.9985	2.4471	2.9128	3.5644	4.0900
	21	1.9819	2.4205	2.8740	3.5056	4.0128
	22	1.9668	2.3965	2.8392	3.4530	3.9440
	23	1.9531	2.3748	2.8077	3.4057	3.8822
	24	1.9407	2.3551	2.7791	3.3629	3.8264
	25	1.9292	2.3371	2.7531	3.3239	3.7758
	30	1.8841	2.2662	2.6513	3.1726	3.5801
	35	1.8524	2.2167	2.5807	3.0687	3.4466
	40	1.8289	2.1802	2.5289	2.9930	3.3498
	45	1.8289	2.1521	2.4892	2.9353	3.2764
	50	1.7963	2.1299	2.4579	2.8900	3.2189
	60	1.7748	2.0970	2.4117	2.8233	3.1344
	70	1.7596	2.0737	2.3791	2.7765	3.0755
	80	1.7483	2.0564	2.3549	2.7420	3.0320
	100	1.7324	2.0323	2.3215	2.6943	2.9722
	120	1.7220	2.0164	2.2994	2.6629	2.9330
	150	1.7115	2.0006	2.2775	2.6319	2.8942
	200	1.7011	1.9849	2.2558	2.6012	2.8560
	500	1.6825	1.9569	2.2172	2.5469	2.7885
	+∞	1.6702	1.9384	2.1918	2.5113	2.7444

contd...

contd...

v_1	v_2	0.9	0.95	0.975	0.99	0.995
9	1	59.858	240.54	963.28	6022.5	24091
	2	9.3805	19.385	39.387	99.388	199.39
	3	5.2400	8.8123	14.473	27.345	43.882
	4	3.9357	5.9988	8.9047	14.659	21.139
	5	3.3163	4.7725	6.6811	10.158	13.772
	6	2.9577	4.0990	5.5234	7.9761	10.391
	7	2.7247	3.6767	4.8232	6.7188	8.5138
	8	2.5612	3.3881	4.3572	5.9106	7.3386
	9	2.4403	3.1789	4.0260	5.3511	6.5411
	10	2.3473	3.0204	3.7790	4.9424	5.9676
	11	2.2735	2.8962	3.5879	4.6315	5.5368
	12	2.2135	2.7964	3.4358	4.3875	5.2021
	13	2.1638	2.7144	3.3120	4.1911	4.9351
	14	2.1220	2.6458	3.2093	4.0297	4.7173
	15	2.0862	2.5876	3.1227	3.8948	4.5364
	16	2.0553	2.5377	3.0488	3.7804	4.3838
	17	2.0284	2.4943	2.9849	3.6822	4.2535
	18	2.0047	2.4563	2.9291	3.5971	4.1410
	19	1.9836	2.4227	2.8801	3.5225	4.0428
	20	1.9649	2.3928	2.8365	3.4567	3.9564
	21	1.9480	2.3660	2.7977	3.3981	3.8799
	22	1.9327	2.3419	2.7628	3.3458	3.8116
	23	1.9189	2.3201	2.7313	3.2986	3.7502
	24	1.9063	2.3002	2.7027	3.2560	3.6949
	25	1.8947	2.2821	2.6766	3.2172	3.6447
	30	1.8490	2.2107	2.5746	3.0665	3.4505
	35	1.8168	2.1608	2.5039	2.9630	3.3180
	40	1.7929	2.1240	2.4519	2.8876	3.2220
	45	1.7745	2.0958	2.4122	2.8301	3.1492
	50	1.7598	2.0734	2.3808	2.7850	3.0920
	60	1.7380	2.0401	2.3344	2.7185	3.0083
	70	1.7225	2.0166	2.3017	2.6719	2.9498
	80	1.7110	1.9991	2.2775	2.6374	2.9066
	100	1.6949	1.9748	2.2439	2.5898	2.8472
	120	1.6842	1.9588	2.2217	2.5586	2.8083
	150	1.6736	1.9428	2.1998	2.5277	2.7698
	200	1.6630	1.9269	2.1780	2.4971	2.7319
	500	1.6441	1.8986	2.1392	2.4429	2.6649
	$+\infty$	1.6315	1.8799	2.1136	2.4073	2.6210
10	1	60.195	241.88	968.63	6055.8	24224
	2	9.3916	19.396	39.398	99.399	199.40
	3	5.2304	8.7855	14.419	27.229	43.686
	4	3.9199	5.9644	8.8439	14.546	20.967
	5	3.2974	4.7351	6.6192	10.051	13.618
	6	2.9336	4.0600	5.4613	7.8741	10.250
	7	2.7025	3.6365	4.7611	6.6201	8.3803
	8	2.5380	3.3472	4.2951	5.8143	7.2106
	9	2.4163	3.1373	3.9639	5.2565	6.4172
	10	2.3226	2.9782	3.7168	4.8491	5.8467
	11	2.2482	2.8536	3.5257	4.5393	5.4183
	12	2.1878	2.7534	3.3736	4.2961	5.0855
	13	2.1376	2.6710	3.2497	4.1003	4.8199
	14	2.0954	2.6022	3.1469	3.9394	4.6034

v_1	v_2	0.9	0.95	0.975	0.99	0.995
	15	2.0593	2.5437	3.0602	3.8049	4.4235
	16	2.0281	2.4935	2.9862	3.6909	4.2719
	17	2.0009	2.4499	2.9222	3.5931	4.1424
	18	1.9770	2.4117	2.8664	3.5082	4.0305
	19	1.9557	2.1779	2.8172	3.4338	3.9329
	20	1.9367	2.3479	2.7737	3.3682	3.8470
	21	1.9197	2.3210	2.7348	3.3098	3.7709
	22	1.9043	2.2967	2.6998	3.2576	3.7030
	23	1.8903	2.2747	2.6682	3.2106	3.6420
	24	1.8775	2.2547	2.6396	3.1681	3.5870
	25	1.8658	2.2365	2.6135	3.1294	3.5370
	30	1.8195	2.1646	2.5112	2.9791	3.3440
	35	1.7869	2.1143	2.4403	2.8758	3.2123
	40	1.7627	2.0772	2.3882	2.8005	3.1167
	45	1.7440	2.0487	2.3483	2.7432	3.0443
	50	1.7291	2.0261	2.3168	2.6981	2.9875
	60	1.7070	1.9926	2.2702	2.6318	2.9042
	70	1.6913	1.9689	2.2374	2.5852	2.8460
	80	1.6796	1.9512	2.2130	2.5508	2.8031
	100	1.6632	1.9267	2.1793	2.5033	2.7440
	120	1.6524	1.9105	2.1570	2.4721	2.7052
	150	1.6416	1.8943	2.1349	2.4412	2.6669
	200	1.6308	1.8783	2.1130	2.4106	2.6292
	500	1.6115	1.8496	2.0740	2.3565	2.5625
	$+\infty$	1.5987	1.8307	2.0483	2.3209	2.5188
11	1	60.473	242.98	973.03	6083.3	24334
	2	9.4006	19.405	39.407	99.408	199.41
	3	5.2224	8.7633	14.374	27.133	43.524
	4	3.9067	5.9358	8.7935	14.452	20.824
	5	3.2816	4.7040	6.5678	9.9626	13.491
	6	2.9195	4.0274	5.4098	7.7896	10.133
	7	2.6839	3.6030	4.7095	6.5382	8.2697
	8	2.5186	3.3130	4.2434	5.7343	7.1045
	9	2.3961	3.1025	3.9121	5.1779	6.3142
	10	2.3018	2.9430	3.6649	4.7715	5.7462
	11	2.2269	2.8179	3.4737	4.4624	5.3197
	12	2.1660	2.7173	3.3215	4.2198	4.9884
	13	2.1155	2.6347	3.1975	4.0245	4.7240
	14	2.0729	2.5655	3.0946	3.8640	4.5085
	15	2.0366	2.5068	3.0078	3.7299	4.3295
	16	2.0051	2.4564	2.9337	3.6162	4.1785
	17	1.9777	2.4126	2.8696	3.5185	4.0496
	18	1.9535	2.3742	2.8137	3.4338	3.9382
	19	1.9321	2.3402	2.7645	3.3596	3.8410
	20	1.9129	2.3100	2.7209	3.2941	3.7555
	21	1.8956	2.2829	2.6819	3.2359	3.6798
	22	1.8801	2.2585	2.6469	3.1837	3.6122
	23	1.8659	2.2364	2.6152	3.1368	3.5515
	24	1.8530	2.2163	2.5865	3.0944	3.4967
	25	1.8412	2.1979	2.5603	3.0558	3.4470
	30	1.7944	2.1256	2.4577	2.9057	3.2547
	35	1.7614	2.0750	2.3866	2.8026	3.1236

contd...

contd...

v_1	v_2	0.9	0.95	0.975	0.99	0.995
	40	1.7369	2.0376	2.3343	2.7274	3.0284
	45	1.7180	2.0088	2.2943	2.6701	2.9563
	50	1.7029	1.9861	2.2627	2.6250	2.8997
	60	1.6805	1.9522	2.2159	2.5587	2.8166
	70	1.6645	1.9283	2.1829	2.5122	2.7587
	80	1.6526	1.9105	2.1584	2.4777	2.7159
	100	1.6360	1.8857	2.1245	2.4302	2.6570
	120	1.6250	1.8693	2.1021	2.3990	2.6183
	150	1.6140	1.8530	2.0799	2.3681	2.5802
	200	1.6031	1.8368	2.0578	2.3375	2.5425
	500	1.5835	1.8078	2.0186	2.2833	2.4760
	+∞	1.5705	1.7886	1.9927	2.2477	2.4324
12	1	60.705	243.91	976.71	6106.3	24426
	2	9.4081	19.413	39.415	99.416	199.42
	3	5.2156	8.7446	14.337	27.052	43.387
	4	3.8955	5.9117	8.7512	14.374	20.705
	5	3.2682	4.6777	6.5245	9.8883	13.384
	6	2.9047	3.9999	5.3662	7.7183	10.034
	7	2.6681	3.5747	4.6658	6.4691	8.1764
	8	2.5020	3.2839	4.1997	5.6667	7.0149
	9	2.3789	3.0729	3.8682	5.1114	6.2274
	10	2.2841	2.9130	3.6209	4.7059	5.6613
	35	1.7869	2.1143	2.4403	2.8758	3.2123
	11	2.2087	2.7876	3.4296	4.3974	5.2363
	12	2.1474	2.6866	3.2773	4.1553	4.9062
	13	2.0966	2.6037	3.1532	3.9603	4.6429
	14	2.0537	2.5342	3.0502	3.8001	4.4281
	15	2.0171	2.4753	2.9633	3.6662	4.2497
	16	1.9854	2.4247	2.8890	3.5527	4.0994
	17	1.9577	2.3807	2.8249	3.4552	3.9709
	18	1.9333	2.3421	2.7689	3.3706	3.8599
	19	1.9117	2.3080	2.7196	3.2965	3.7631
	20	1.8924	2.2776	2.6758	3.2311	3.6779
	21	1.8750	2.2504	2.6368	3.1730	3.6024
	22	1.8593	2.2258	2.6017	3.1209	3.5350
	23	1.8450	2.2036	2.5699	3.0740	3.4745
	24	1.8319	2.1834	2.5411	3.0316	3.4199
	25	1.8200	2.1649	2.5149	2.9931	3.3704
	30	1.7727	2.0921	2.4120	2.8431	3.1787
	35	1.7394	2.0411	2.3406	2.7400	3.0480
	40	1.7146	2.0035	2.2882	2.6648	2.9531
	45	1.6954	1.9745	2.2480	2.6076	2.8811
	50	1.6802	1.9515	2.2162	2.5625	2.8247
	60	1.6574	1.9174	2.1692	2.4961	2.7419
	70	1.6413	1.8932	2.1361	2.4496	2.6840
	80	1.6292	1.8753	2.1115	2.4151	2.6413
	100	1.6124	1.8503	2.0773	2.3676	2.5825
	120	1.6012	1.8337	2.0548	2.3363	2.5439
	150	1.5901	1.8172	2.0325	2.3053	2.5059
	200	1.5789	1.8008	2.0103	2.2747	2.4683
	500	1.5590	1.7715	1.9708	2.2204	2.4018
	+∞	1.5458	1.7522	1.9447	2.1847	2.3583

v_1	v_2	0.9	0.95	0.975	0.99	0.995
13	1	60.903	244.69	979.84	6125.9	24505
	2	9.4145	19.419	39.421	99.422	199.42
	3	5.2098	8.7287	14.304	26.983	43.271
	4	3.8859	5.8911	8.7150	14.307	20.603
	5	3.2567	4.6552	6.4876	9.8248	13.293
	6	2.8920	3.9764	5.3290	7.6575	9.9501
	7	2.6545	3.5503	4.6285	6.4100	8.0967
	8	2.4876	3.2590	4.1622	5.6089	6.9384
	9	2.3640	3.0475	3.8306	5.0545	6.1530
	10	2.2687	2.8872	3.5832	4.6496	5.5887
	11	2.1930	2.7614	3.3917	4.3416	5.1649
	12	2.1313	2.6602	3.2393	4.0999	4.8358
	13	2.0802	2.5769	3.1150	3.9052	4.5733
	14	2.0370	2.5073	3.0119	3.7452	4.3591
	15	2.0001	2.4481	2.9249	3.6115	4.1813
	16	1.9682	2.3973	2.8506	3.4981	4.0314
	17	1.9404	2.3531	2.7863	3.4007	3.9033
	18	1.9158	2.3143	2.7302	3.3162	3.7926
	19	1.8940	2.2800	2.6808	3.2422	3.6961
	20	1.8745	2.2495	2.6369	3.1769	3.6111
	21	1.8570	2.2222	2.5978	3.1187	3.5358
	22	1.8411	2.1975	2.5626	3.0667	3.4686
	23	1.8267	2.1752	2.5308	3.0199	3.4083
	24	1.8136	2.1548	2.5019	2.9775	3.3538
	25	1.8015	2.1362	2.4756	2.9389	3.3044
	30	1.7538	2.0630	2.3724	2.7890	3.1132
	35	1.7201	2.0117	2.3008	2.6859	2.9827
	40	1.6950	1.9738	2.2481	2.6107	2.8880
	45	1.6757	1.9446	2.2078	2.5534	2.8162
	50	1.6602	1.9214	2.1758	2.5083	2.7599
	60	1.6372	1.8870	2.1286	2.4419	2.6771
	70	1.6209	1.8627	2.0953	2.3953	2.6193
	80	1.6086	1.8445	2.0706	2.3608	2.5767
	100	1.5916	1.8193	2.0363	2.3132	2.5180
	120	1.5803	1.8026	2.0136	2.2818	2.4794
	150	1.5690	1.7859	1.9911	2.2508	2.4413
	200	1.5577	1.7694	1.9688	2.2201	2.4038
	500	1.5374	1.7398	1.9290	2.1656	2.3373
	+∞	1.5240	1.7202	1.9027	2.1299	2.2938
14	1.	61.073	245.36	982.53	6142.7	24572
	2	9.4200	19.424	39.427	99.428	199.43
	3	5.2047	8.7149	14.277	26.924	43.172
	4	3.8776	5.8733	8.6838	14.249	20.515
	5	3.2468	4.6358	6.4556	9.7700	13.215
	6	2.8809	3.9559	5.2968	7.6049	9.8774
	7	2.6426	3.5292	4.5961	6.3590	8.0279
	8	2.4752	3.2374	4.1297	5.5589	6.8721
	9	2.3510	3.0255	3.7980	5.0052	6.0887
	10	2.2553	2.8647	3.5504	4.6008	5.5257
	11	2.1792	2.7386	3.3588	4.2932	5.1031
	12	2.1173	2.6371	3.2062	4.0518	4.7748
	13	2.0658	2.5536	3.0819	3.8573	4.5129
	14	2.0224	2.4837	2.9786	3.6975	4.2993

contd...

contd...

v_1	v_2	0.9	0.95	0.975	0.99	0.995
	15	1.9853	2.4244	2.8915	3.5639	4.1219
	16	1.9532	2.3733	2.8170	3.4506	3.9723
	17	1.9252	2.3290	2.7526	3.3533	3.8445
	18	1.9004	2.2900	2.6964	3.2689	3.7341
	19	1.8785	2.2556	2.6469	3.1949	3.6378
	20	1.8588	2.2250	2.6030	3.1296	3.5530
	21	1.8412	2.1975	2.5638	3.0715	3.4779
	22	1.8252	2.1727	2.5285	3.0195	3.4108
	23	1.8107	2.1502	2.4966	2.9727	3.3506
	24	1.7974	2.1298	2.4677	2.9303	3.2962
	25	1.7853	2.1111	2.4413	2.8917	3.2469
	30	1.7371	2.0374	2.3378	2.7418	3.0560
	35	1.7031	1.9858	2.2659	2.6387	2.9258
	40	1.6778	1.9476	2.2130	2.5634	2.8312
	45	1.6582	1.9182	2.1725	2.5060	2.7595
	50	1.6426	1.8949	2.1404	2.4609	2.7032
	60	1.6193	1.8602	2.0929	2.3943	2.6205
	70	1.6028	1.8357	2.0595	2.3477	2.5627
	80	1.5904	1.8174	2.0346	2.3131	2.5201
	100	1.5731	1.7919	2.0001	2.2654	2.4614
	120	1.5617	1.7750	1.9773	2.2339	2.4228
	150	1.5502	1.7582	1.9546	2.2028	2.3847
	200	1.5388	1.7415	1.9322	2.1721	2.3472
	500	1.5182	1.7116	1.8921	2.1174	2.2806
	+∞	1.5046	1.6918	1.8656	2.0815	2.2371
15	1	61.220	245.95	984.87	6157.3	24630
	2	9.4247	19.429	39.431	99.433	199.43
	3	5.2003	8.7029	14.253	26.872	43.085
	4	3.8704	5.8578	8.6565	14.198	20.438
	5	3.2380	4.6188	6.4277	9.7222	13.146
	6	2.8712	3.9381	5.2687	7.5590	9.8140
	7	2.6322	3.5107	4.5678	6.3143	7.9678
	8	2.4642	3.2184	4.1012	5.5151	6.8143
	9	2.3396	3.0061	3.7694	4.9621	6.0325
	10	2.2435	2.8450	3.5217	4.5581	5.4707
	11	2.1671	2.7186	3.3299	4.2509	5.0489
	12	2.1049	2.6169	3.1772	4.0096	4.7213
	13	2.0532	2.5331	3.0527	3.8154	4.4600
	14	2.0095	2.4630	2.9493	3.6557	4.2468
	15	1.9722	2.4034	2.8621	3.5222	4.0698
	16	1.9399	2.3522	2.7875	3.4089	3.9205
	17	1.9117	2.3077	2.7230	3.3117	3.7929
	18	1.8868	2.2686	2.6667	3.2273	3.6827
	19	1.8647	2.2341	2.6171	3.1533	3.5866
	20	1.8449	2.2033	2.5731	3.0880	3.5020
	21	1.8271	2.1757	2.5338	3.0300	3.4270
	22	1.8111	2.1508	2.4984	2.9779	3.3600
	23	1.7964	2.1282	2.4665	2.9311	3.2999
	24	1.7831	2.1077	2.4374	2.8887	3.2456
	25	1.7708	2.0889	2.4110	2.8502	3.1963
	30	1.7223	2.0148	2.3072	2.7002	3.0057
	35	1.6880	1.9629	2.2350	2.5970	2.8756
	40	1.6624	1.9245	2.1819	2.5216	2.7811
	45	1.6426	1.8949	2.1412	2.4642	2.7094

v_1	v_2	0.9	0.95	0.975	0.99	0.995
	50	1.6269	1.8714	2.1090	2.4190	2.6531
	60	1.6034	1.8364	2.0613	2.3523	2.5705
	70	1.5866	1.8117	2.0277	2.3055	2.5127
	80	1.5741	1.7932	2.0026	2.2709	2.4700
	100	1.5566	1.7675	1.9679	2.2230	2.4113
	120	1.5450	1.7505	1.9450	2.1915	2.3727
	150	1.5334	1.7335	1.9222	2.1603	2.3346
	200	1.5218	1.7166	1.8996	2.1294	2.2970
	500	1.5010	1.6864	1.8592	2.0746	2.2304
	+∞	1.4871	1.6664	1.8326	2.0385	2.1868
16	1	61.350	246.46	986.92	6170.1	24681
	2	9.4289	19.433	39.435	99.437	199.44
	3	5.1964	8.6923	14.232	26.827	43.008
	4	3.8639	5.8441	8.6326	14.154	20.371
	5	3.2303	4.6038	6.4032	9.6802	13.086
	6	2.8626	3.9223	5.2439	7.5186	9.7582
	7	2.6230	3.4944	4.5428	6.2750	7.9148
	8	2.4545	3.2016	4.0761	5.4766	6.7633
	9	2.3295	2.9890	3.7441	4.9240	5.9829
	10	2.2330	2.8276	3.4963	4.5204	5.4221
	11	2.1563	2.7009	3.3044	4.2134	5.0011
	12	2.0938	2.5989	3.1515	3.9724	4.6741
	13	2.0419	2.5149	3.0269	3.7783	4.4132
	14	1.9981	2.4446	2.9234	3.6187	4.2005
	15	1.9605	2.3849	2.8360	3.4852	4.0237
	16	1.9281	2.3335	2.7614	3.3720	3.8747
	17	1.8997	2.2888	2.6968	3.2748	3.7473
	18	1.8747	2.2496	2.6404	3.1904	3.6373
	19	1.8524	2.2149	2.5907	3.1165	3.5412
	20	1.8325	2.1840	2.5465	3.0512	3.4568
	21	1.8146	2.1563	2.5071	2.9931	3.3818
	22	1.7984	2.1313	2.4717	2.9411	3.3150
	23	1.7837	2.1086	2.4396	2.8943	3.2549
	24	1.7703	2.0880	2.4105	2.8519	3.2007
	25	1.7579	2.0691	2.3840	2.8133	3.1515
	30	1.7090	1.9946	2.2799	2.6632	2.9611
	35	1.6744	1.9424	2.2075	2.5599	2.8310
	40	1.6486	1.9037	2.1542	2.4844	2.7365
	45	1.6287	1.8740	2.1133	2.4269	2.6648
	50	1.6128	1.8503	2.0810	2.3816	2.6086
	60	1.5890	1.8151	2.0330	2.3148	2.5259
	70	1.5721	1.7902	1.9992	2.2679	2.4681
	80	1.5594	1.7716	1.9741	2.2332	2.4254
	100	1.5418	1.7456	1.9391	2.1852	2.3666
	120	1.5300	1.7285	1.9161	2.1536	2.3280
	150	1.5182	1.7113	1.8931	2.1223	2.2898
	200	1.5065	1.6943	1.8704	2.0913	2.2521
	500	1.4854	1.6638	1.8297	2.0362	2.1854
	+∞	1.4714	1.6435	1.8028	2.0000	2.1417
17	1	61.464	246.92	988.73	6181.4	24727
	2	9.4325	19.437	39.439	99.440	199.44
	3	5.1929	8.6829	14.213	26.787	42.941
	4	3.8582	5.8320	8.6113	14.115	20.311

contd...

contd...

v_1	v_2	0.9	0.95	0.975	0.99	0.995
	5	3.2234	4.5904	6.3814	9.6429	13.033
	6	2.8550	3.9083	5.2218	7.4827	9.7086
	7	2.6148	3.4799	4.5206	6.2401	7.8678
	8	2.4458	3.1867	4.0538	5.4423	6.7180
	9	2.3205	2.9737	3.7216	4.8902	5.9388
	10	2.2237	2.8120	3.4737	4.4869	5.3789
	11	2.1467	2.6851	3.2816	4.1801	4.9586
	12	2.0839	2.5828	3.1286	3.9392	4.6321
	13	2.0318	2.4987	3.0039	3.7452	4.3716
	14	1.9878	2.4282	2.9003	3.5857	4.1592
	15	1.9501	2.3683	2.8128	3.4523	3.9827
	16	1.9175	2.3167	2.7380	3.3391	3.8338
	17	1.8889	2.2719	2.6733	3.2419	3.7066
	18	1.8638	2.2:125	2.6168	3.1575	3.5967
	19	1.8414	2.1977	2.5670	3.0836	3.5008
	20	1.8214	2.1667	2.5228	3.0183	3.4164
	21	1.8034	2.1389	2.4833	2.9602	3.3416
	22	1.7871	2.1138	2.4478	2.9082	3.2748
	23	1.7723	2.0910	2.4157	2.8613	3.2148
	24	1.7587	2.0703	2.3865	2.8189	3.1606
	25	1.7463	2.0513	2.3599	2.7803	3.1114
	30	1.6970	1.9765	2.2554	2.6301	2.9211
	35	1.6622	1.9240	2.1828	2.5266	2.7911
	40	1.6362	1.8851	2.1293	2.4511	2.6966
	45	1.6161	1.8551	2.0883	2.3935	2.6249
	50	1.6000	1.8313	2.0558	2.3481	2.5686
	60	1.5760	1.7959	2.0076	2.2811	2.4859
	70	1.5589	1.7708	1.9736	2.2341	2.4281
	80	1.5461	1.7520	1.9483	2.1993	2.3854
	100	1.5283	1.7259	1.9132	2.1511	2.3265
	120	1.5164	1.7085	1.8900	2.1194	2.2878
	150	1.5045	1.6913	1.8669	2.0880	2.2496
	200	1.4926	1.6741	1.8440	2.0569	2.2118
	500	1.4712	1.6432	1.8030	2.0016	2.1449
	+∞	1.4570	1.6228	1.7759	1.9652	2.1011
18	1	61.566	247.32	990.35	6191.5	24767
	2	9.4358	19.440	39.442	99.444	199.44
	3	5.1898	8.6745	14.196	26.751	42.880
	4	3.8531	5.8211	8.5924	14.080	20.258
	5	3.2172	4.5785	6.3619	9.6096	12.985
	6	2.8481	3.8957	5.2021	7.4507	9.6644
	7	2.6074	3.4669	4.5008	6.2089	7.8258
	8	2.4380	3.1733	4.0338	5.4116	6.6775
	9	2.3123	2.9600	3.7015	4.8599	5.8994
	10	2.2153	2.7980	3.4534	4.4569	5.3403
	11	2.1380	2.6709	3.2612	4.1503	4.9205
	12	2.0750	2.5684	3.1081	3.9095	4.5945
	13	2.0227	2.4841	2.9832	3.7156	4.3344
	14	1.9785	2.4134	2.8795	3.5561	4.1221
	15	1.9407	2.3533	2.7919	3.4228	3.9459
	16	1.9079	2.3016	2.7170	3.3096	3.7972
	17	1.8792	2.2567	2.6522	3.2124	3.6701
	18	1.8539	2.2172	2.5956	3.1280	3.5603

v_1	v_2	0.9	0.95	0.975	0.99	0.995
	19	1.8314	2.1823	2.5457	3.0541	3.4645
	20	1.8113	2.1511	2.5014	2.9887	3.3802
	21	1.7932	2.1232	2.4618	2.9306	3.3054
	22	1.7768	2.0980	2.4262	2.8786	3.2387
	23	1.7619	2.0751	2.3940	2.8317	3.1787
	24	1.7483	2.0543	2.3648	2.7892	3.1246
	25	1.7358	2.0353	2.3381	2.7506	3.0754
	30	1.6862	1.9601	2.2334	2.6003	2.8852
	35	1.6511	1.9073	2.1605	2.4967	2.7551
	40	1.6249	1.8682	2.1068	2.4210	2.6607
	45	1.6046	1.8381	2.0656	2.3633	2.5889
	50	1.5884	1.8141	2.0330	2.3178	2.5326
	60	1.5642	1.7784	1.9846	2.2507	2.4498
	70	1.5470	1.7531	1.9504	2.2036	2.3919
	80	1.5340	1.7342	1.9250	2.1686	2.3492
	100	1.5160	1.7079	1.8897	2.1203	2.2902
	120	1.5039	1.6904	1.8663	2.0885	2.2514
	150	1.4919	1.6730	1.8431	2.0570	2.2131
	200	1.4799	1.6556	1.8200	2.0257	2.1753
	500	1.4583	1.6245	1.7787	1.9702	2.1082
	+∞	1.4439	1.6038	1.7515	1.9336	2.0642
19	1	61.658	247.69	991.80	6200.6	24803
	2	9.4387	19.443	39.445	99.447	199.45
	3	5.1870	8.6670	14.181	26.719	42.826
	4	3.8485	5.8114	8.5753	14.048	20.210
	5	3.2117	4.5678	6.3444	9.5797	12.942
	6	2.8419	3.8844	5.1844	7.4219	9.6247
	7	2.6008	3.4551	4.4829	6.1808	7.7881
	8	2.4310	3.1613	4.0158	5.3840	6.6411
	9	2.3050	2.9477	3.6833	4.8327	5.8639
	10	2.2077	2.7854	3.4351	4.4299	5.3055
	11	2.1302	2.6581	3.2428	4.1234	4.8863
	12	2.0670	2.5554	3.0896	3.8827	4.5606
	13	2.0145	2.4709	2.9646	3.6888	4.3008
	14	1.9701	2.4000	2.8607	3.5294	4.0888
	15	1.9321	2.3398	2.7730	3.3961	3.9127
	16	1.8992	2.2880	2.6980	3.2829	3.7641
	17	1.8704	2.2429	2.6331	3.1857	3.6372
	18	1.8450	2.2033	2.5764	3.1013	3.5275
	19	1.8224	2.1683	2.5265	3.0274	3.4318
	20	1.8022	2.1370	2.4821	2.9620	3.3475
	21	1.7840	2.1090	2.4424	2.9039	3.2728
	22	1.7675	2.0837	2.4067	2.8518	3.2060
	23	1.7525	2.0608	2.3745	2.8049	3.1461
	24	1.7388	2.0399	2.3452	2.7624	3.0920
	25	1.7263	2.0207	2.3184	2.7238	3.0429
	30	1.6763	1.9452	2.2134	2.5732	2.8526
	35	1.6410	1.8922	2.1403	2.4695	2.7226
	40	1.6146	1.8529	2.0864	2.3937	2.6281
	45	1.5941	1.8226	2.0450	2.3359	2.5563

contd...

contd...

v_1	v_2	0.9	0.95	0.975	0.99	0.995
	50	1.5778	1.7985	2.0122	2.2903	2.4999
	60	1.5534	1.7625	1.9636	2.2230	2.4171
	70	1.5360	1.7371	1.9293	2.1758	2.3591
	80	1.5230	1.7180	1.9037	2.1408	2.3163
	100	1.5047	1.6915	1.8682	2.0923	2.2572
	120	1.4926	1.6739	1.8447	2.0604	2.2183
	150	1.4804	1.6563	1.8213	2.0287	2.1800
	200	1.4683	1.6388	1.7981	1.9973	2.1420
	500	1.4464	1.6074	1.7566	1.9415	2.0748
	+∞	1.4318	1.5865	1.7291	1.9048	2.0306
20	1	61.740	248.01	993.10	6208.7	24836
	2	9.4413	19.446	39.448	99.449	199.45
	3	5.1845	8.6602	14.167	26.690	42.778
	4	3.8443	5.8025	8.5599	14.020	20.167
	5	3.2067	4.5581	6.3286	9.5526	12.903
	6	2.8363	3.8742	5.1684	7.3958	9.5888
	7	2.5947	3.4445	4.4667	6.1554	7.7540
	8	2.4246	3.1503	3.9995	5.3591	6.6082
	9	2.2983	2.9365	3.6669	4.8080	5.8318
	10	2.2007	2.7740	3.4185	4.4054	5.2740
	11	2.1230	2.6464	3.2261	4.0990	4.8552
	12	2.0597	2.5436	3.0728	3.8584	4.5299
	13	2.0070	2.4589	2.9477	3.6646	4.2703
	14	1.9625	2.3879	2.8437	3.5052	4.0585
	15	1.9243	2.3275	2.7559	3.3719	3.8826
	16	1.8913	2.2756	2.6808	3.2587	3.7342
	17	1.8624	2.2304	2.6158	3.1615	3.6073
	18	1.8368	2.1906	2.5590	3.0771	3.4977
	19	1.8142	2.1555	2.5089	3.0031	3.4020
	20	1.7938	2.1242	2.4645	2.9377	3.3178
	21	1.7756	2.0960	2.4247	2.8796	3.2431
	22	1.7590	2.0707	2.3890	2.8274	3.1764
	23	1.7439	2.0476	2.3567	2.7805	3.1165
	24	1.7302	2.0267	2.3273	2.7380	3.0624
	25	1.7175	2.0075	2.3005	2.6993	3.0133
	30	1.6673	1.9317	2.1952	2.5487	2.8230
	35	1.6317	1.8784	2.1218	2.4448	2.6930
	40	1.6052	1.8389	2.0677	2.3689	2.5984
	45	1.5846	1.8084	2.0262	2.3109	2.5266
	50	1.5681	1.7841	1.9933	2.2652	2.4702
	60	1.5435	1.7480	1.9445	2.1978	2.3872
	70	1.5259	1.7223	1.9100	2.1504	2.3291
	80	1.5128	1.7032	1.8843	2.1153	2.2862
	100	1.4943	1.6764	1.8486	2.0666	2.2270
	120	1.4821	1.6587	1.8249	2.0346	2.1881
	150	1.4698	1.6410	1.8014	2.0028	2.1496
	200	1.4575	1.6233	1.7780	1.9713	2.1116
	500	1.4354	1.5916	l.7362	1.9152	2.0441
	+∞	1.4206	1.5705	1.7085	1.8783	1.9998
21	1	61.815	248.31	994.29	6216.1	24866
	2	9.4437	19.448	39.450	99.452	199.45
	3	5.1822	8.6540	14.155	26.664	42.733
	4	3.8405	5.7945	8.5460	13.994	20.128
	5	3.2021	4.5493	6.3142	9.5281	12.868

v_1	v_2	0.9	0.95	0.975	0.99	0.995
	6	2.8312	3.8649	5.1538	7.3722	9.5562
	7	2.5892	3.4349	4.4520	6.1324	7.7230
	8	2.4188	3.1404	3.9846	5.3364	6.5783
	9	2.2922	2.9263	3.6520	4.7856	5.8027
	10	2.1944	2.7636	3.4035	4.3831	5.2454
	11	2.1165	2.6358	3.2109	4.0769	4.8270
	12	2.0530	2.5328	3.0575	3.8363	4.5020
	13	2.0001	2.4479	2.9322	3.6425	4.2426
	14	1.9555	2.3768	2.8282	3.4832	4.0310
	15	1.9172	2.3163	2.7403	3.3498	3.8552
	16	1.8840	2.2642	2.6651	3.2367	3.7069
	17	1.8550	2.2189	2.6000	3.1394	3.5801
	18	1.8294	2.1791	2.5431	3.0550	3.4705
	19	1.8066	2.1438	2.4930	2.9810	3.3749
	20	1.7862	2.1124	2.4484	2.9156	3.2907
	21	1.7678	2.0842	2.4086	2.8574	3.2160
	22	1.7512	2.0587	2.3728	2.8052	3.1494
	23	1.7360	2.0356	2.3404	2.7583	3.0895
	24	1.7222	2.0146	2.3109	2.7157	3.0354
	25	1.7095	1.9953	2.2840	2.6770	2.9862
	30	1.6590	1.9192	2.1785	2.5262	2.7960
	35	1.6232	1.8657	2.1049	2.4222	2.6659
	40	1.5965	1.8260	2.0506	2.3461	2.5713
	45	1.5757	1.7953	2.0089	2.2880	2.4994
	50	1.5592	1.7709	1.9759	2.2423	2.4429
	60	1.5343	1.7346	1.9269	2.1747	2.3598
	70	1.5166	1.7088	1.8922	2.1271	2.3017
	80	1.5034	1.6895	1.8664	2.0919	2.2587
	100	1.4848	1.6626	1.8305	2.0431	2.1993
	120	1.4724	1.6447	1.8067	2.0109	2.1603
	150	1.4600	1.6268	1.7830	1.9790	2.1218
	200	1.4476	1.6090	1.7595	1.9474	2.0836
	500	1.4252	1.5770	1.7174	1.8910	2.0159
	+∞	1.4102	1.5557	1.6895	1.8539	1.9715
22	1	61.883	248.58	995.36	6222.8	24892
	2	9.4458	19.450	39.452	99.454	199.45
	3	5.1801	8.6484	14.144	26.640	42.693
	4	3.8371	5.7872	8.5332	13.970	20.093
	5	3.1979	4.5413	6.3011	9.5058	12.836
	6	2.8266	3.8564	5.1406	7.3506	9.5264
	7	2.5842	3.4260	4.4386	6.1113	7.6947
	8	2.4135	3.1313	3.9711	5.3157	6.5510
	9	2.2867	2.9169	3.6383	4.7651	5.7760
	10	2.1887	2.7541	3.3897	4.3628	5.2192
	11	2.1106	2.6261	3.1970	4.0566	4.8012
	12	2.0469	2.5229	3.0434	3.8161	4.4765
	13	1.9939	2.4379	2.9181	3.6224	4.2173
	14	1.9490	2.3667	2.8139	3.4630	4.0058
	15	1.9106	2.3060	2.7260	3.3297	3.8301
	16	1.8774	2.2538	2.6507	3.2165	3.6819
	17	1.8482	2.2084	2.5855	3.1192	3.5552
	18	1.8225	2.1685	2.5285	3.0348	3.4456
	19	1.7997	2.1331	2.4783	2.9607	3.3500

contd...

contd...

v_1	v_2	0.9	0.95	0.975	0.99	0.995
	20	1.7792	2.1016	2.4337	2.8953	3.2659
	21	1.7607	2.0733	2.3938	2.8370	3.1912
	22	1.7440	2.0478	2.3579	2.7849	3.1246
	23	1.7288	2.0246	2.3254	2.7378	3.0647
	24	1.7149	2.0035	2.2959	2.6953	3.0106
	25	1.7021	1.9842	2.2690	2.6565	2.9615
	30	1.6514	1.9077	2.1631	2.5055	2.7712
	35	1.6154	1.8540	2.0893	2.4014	2.6410
	40	1.5884	1.8141	2.0349	2.3252	2.5463
	45	1.5676	1.7833	1.9930	2.2670	2.4744
	50	1.5509	1.7588	1.9599	2.2211	2.4178
	60	1.5259	1.7222	1.9106	2.1533	2.3346
	70	1.5080	1.6962	1.8758	2.1057	2.2764
	80	1.4947	1.6768	1.8499	2.0703	2.2333
	100	1.4759	1.6497	1.8138	2.0214	2.1738
	120	1.4634	1.6317	1.7899	1.9891	2.1347
	150	1.4509	1.6137	1.7661	1.9570	2.0961
	200	1.4383	1.5958	1.7424	1.9252	2.0578
	500	1.4157	1.5635	1.7000	1.8686	1.9899
	+∞	1.4006	1.5420	1.6719	1.8313	1.9453
23	1	61.945	248.83	996.35	6229.0	24917
	2	9.4478	19.452	39.454	99.456	199.46
	3	5.1781	8.6432	14.134	26.618	42.656
	4	3.8339	5.7805	8.5216	13.949	20.060
	5	3.1941	4.5339	6.2891	9.4853	12.807
	6	2.8223	3.8486	5.1284	7.3309	9.4992
	7	2.5796	3.4179	4.4263	6.0921	7.6688
	8	2.4086	3.1229	3.9587	5.2967	6.5260
	9	2.2816	2.9084	3.6257	4.7463	5.7516
	10	2.1833	2.7453	3.3770	4.3441	5.1953
	11	2.1051	2.6172	3.1843	4.0380	4.7775
	12	2.0412	2.5139	3.0306	3.7976	4.4530
	13	1.9881	2.4287	2.9052	3.6038	4.1940
	14	1.9431	2.3573	2.8009	3.4445	3.9827
	15	1.9046	2.2966	2.7128	3.3111	3.8071
	16	1.8712	2.2443	2.6374	3.1979	3.6589
	17	1.8420	2.1987	2.5721	3.1006	3.5323
	18	1.8162	2.1587	2.5151	3.0161	3.4228
	19	1.7932	2.1233	2.4648	2.9421	3.3272
	20	1.7727	2.0917	2.4201	2.8766	3.2431
	21	1.7541	2.0633	2.3801	2.8183	3.1684
	22	1.7374	2.0377	2.3442	2.7661	3.1018
	23	1.7221	2.0144	2.3116	2.7191	3.0419
	24	1.7081	1.9932	2.2821	2.6765	2.9878
	25	1.6953	1.9738	2.2551	2.6377	2.9387
	30	1.6443	1.8972	2.1490	2.4865	2.7483
	35	1.6081	1.8432	2.0750	2.3822	2.6181
	40	1.5810	1.8031	2.0203	2.3059	2.5233
	45	1.5600	1.7722	1.9784	2.2476	2.4513
	50	1.5432	1.7475	1.9451	2.2016	2.3947
	60	1.5180	1.7108	1.8956	2.1336	2.3114
	70	1.5000	1.6846	1.8606	2.0858	2.2530
	80	1.4866	1.6651	1.8346	2.0504	2.2098
	100	1.4677	1.6378	1.7983	2.0012	2.1502

v_1	v_2	0.9	0.95	0.975	0.99	0.995
	120	1.4550	1.6197	1.7743	1.9688	2.1110
	150	1.4424	1.6015	1.7503	1.9367	2.0723
	200	1.4297	1.5834	1.7265	1.9047	2.0339
	500	1.4069	1.5509	1.6838	1.8479	1.9657
	+∞	1.3916	1.5292	1.6555	1.8104	1.9209
24	1	62.002	249.05	997.25	6234.6	24940
	2	9.4496	19.454	39.456	99.458	199.46
	3	5.1764	8.6385	14.124	26.598	42.622
	4	3.8310	5.7744	8.5109	13.929	20.030
	5	3.1905	4.5272	6.2780	9.4665	12.780
	6	2.8183	3.8415	5.1172	7.3127	9.4742
	7	2.5753	3.4105	4.4150	6.0743	7.6450
	8	2.4041	3.1152	3.9472	5.2793	6.5029
	9	2.2768	2.9005	3.6142	4.7290	5.7292
	10	2.1784	2.7372	3.3654	4.3269	5.1732
	11	2.1000	2.6090	3.1725	4.0209	4.7557
	12	2.0360	2.5055	3.0187	3.7805	4.4314
	13	1.9827	2.4202	2.8932	3.5868	4.1726
	14	1.9377	2.3487	2.7888	3.4274	3.9614
	15	1.8990	2.2878	2.7006	3.2940	3.7859
	16	1.8656	2.2354	2.6252	3.1808	3.6378
	17	1.8362	2.1898	2.5598	3.0835	3.5112
	18	1.8103	2.1497	2.5027	2.9990	3.4017
	19	1.7873	2.1141	2.4523	2.9249	3.3062
	20	1.7667	2.0825	2.4076	2.8594	3.2220
	21	1.7481	2.0540	2.3675	2.8010	3.1474
	22	1.7312	2.0283	2.3315	2.7488	3.0807
	23	1.7159	2.0050	2.2989	2.7017	3.0208
	24	1.7019	1.9838	2.2693	2.6591	2.9667
	25	1.6890	1.9643	2.2422	2.6203	2.9176
	30	1.6377	1.8874	2.1359	2.4689	2.7272
	35	1.6013	1.8332	2.0617	2.3645	2.5969
	40	1.5741	1.7929	2.0069	2.2880	2.5020
	45	1.5530	1.7618	1.9647	2.2296	2.4299
	50	1.5361	1.7371	1.9313	2.1835	2.3732
	60	1.5107	1.7001	1.8817	2.1154	2.2898
	70	1.4926	1.6738	1.8466	2.0674	2.2313
	80	1.4790	1.6542	1.8204	2.0318	2.1881
	100	1.4600	1.6267	1.7839	1.9826	2.1283
	120	1.4472	1.6084	1.7597	1.9500	2.0890
	150	1.4345	1.5902	1.7356	1.9177	2.0501
	200	1.4217	1.5720	1.7117	1.8857	2.0116
	500	1.3986	1.5392	1.6687	1.8285	1.9432
	+∞	1.3832	1.5173	1.6402	1.7908	1.8983
25	1	62.055	249.26	998.08	6239.8	24960
	2	9.4513	19.456	39.458	99.459	199.46
	3	5.1747	8.6341	14.115	26.579	42.591
	4	3.8283	5.7687	8.5010	13.911	20.002
	5	3.1873	4.5209	6.2679	9.4491	12.755
	6	2.8147	3.8348	5.1069	7.2960	9.4511
	7	2.5714	3.4036	4.4045	6.0580	7.6230
	8	2.3999	3.1081	3.9367	5.2631	6.4817
	9	2.2725	2.8932	3.6035	4.7130	5.7084

contd...

contd...

v_1	v_2	0.9	0.95	0.975	0.99	0.995
	10	2.1739	2.7298	3.3546	4.3111	5.1528
	11	2.0953	2.6014	3.1616	4.0051	4.7356
	12	2.0312	2.4977	3.0077	3.7647	4.4115
	13	1.9778	2.4123	2.8821	3.5710	4.1528
	14	1.9326	2.3407	2.7777	3.4116	3.9417
	15	1.8939	2.2797	2.6894	3.2782	3.7662
	16	1.8603	2.2272	2.6138	3.1650	3.6182
	17	1.8309	2.1815	2.5484	3.0676	3.4916
	18	1.8049	2.1413	2.4912	2.9831	3.3822
	19	1.7818	2.1057	2.4408	2.9089	3.2867
	20	1.7611	2.0739	2.3959	2.8434	3.2025
	21	1.7424	2.0454	2.3558	2.7850	3.1279
	22	1.7255	2.0196	2.3198	2.7328	3.0613
	23	1.7101	1.9963	2.2871	2.6856	3.0014
	24	1.6960	1.9750	2.2574	2.6430	2.9472
	25	1.6831	1.9554	2.2303	2.6041	2.8981
	30	1.6316	1.8782	2.1237	2.4526	2.7076
	35	1.5950	1.8239	2.0493	2.3480	2.5772
	40	1.5677	1.7835	1.9943	2.2714	2.4823
	45	1.5464	1.7522	1.9521	2.2129	2.4101
	50	1.5294	1.7273	1.9186	2.1667	2.3533
	60	1.5039	1.6902	1.8687	2.0984	2.2697
	70	1.4857	1.6638	1.8334	2.0503	2.2112
	80	1.4720	1.6440	1.8071	2.0146	2.1678
	100	1.4528	1.6163	1.7705	1.9652	2.1080
	120	1.4399	1.5980	1.7462	1.9325	2.0686
	150	1.4271	1.5796	1.7220	1.9001	2.0295
	200	1.4142	1.5612	1.6978	1.8679	1.9909
	500	1.3909	1.5282	1.6546	1.8105	1.9223
	+∞	1.3753	1.5061	1.6259	1.7726	1.8771
30	1	62.265	250.10	1001.4	6260.6	25044
	2	9.4579	19.462	39.465	99.466	199.47
	3	5.1681	8.6166	14.081	26.505	42.466
	4	3.8174	5.7459	8.4613	13.838	19.892
	5	3.1741	4.4957	6.2269	9.3793	12.656
	6	2.8000	3.8082	5.0652	7.2285	9.3582
	7	2.5555	3.3758	4.3624	5.9920	7.5345
	8	2.3830	3.0794	3.8940	5.1981	6.3961
	9	2.2547	2.8637	3.5604	4.6486	5.6248
	10	2.1554	2.6996	3.3110	4.2469	5.0706
	11	2.0762	2.5705	3.1176	3.9411	4.6543
	12	2.0115	2.4663	2.9633	3.7008	4.3309
	13	1.9576	2.3803	2.8372	3.5070	4.0727
	14	1.9119	2.3082	2.7324	3.3476	3.8619
	15	1.8728	2.2468	2.6437	3.2141	3.6867
	16	1.8388	2.1938	2.5678	3.1007	3.5389
	17	1.8090	2.1477	2.5020	3.0032	3.4124
	18	1.7827	2.1071	2.4445	2.9185	3.3030
	19	1.7592	2.0712	2.3937	2.8442	3.2075
	20	1.7382	2.0391	2.3486	2.7785	3.1234
	21	1.7193	2.0102	2.3082	2.7200	3.0488
	22	1.7021	1.9842	2.2718	2.6675	2.9821
	23	1.6864	1.9605	2.2389	2.6202	2.9221

v_1	v_2	0.9	0.95	0.975	0.99	0.995
	24	1.6721	1.9390	2.2090	2.5773	2.8679
	25	1.6589	1.9192	2.1816	2.5383	2.8187
	30	1.6065	1.8409	2.0739	2.3860	2.6278
	35	1.5691	1.7856	1.9986	2.2806	2.4969
	40	1.5411	1.7444	1.9429	2.2034	2.4015
	45	1.5193	1.7126	1.9000	2.1443	2.3288
	50	1.5018	1.6872	1.8659	2.0976	2.2717
	60	1.4755	1.6491	1.8152	2.0285	2.1874
	70	1.4567	1.6220	1.7792	1.9797	2.1283
	80	1.4426	1.6017	1.7523	1.9435	2.0845
	100	1.4227	1.5733	1.7148	1.8933	2.0239
	120	1.4094	1.5543	1.6899	1.8600	1.9840
	150	1.3960	1.5164	1.6651	1.8270	1.9444
	200	1.3826	1.4824	1.6403	1.7941	1.9051
	500	1.3582	1.4821	1.5957	1.7353	1.8352
	+∞	1.3419	1.4591	1.5660	1.6964	1.7891
35	1	62.416	250.69	1003.8	6275.6	25103
	2	9.4627	19.467	39.469	99.471	199.47
	3	5.1633	8.6039	14.055	26.451	42.376
	4	3.8096	5.7294	8.4327	13.785	19.812
	5	3.1645	4.4775	6.1973	9.3291	12.584
	6	2.7893	3.7889	5.0352	7.1799	9.2913
	7	2.5439	3.3557	4.3319	5.9444	7.4707
	8	2.3707	3.0586	3.8632	5.1512	6.3343
	9	2.2418	2.8422	3.5292	4.6020	5.5643
	10	2.1420	2.6776	3.2794	4.2005	5.0110
	11	2.0623	2.5480	3.0856	3.8948	4.5955
	12	1.9971	2.4433	2.9309	3.6544	4.2725
	13	1.9428	2.3570	2.8046	3.4606	4.0146
	14	1.8968	2.2845	2.6994	3.3010	3.8040
	15	1.8573	2.2227	2.6104	3.1674	3.6289
	16	1.8230	2.1694	2.5342	3.0539	3.4811
	17	1.7929	2.1229	2.4681	2.9563	3.3547
	18	1.7663	2.0821	2.4103	2.8714	3.2453
	19	1.7426	2.0458	2.3593	2.7969	3.1498
	20	1.7213	2.0135	2.3139	2.7310	3.0656
	21	1.7021	1.9844	2.2733	2.6723	2.9909
	22	1.6847	1.9581	2.2366	2.6197	2.9241
	23	1.6689	1.9342	2.2035	2.5722	2.8641
	24	1.6544	1.9124	2.1733	2.5292	2.8098
	25	1.6410	1.8924	2.1458	2.4900	2.7605
	30	1.5877	1.8132	2.0372	2.3369	2.5691
	35	1.5497	1.7571	1.9611	2.2309	2.4377
	40	1.5211	1.7154	1.9047	2.1531	2.3418
	45	1.4989	1.6830	1.8613	2.0934	2.2687
	50	1.4810	1.6571	1.8267	2.0463	2.2112
	60	1.4541	1.6183	1.7752	1.9764	2.1263
	70	1.4348	1.5906	1.7386	1.9271	2.0666
	80	1.4203	1.5699	1.7112	1.8904	2.0223
	100	1.3998	1.5407	1.6729	1.8393	1.9610
	120	1.3861	1.5213	1.6475	1.8055	1.9205
	150	1.3723	1.5018	1.6220	1.7719	1.8803
	200	1.3583	1.4822	1.5966	1.7383	1.8404
	500	1.3331	1.4467	1.5508	1.6783	1.7692
	+∞	1.3160	1.4229	1.5201	1.6383	1.7221

contd...

contd...

v_1	v_2	0.9	0.95	0.975	0.99	0.995
40	1	62.529	251.14	1005.6	6286.8	25148
	2	9.4662	19.471	39.473	99.474	199.47
	3	5.1597	8.5944	14.037	26.411	42.308
	4	3.8036	5.7170	8.4111	3.745	19.752
	5	3.1573	4.4638	6.1750	9.2912	12.530
	6	2.7812	3.7743	5.0125	7.1432	9.2408
	7	2.5351	3.3404	4.3089	5.9084	7.4224
	8	2.3614	3.0428	3.8398	5.1156	6.2875
	9	2.2320	2.8259	3.5055	4.5666	5.5186
	10	2.1317	2.6609	3.2554	4.1653	4.9659
	11	2.0516	2.5309	3.0613	3.8596	4.5508
	12	1.9861	2.4259	2.9063	3.6192	4.2282
	13	1.9315	2.3392	2.7797	3.4253	3.9704
	14	1.8852	2.2664	2.6742	3.2656	3.7600
	15	1.8454	2.2043	2.5850	3.1319	3.5850
	16	1.8108	2.1507	2.5085	3.0182	3.4372
	17	1.7805	2.1040	2.4422	2.9205	3.3108
	18	1.7537	2.0629	2.3842	2.8354	3.2014
	19	1.7298	2.0264	2.3329	2.7608	3.1058
	20	1.7083	1.9938	2.2873	2.6947	3.0215
	21	1.6890	1.9645	2.2465	2.6359	2.9467
	22	1.6714	1.9380	2.2097	2.5831	2.8799
	23	1.6554	1.9139	2.1763	2.5335	2.8197
	24	1.6407	1.8920	2.1460	2.4923	2.7654
	25	1.6272	1.8718	2.1183	2.4530	2.7160
	30	1.5732	1.7918	2.0089	2.2992	2.5241
	35	1.5346	1.7351	1.9321	2.1926	2.3922
	40	1.5056	1.6928	1.8752	2.1142	2.2958
	45	1.4830	1.6599	1.8313	2.0542	2.2224
	50	1.4648	1.6337	1.7963	2.0066	2.1644
	60	1.4373	1.5943	1.7440	1.9360	2.0789
	70	1.4176	1.5661	1.7069	1.8861	2.0186
	80	1.4027	1.5449	1.6790	1.8489	1.9739
	100	1.3817	1.5151	1.6401	1.7972	1.9119
	120	1.3676	1.4952	1.6141	1.7628	1.8709
	150	1.3534	1.4752	1.5882	1.7286	1.8302
	200	1.3390	1.4551	1.5621	1.6945	1.7897
	500	1.3129	1.4186	1.5151	1.6332	1.7172
	$+\infty$	1.2951	1.3940	1.4835	1.5923	1.6691
45	1	62.617	251.49	1007.0	6295.5	25183
	2	9.4690	19.474	39.476	99.477	199.48
	3	5.1569	8.5870	14.022	26.379	42.255
	4	3.7990	5.7073	8.3943	13.714	19.705
	5	3.1517	4.4530	6.1576	9.2616	12.487
	6	2.7748	3.7629	4.9947	7.1145	9.2014
	7	2.5282	3.3285	4.2908	5.8803	7.3847
	8	2.3540	3.0304	3.8215	5.0878	6.2510
	9	2.2242	2.8131	3.4869	4.5390	5.4827
	10	2.1236	2.6477	3.2366	4.1377	4.9306
	11	2.0432	2.5174	3.0422	3.8320	4.5158
	12	1.9774	2.4121	2.8870	3.5915	4.1934
	13	1.9225	2.3252	2.7601	3.3976	3.9358
	14	1.8760	2.2521	2.6544	3.2378	3.7254
	15	1.8360	2.1897	2.5650	3.1039	3.5504
	16	1.8012	2.1360	2.4883	2.9902	3.4026
	17	1.7707	2.0890	2.4218	2.8922	3.2762
	18	1.7437	2.0477	2.3635	2.8071	3.1667
	19	1.7196	2.0110	2.3121	2.7323	3.0711
	20	1.6980	1.9783	2.2663	2.6661	2.9868
	21	1.6785	1.9488	2.2253	2.6071	2.9119
	22	1.6608	1.9221	2.1883	2.5542	2.8449
	23	1.6446	1.8979	2.1548	2.5065	2.7847
	24	1.6298	1.8757	2.1243	2.4632	2.7303
	25	1.6161	1.8554	2.0964	2.4237	2.6808
	30	1.5616	1.7748	1.9864	2.2693	2.4884
	35	1.5226	1.7175	1.9090	2.1622	2.3560
	40	1.4932	1.6748	1.8516	2.0833	2.2593
	45	1.4702	1.6415	1.8073	2.0228	2.1854
	50	1.4517	1.6149	1.7719	1.9749	2.1272
	60	1.4238	1.5749	1.7191	1.9037	2.0410
	70	1.4037	1.5463	1.6814	1.8533	1.9803
	80	1.3885	1.5247	1.6532	1.8157	1.9352
	100	1.3670	1.4944	1.6136	1.7633	1.8725
	120	1.3526	1.4741	1.5872	1.7284	1.8310
	150	1.3380	1.4536	1.5607	1.6937	1.7898
	200	1.3232	1.4330	1.5341	1.6590	1.7487
	500	1.2963	1.3955	1.4860	1.5964	1.6750
	$+\infty$	1.2779	1.3701	1.4536	1.5546	1.6259
50	1	62.688	251.77	1008.1	6302.5	25211
	2	9.4712	19.476	39.478	99.479	199.48
	3	5.1546	8.5810	14.010	26.354	42.213
	4	3.7952	5.6995	8.3808	13.690	19.667
	5	3.1471	4.4444	6.1436	9.2378	12.454
	6	2.7697	3.7537	4.9804	7.0915	9.1697
	7	2.5226	3.3189	4.2763	5.8577	7.3544
	8	2.3481	3.0204	3.8067	5.0654	6.2215
	9	2.2180	2.8028	3.4719	4.5167	5.4539
	10	2.1171	2.6371	3.2214	4.1155	4.9022
	11	2.0364	2.5066	3.0268	3.8097	4.4876
	12	1.9704	2.4010	2.8714	3.5692	4.1653
	13	1.9153	2.3138	2.7443	3.3752	3.9078
	14	1.8686	2.2405	2.6384	3.2153	3.6975
	15	1.8284	2.1780	2.5488	3.0814	3.5225
	16	1.7934	2.1240	2.4719	2.9675	3.3747
	17	1.7628	2.0769	2.4053	2.8694	3.2482
	18	1.7356	2.0354	2.3468	2.7841	3.1387
	19	1.7114	1.9986	2.2952	2.7093	3.0430
	20	1.6896	1.9656	2.2493	2.6430	2.9586
	21	1.6700	1.9360	2.2081	2.5838	2.8837
	22	1.6521	1.9092	2.1710	2.5308	2.8167
	23	1.6358	1.8848	2.1374	2.4829	2.7564
	24	1.6209	1.8625	2.1067	2.4395	2.7018
	25	1.6072	1.8421	2.0787	2.3999	2.6522
	30	1.5522	1.7609	1.9681	2.2450	2.4594
	35	1.5127	1.7032	1.8902	2.1374	2.3266
	40	1.4830	1.6600	1.8324	2.0581	2.2295
	45	1.4597	1.6264	1.7876	1.9972	2.1553

contd...

contd...

v_1	v_2	0.9	0.95	0.975	0.99	0.995
	50	1.4409	1.5995	1.7520	1.9490	2.0967
	60	1.4126	1.5590	1.6985	1.8772	2.0100
	70	1.3922	1.5300	1.6604	1.8263	1.9488
	80	1.3767	1.5081	1.6318	1.7883	1.9033
	100	1.3548	1.4772	1.5917	1.7353	1.8400
	120	1.3400	1.4565	1.5649	1.7000	1.7981
	150	1.3251	1.4357	1.5379	1.6648	1.7563
	200	1.3100	1.4146	1.5108	1.6295	1.7147
	500	1.2823	1.3762	1.4616	1.5658	1.6398
	+∞	1.2633	1.3501	1.4284	1.5231	1.5898
60	1	62.794	252.20	1009.8	6313.0	25253
	2	9.4746	19.479	39.481	99.482	199.48
	3	5.1512	8.5720	13.992	26.316	42.149
	4	3.7896	5.6877	8.3604	13.652	19.611
	5	3.1402	4.4314	6.1225	9.2020	12.402
	6	2.7620	3.7398	4.9589	7.0567	9.1219
	7	2.5142	3.3043	4.2544	5.8236	7.3088
	8	2.3391	3.0053	3.7844	5.0316	6.1772
	9	2.2085	2.7872	3.4493	4.4831	5.4104
	10	2.1072	2.6211	3.1984	4.0819	4.8592
	11	2.0261	2.4901	3.0035	3.7761	4.4450
	12	1.9597	2.3842	2.8478	3.5355	4.1229
	13	1.9043	2.2966	2.7204	3.3413	3.8655
	14	1.8572	2.2229	2.6142	3.1813	3.6552
	15	1.8168	2.1601	2.5242	3.0471	3.4803
	16	1.7816	2.1058	2.4471	2.9330	3.3324
	17	1.7506	2.0584	2.3801	2.8348	3.2058
	18	1.7232	2.0166	2.3214	2.7493	3.0962
	19	1.6988	1.9795	2.2696	2.6742	3.0004
	20	1.6768	1.9464	2.2234	2.6077	2.9159
	21	1.6569	1.9165	2.1819	2.5484	2.8408
	22	1.6389	1.8894	2.1446	2.4951	2.7736
	23	1.6224	1.8648	2.1107	2.4471	2.7132
	24	1.6073	1.8424	2.0799	2.4035	2.6585
	25	1.5934	1.8217	2.0516	2.3637	2.6088
	30	1.5376	1.7396	1.9400	2.2079	2.4151
	35	1.4975	1.6811	1.8613	2.0994	2.2816
	40	1.4672	1.6373	1.8028	2.0194	2.1838
	45	1.4434	1.6031	1.7574	1.9579	2.1090
	50	1.4242	1.5757	1.7211	1.9090	2.0499
	60	1.3952	1.5343	1.6668	1.8363	1.9622
	70	1.3742	1.5046	1.6279	1.7846	1.9002
	80	1.3583	1.4821	1.5987	1.7459	1.8540
	100	1.3356	1.4504	1.5575	1.6918	1.7896
	120	1.3203	1.4290	1.5299	1.6557	1.7469
	150	1.3048	1.4074	1.5022	1.6195	1.7041
	200	1.2891	1.3856	1.4742	1.5833	1.6614
	500	1.2600	1.3455	1.4231	1.5174	1.5843
	+∞	1.2400	1.3180	1.3883	1.4730	1.5325
70	1	62.870	252.50	1011.0	6320.6	25283
	2	9.4769	19.481	39.484	99.485	199.49
	3	5.1487	8.5656	13.979	26.289	42.104
	4	3.7855	5.6793	8.3458	13.625	19.570
	5	3.1353	4.4220	6.1074	9.1763	12.366
	6	2.7564	3.7298	4.9434	7.0318	9.0877
	7	2.5082	3.2939	4.2386	5.7991	7.2760
	8	2.3326	2.9944	3.7684	5.0073	6.1453
	9	2.2017	2.7760	3.4330	4.4589	5.3791
	10	2.1000	2.6095	3.1818	4.0577	4.8283
	11	2.0187	2.4782	2.9867	3.7518	4.4143
	12	1.9520	2.3720	2.8307	3.5111	4.0924
	13	1.8963	2.2841	2.7030	3.3168	3.8350
	14	1.8490	2.2102	2.5966	3.1567	3.6248
	15	1.8083	2.1472	2.5064	3.0224	3.4498
	16	1.7729	2.0926	2.4291	2.9082	3.3018
	17	1.7418	2.0450	2.3619	2.8097	3.1752
	18	1.7142	2.0030	2.3030	2.7241	3.0655
	19	1.6896	1.9657	2.2509	2.6488	2.9695
	20	1.6674	1.9323	2.2045	2.5822	2.8849
	21	1.6474	1.9023	2.1629	2.5227	2.8097
	22	1.6292	1.8751	2.1254	2.4693	2.7424
	23	1.6125	1.8503	2.0913	2.4210	2.6818
	24	1.5973	1.8276	2.0603	2.3773	2.6270
	25	1.5833	1.8069	2.0319	2.3373	2.5772
	30	1.5269	1.7240	1.9195	2.1808	2.3829
	35	1.4862	1.6649	1.8402	2.0716	2.2488
	40	1.4555	1.6205	1.7810	1.9911	2.1504
	45	1.4313	1.5859	1.7351	1.9290	2.0751
	50	1.4119	1.5580	1.6984	1.8797	2.0155
	60	1.3822	1.5160	1.6433	1.8061	1.9269
	70	1.3608	1.4857	1.6038	1.7537	1.8642
	80	1.3444	1.4628	1.5740	1.7144	1.8174
	100	1.3212	1.4303	1.5320	1.6594	1.7521
	120	1.3055	1.4083	1.5038	1.6226	1.7086
	150	1.2895	1.3861	1.4753	1.5856	1.6651
	200	1.2731	1.3636	1.4465	1.5485	1.6215
	500	1.2428	1.3220	1.3937	1.4807	1.5423
	+∞	1.2218	1.2933	1.3575	1.4346	1.4888
80	1	62.927	252.72	1011.9	6326.2	25306
	2	9.4787	19.483	39.485	99.487	199.49
	3	5.1469	8.5607	13.970	26.269	42.070
	4	3.7825	5.6730	8.3349	13.605	19.540
	5	3.1316	4.4150	6.0960	9.1570	12.338
	6	2.7522	3.7223	4.9318	7.0130	9.0619
	7	2.5036	3.2860	4.2268	5.7806	7.2513
	8	2.3277	2.9862	3.7563	4.9890	6.1213
	9	2.1965	2.7675	3.4207	4.4407	5.3555
	10	2.0946	2.6008	3.1694	4.0394	4.8050
	11	2.0130	2.4692	2.9740	3.7335	4.3912
	12	1.9461	2.3628	2.8178	3.4928	4.0693
	13	1.8903	2.2747	2.6900	3.2984	3.8120
	14	1.8428	2.2006	2.5833	3.1381	3.6017
	15	1.8019	2.1373	2.4930	3.0037	3.4267
	16	1.7664	2.0826	2.4154	2.8893	3.2787
	17	1.7351	2.0348	2.3481	2.7908	3.1520
	18	1.7073	1.9927	2.2890	2.7050	3.0422
	19	1.6826	1.9552	2.2368	2.6296	2.9462

contd...

contd...

v_1	v_2	0.9	0.95	0.975	0.99	0.995
	20	1.6603	1.9217	2.1902	2.5628	2.8614
	21	1.6401	1.8915	2.1485	2.5032	2.7861
	22	1.6218	1.8641	2.1108	2.4496	2.7187
	23	1.6051	1.8392	2.0766	2.4013	2.6581
	24	1.5897	1.8164	2.0454	2.3573	2.6031
	25	1.5755	1.7955	2.0169	2.3173	2.5532
	30	1.5187	1.7121	1.9039	2.1601	2.3584
	35	1.4776	1.6525	1.8240	2.0505	2.2237
	40	1.4465	1.6077	1.7644	1.9694	2.1249
	45	1.4221	1.5726	1.7181	1.9069	2.0491
	50	1.4023	1.5445	1.6810	1.8571	1.9891
	60	1.3722	1.5019	1.6252	1.7828	1.8998
	70	1.3503	1.4711	1.5851	1.7298	1.8365
	80	1.3337	1.4477	1.5549	1.6901	1.7892
	100	1.3100	1.4146	1.5122	1.6342	1.7231
	120	1.2938	1.3922	1.4834	1.5968	1.6789
	150	1.2774	1.3694	1.4543	1.5592	1.6347
	200	1.2605	1.3463	1.4248	1.5212	1.5902
	500	1.2292	1.3033	1.3704	1.4517	1.5091
	+∞	1.2072	1.2735	1.3329	1.4041	1.4540
100	1	63.007	253.04	1013.2	6334.1	25337
	2	9.4812	19.486	39.488	99.489	199.49
	3	5.1443	8.5539	13.956	26.240	42.022
	4	3.7782	5.6641	8.3195	13.577	19.497
	5	3.1263	4.4051	6.0800	9.1299	12.300
	6	2.7463	3.7117	4.9154	6.9867	9.0257
	7	2.4971	3.2749	4.2101	5.7547	7.2165
	8	2.3208	2.9747	3.7393	4.9633	6.0875
	9	2.1892	2.7556	3.4034	4.4150	5.3223
	10	2.0869	2.5884	3.1517	4.0137	4.7721
	11	2.0050	2.4566	2.9561	3.7077	4.3585
	12	1.9379	2.3498	2.7996	3.4668	4.0368
	13	1.8817	2.2614	2.6715	3.2723	3.7795
	14	1.8340	2.1870	2.5646	3.1118	3.5692
	15	1.7929	2.1234	2.4739	2.9772	3.3941
	16	1.7570	2.0685	2.3961	2.8627	3.2460
	17	1.7255	2.0204	2.3285	2.7639	3.1192
	18	1.6976	1.9780	2.2692	2.6779	3.0093
	19	1.6726	1.9403	2.2167	2.6023	2.9131
	20	1.6501	1.9066	2.1699	2.5353	2.8282
	21	1.6298	1.8761	2.1280	2.4755	2.7527
	22	1.6113	1.8486	2.0901	2.4217	2.6852
	23	1.5944	1.8234	2.0557	2.3732	2.6243
	24	1.5788	1.8005	2.0243	2.3291	2.5692
	25	1.5645	1.7794	1.9955	2.2888	2.5191
	30	1.5069	1.6950	1.8816	2.1307	2.3234
	35	1.4653	1.6347	1.8009	2.0202	2.1880
	40	1.4336	1.5892	1.7405	1.9383	2.0884
	45	1.4087	1.5536	1.6935	1.8751	2.0119
	50	1.3885	1.5249	1.6558	1.8248	1.9512
	60	1.3576	1.4814	1.5990	1.7493	1.8609
	70	1.3352	1.4498	1.5581	1.6954	1.7966
	80	1.3180	1.4259	1.5271	1.6548	1.7484
	100	1.2934	1.3917	1.4833	1.5977	1.6809
	120	1.2767	1.3685	1.4536	1.5592	1.6357
	150	1.2595	1.3448	1.4234	1.5204	1.5901
	200	1.2418	1.3206	1.3927	1.4811	1.5442
	500	1.2086	1.2753	1.3356	1.4084	1.4598
	+∞	1.1850	1.2434	1.2956	1.3581	1.4017
120	1	63.061	253.25	1014.0	6339.4	25359
	2	9.4829	19.487	39.490	99.491	199.49
	3	5.1425	8.5494	13.947	26.221	41.989
	4	3.7753	5.6581	8.3092	13.558	19.468
	5	3.1228	4.3985	6.0693	9.1118	12.274
	6	2.7423	3.7047	4.9044	6.9690	9.0015
	7	2.4928	3.2674	4.1989	5.7373	7.1933
	8	2.3162	2.9669	3.7279	4.9461	6.0649
	9	2.1843	2.7475	3.3918	4.3978	5.3001
	10	2.0818	2.5801	3.1399	3.9965	4.7501
	11	1.9997	2.4480	2.9441	3.6904	4.3367
	12	1.9323	2.3410	2.7874	3.4494	4.0149
	13	1.8759	2.2524	2.6590	3.2548	3.7577
	14	1.8280	2.1778	2.5519	3.0942	3.5473
	15	1.7867	2.1141	2.4611	2.9595	3.3722
	16	1.7507	2.0107	2.3153	2.8477	3.2240
	17	1.7191	2.0107	2.3153	2.7459	3.0971
	18	1.6910	1.9681	2.2558	2.6597	2.9871
	19	1.6659	1.9302	2.2032	2.5839	2.8908
	20	1.6433	1.8963	2.1562	2.5168	2.8058
	21	1.6228	1.8657	2.1141	2.4568	2.7302
	22	1.6041	1.8380	2.0760	2.4029	2.6625
	23	1.5871	1.8128	2.0415	2.3542	2.6015
	24	1.5715	1.7896	2.0099	2.3100	2.5463
	25	1.5570	1.7684	1.9811	2.2696	2.4961
	30	1.4989	1.6835	1.8664	2.1108	2.2998
	35	1.4568	1.6226	1.7851	1.9996	2.1637
	40	1.4248	1.5766	1.7242	1.9172	2.0636
	45	1.3995	1.5406	1.6767	1.8535	1.9865
	50	1.3789	1.5115	1.6386	1.8026	1.9254
	60	1.3476	1.4673	1.5810	1.7263	1.8341
	70	1.3246	1.4351	1.5394	1.6717	1.7691
	80	1.3071	1.4107	1.5079	1.6305	1.7203
	100	1.2819	1.3757	1.4631	1.5723	1.6516
	120	1.2646	1.3519	1.4327	1.5330	1.6055
	150	1.2468	1.3275	1.4017	1.4932	1.5590
	200	1.2285	1.3024	1.3700	1.4527	1.5118
	500	1.1936	1.2551	1.3105	1.3774	1.4245
	+∞	1.1686	1.2214	1.2684	1.3246	1.3637

contd...

contd...

v_1	v_2	0.9	0.95	0.975	0.99	0.995
150	1	63.114	253.46	1014.9	6344.7	25380
	2	9.4846	19.489	39.491	99.492	199.49
	3	5.1408	8.5448	13.938	26.202	41.957
	4	3.7724	5.6521	8.2988	13.539	19.440
	5	3.1193	4.3918	6.0586	9.0936	12.248
	6	2.7383	3.6976	4.8934	6.9513	8.9772
	7	2.4884	3.2600	4.1877	5.7199	7.1700
	8	2.3115	2.9591	3.7165	4.9287	6.0422
	9	2.1793	2.7394	3.3801	4.3805	5.2778
	10	2.0766	2.5718	3.1280	3.9792	4.7280
	11	1.9942	2.4394	2.9320	3.6730	4.3147
	12	1.9266	2.3322	2.7750	3.4319	3.9930
	13	1.8701	2.2434	2.6465	3.2371	3.7357
	14	1.8220	2.1686	2.5392	3.0764	3.5254
	15	1.7805	2.1046	2.4482	2.9415	3.3501
	16	1.7444	2.0492	2.3700	2.8267	3.2019
	17	1.7126	2.0008	2.3020	2.7276	3.0748
	18	1.6843	1.9581	2.2423	2.6413	2.9647
	19	1.6590	1.9200	2.1895	2.5654	2.8683
	20	1.6363	1.8860	2.1424	2.4981	2.7832
	21	1.6157	1.8552	2.1001	2.4379	2.7075
	22	1.5969	1.8273	2.0618	2.3839	2.6396
	23	1.5797	1.8019	2.0271	2.3350	2.5785
	24	1.5640	1.7787	1.9954	2.2906	2.5232
	25	1.5494	1.7573	1.9664	2.2501	2.4727
	30	1.4907	1.6717	1.8510	2.0905	2.2758
	35	1.4482	1.6102	1.7691	1.9787	2.1391
	40	1.4157	1.5637	1.7076	1.8956	2.0383
	45	1.3900	1.5272	1.6596	1.8313	1.9607
	50	1.3691	1.4977	1.6210	1.7799	1.8989
	60	1.3372	1.4527	1.5625	1.7027	1.8067
	70	1.3137	1.4200	1.5202	1.6472	1.7408
	80	1.2957	1.3949	1.4880	1.6053	1.6912
	100	1.2698	1.3591	1.4422	1.5459	1.6213
	120	1.2519	1.3345	1.4109	1.5057	1.5741
	150	1.2335	1.3093	1.3789	1.4647	1.5264
	200	1.2143	1.2832	1.3460	1.4229	1.4777
	500	1.1775	1.2334	1.2836	1.3442	1.3868
	+∞	1.1505	1.1972	1.2387	1.2881	1.3224
200	1	63.167	253.68	1015.7	6350.0	25401
	2	9.4862	19.491	39.493	99.494	199.49
	3	5.1390	8.5402	13.929	26.183	41.925
	4	3.7695	5.6461	8.2885	13.520	19.411
	5	3.1157	4.3851	6.0478	9.0754	12.222
	6	2.7343	3.6904	4.8824	6.9336	8.9528
	7	2.4841	3.2525	4.1764	5.7024	7.1466
	8	2.3068	2.9513	3.7050	4.9114	6.0194
	9	2.1744	2.7313	3.3684	4.3631	5.2554
	10	2.0713	2.5634	3.1161	3.9617	4.7058
	11	1.9888	2.4308	2.9198	3.6555	4.2926
	12	1.9210	2.3233	2.7626	3.4143	3.9709
	13	1.8642	2.2343	2.6339	3.2194	3.7136
	14	1.8159	2.1592	2.5264	3.0585	3.5032
	17	1.7060	1.9909	2.2886	2.7092	3.0524
	18	1.6775	1.9479	2.2287	2.6227	2.9421
	19	1.6521	1.9097	2.1757	2.5467	2.8456
	20	1.6292	1.8755	2.1284	2.4792	2.7603
	21	1.6085	1.8446	2.0859	2.4189	2.6845
	22	1.5896	1.8165	2.0475	2.3646	2.6165
	23	1.5723	1.7909	2.0126	2.3156	2.5552
	24	1.5563	1.7675	1.9807	2.2710	2.4997
	25	1.5417	1.7460	1.9515	2.2303	2.4492
	30	1.4824	1.6597	1.8354	2.0700	2.2514
	35	1.4393	1.5976	1.7527	1.9574	2.1140
	40	1.4064	1.5505	1.6906	1.8737	2.0125
	45	1.3803	1.5135	1.6420	1.8087	1.9342
	50	1.3590	1.4835	1.6029	1.7567	1.8719
	60	1.3264	1.4377	1.5435	1.6784	1.7785
	70	1.3024	1.4042	1.5003	1.6220	1.7116
	80	1.2839	1.3786	1.4674	1.5792	1.6611
	100	1.2571	1.3416	1.4203	1.5184	1.5897
	120	1.2385	1.3162	1.3880	1.4770	1.5413
	150	1.2193	1.2899	1.3548	1.4347	1.4921
	200	1.1991	1.2626	1.3204	1.3912	1.4416
	500	1.1598	1.2096	1.2543	1.3081	1.3459
	+∞	1.1301	1.1700	1.2053	1.2472	1.2763
500	1	63.264	254.06	1017.2	6359.5	25439
	2	9.4892	19.494	39.496	99.497	199.50
	3	5.1358	8.5320	13.913	26.148	41.867
	4	3.7642	5.6353	8.2698	13.486	19.359
	5	3.1093	4.3731	6.0283	9.0424	12.175
	6	2.7270	3.6775	4.8625	6.9015	8.9088
	7	2.4761	3.2389	4.1560	5.6707	7.1044
	8	2.2983	2.9371	3.6842	4.8799	5.9782
	9	2.1653	2.7166	3.3471	4.3317	5.2148
	10	2.0618	2.5481	3.0944	3.9302	4.6656
	11	1.9788	2.4151	2.8977	3.6238	4.2525
	12	1.9106	2.3071	2.7401	3.3823	3.9309
	13	1.8535	2.2176	2.6109	3.1871	3.6735
	14	1.8048	2.1422	2.5030	3.0260	3.4630
	15	1.7628	2.0776	2.4114	2.8906	3.2875
	16	1.7262	2.0217	2.3326	2.7752	3.1389
	17	1.6939	1.9727	2.2640	2.6757	3.0115
	18	1.6651	1.9294	2.2038	2.5889	2.9010
	19	1.6394	1.8909	2.1504	2.5124	2.8042
	20	1.6162	1.8562	2.1027	2.4446	2.7186
	21	1.5952	1.8250	2.0599	2.3840	2.6425
	22	1.5760	1.7966	2.0211	2.3294	2.5742
	23	1.5585	1.7708	1.9859	2.2800	2.5126
	24	1.5423	1.7470	1.9537	2.2351	2.4568
	25	1.5274	1.7252	1.9242	2.1941	2.4059
	30	1.4670	1.6375	1.8065	2.0321	2.2066
	35	1.4229	1.5742	1.7224	1.9180	2.0676
	40	1.3890	1.5260	1.6590	1.8329	1.9647
	45	1.3621	1.4879	1.6092	1.7666	1.8850
	50	1.3400	1.4569	1.5689	1.7133	1.8214

contd...

contd...

v_1	v_2	0.9	0.95	0.975	0.99	0.995
	60	1.3060	1.4093	1.5075	1.6327	1.7256
	70	1.2807	1.3743	1.4625	1.5743	1.6565
	80	1.2611	1.3472	1.4280	1.5296	1.6041
	100	1.2324	1.3079	1.3781	1.4656	1.5291
	120	1.2122	1.2804	1.3434	1.4215	1.4778
	150	1.1910	1.2516	1.3073	1.3757	1.4248
	200	1.1683	1.2211	1.2691	1.3277	1.3694
	500	1.1216	1.1587	1.1918	1.2317	1.2596
	$+\infty$	1.0819	1.1063	1.1277	1.1530	1.1704
$+\infty$	1	63.328	254.31	1018.3	6365.9	25464
	2	9.4912	19.496	39.498	99.499	199.50
	3	5.1337	8.5264	13.902	26.125	41.828
	4	3.7607	5.6281	8.2573	13.463	19.325
	5	3.1050	4.3650	6.0153	9.0204	12.144
	6	2.7222	3.6689	4.8491	6.8800	8.8793
	7	2.4708	3.2298	4.1423	5.6495	7.0760
	8	2.2926	2.9276	3.6702	4.8588	5.9506
	9	2.1592	2.7067	3.3329	4.3105	5.1875
	10	2.0554	2.5379	3.0798	3.9090	4.6385
	11	1.9721	2.4045	2.8828	3.6024	4.2255
	12	1.9036	2.2962	2.7249	3.3608	3.9039
	13	1.8462	2.2064	2.5955	3.1654	3.6465
	14	1.7973	2.1307	2.4872	3.0040	3.4359
	15	1.7551	2.0658	2.3953	2.8684	3.2602
	16	1.7182	2.0096	2.3163	2.7528	3.1115
	17	1.6856	1.9604	2.2474	2.6530	2.9839
	18	1.6567	1.9168	2.1869	2.5660	2.8732
	19	1.6308	1.8780	2.1333	2.4893	2.7762
	20	1.6074	1.8432	2.0853	2.4212	2.6904
	21	1.5862	1.8117	2.0422	2.3603	2.6140
	22	1.5668	1.7831	2.0032	2.3055	2.5455
	23	1.5490	1.7570	1.9677	2.2558	2.4837
	24	1.5327	1.7330	1.9353	2.2107	2.4276
	25	1.5176	1.7110	1.9055	2.1694	2.3765
	30	1.4564	1.6223	1.7867	2.0062	2.1760
	35	1.4115	1.5580	1.7016	1.8910	2.0359
	40	1.3769	1.5089	1.6371	1.8047	1.9318
	45	1.3493	1.4700	1.5864	1.7374	1.8510
	50	1.3267	1.4383	1.5452	1.6831	1.7863
	60	1.2915	1.3893	1.4821	1.6006	1.6885
	70	1.2652	1.3529	1.4357	1.5404	1.6176
	80	1.2446	1.3247	1.3997	1.4942	1.5634
	100	1.2142	1.2832	1.3473	1.4272	1.4853
	120	1.1926	1.2539	1.3104	1.3805	1.4311
	150	1.1694	1.2226	1.2714	1.3314	1.3744
	200	1.1439	1.1885	1.2290	1.2785	1.3137
	500	1.0871	1.1132	1.1365	1.1644	1.1840
	$+\infty$	1.0000	1.0000	1.0000	1.0000	1.0000

Table A12: Nonparametric tests

Rejection regions of the Wilcoxon signed-rank test (one sample)

The table below contains the end points of the rejection regions for the Wilcoxon signed-rank test for inference about the median η of a symmetric distribution.

Denote by ω_- the rank sum of the observations less than η_0, and denote by ω_+ the rank sum of the observations greater than η_0.

$H_0: \eta \leq \eta_0$ vs $H_1 \eta > \eta_0$ (one-sided): Reject H_0 if ω_- is not larger than the tabulated value.
$H_0: \eta \geq \eta_0$ vs $H_1 \eta > \eta_0$ (one-sided): Reject H_0 if ω_+ is not larger than the tabulated value.
$H_0: \eta = \eta_0$ vs $H_1 \eta \neq \eta_0$ (two-sided): Reject H_0 if $\{\omega_+, \omega_-\}$ is not larger than the tabulated value.

	size α (one-sided)					size α (one-sided)					size α (one-sided)			
	5%	2.5%	1%	0.5%		5%	2.5%	1%	0.5%		5%	2.5%	1%	0.5%
	size α (two-sided)					size α (two-sided)					size α (two-sided)			
n	10%	5%	2%	1%	*n*	10%	5%	2%	1%	*n*	10%	5%	2%	1%
1	–	–	–	–	31	163	147	130	118	61	715	672	623	589
2	–	–	–	–	32	175	159	140	128	62	741	697	646	611
3	–	–	–	–	33	187	170	151	138	63	767	721	669	634
4	–	–	–	–	34	200	182	162	148	64	793	747	693	657
5	0	–	–	–	35	213	195	173	159	65	820	772	718	681
6	2	0	–	–	36	227	208	185	171	66	847	798	742	705
7	3	2	0	–	37	241	221	198	182	67	875	825	768	729
8	5	3	1	0	38	256	235	211	194	68	903	852	793	754
9	8	5	3	1	39	271	249	224	207	69	931	879	819	779
10	10	8	5	3	40	286	264	238	220	70	960	907	846	805
11	13	10	7	5	41	302	279	252	233	71	990	936	873	831
12	17	13	9	7	42	319	294	266	247	72	1020	964	901	858
13	21	17	12	9	43	336	310	281	261	73	1050	994	928	884
14	25	21	15	12	44	353	327	296	276	74	1081	1023	957	912
15	30	25	19	15	45	371	343	312	291	75	1112	1053	986	940
16	35	29	23	19	46	389	361	328	307	76	1144	1084	1015	968
17	41	34	27	23	47	407	378	345	322	77	1176	1115	1044	997
18	47	40	32	27	48	426	396	362	339	78	1209	1147	1075	1026
19	53	46	37	32	49	446	415	379	355	79	1242	1179	1105	1056
20	60	52	43	37	50	466	434	397	373	80	1276	1211	1136	1086
21	67	58	49	42	51	486	453	416	390	81	1310	1244	1168	1116
22	75	65	55	48	52	507	473	434	408	82	1345	1277	1200	1147
23	83	73	62	54	53	529	494	454	427	83	1380	1311	1232	1178
24	91	81	69	61	54	550	514	473	445	84	1415	1345	1265	1210
25	100	89	76	68	55	573	536	493	465	85	1451	1380	1298	1242
26	110	98	84	75	56	595	557	514	484	86	1487	1415	1332	1275
27	119	107	92	83	57	618	579	535	504	87	1524	1451	1366	1308
28	130	116	101	91	58	642	602	556	525	88	1561	1487	1400	1342
29	140	126	110	100	59	666	625	578	546	89	1599	1523	1435	1376
30	151	137	120	109	60	690	648	600	567	90	1638	1560	1471	1410

Rejection regions of the Mann-Whitneyl/Wilcoxon two-sample test

The table below contains the end points of the rejection regions for the Mann-Whitney test for inference about the medians η_1 and η_2 of two translated symmetric distributions based on two samples of size n_1 and n_2, respectively.

Denote by r_1 and r_2 the rank sums obtained for the observations from the first and the second sample. Define $u_1 = r_1 - \frac{n_1(n_1+1)}{2}$ and $u_2 = r_2 - \frac{n_2(n_2+1)}{2}$.

$H_0: \eta_1 \leq \eta_0$ vs $H_1 \eta_1 > \eta_2$ (one-sided): Reject H_0 if u_2 is not larger than the tabulated value.
$H_0: \eta_1 \geq \eta_0$ vs $H_1 \eta_1 > \eta_2$ (one-sided): Reject H_0 if u_1 is not larger than the tabulated value.
$H_0: \eta_1 = \eta_0$ vs $H_1 \eta_1 \neq \eta_2$ (two-sided): Reject H_0 if min $\{u_1, u_2\}$ is not larger than the tabulated value.

"–" indicates that H_0 is never rejected for the chosen size α and sample sizes n_1 and n_2.

Rejection regions of the Mann-Whitney/Wilcoxon two-sample test (size α : 5% one-sided, 10% two-sided)

	n_2																							
n_1	2	3	4	5	6	7	8	9	10	11	12	13	14	15	16	17	18	19	20	21	22	23	24	25
2	-	-		0	0	0	1	1	1	1	2	2	2	3	3	3	4	*4*	*4*	5	5	5	6	6
3	-	-	0	1	2	2	3	3	4	5	5	6	7	7	8	9	9	10	11	11	12	13	13	14
4	-	0		2	3	*4*	5	6	7	8	9	10	11	12	14	15	16	17	18	19	20	21	22	23
5	0	I	2	4	5	6	8	9	11	12	13	15	16	18	19	20	22	23	25	26	28	29	30	32
6	0	2	3	5	7	8	10	12	14	16	17	19	21	23	25	26	28	30	32	34	36	37	39	41
7	0	2	4	6	8	11	13	15	17	19	21	24	26	28	30	33	35	37	39	41	44	*46*	48	50
8	1	3	5	8	10	13	15	18	20	23	26	28	31	33	36	39	41	44	47	49	52	54	57	60
9	1	3	6	9	12	15	18	21	24	27	30	33	36	39	42	45	48	51	54	57	60	63	66	69
10	1	*4*	7	11	14	17	20	24	27	31	34	37	41	44	48	51	55	58	62	65	68	72	75	79
11	1	5	8	12	16	19	23	27	31	34	38	42	46	50	54	57	61	65	69	73	77	81	85	89
12	2	5	9	13	17	21	26	30	34	38	42	47	51	55	60	*64*	68	72	77	81	85	90	94	98
13	2	6	10	15	19	24	28	33	37	42	47	51	56	61	65	70	75	80	84	89	94	98	103	108
14	2	7	11	16	21	26	31	36	41	46	51	56	61	66	71	77	82	87	92	97	102	107	113	118
15	3	7	12	18	23	28	33	39	44	50	55	61	66	72	77	83	88	94	100	105	111	116	122	128
16	3	8	14	19	25	30	36	42	48	54	60	65	71	77	83	89	95	101	107	113	119	125	131	137
17	3	9	15	20	26	33	39	45	51	57	*64*	70	77	83	89	96	102	109	115	121	128	134	141	147
18	4	9	16	22	28	35	41	48	55	61	68	75	82	88	95	102	109	116	123	130	136	143	150	157
19	4	10	17	23	30	37	44	51	58	65	72	80	87	94	101	109	116	123	130	138	145	152	160	167
20	4	11	18	25	32	39	47	54	62	69	77	84	92	100	107	115	123	130	138	146	154	161	169	177
21	5	11	19	26	34	41	49	57	65	73	81	89	97	105	113	121	130	138	146	154	162	170	179	187
22	5	12	20	28	36	44	52	60	68	77	85	94	102	111	119	128	136	145	154	162	171	179	188	197
23	5	13	21	29	37	46	54	63	72	81	90	98	107	116	125	134	143	152	161	170	179	189	198	207
24	6	13	22	30	39	48	57	66	75	85	94	103	113	122	131	141	150	160	169	179	188	198	207	217
25	6	14	23	32	41	50	60	69	79	89	98	108	118	128	137	147	157	167	177	187	197	207	217	227

Rejection regions of the Mann-Whitney/Wilcoxon two-sample test (size α : 2.5% one-sided, 5% two-sided)

	n_2																							
n_1	2	3	4	5	6	7	8	9	10	11	12	13	14	15	16	17	18	19	20	21	22	23	24	25
2	–	–	–	–	–	–	0	0	0	0	1	1	1	1	1	2	2	2	2	3	3	3	3	3
3	–	–	–	0	1	1	2	2	3	3	4	4	5	5	6	6	7	7	8	8	9	9	10	10
4	–	–	0	1	2	3	4	4	5	6	7	8	9	10	11	11	12	13	14	15	16	17	17	18
5	–	0	1	2	3	5	6	7	8	9	11	12	13	14	15	17	18	19	20	22	23	24	25	27
6	–	1	2	3	5	6	8	10	11	13	14	16	17	19	21	22	24	25	27	29	30	32	33	35
7	–	1	3	5	6	8	10	12	14	16	18	20	22	24	26	28	30	32	34	36	38	40	42	44
8	0	2	4	6	8	10	13	15	17	19	22	24	26	29	31	34	36	38	41	43	45	48	50	53
9	0	2	4	7	10	12	15	17	20	23	26	28	31	34	37	39	42	45	48	50	53	56	59	62
10	0	3	5	8	11	14	17	20	23	26	29	33	36	39	42	45	48	52	55	58	61	64	67	71
11	0	3	6	9	13	16	19	23	26	30	33	37	40	44	47	51	55	58	62	65	69	73	76	80
12	1	4	7	11	14	18	22	26	29	33	37	41	45	49	53	57	61	65	69	73	77	81	85	89
13	1	4	8	12	16	20	24	28	33	37	41	45	50	54	59	63	67	72	76	80	85	89	94	98
14	1	5	9	13	17	22	26	31	36	40	45	50	55	59	64	69	74	78	83	88	93	98	102	107
15	1	5	10	14	19	24	29	34	39	44	49	54	59	64	70	75	80	85	90	96	101	106	111	117
16	1	6	11	15	21	26	31	37	42	47	53	59	64	70	75	81	86	92	98	103	109	115	120	126
17	2	6	11	17	22	28	34	39	45	51	57	63	69	75	81	87	93	99	105	111	117	123	129	135
18	2	7	12	18	24	30	36	42	48	55	61	67	74	80	86	93	99	106	112	119	125	132	138	145
19	2	7	13	19	25	32	38	45	52	58	65	72	78	85	92	99	106	113	119	126	133	140	147	154
20	2	8	14	20	27	34	41	48	55	62	69	76	83	90	98	105	112	119	127	134	141	149	156	163
21	3	8	15	22	29	36	43	50	58	65	73	80	88	96	103	111	119	126	134	142	150	157	165	173
22	3	9	16	23	30	38	45	53	61	69	77	85	93	101	109	117	125	133	141	150	158	166	174	182
23	3	9	17	24	32	40	48	56	*64*	73	81	89	98	106	115	123	132	140	149	157	166	175	183	192
24	3	10	17	25	33	42	50	59	67	76	85	94	102	111	120	129	138	147	156	165	174	183	192	201
25	3	10	18	27	35	44	53	62	71	80	89	98	107	117	126	135	145	154	163	173	182	192	201	211

Rejection regions of the Mann-Whitney/Wilcoxon two-sample test (size α : 1% one-sided, 2% two-sided)

	n_2																							
n_1	2	3	4	5	6	7	8	9	10	11	12	13	14	15	16	17	18	19	20	21	22	23	24	25
2	–	–	–	–	–	–	–	–	–	–	–	0	0	0	0	0	0	1	1	1	l	1	1	1
3	–	–	–	–	–	0	0	1	1	1	2	2	2	3	3	4	4	4	5	5	5	6	6	7
4	–	–	–	0	1	1	2	3	3	4	5	5	6	7	7	8	9	9	10	11	11	12	13	13
5	–	–	0	1	2	3	4	5	6	7	8	9	10	11	12	13	14	15	16	17	18	19	20	21
6			1	2	3	4	6	7	8	9	11	12	13	15	16	18	19	20	22	23	24	26	27	29
7	–	0	1	3	4	6	7	9	11	12	14	16	17	19	21	23	24	26	28	30	31	33	35	36
8	–	0	2	4	6	7	9	11	13	15	17	20	22	24	26	28	30	32	34	36	38	40	42	45
9	–	1	3	5	7	9	11	14	16	18	21	23	26	28	31	33	36	38	40	43	45	48	50	53
10	–	1	3	6	8	11	13	16	19	22	24	27	30	33	36	38	41	44	47	50	53	55	58	61
11	–	1	4	7	9	12	15	18	22	25	28	31	34	37	41	44	47	50	53	57	60	63	66	70
12	–	2	5	8	11	14	17	21	24	28	31	35	38	42	46	49	53	56	60	64	67	71	75	78
13	0	2	5	9	12	16	20	23	27	31	35	39	43	47	51	55	59	63	67	71	75	79	83	87
14	0	2	6	10	13	17	22	26	30	34	38	43	47	51	56	60	65	69	73	78	82	87	91	95
15	0	3	7	11	15	19	24	28	33	37	42	47	51	56	61	66	70	75	80	85	90	94	99	104
16	0	3	7	12	16	21	26	31	36	41	46	51	56	61	66	71	76	82	87	92	97	102	108	113
17	0	4	8	13	18	23	28	33	38	44	49	55	60	66	71	77	82	88	93	99	105	110	116	122
18	0	4	9	14	19	24	30	36	41	47	53	59	65	70	76	82	88	94	100	106	112	118	124	130
19	1	4	9	15	20	26	32	38	44	50	56	63	69	75	82	88	94	101	107	113	120	126	133	139
20	1	5	10	16	22	28	34	40	47	53	60	67	73	80	87	93	100	107	114	121	127	134	141	148
21	1	5	11	17	23	30	36	43	50	57	64	71	78	85	92	99	106	113	121	128	135	142	150	157
22	1	5	11	18	24	31	38	45	53	60	67	75	82	90	97	105	112	120	127	135	143	150	158	166
23	1	6	12	19	26	33	40	48	55	63	71	79	87	94	102	110	118	126	134	142	150	158	167	175
24	1	6	13	20	27	35	42	50	58	66	75	83	91	99	108	116	124	133	141	150	158	167	175	184
25	1	7	13	21	29	36	45	53	61	70	78	87	95	104	113	122	130	139	148	157	166	175	184	192

Rejection regions of the Mann-WhitneylWilcoxon two-sample test (size α : 0.5% one-sided, 1% two-sided)

	n_2																							
n_1	2	3	4	5	6	7	8	9	10	11	12	13	14	15	16	17	18	19	20	21	22	23	24	25
2	–	–	–	–	–	–	–	–	–	–	–	–	–	–	–	–	–	0	0	0	0	0	0	0
3	–	–	–	–	–	–		0	0	0	1	1		2	2	2	2	3	3	3	4	4	4	5
4	–	–	–	–	0	0	1	1	2	2	3	3	4	5	5	6	6	7	8	8	9	9	10	10
5	–	–	–	0	1	1	2	3	4	5	6	7	7	8	9	10	11	12	13	14	14	15	16	17
6	–	–	0	1	2	3	4	5	6	7	9	10	11	12	13	15	16	17	18	19	21	22	23	24
7	–	–	0	1	3	4	6	7	9	10	12	13	15	16	18	19	21	22	24	25	27	29	30	32
8	-	–	1	2	4	6	7	9	11	13	15	17	18	20	22	24	26	28	30	32	34	35	37	39
9	–	0	1	3	5	7	9	11	13	16	18	20	22	24	27	29	31	33	36	38	40	43	45	47
10	–	0	2	4	6	9	11	13	16	18	21	24	26	29	31	34	37	39	42	44	47	50	52	55
11	–	0	2	5	7	10	13	16	18	21	24	27	30	33	36	39	42	45	48	51	54	57	60	63
12	–	1	3	6	9	12	15	18	21	24	27	31	34	37	41	44	47	51	54	58	61	64	68	71
13	–	1	3	7	10	13	17	20	24	27	31	34	38	42	45	49	53	57	60	64	68	72	75	79
14	–	1	4	7	11	15	18	22	26	30	34	38	42	46	50	54	58	63	67	71	75	79	83	87
15	–	2	5	8	12	16	20	24	29	33	37	42	46	51	55	60	64	69	73	78	82	87	91	96
16	–	2	5	9	13	18	22	27	31	36	41	45	50	55	60	65	70	74	79	84	89	94	99	104
17	–	2	6	10	15	19	24	29	34	39	44	49	54	60	65	70	75	81	86	91	96	102	107	112
18	–	2	6	11	16	21	26	31	37	42	47	53	58	64	70	75	81	87	92	98	104	109	115	121
19	0	3	7	12	17	22	28	33	39	45	51	57	63	69	74	81	87	93	99	105	111	117	123	129
20	0	3	8	13	18	24	30	36	42	48	54	60	67	73	79	86	92	99	105	112	118	125	131	138
21	0	3	8	14	19	25	32	38	44	51	58	64	71	78	84	91	98	105	112	118	125	132	139	146
22	0	4	9	14	21	27	34	40	47	54	61	68	75	82	89	96	104	111	118	125	133	140	147	155
23	0	4	9	15	22	29	35	43	50	57	64	72	79	87	94	102	109	117	125	132	140	148	155	163
24	0	4	10	16	23	30	37	45	52	60	68	75	83	91	99	107	115	123	131	139	147	155	164	172
25	0	5	10	17	24	32	39	47	55	63	71	79	87	96	104	112	121	129	138	146	155	163	172	180

References

1. Alligood MR, Tomey AM. Nursing theory: Utilization and application. 2nd ed. Missouri: Mosby; 2002.
2. American Psychological Association. APA style. 2013. Retrieved from http://www.apastyle.org/.
3. Arora PN, Arora S, Arora A. Elements of Statistical Methods. New Delhi: S Chand & Company Ltd; 2009.
4. Bowling A. Research methods in health: Investigating health and health sciences. Philadelphia: Open University Press; 1997.
5. Boylan J, Alderdice FA, McGowan JE, et al. Behavioural outcomes of 3 years of age among late preterm infants admitted to neonatal intensive care: a cohort study. Arch Dis Child Fetal Neonatal Ed. *2014;99(5):F359-65.*
6. Burns N, Grove SK. Understanding nursing research: Building evidence-based practice. 4th ed. Noida: Elsevier; 2007.
7. Census and Survey Processing System (CSPro). (n.d.). Retrieved from http://www.census.gov/population/international/software/cspro/
8. Chandraiah P. Nursing research and statistics. Hyderabad: Florence Publishers; 2010.
9. Charalambous A, Kaite C. Undergraduate nursing students caring for cancer patients: hermeneutic phenomenological insights of their experiences. BMC Health Service Research. 2013;13:63.
10. Cheranmadevi P. A study to assess the effectiveness of ice massage on knee pain among women with osteoarthritis in selected hospital, Chennai. Unpublished dissertation. The Tamil Nadu Dr MGR Medical University, Chennai; 2012.
11. Cochrane Library. 2013. Retrieved from http://www.thecochranelibrary.com/view/0/index.html.
12. Cormack DFS. The research process in nursing. 4th ed. Blackwell Science; 2000.
13. Dal U, Sarpkaya D. Knowledge and psychomotor skills of nursing students in North Cyprus in the area of cardiopulmonary resuscitation. Pak J Med Sci. 2013;29(4):966-71.
14. Daniel WW. Biostatistics: A foundation for analysis in the health sciences. 7th ed. John Wiley & Sons; 2000.
15. Defeyter MA, Russo R. The effect of breakfast cereal consumption on adolescents› cognitive performance and mood. Front Hum Neurosci. 2013;7:789.

16. de Leeuw JR, de Bruijn M, de Weert-van Oene GH, et al. Internet and game behaviour at a secondary school and a newly developed health promotion programme: a prospective study. BMC Public Health. 2010;10:544.
17. Dempsey PA, Dempsey AD. Using nursing research process: Critical evaluation and utilization. 5th ed. Philadelphia: Lippincott; 2000.
18. Devís-Devís J, Peiró-Velert C, Beltrán-Carrillo VJ, et al. Screen media time usage of 12–16 year-old Spanish school adolescents: Effects of personal and socioeconomic factors, season and type of day. J Adolesc. 2009;32(2):213-31.
19. Divya T. A study to assess the psychosocial problems and coping measures adopted by the mothers of children with autism in selected special schools in Chennai. Unpublished dissertation. The Tamil Nadu Dr MGR Medical University, Chennai; 2013.
20. Einarsdottir J. Happiness in the neonatal intensive care unit: Merits of ethnographic fieldwork. Int J Qual Stud Health Well-being. 2012;7:10.3402.
21. Epi Info. 2013. Retrieved from http://www.cdc.gov/epiinfo.
22. Fain J. Understanding and applying nursing research: A textbook & workbook. 2nd ed. Philadelphia: FA Davis Company; 2004.
23. Frank H, Althoen SC. Statistics: Concepts and applications. New York: Cambridge University Press; 1995.
24. Gayathri R, Kumar A, Ramakrishnan. Cognitive behaviour therapy for childhood depression- A case study. Progressive outlook (Quarterly Vol.: 1-B (Special Issue-Apr. 2013), 379-387.
25. George JB. Nursing theories: The base for professional nursing practice. 6th ed. New Delhi: Dorling Kindersley (India) Pvt Ltd; 2011.
26. Gillis A, Jackson W. Research for nurse: Methods and interpretation. Philadelphia: FA Davis Company; 2002.
27. Gormely DK, Kennerly S. Predictors of turnover intention in nurse faculty. J Nurs Educ. 2011;50(4):190-6.
28. Goyal A, Sharma A, Gaur T, et al. Impact of dental fear on oral health-related quality of life among school going and non-school going children in Udaipur city: A cross-sectional study. Contemp Clin Dent. 2014;5(1):42-48.
29. Gremigni P, Cappelli G. Psychosocial well-being after kidney transplantation: A matched-pair case-control study. J Health Psychol. 2016;21(5):599-606.
30. Heiman GW. Understanding research methods and statistics: An integrated introduction for psychology. New York: Houghton Mifflin Company; 1998.
31. Hosseinit H, Abdi F. Experiences of vasectomy: A Phenomenological study. N Am J Med Sci. 2012;4(12):619-23.
32. Hott JR, Budin WC. Notter's essentials of nursing research. 6th ed. New York: Springer Publishing Company; 2006.

33. Hounsgaard L, Augustussen M, Moller H, et al. Women's perspectives on illness when being screened for cervical cancer. International Journal of Circumpolar Health. 2013;72.
34. Immonen I. Nursing during world war II: Finnmark county, Northern Norway. International Journal of Circumpolar Health.2013;25, 72:20278.
35. Indian Council of Medical Research. Ethical guidelines for biomedical research on human participants. 2006. Retrieved from http://icmr.nic.in/ethical_guidelines.pdf.
36. Janardhan P. Assessment of the client factors influencing the success of embryo transfer among clients who had undergone embryo transfer between 2003–2005 in GG hospital, Chennai. Unpublished dissertation. The Tamil Nadu Dr MGR Medical University, Chennai; 2008.
37. Jang GJ, Kim SH. Effects of breast-feeding education and support services on breast-feeding rates and infant's growth. J Korean Acad Nurs. 2010;40(2):277-86.
38. Jeya Bharathi S. The use of positive therapy to enhance the general wellbeing among prisoners. Dimensions of Violations and Victimizations. Tirunelveli, Manonmaniam Sundaranar Universit; 2012.
39. Kothari CR. Research methodology: Methods and techniques. 2nd revised ed. New Delhi: New Age International Publishers; 2011.
40. Krishnaswami OR, Ranganathan M. Methodology of research in social sciences. Mumbai: Himalaya Publishing House; 2009.
41. Kumar R. Research Methodology: A Step by Step Guide for Beginners. New Delhi: Sage Publications; 2005.
42. Laavanya PV. Adolescents' perception of bodily change: A phenomenological study *Progressive Outlook,* (Quarterly Vol.: 1-B (Special Issue-Apr. 2013), 438-444.
43. Lin MH, Huang SJ, Shih WM. Effects of an anti-smoking program to prevent lung cancer among urban aboriginals in Taiwan. Asian Pac J Cancer Prev. 2013;14(11):6451-7.
44. Lundgren I, Wahlberg V. The Experience of Pregnancy: A Hermeneutical/Phenomenological Study. J Perinat Educ. 1999;8(3):12-20.
45. Mademe G. (n.d.). Retrieved from http://www.scribd.com/doc/16739725/Research-Problem-Hypotheses-and-Variables#force_seo
46. Mahajan BK. Methods in Biostatistics. 6th ed. New Delhi: Jaypee Brothers Medical Publishers Ltd; 2004.
47. McEwen M, Wills EM. Theoretical basis for nursing. 3rd ed. Philadelphia: Lippincott Williams & Wilkins; 2011.
48. McGilton KS, Davis A, Mahomed N, et al. An inpatient rehabilitation model of care targeting patients with cognitive impairment. BMC Geriatric. 2012;12:21.
49. McNiesh SG. The lived experience of students in an accelerated nursing program: Intersecting factors that influence experiential learning. J Nurs Educ. 2011;50(4):197-203.

50. MedInd. 2013. Retrieved from http://www.medindia.net/
51. Metz AM, Cech EA, Babcock T, et al. Effects of Formal and Informal support structures on the motivation of Native American students in nursing. J Nurs Educ. 2011;50(7):388-94.
52. Morse JM, Field PA. Nursing Research: The Application of Qualitative Approaches. 2nd ed. London: Chapman and Hall; 1996.
53. Mull DS, Agran PF, Winn DG, et al. Household poisoning exposure among children of Mexican-born mothers: an ethnographic study. West J Med. 1999;171(1):16-9.
54. Mulhall A, May AL. Nursing research: Dissemination and implementation. London: Churchill Livingstone; 1999.
55. Nanchahal K, Townsend J, Letley L, et al. Weight-management interventions in primary care: a pilot randomised controlled trial. Br J Gen Pract. 2009;59(562):157-66.
56. Nieswiadomy RM. Foundations of Nursing Research. 5th ed. New Delhi: Dorling Kindersley (India) Pvt. Ltd; 2008.
57. Nguyen DN, Zierler B, Nguyen HQ. A survey of nursing faculty needs for training in use of new technologies for education and practice. J Nurs Educ. 2011;50(4):181-9.
58. Parker ME. Nursing theories and nursing practice. 2nd ed. New Delhi: Jaypee Brothers Medical Publishers Ltd; 2007.
59. Parahoo K. Nursing Research: Principles, process and issues. 2nd ed. London: Palgrave; 2006.
60. Pillai RSN, Bagavathi. Statistics: Theory and practice. New Delhi: S Chand & Company Pvt Ltd; 2013.
61. Polit DF, Beck CT. Essentials of nursing research. 7th ed. New Delhi: Wolters Kluwer (India) Pvt. Ltd; 2010.
62. Prabha J. A study to assess the knowledge and attitude towards safety behavior among adolescents in selected settings, Chennai. Unpublished dissertation. The Tamil Nadu Dr MGR Medical University, Chennai; 2013.
63. Prathima S. Caregivers perception on emotional problems in children living with HIV/AIDS. *Progressive Outlook,* (Quarterly Vol.: 1-B (Special Issue-Apr. 2013), 363-370.
64. PubMed Central. 2013. Retrieved from http://www.ncbi.nlm.nih.gov/pmc/
65. Reed PG, Shearer NC, Nicoll LH. Perspectives of nursing theory. 4th ed. Lippincott: Williams & Wilkins; 2004.
66. Research. 2013, November, 10. Retrieved from http://en.wikipedia.org/wiki/Research
67. Research. 2014. Retrieved from http://www.merriam-webster.com/dictionary/research
68. Rose Marie. Foundations of nursing research. 5th ed. New Delhi, DK (India) Pvt. Ltd; 2008.

69. Saly Stains. A study to assess the minor health problems in under-five children and the health seeking measures followed by mothers in selected areas in Chennai. Unpublished dissertation. The Tamil Nadu Dr MGR Medical University, Chennai; 2013.
70. Satish L. A study to assess the effectiveness of video assisted teaching program on knowledge on basic life support among students studying in polytechnic colleges in Chennai. Unpublished dissertation. The Tamil Nadu Dr MGR Medical University, Chennai; 2012.
71. Sankara Narayanan R. (2013). An experimental study assessing the impact of group counseling intervention to impart knowledge on reproductive health among adolescent school girls. Progressive Outlook, (Quarterly Vol.: 1-B (Special Issue-Apr. 2013), 413-418.
72. Schlimme JE. Sense of self-determination and the suicidal experience. A phenomenological approach. Med Health Care Philos. 2013;16(2):211-23.
73. Shrikhande SN, Zodpey SP, Negandhi H. A case control study examining association between infectious agents and acute myocardial infarction. Indian J Public Health. 2014;58(2):106-9.
74. Smid M, Bourgois P, Auerswald CL. The challenge of pregnancy among homeless youth: Reclaiming a lost opportunity. J Health Care Poor Underserved. 2010;21(2 Suppl):140-56.
75. Smith P. Research mindedness for practice: An interactive approach for nursing and health care. Churchill Livingstone; 1997.
76. Smith P. Nursing research: Setting new agendas. London: Arnold; 1998.
77. Sneha Mercy R. A study to assess knowledge on early identification and prevention of behavioral problems in children among teachers in selected schools in Chennai. Unpublished dissertation. The Tamil Nadu Dr MGR Medical University, Chennai; 2013.
78. Sowndaram CS. (2013). Effectiveness of psychosocial intervention enhancing the mental health of the adolescents. Progressive Outlook, (Quarterly Vol.: 1-B (Special Issue-Apr. 2013), 358-362.
79. Straus L, Munguambe K, Bassat Q, et al. Inherent illnesses and attacks: an ethnographic study of interpretations of childhood Acute Respiratory Infections (ARIs) in Manhiça, southern Mozambique. BMC Public Health. 2011;11:556.
80. Streubert HJ, Carpenter DR. Quantitative research in nursing: Advancing the humanistic imperative. 5th ed. Lippincott Williams & Wilkins; 2011.
81. Sudha R. A study to evaluate the effectiveness of structured teaching program on knowledge on management of malnutrition in children among mothers of malnourished under-five children in two selected villages at Porur, Chennai. Unpublished dissertation, The Tamil Nadu Dr MGR Medical University, Chennai; 2002.
82. Sudha R, Shekhar B. Anti-ragging: Awareness and attitude among college students. Social Welfare. 2009;6-9.

83. Sudha R. (2011). Awareness of the mothers regarding child abuse and neglect, The Nursing Journal of India, Vol. CII No.5. Retrieved from http://www.tnaionline.org/thenursing.htm.
84. Sudha R. Effect of playing violent video games on children. Nightingale Nursing Times. 2011;7,10-11,63–65.
85. Sudha R, Shekhar B. Playing violent video games. Health Action. 2011;33-35.
86. Sudha R. Victimization of freshmen in colleges. Dimensions of Violations & Victimization, Tirunelveli, Manonmaniam Sundaranar University; 2012.
87. Sudha R, Shekhar B. Violent video game playing and its impact on physiological variables: A study among adolescents in Chennai. *Progressive Outlook,* (Quarterly Vol.: 1-B (Special Issue-Apr. 2013), 456-464.
88. Sudha R. (2013). Adolescent boys' food practice-A descriptive study. *TNNMC Journal of Pediatric Nursing, 1,* 7-10.
89. Sudha R, Shekhar B. Victims of Interactive Media. Tirunelveli: Publication Division, Manonmaniam Sundaranar University; 2013.
90. Sundaram B, Siddegowda YS. (2013). Major correlates of language and cognitive development of toddlers. Progressive Outlook, (Quarterly Vol.: 1-B (Special Issue-Apr. 2013),421-426.
91. Sundar Rao PSS, Richard J. Introduction to biostatistics and research methods. 4th ed. New Delhi: Prentice-Hall of India Pvt Ltd; 2008.
92. Thomas DG, A Sudha, Shekhar B. Transgender victimization. Dimensions of Violations & Victimization, Tirunelveli, Manonmaniam Sundaranar University; 2012.
93. Tripathi PC. A textbook of research methodology in social sciences. 6th revised and enlarged ed. New Delhi: Sultan Chand & Sons; 2010.
94. Troy PH, Wyness LA, McAuliffe E. Nurses' experiences of recruitment and migration from developing countries: a phenomenological approach. Hum Resour Health. 2007;5:15.
95. Universal Declaration of Human Rights. Retrieved from www.ohchr.org/en/udhr/documents/udhr_Translations/eng.pdf
96. Vermandel A, Weyler J, De wachter S, et al. Toilet training of healthy young toddlers: A randomized trial between a daytime wetting alarm and timed potty training. J Dev Behav Pediatr. 2008;29(3):191-6.
97. Vital Statistics. 2011. Retrieved from http://www.censusindia.gov.in/2011-Common/VitalStatistics.html.
98. Waller A, Girgis A, Johnson C, et al. Facilitating needs based cancer care for people with a chronic disease: Evaluation of an intervention using a multi-centre interrupted time series design. BMC Palliat Care. 2010;9:2.
99. Wang YM, Shu BC, Fetzer S, et al. Parenting style of women who conceived using in vitro fertilization: a meta-analysis. J Nurs Res. 2014;22(2):69-80.
100. Whitaker R, Ballard C, Stafford J, et al. Feasibility study of an optimised person-centered intervention to improve mental health and reduce antipsychotics amongst people with dementia in care homes: Study protocol for a randomised controlled trial. Trials. 2013;14:13.

101. Wolf A, Ekman I, Dellenborg L. Everyday practices at the medical ward: A 16-month ethnographic field study. BMC Health Services Research. 2012;12:184.
102. Wood GB, Haber J. Nursing research. 7th ed. St. Louis: Moshy Elsevier; 2010.
103. Wood GB, Haber J. Nursing research: Methods and critical appraisal, and utilization. Missouri: Mosby; 2006.
104. Wu DS, Hu J, McCoy TP, et al. The effects of a breastfeeding self-efficacy intervention on short-term breastfeeding outcomes among primiparous mothers in Wuhan, China. J Adv Nurs. 2014;70(8):1867-79.
105. Yoo JS, Jeon MY, Kim CG. Effects of a fall prevention program on falls in frail elders living at home in rural communities. J Korean Acad Nurs. 2013;43(5):613-25.
106. Young A, Taylor SG, Renpenning KM. Connections: Nursing research, theory and practice. Missouri: Mosby; 2001.

Index

Page numbers followed by *f* and *t* refer to figure and table, respectively.

D

S